1997 Red Book.

REPORT OF THE COMMITTEE
ON INFECTIOUS DISEASES
TWENTY-FOURTH EDITION

Author: Committee on Infectious Diseases
          American Academy of Pediatrics

          Georges Peter, MD, Editor

          Caroline B. Hall, MD, Associate Editor
          Neal A. Halsey, MD, Associate Editor
          S. Michael Marcy, MD, Associate Editor
          Larry K. Pickering, MD, Associate Editor

          Walter A. Orenstein, MD
          Centers for Disease Control and Prevention, Liaison

          American Academy of Pediatrics
          PO Box 927
          141 Northwest Point Blvd
          Elk Grove Village, IL 60009-0927

Suggested Citation: American Academy of Pediatrics. [chapter title]. In: Peter G, ed. *1997 Red Book: Report of the Committee on Infectious Diseases.* 24th ed. Elk Grove Village, IL: American Academy of Pediatrics; 1997: [page number]

24th Edition
1st Edition–1938
2nd Edition–1939
3rd Edition–1940
4th Edition–1942
5th Edition–1943
6th Edition–1944
7th Edition–1945
8th Edition–1947
9th Edition–1951
10th Edition–1952
11th Edition–1955
12th Edition–1957
13th Edition–1961
14th Edition–1964
15th Edition–1966
16th Edition–1970
16th Edition Revised–1971
17th Edition–1974
18th Edition–1977
19th Edition–1982
20th Edition–1986
21st Edition–1988
22nd Edition–1991
23rd Edition–1994

Library of Congress Catalog Card No.: 97-93785
ISBN No.: 0-910761-85-X
MA0001

Quantity prices on request. Address all inquiries to:
American Academy of Pediatrics
PO Box 927, 141 Northwest Point Blvd
Elk Grove Village, IL 60009-0927

The recommendations in this publication do not indicate an exclusive course of treatment or serve as a standard of medical care. Variations, taking into account individual circumstances, may be appropriate.

Committee on Infectious Diseases 1994–1997

Neal A. Halsey, MD, Chairperson 1995–1997
Caroline Breese Hall, MD, Chairperson 1991–1995

Jon S. Abramson, MD

P. Joan Chesney, MD

Margaret C. Fisher, MD

Michael A. Gerber, MD

Donald S. Gromisch, MD

Steve Kohl, MD

S. Michael Marcy, MD

Melvin I. Marks, MD

Dennis L. Murray, MD

George Nankervis, PhD, MD

James C. Overall, Jr, MD

Gary D. Overturf, MD

Larry K. Pickering, MD

Russell W. Steele, MD

Richard J. Whitley, MD

Ram Yogev, MD

Georges Peter, MD, *Ex Officio*

Liaison Representatives

Ruth L. Berkelman, MD, Centers for Disease Control and Prevention

Robert Breiman, MD, National Vaccine Program Office

Stephen C. Hadler, MD, Centers for Disease Control and Prevention

M. Carolyn Hardegree, MD, Food and Drug Administration

Richard F. Jacobs, MD, American Thoracic Society

Noni E. MacDonald, MD, Canadian Pediatric Society

Walter A. Orenstein, MD, Centers for Disease Control and Prevention

N. Regina Rabinovich, MD, National Institutes of Health

Benjamin Schwartz, MD, Centers for Disease Control and Prevention

Consultants to the Editors

Thomas Cleary, MD

Leigh Grossman Donowitz, MD

John S. Finlayson, PhD

Edgar K. Marcuse, MD, MPH

George H. McCracken, Jr, MD

Christian Patrick, MD, PhD

Catherine M. Wilfert, MD

Collaborators

On behalf of the American Academy of Pediatrics, the Committee gratefully acknowledges the invaluable assistance provided by the following individuals who served as contributors and reviewers in the preparation of this edition of the *Red Book*. Their expertise, critical review, and cooperation are essential in the Committee's continuing review and revisions of its recommendations for the management, control, and prevention of infectious diseases in children.

Every attempt has been made to recognize all those who contributed to this edition of the *Red Book*; the Academy regrets any omissions that may have occurred.

David G. Addiss, MD, Centers for Disease Control and Prevention, Atlanta, GA
Mercedes Albuerne, MD, Food and Drug Administration, Bethesda, MD
John Alexander, MD, Food and Drug Administration, Bethesda, MD
Miriam J. Alter, PhD, Centers for Disease Control and Prevention, Atlanta, GA
Larry J. Anderson, MD, Centers for Disease Control and Prevention, Atlanta, GA
Frederick J. Angulo, DVM, Centers for Disease Control and Prevention, Atlanta, GA
Bascom Anthony, MD, Food and Drug Administration, Bethesda, MD
Juan Arciniega, MD, Food and Drug Administration, Bethesda, MD
Nancy H. Arden, MD, Centers for Disease Control and Prevention, Atlanta, GA
Stephen S. Arnon, MD, California Department of Health Services, Berkeley, CA
William L. Atkinson, MD, MPH, Centers for Disease Control and Prevention, Atlanta, GA
Francisco M. Averhoff, MD, Centers for Disease Control and Prevention, Atlanta, GA
Carol J. Baker, MD, Baylor College of Medicine, Houston, TX
Julia Barrett, MD, Food and Drug Administration, Bethesda, MD
Margaret Bash, MD, Food and Drug Administration, Bethesda, MD
Judy Beeler, MD, Food and Drug Administration, Bethesda, MD
David M. Bell, MD, Centers for Disease Control and Prevention, Atlanta, GA
Thomas A. Bell, MD, MPH, Cowlitz County Health Department, Longview, WA
Martin J. Blaser, MD, Vanderbilt University School of Medicine, Nashville, TN
Dean A. Blumberg, MD, University of California, Los Angeles Medical Center, Los Angeles, CA
Andrew Bonwit, MD, Food and Drug Administration, Bethesda, MD
David Bostwick, MD, Food and Drug Administration, Bethesda, MD
Thomas G. Boyce, MD, Centers for Disease Control and Prevention, Atlanta, GA
Michael Brennan, MD, Food and Drug Administration, Bethesda, MD
Philip A. Brunell, MD, Cedars Sinai Medical Center, Los Angeles, CA
Thomas Bull, MD, Food and Drug Administration, Bethesda, MD
Gilbert M. Burnham, MD, PhD, Johns Hopkins School of Hygiene and Public Health, Baltimore, MD

Jay C. Butler, MD, Centers for Disease Control and Prevention, Atlanta, GA

Daniel T. Casto, PharmD, University of Texas Health Science Center at San Antonio, San Antonio, TX

Stanley W. Chapman, MD, University of Mississippi, School of Medicine, Jackson, MS

Robert T. Chen, MD, Centers for Disease Control and Prevention, Atlanta, GA

James D. Cherry, MD, University of California, Los Angeles, CA

Joseph Church, MD, Children's Hospital of Los Angeles, CA

Stephen L. Cochi, MD, Centers for Disease Control and Prevention, Atlanta, GA

Mitchel Cohen, MD, Centers for Disease Control and Prevention, Atlanta, GA

Daniel Colley, MD, Centers for Disease Control and Prevention, Atlanta, GA

Frank Collins, MD, Food and Drug Administration, Bethesda, MD

Kimberly A. Cook, MD, MSPH, Centers for Disease Control and Prevention, Atlanta, GA

Philip Coyne, MD, Food and Drug Administration, Bethesda, MD

Therese Cvetkovich, MD, Food and Drug Administration, Bethesda, MD

Antonio D'Allesandro, MD, Tulane University, New Orleans, LA

Adnan S. Dajani, MD, Wayne State University School of Medicine, Detroit, MI

Robert S. Daum, MD, University of Chicago, Chicago, IL

Jeffrey P. Davis, MD, Bureau of Public Health, Madison, WI

David T. Dennis, MD, MPH, Centers for Disease Control and Prevention, Atlanta, GA

Franklin Desposito, MD, University of Medicine and Dentistry, Newark, NJ

Rosamund Dewart, MD, Centers for Disease Control and Prevention, Atlanta, GA

Vance Dietz, MD, MPH, Centers for Disease Control and Prevention, Atlanta, GA

Dennis M. Dixon, MD, Centers for Disease Control and Prevention, Atlanta, GA

Steven Ducatman, MD, Kaiser Permanente Health Care Program, Los Angeles, CA

Clare A. Dykewicz, MD, MPH, Centers for Disease Control and Prevention, Atlanta, GA

Moraven S. Edwards, MD, Baylor College of Medicine, Houston, TX

Joseph J. Esposito, PhD, Centers for Disease Control and Prevention, Atlanta, GA

Gary Euler, PhD, Centers for Disease Control and Prevention, Atlanta, GA

Geoffrey Evans, MD, Food and Drug Administration, Bethesda, MD

Karen Farizo, MD, Food and Drug Administration, Bethesda, MD

David Feigal, MD, Food and Drug Administration, Bethesda, MD

Stephen Feinstone, MD, Food and Drug Administration, Bethesda, MD

Patricia Ferrieri, MD, American Heart Association, Dallas, TX

John Marc Fischer, MD, Centers for Disease Control and Prevention, Atlanta, GA

Patricia M. Flynn, MD, St. Jude Children's Research Hospital, Memphis, TN

Julie Francis, MD, Children's Hospital and Medical Center, Seattle, WA

Carl Frasch, MD, Food and Drug Administration, Bethesda, MD

Judy M. Gantt, Centers for Disease Control and Prevention, Atlanta, GA

Julia S. Garner, RN, MN, Centers for Disease Control and Prevention, Atlanta, GA

Lawrence M. Gartner, MD, University of Chicago, Chicago, IL

Robert P. Gaynes, MD, Centers for Disease Control and Prevention, Atlanta, GA

Antonia Geber, MD, Food and Drug Administration, Bethesda, MD

Anne Gershon, MD, Columbia University, New York, NY

Scott Giebink, MD, University of Minnesota, Minneapolis, MN
Ann E. Giesel, MD, University of Washington, Seattle, WA
Jacqueline Gindler, MD, Centers for Disease Control and Prevention, Atlanta, GA
Roger I. Glass, MD, Centers for Disease Control and Prevention, Atlanta, GA
Karen Goldenthal, MD, Food and Drug Administration, Bethesda, MD
Ellie J.C. Goldstein, MD, University of California Los Angeles, School of Medicine,
     Los Angeles, CA
Elizabeth Gordon, MD, Food and Drug Administration, Bethesda, MD
Eve H. Gordon, MD, Kaiser Permanente Health Care Program, Los Angeles, CA
Philip J. Goscienski, MD, University of San Diego Medical Center, San Diego, CA
Giora Gottesman, MD, Cedars-Sinai Medical Center, Los Angeles, CA
David P. Greenberg, MD, Children's Hospital of Pittsburgh, Pittsburgh, PA
Patricia M. Griffin, MD, Centers for Disease Control and Prevention, Atlanta, GA
Jay L. Grosfeld, MD, Indiana University Medical Center, Indianapolis, IN
Duane J. Gublir, ScD, Centers for Disease Control and Prevention, Atlanta, GA
Rana A. Hajjeh, MD, Centers for Disease Control and Prevention, Atlanta, GA
Holli Hamilton, MD, Food and Drug Administration, Bethesda, MD
Celine Hanson, MD, Centers for Disease Control and Prevention, Atlanta, GA
Charles Hatheway, MD, Centers for Disease Control and Prevention, Atlanta, GA
Kenneth L. Herrmann, MD, Centers for Disease Control and Prevention,
     Atlanta, GA
Barbara L. Herwaldt, MD, MPH, Centers for Disease Control and Prevention,
     Atlanta, GA
John C. Hierholzer, PhD, Centers for Disease Control and Prevention, Atlanta, GA
David R. Hill, MD, DTM&H, University of Connecticut School of Medicine,
     Farmington, CT
Sandra Holmes, PhD, Center for Pediatric Research, Norfolk, VA
Robert Hopkins, MD, Food and Drug Administration, Bethesda, MD
Sonja S. Hutchins, MD, MPH, Centers for Disease Control and Prevention,
     Atlanta, GA
Hamid S. Jafari, MD, Centers for Disease Control and Prevention, Atlanta, GA
Deborah Jansen, MD, Food and Drug Administration, Bethesda, MD
William R. Jarvis, MD, Centers for Disease Control and Prevention, Atlanta, GA
John Jereb, MD, Centers for Disease Control and Prevention, Atlanta, GA
Robert E. Johnson, MD, MPH, Centers for Disease Control and Prevention,
     Atlanta, GA
Elaine C. Jong, MD, University of Washington Medical Center, Seattle, WA
Dennis D. Juranek, DVM, Centers for Disease Control and Prevention, Atlanta, GA
Edward L. Kaplan, MD, University of Minnesota, School of Medicine,
     Minneapolis, MN
Sheldon L. Kaplan, MD, Baylor College of Medicine, Houston, TX
Ruth A. Karron, MD, Johns Hopkins University School of Hygiene and Public
     Health, Baltimore, MD
Samuel L. Katz, MD, Duke University School of Medicine, Durham, NC
Richard Kenney, MD, Food and Drug Administration, Bethesda, MD
Rima F. Khabbaz, MD, Centers for Disease Control and Prevention, Atlanta, GA
Dennis Kopecko, MD, Food and Drug Administration, Bethesda, MD

Peter J. Krause, MD, University of Connecticut School of Medicine, Hartford, CT

Phillip Krause, MD, Food and Drug Administration, Bethesda, MD

Sandra A. Larsen, MD, Centers for Disease Control and Prevention, Atlanta, GA

Ruth A. Lawrence, MD, Strong Memorial Hospital, Rochester, NY

Brad Leissa, MD, Food and Drug Administration, Bethesda, MD

David LePay, MD, Food and Drug Administration, Bethesda, MD

Roland Levandowski, MD, Food and Drug Administration, Bethesda, MD

Jay M. Lieberman, MD, University of California Los Angeles Center for Vaccine Research, Torrance, CA

M. Dale Little, PhD, Tulane University, New Orleans, LA

Sarah S. Long, MD, St. Christopher's Hospital for Children, Philadelphia, PA

Dan Lucey, MD, Food and Drug Administration, Bethesda, MD

Ronald Lundquist, MD, Food and Drug Administration, Bethesda, MD

Freyja Lynn, MD, Food and Drug Administration, Bethesda, MD

H. Trent MacKay, MD, MPH, Centers for Disease Control and Prevention, Atlanta, GA

Brian Mahy, PhD, ScD, Centers for Disease Control and Prevention, Atlanta, GA

Samuel D. Maldonado, MD, Food and Drug Administration, Bethesda, MD

Susan Maloney, MD, Food and Drug Administration, Bethesda, MD

Harold S. Margolis, MD, Centers for Disease Control and Prevention, Atlanta, GA

Wilbert Mason, MD, University of Southern California School of Medicine, Los Angeles, CA

David O. Matson, MD, PhD, Children's Hospital of The King's Daughters and Eastern Virginia Medical School, Norfolk, VA

Emily McClure, MD, MPH, Centers for Disease Control and Prevention, Atlanta, GA

Katherine L. McDonald, MD, Minnesota Department of Health, Minneapolis, MN

Kelly T. McKee, Jr, MD, MPH, Womack Army Medical Center, Fort Bragg, NC

Julia A. McMillan, MD, Johns Hopkins University School of Medicine, Baltimore, MD

Michael M. McNeil, MD, MPH, Centers for Disease Control and Prevention, Atlanta, GA

Bruce Meade, MD, Food and Drug Administration, Bethesda, MD

Kristen J. Mertz, MD, Centers for Disease Control and Prevention, Atlanta, GA

Karen Midthun, MD, Food and Drug Administration, Bethesda, MD

Mark A. Miller, MD, Centers for Disease Control and Prevention, Atlanta, GA

Charles D. Mitchell, MD, University of Miami School of Medicine, Miami, FL

Douglas K. Mitchell, MD, Eastern Virginia Medical School, Norfolk, VA

John F. Modlin, MD, Dartmouth Medical School, Lebanon, NH

Nasim Moledina, MD, Food and Drug Administration, Bethesda, MD

Anne C. Moore, MD, PhD, Centers for Disease Control and Prevention, Atlanta, GA

John S. Moran, MD, Centers for Disease Control and Prevention, Atlanta, GA

Sheldon Morris, MD, Food and Drug Administration, Bethesda, MD

Ardythe L. Morrow, MD, Eastern Virginia Medical School, Norfolk, VA

James P. Nataro, MD, PhD, University of Maryland School of Medicine, Baltimore, MD

Thomas R. Navin, Centers for Disease Control and Prevention, Atlanta, GA

Kenard E. Nelson, MD, Johns Hopkins University, Baltimore, MD

Thomas B. Nutman, MD, Centers for Disease Control and Prevention, Atlanta, GA

Karen Olness, MD, University Hospital of Cleveland, Cleveland, OH

James G. Olson, PhD, MPH, Centers for Disease Control and Prevention,
    Atlanta, GA

Margaret J. Oxtoby, MD, Centers for Disease Control and Prevention, Atlanta, GA

Mark Pallansch, PhD, Centers for Disease Control and Prevention, Atlanta, GA

Demosthenes Pappagianis, MD, University of California, Davis School of Medicine,
    Davis, CA

Peter Patriarca, MD, Food and Drug Administration, Bethesda, MD

Andrew Pavia, MD, University of Utah, Salt Lake City, UT

Richard D. Pearson, MD, University of Virginia School of Medicine,
    Charlottesville, VA

Bradley A. Perkins, MD, Centers for Disease Control and Prevention, Atlanta, GA

Seleda Perryman, MD, Centers for Disease Control and Prevention, Atlanta, GA

Clarence J. Peters, MD, Centers for Disease Control and Prevention, Atlanta, GA

Lynelle Phillips, MD, Centers for Disease Control and Prevention, Atlanta, GA

Stanley Plotkin, MD, Pasteur-Merieux Serums et Vaccins, Marnes-la-Coquette, France

Christopher Plowe, MD, University of Maryland, Baltimore, MD

Douglas Pratt, MD, Food and Drug Administration, Bethesda, MD

Neil S. Prose, MD, Duke University Medical Center, Durham, NC

Alexander Rakowsky, MD, Food and Drug Administration, Bethesda, MD

Mobeen Hasan Rathore, MD, University of Florida Health Science Center,
    Jacksonville, FL

Stephen C. Redd, MD, Centers for Disease Control and Prevention, Atlanta, GA

Susan E. Reef, MD, Centers for Disease Control and Prevention, Atlanta, GA

Russell L. Regnery, PhD, Centers for Disease Control and Prevention, Atlanta, GA

Frank O. Richards, Jr, MD, Centers for Disease Control and Prevention, Atlanta, GA

Rosemary Roberts, MD, Food and Drug Administration, Bethesda, MD

Theresa Romani, MD, Food and Drug Administration, Bethesda, MD

Lorry G. Rubin, MD, Schneider Children's Hospital, New Hyde Park, NY

Andrea S. Ruff, MD, Johns Hopkins University, Baltimore, MD

Charles E. Rupprecht, MD, Centers for Disease Control and Prevention,
    Atlanta, GA

Peter M. Schantz, VMD, Centers for Disease Control and Prevention, Atlanta, GA

Walter W. Schluter, MD, MSPH, Centers for Disease Control and Prevention,
    Atlanta, GA

Lawrence B. Schonberger, MD, MPH, Centers for Disease Control and Prevention,
    Atlanta, GA

Anne Schuchat, MD, Centers for Disease Control and Prevention, Atlanta, GA

Mary-Ann B. Shafer, MD, University of California at San Francisco, San
    Francisco, CA

Craig N. Shapiro, MD, Centers for Disease Control and Prevention, Atlanta, GA

Eugene D. Shapiro, MD, Yale University School of Medicine, Boston, MA

Stanford T. Shulman, MD, Children's Memorial Hospital, Chicago, IL

Jane D. Siegel, MD, University of Texas Southwestern Medical Center, Dallas, TX

Robert J. Simonds, MD, Centers for Disease Control and Prevention, Atlanta, GA

Lawrence M. Slutsker, MD, MPH, Centers for Disease Control and Prevention, Atlanta, GA

Steven L. Solomon, MD Centers for Disease Control and Prevention, Atlanta, GA

Janice Soreth, MD, Food and Drug Administration, Bethesda, MD

Richard A. Spiegel, DVM, MPH, Centers for Disease Control and Prevention, Atlanta, GA

Joseph W. St Geme, III, MD, Washington University School of Medicine, St. Louis, MO

Jeffrey Starke, MD, Baylor College of Medicine, Houston, TX

Mark C. Steinhoff, MD, Johns Hopkins University, Baltimore, MD

William Stevens, MD, Food and Drug Administration, Bethesda, MD

John A. Stewart, MD, Centers for Disease Control and Prevention, Atlanta, GA

Katherine M. Stone, MD, Centers for Disease Control and Prevention, Atlanta, GA

Howard Z. Streicher, MD, Food and Drug Administration, Bethesda, MD

Raymond A. Strikas, MD, Centers for Disease Control and Prevention, Atlanta, GA

Roland W. Sutter, MD, MPH, TM, Centers for Disease Control and Prevention, Atlanta, GA

Howard Taras, MD University of California, San Diego, CA

Katherine Taubert, PhD, American Heart Association, Dallas, TX

Robert V. Tauxe, MD, MPH, Centers for Disease Control and Prevention, Atlanta, GA

Fred C. Tenover, PhD, Centers for Disease Control and Prevention, Atlanta, GA

Margaret Tipple, MD, Centers for Disease Control and Prevention, Atlanta, GA

Theodore F. Tsai, MD, Centers for Disease Control and Prevention, Atlanta, GA

Paul Turkeltaub, MD, Food and Drug Administration, Bethesda, MD

Jessica Tuttle, MD, Centers for Disease Control and Prevention, Atlanta, GA

Julianne Valianncourt, MD, Food and Drug Administration, Bethesda, MD

Frederik van Loon, MD, PhD, MPH, Centers for Disease Control and Prevention, Atlanta, GA

Govinda S. Visvesvara, PhD, Centers for Disease Control and Prevention, Atlanta, GA

Charles Vitek, MD, MPH, Centers for Disease Control and Prevention, Atlanta, GA

Ellen Wald, MD, Children's Hospital of Pittsburgh, Pittsburgh, PA

Richard J. Wallace, Jr, MD, University of Texas Health Center, Tyler, TX

Susan Wasner, MD, Centers for Disease Control and Prevention, Atlanta, GA

Judy Wasserheit, MD, Centers for Disease Control and Prevention, Atlanta, GA

John C. Watson, MD, MPH, Centers for Disease Control and Prevention, Atlanta, GA

Geoffrey A. Weinberg, MD, University of Rochester School of Medicine, Rochester, NY

Carol Weiss, MD, Food and Drug Administration, Bethesda, MD

Jay D. Wenger, MD, Centers for Disease Control and Prevention, Atlanta, GA

Melinda Wharton, MD, Centers for Disease Control and Prevention, Atlanta, GA

Edward J. Young, MD, Baylor College of Medicine, Houston, TX

Jane R. Zucker, MD, MSc, Centers for Disease Control and Prevention, Atlanta, GA

Committee on Infectious Diseases, 1995–1996

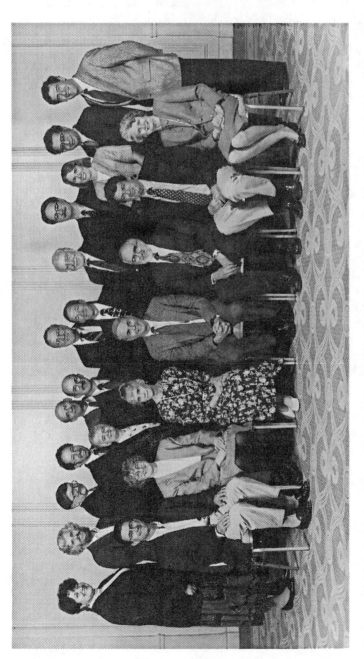

Front row: Melvin I. Marks, P. Joan Chesney, Caroline B. Hall, Georges Peter, Neal A. Halsey, S. Michael Marcy, M. Carolyn Hardegree

Second row: N. Regina Rabinovich, Stephen C. Hadler, Dennis L. Murray, Walter A. Orenstein, Noni E. MacDonald, Ram Yogev, Michael A. Gerber, Donald S. Gromisch, James C. Overall, Jr, Richard J. Whitley, Richard F. Jacobs, Ruth L. Berkelman, Samuel D. Maldonado, Robert Breiman

Not pictured: Larry K. Pickering and Steve Kohl

Dedication

Everything changes, especially in the *Red Book*. A large amount of new information is generated in the 3-year interval between editions that has an impact on the diagnosis, treatment, and prevention of infectious diseases in children. Georges Peter, MD, deserves enormous credit for organizing and incorporating this new information into the 1997 edition of the *Red Book* as well as in four previous editions. Georges' intense scrutiny of each chapter of each edition has improved the content, consistency in writing style, and clarity of presentation.

Georges has announced that this edition will be his last, despite many pleas for him to continue as editor of the *Red Book*. For 15 years he has contributed not only to the writing and editing of the *Red Book*, but also to the development of virtually every Committee on Infectious Diseases policy statement. His sage advice has been sincerely appreciated by current and former members of the Academy and the Committee; his many contributions will be sorely missed.

Filling the void when Georges leaves will be a challenge for two main reasons; the health care environment is changing very rapidly and Georges Peter has been a wonderful *Red Book* editor.

Preface

The practice of pediatrics is changing at an ever-increasing pace. Providers of pediatric care face not only a rapidly changing knowledge base, but also increasing economic and time constraints that affect the delivery of health care services. The Academy and other organizations are developing systems that allow electronic access to information that is pertinent to the health of children. Future editions of the *Red Book* are highly likely to be even more easily accessed electronically. Nevertheless, the ability to obtain information quickly about common and unusual infectious diseases affecting children from a small, easily identifiable, frequently updated compendium of information like the *Red Book* continues to be an important tool for pediatricians and other health care providers.

The Committee on Infectious Diseases is dedicated to providing practitioners with the most up-to-date and highest quality information available. The process of preparing a new edition starts $2\frac{1}{2}$–3 years prior to the publication date. Advice and information are obtained from many experts as evidenced by the lengthy list of contributors. We are especially indebted to the many contributors from other Academy committees, the Centers for Disease Control and Prevention, the Food and Drug Administration, the National Institutes of Health, the World Health Organization, and many other organizations that have made this edition possible. In addition, many suggestions made by individual Academy members to improve the presentation or wording on specific issues have been taken into account under the able leadership of Georges Peter, MD, and the Associate Editors.

As noted in previous editions of the *Red Book*, some omissions and errors are inevitable in a book of this type. We hope that Academy members will continue to actively assist the Committee by suggesting specific ways to improve the quality of future editions.

Neal A. Halsey, MD, FAAP
Chairman, Committee on Infectious Diseases

Introduction

The Committee on Infectious Diseases is responsible for formulating and revising guidelines of the American Academy of Pediatrics for the control of infectious diseases in children. At intervals of approximately 3 years, the Committee reviews and revises all of its recommendations and issues a composite summary, *Red Book: Report of the Committee on Infectious Diseases.* These recommendations represent consensuses developed by the members of the Committee in conjunction with liaison representatives from the Centers for Disease Control and Prevention, the Food and Drug Administration, the National Institutes of Health, the National Vaccine Program, and the Canadian Paediatric Society, *Red Book* consultants, and numerous collaborators whose expert advice the Committee solicited. This edition is based on information available as of December 1996.

Unanswered scientific questions, the complexity of medical practice, new information, and inevitable differences of opinion among experts result in inherent limitations of the *Red Book.* In the context of these limitations, the Committee endeavors to provide current, relevant and defensible recommendations for the prevention and management of infectious diseases in children. In some cases, other committees and experts may differ in their interpretation of the data and resulting recommendations. In some instances, no single recommendation can be made as several options for management are equally acceptable.

In making its recommendations, the Committee acknowledges these differences in viewpoints by judicious use of the phrases "most experts recommend..." and "some experts recommend..." Both phrases indicate valid recommendations but the first signifies more support among experts, and the second, less support. Hence, "some experts recommend..." indicates a minority view that is based on data and/or experience and is sufficiently valid to warrant consideration.

Inevitably in clinical practice, questions arise that cannot be answered on the basis of currently available data. In such cases, the Committee attempts to provide guidelines and information that in conjunction with clinical judgment will facilitate well-reasoned decisions. We welcome questions, different perspectives and alternative recommendations, as the resulting dialogue helps the Committee in its continuing review and periodic revisions of the *Red Book.* Through this process, the Committee seeks to provide a practical and authoritative guide for physicians in their care of children.

To aid physicians and other health care providers in assimilating current changes in the recommendations in the *Red Book,* a list of major changes has been compiled (see Summary of Major Changes, p xxiii). However, this listing does not include many changes of lesser importance and health care providers should consult individual chapters and sections of the book for further guidelines. In addition, new information inevitably begins to outdate some recommendations in the *Red Book,* even in the year of its publication, and necessitates that health care providers remain informed of new developments and resulting changes in recommendations. Between editions, the Academy publishes new recommendations from the Committee in *Pediatrics* and/or in *AAP News*.

Physicians in using antimicrobials should review the package inserts (product labels) prepared by the manufacturers, particularly for information concerning contraindications and adverse reactions. No attempt has been made in the *Red Book* to provide this information, since it is readily available in the *Physicians' Desk Reference*. As in previous editions, recommended dosage schedules for antimicrobials are given (see Section 5, Antimicrobials and Related Therapy). Recommendations in the *Red Book* for drug dosages may differ from those of the manufacturer in the product label. Physicians also should be familiar with the information in the product label for vaccines and immune globulins as well as the recommendations of other committees (see Sources of Vaccine Information, p 1).

This book could not have been prepared without the dedicated professional and administrative competence of Dr Edgar O. Ledbetter, Director of the Department of Maternal, Child and Adolescent Health at the Academy. His wise counsel and support throughout the detailed 3-year process of preparation of this edition of the *Red Book* is very much appreciated. His staff has been equally invaluable in their committed work and contributions, particularly Vida Urba Schwartz, Project Manager, who served as the administrative director for the Committee and coordinated the preparation of the *Red Book*, and of Barbara A. Scotese, the AAP Senior Medical Copy Editor. Special thanks are given to Charlotte A. Gauthier, secretary to the Editor, for her work, patience and support. They are the unsung heroes of this edition who deserve the gratitude of those who use the *Red Book*. As Editor, I also am indebted to the Associate Editors, Drs Caroline Breese Hall (the previous Chairperson of the Committee), Neal A. Halsey, S. Michael Marcy, and Larry K. Pickering for their expertise, tireless work, and immense contributions in their editorial and Committee work. Members of the Committee also gave countless hours and deserve appropriate recognition for their dedication, revisions, and reviews. As a Committee, we particularly appreciate the guidance and dedication of the current Committee Chairperson, Dr Neal A Halsey, whose immense knowledge, energy, dedication, and leadership are reflected in the quality and productivity of the Committee's work.

These individuals are only a few of the many contributors whose professional work and commitment have been not only integral but also essential in the Committee's preparation of the *Red Book*.

Georges Peter, MD
Editor

Table of Contents

SECTION 2
RECOMMENDATIONS FOR CARE OF CHILDREN
IN SPECIAL CIRCUMSTANCES

SECTION 3
SUMMARIES OF INFECTIOUS DISEASES

Summary of Major Changes in the 1997 *Red Book*

Major changes in recommendations and related information concerning pediatric infectious diseases are summarized as follows:

1. **Immunization Schedule** (see Fig 1.1, p 18). The 1997 schedule for routine childhood immunizations is given. Recent changes, which are reviewed in detail in the disease-specific chapters, concern recommendations for poliovirus vaccination, use of acellular pertussis vaccine in infants, varicella vaccine, and the recommended age for the second dose of MMR. A routine visit at 11 to 12 years of age for review and administration of vaccines necessary for adolescents is now recommended (see also Adolescent and College Populations, p 63). The footnotes in the schedule (see Fig 1.1, p 18) include further guidelines, including generic recommendations for the use of combination vaccines. This schedule is revised yearly and, accordingly, will be updated in early 1998.

2. **Guidelines on Active Immunization** (see Section 1). New recommendations include revised contraindications for MMR vaccination of egg-allergic children (see Hypersensitivity Reactions to Vaccine Constituents, p 32) and of HIV-infected patients with severe immunosuppression (see Immunodeficient and Immunosuppressed Children, p 50); guidelines for live-virus vaccination in children who are or who have recently received high doses of corticosteroids (see Immunodeficient and Immunosuppressed Children, p 51); generic precautions for patient observation after vaccination (see Vaccine Administration, p 8); guidelines for administrations of vaccine in recent recipients of an immune globulin product (see Active Immunization of Persons Who Recently Received Immune Globulin, p 23) and management of anaphylaxis (see Treatment of Anaphylactic Reactions, p 45). The guidelines for immunization for foreign travel have been updated to include the recently licensed hepatitis A and typhoid fever vaccines (see Foreign Travel, p 68).

3. **Infection Control for Hospitalized Children** (see p 100). The new recommendations for isolation precautions of children issued by the Centers for Disease Control and Prevention (CDC) in 1996 are summarized and information is provided to aid in the implementation of these recommendations in hospitalized pediatric patients. In the disease-specific chapters in Section 3, the recommendations in *Isolation of the Hospitalized Patient* are based on the new CDC system for precautions.

4. ***Escherichia coli* diarrhea.** Recent information on *E coli* 0157:H7 infection and its complication of hemolytic-uremic syndrome are summarized (see p 204).

5. **Ehrlichiosis.** New information on the epidemiology, diagnosis, and treatment of this emerging rickettsial infection is given (see p 196).

6. **Hepatitis A.** This chapter has been extensively revised and includes the AAP recommendations on the indications and related information concerning hepatitis A vaccines (see p 237) as well as current indications for passive immunoprophylaxis, including postexposure prophylaxis (see p 241).

7. **Hepatitis B.** Changes include increased emphasis on universal immunization of adolescents (see p 247), revised recommendations for immunoprophylaxis of premature infants born of mothers with chronic hepatitis B infection or whose serum hepatitis B surface antigen (HBsAg) status is not known at birth (see p 256), current vaccine schedules (see p 258), and recommended vaccine dosages at different ages (see Table 3.16, p 252). Guidelines also have been provided on the management of children and adolescents who are chronically infected, ie, HBsAg carriers (see p 260). Since the recommendations for immunoprophylaxis are complex, health care providers should review the immunization recommendations in detail for current information.

8. **Hepatitis C** (see p 260). Considerable new information on the epidemiology, diagnosis, and management of hepatitis C virus (HCV) infection has accumulated since publication of the 1994 *Red Book*. As a result, this chapter has been extensively revised and includes recommendations on the management of infants born of women who are HCV-infected, serological testing, management of patients with chronic HCV infection, and counseling of these patients.

9. **HIV Infection.** Continuing new developments and information about HIV infection have necessitated extensive revision of this chapter, which physicians and other providers involved in the care of children and adolescents with HIV infection should review in detail. Major changes include the 1994 pediatric classification system (see Table 3.22, p 282), guidelines for serological testing (see p 288), antiretroviral therapy (see p 290), indications for chemoprophylaxis of *Pneumocystis carinii* pneumonia (see p 293), indications for MMR and other vaccines (see p 294), recommendations for chemoprophylaxis to reduce perinatal HIV transmission (see p 296), and indications for postexposure prophylaxis (see p 302). Because the management of HIV infection is evolving rapidly, some of these recommendations in the 1997 *Red Book* will be outdated before the next edition is published and new recommendations should be anticipated.

10. **Prevention of Opportunistic Infections in Children and Adolescents With HIV Infection.** The 1995 guidelines of the United States Public Health Service and the Infectious Disease Society of America,* which have been endorsed by the AAP, have been incorporated into the disease-specific chapters in Section 3, as related to pediatric patients. These infections include *Pneumocystis carinii* pneumonia, toxoplasmic encephalitis, *Mycobacterium avium* complex (MAC) infection, *Candida albicans,* and other fungal infections.

11. **Lyme Disease.** New recommendations on diagnostic testing (see p 330) and treatment (see p 331) are given.

12. **Malaria.** Recommendations on chemoprophylaxis (see p 339) and treatment (see p 336) have been updated.

---

* Centers for Disease Control and Prevention. USPHS/IDSA guidelines for the prevention of opportunistic infections in persons infected with human immunodeficiency virus: a summary. *MMWR.* 1995;44(No. RR-8):1-34.

13. **Meningococcal Infections.** The 1996 AAP guidelines on diagnostic tests (see p 358), indications, and regimens for chemoprophylaxis for contacts (see p 359), and recommendations for meningococcal vaccination (see p 361) are given.

14. **Measles.** New immunization recommendations concern the routine age for the second dose of MMR vaccine (see p 349); precautions and contraindications to vaccination, including for egg-allergic children, steroid recipients, children with HIV infection, and vaccine-associated thrombocytopenia (see p 352), and the recommended intervals after receipt of immune globulin preparations before vaccination (see p 352). Relevant revisions also are included in the mumps (see p 366) and rubella (see p 456) chapters.

15. **Pertussis.** Recommendations for vaccination against pertussis have been revised significantly as the result of approval of acellular pertussis vaccines, given as DTaP, for use in the primary immunization of infants (see p 397). Other changes include the updated AAP assessment of the role of DTP in neurological disorders temporally associated with pertussis vaccination (see p 405) and guidelines on the management of school outbreaks of pertussis (see p 397).

16. ***Pneumocystis carinii* Infections.** The indications for chemoprophylaxis in HIV-infected infants and children have been revised (see p 421).

17. **Pneumococcal Infections.** Major changes include the 1997 AAP recommendations for antimicrobial therapy of suspected or proven *Streptococcus pneumoniae* meningitis (see p 413). The emergence of antimicrobial-resistant pneumococcal infections has necessitated new guidelines for the treatment of invasive pneumococcal infections that should be reviewed in detail. Indications for pneumococcal vaccination and revaccination also have been revised (see p 417).

18. **Poliovirus Infections.** Expanded use of inactivated poliovirus vaccine (IPV) is recommended by the AAP and the Advisory Committee on Immunization Practices (ACIP) of the CDC. Current AAP recommendations for poliovirus vaccination, as well as those of the ACIP, are given (see p 430).

19. **Rabies.** The epidemiology of rabies in animals in the United States (see p 435) and resulting recommendations for immunoprophylaxis for persons exposed to potentially or known rabid animals (see p 439) are provided.

20. **Respiratory Syncytial Virus.** The revised AAP recommendations on indications for ribavirin therapy (see p 445) and recently issued guidelines for immunoprophylaxis of high-risk infants with RSV receive RSV-IGIV (see p 446) are included.

21. ***Salmonella* Infections.** Since publication of the 1994 *Red Book*, a third typhoid fever vaccine has been licensed for use in children. Guidelines for use of these three vaccines are summarized (see p 466).

22. **Group A Streptococcal Infections (GAS).** Current recommendations on the diagnosis and therapy of GAS pharyngitis are given (see p 486). Information on the diagnosis and management of invasive GAS infections also is included in this chapter.

23. **Group B Streptococcal Infections.** The recently revised guidelines for prevention of early onset, neonatal group B streptococcal infections, including indications for screening of pregnant women and for chemoprophylaxis, are given in detail (p 495). The guidelines for management of newborns whose mothers received intrapartum chemoprophylaxis have been considerably expanded.

24. **Tuberculosis.** The AAP recommendations for skin testing of children, as updated in 1996 (see p 546), and revised guidelines on therapy, including duration, are given (see p 547). Since this chapter is extensive and complex, physicians involved in the care of children with suspected or proven tuberculosis should review this chapter for further information.

25. **Diseases Caused By Nontuberculous Mycobacteria.** Recommendations concerning chemoprophylaxis of HIV-infected persons (see p 567) and treatment (see p 566) have been revised.

26. **Varicella-Zoster Infections.** The current AAP recommendations for vaccination, including indications, precautions, and contraindications (see p 573), are included. The guidelines for the use of the vaccine in children who are or have recently received corticosteroids have been revised to be consistent with generic recommendations for live-virus vaccination of steroid recipients (see Immunodeficient and Immunosuppressed Children, p 51).

27. **Tinea Infections** (see p 523). The recommendations for therapy of these infections have been updated.

28. **Antimicrobials and Related Therapy** (see Section 5). The tables on drug dosages and recommendations have been revised to include new drugs and recommendations, including antibacterial, antiviral, antifungal and antiparasitic drugs. Information on the use of fluoroquinolones and tetracyclines in pediatric patients is given. The age for which tetracycline should not be given routinely has been changed from less than 9 years old to less than 8 years old.

29. **Vaccine Injury Table.** The current Table (effective as of March 1997) is reproduced (see p 681).

30. **New Chapters and Tables.**
    - *School health* (see p 93)
    - *Injuries from discarded needles in the community* (see p 120)
    - *Bite wounds* (see p 122)
    - *Chancroid* (see p 166)
    - *Sporotrichosis* (see p 474)
    - *Guidelines for treatment of sexually transmitted diseases in children and adolescents according to syndrome* (see p 623)
    - *MEDWATCH — Medical Products Reporting Program* (see p 665)
    - *Clinical syndromes associated with food-borne diseases* (see p 689)

Every effort has been made to identify major changes in order to aid in adopting new guidelines and recommendations from the 1997 *Red Book* to the care of their patients. However, since no list is likely to be complete and the designation of a change as major can be arbitrary, physicians and other health care providers are urged to review relevant chapters, tables, and sections in the *Red Book*. In addition, since preparation of each edition involves review of the entire book, considerable new information is included which also should be helpful in the diagnosis, management, and prevention of infectious diseases in infants, children, and adolescents.

Active and Passive Immunization

••••••••••••••••••••

PROLOGUE

The ultimate goal of immunization is eradication of disease; the immediate goal is prevention of disease in individuals or groups. To accomplish these goals, physicians must maintain timely immunization, including both active and passive immunoprophylaxis, as a high priority in the care of infants, children, adolescents, and adults. The global eradication of smallpox in 1977 and elimination of poliomyelitis from the Americas in 1991 serve as models for the control of disease through immunization. Both of these accomplishments were achieved by combining an effective immunization program with intense surveillance and effective public health control measures worldwide.

Many infectious diseases can be prevented by immunoprophylaxis. With active immunization, a person is stimulated to develop immunologic defenses against future natural exposure. With passive immunization, a person already exposed, or about to be exposed, to certain infectious agents is given preformed human or animal antibody.

In the United States, immunization has sharply curtailed, or practically eliminated, diphtheria, measles, mumps, pertussis, rubella (congenital and acquired), tetanus, and *Haemophilus influenzae* type b disease. Yet, because these diseases persist in the United States as well as in other countries, immunizations need to be continued. Research on new vaccines involves molecular biologic techniques. Eventually, some of these experimental vaccines will be used routinely. Physicians must regularly update their knowledge about specific vaccines and their use because information about the safety and efficacy of vaccines and recommendations relative to their administration continue to develop after a vaccine is licensed.

Each edition of the *Red Book* gives recommendations for immunization of children and adolescents based on the knowledge, experience, and premises at the time of publication. The recommendations represent a consensus with which reasonable physicians may at times disagree. No claim is made for infallibility, and the Committee acknowledges that individual circumstances may warrant decisions differing from the recommendations given here.

••

SOURCES OF VACCINE INFORMATION

In addition to the *Red Book*, which is published at intervals of approximately 3 years, physicians should utilize the scientific literature and other sources for data or answers to specific questions encountered in practice. Among these sources are the following:
* ***Pediatrics.*** Statements developed by the Committee on Infectious Diseases (COID) and approved by the American Academy of Pediatrics, giving updated recommendations, are published in *Pediatrics* between editions of the *Red Book*. In addition,

articles provide new information on infectious diseases and immunizations. The updated, national immunization schedule is published at least annually in *Pediatrics*, usually in January, as well as in other sources (see Scheduling Immunizations, p 15).

- **AAP News.** Policy statements (or statement summaries) from the COID are often initially published in *AAP News*, the Academy's monthly newspaper, to inform its membership promptly of new recommendations.
- ***Morbidity and Mortality Weekly Report (MMWR).*** Published weekly by the Centers for Disease Control and Prevention (CDC), *MMWR* contains current vaccine recommendations, reports of specific disease activity, and changes in policy statements. Recommendations of the Immunization Practices Advisory Committee (ACIP) of the CDC are published periodically, usually as supplements.
- **Official package inserts (product labels).** Manufacturers provide product-specific information with each vaccine product. This information also is given in the *Physicians' Desk Reference (PDR)*. The product label must be in full compliance with Food and Drug Administration (FDA) regulations pertaining to labeling for prescription, including indications and usage, dosages, routes of administration, clinical pharmacology, contraindications, and adverse reactions. The package insert lists preservatives, stabilizers, antibiotics, adjuvants, and suspending fluids, which may cause inflammation or elicit an allergic response. Health care providers should be familiar with the label for each product they administer.
- ***Health Information for International Travel.*** This useful monograph is published annually by the CDC as a guide to requirements of the various countries for specific immunizations. It also provides information concerning other vaccines recommended for travel in specific areas and other information for travelers. It can be purchased from the Superintendent of Documents, US Government Printing Office, Washington, DC 20402-9235. For further sources of information on international travel, see Foreign Travel (p 68).
- ***Control of Communicable Diseases in Man.*** The American Public Health Association publishes this manual at intervals of approximately 5 years. It contains valuable information about most infectious diseases, their worldwide occurrence, diagnostic and therapeutic information, immunizations, recommendations on isolation, and other control measures for specific diseases. The latest edition was published in 1995. It is available from the American Public Health Association, 1015 Fifteenth St, NW; Washington, DC 20005.
- ***Guide for Adult Immunization.*** This publication by the American College of Physicians (Subscriber Services, Independence Mall, West Sixth Street at Race, Philadelphia, PA 19106-1572) provides useful information about infectious diseases and vaccine recommendations for adults. The most recent edition was published in 1994.

Physicians can consult members of the Committee by phone or letter. Specific questions may be addressed directly to the Academy.*

Consultation and printed material on immunizations can also be obtained from the Voice Information System (VIS)* of the National Immunization Program at the CDC. The VIS provides current information by voice, mail or fax. Specific

---

* See Directory of Telephone Numbers, p 667.

consultations can be obtained by calling the National Immunization Program.* Other resources include the FDA*; infectious disease experts at university affiliated hospitals, medical schools, and/or in private practice, and regional public health departments. Information can be obtained from the latter about current epidemiology of diseases, immunization recommendations, legal requirements, public health policies, foreign travel, and nursery school, child care, and school health concerns.

INFORMING PATIENTS AND PARENTS

Parents and patients should be informed about the benefits and risks of preventive and therapeutic procedures, including immunizations.

The patient, parent, and/or legal guardian should be informed about the benefits to be derived from vaccines in preventing disease in individuals and in the community, and about the risks of those vaccines. Questions should be encouraged so that the information is understood and coercion is avoided.

The National Childhood Vaccine Injury Act of 1986 included requirements for notifying patients and parents in both the private and public sectors about vaccine benefits and risks. This legislation, as subsequently amended, mandates distribution of standardized vaccine information materials (now termed Vaccine Information Statements [VISs]) when administering vaccines for which compensation is available (see Vaccine Injury Table, p 681). Amendments to the original legislation deleted the language that allowed providers who buy their own vaccines the flexibility to develop their own materials. Copies of the current VISs can be obtained from state and local health departments, the CDC, the Academy, and vaccine manufacturers. For vaccines not yet included in the Vaccine Injury Compensation Program, such as *Haemophilus influenzae* type b, hepatitis B, and varicella vaccines (as of December 1996), legally ratified VISs are not available. The CDC has developed "Important Information" statements about these vaccines; these statements are revised periodically and are available from state health departments. The new VISs and "Important Information" statements no longer include space for the parents' or patients' signatures to indicate that they have read and understood the material, although the provider has the option to obtain a signature. Whether or not a signature is obtained, the Academy recommends that physicians document in the chart that the VISs or the "Important Information" statements have been provided and discussed with the parent, legal representative, and/or patient. Health care providers, however, should note in the patient's permanent medical record that the statements were provided at the time of immunization. In addition, the date of administration of the vaccine, the manufacturer and lot number of the vaccine, and the name and business address of the provider administering the vaccine must be recorded in the patient's record (see also Vaccine Safety and Contraindications, p 26).

---

* See Directory of Telephone Numbers, p 667.

ACTIVE IMMUNIZATION

Active immunization involves administration of all or part of a microorganism or a modified product of that microorganism (eg, a toxoid, a purified antigen, or an antigen produced by genetic engineering) to evoke an immunologic response mimicking that of the natural infection but which usually presents little or no risk to the recipient. The immunization can result in antitoxin, anti-invasive, or neutralizing activity, or other types of protective humoral or cellular response in the patient. Some immunizing agents provide complete protection against disease for life, some provide partial protection, and some must be readministered at intervals. The effectiveness of a vaccine or toxoid is assessed by the evidence of protection against the natural disease. Induction of antibodies frequently is an indirect measure of protection, but in some circumstances (eg, in pertussis) the immunologic response correlated with protection is poorly understood, and serum antibody concentrations are not always predictive of protection.

Vaccines incorporating an intact infectious agent may be either live and attenuated, or killed (inactivated). Currently licensed vaccines are listed in Table 1.1 (see p 5). Many viral vaccines contain live-attenuated virus. Although active infection (with replication) ensues after administration of these vaccines, little or no adverse host reaction usually occurs. The vaccines for some viruses and most bacteria are inactivated (killed) or subunit preparations. Inactive agents are incapable of replicating in the host; therefore, these vaccines must contain a sufficient antigenic mass to stimulate the desired response. Maintenance of long-lasting immunity with killed (inactivated) viral or bacterial vaccines often requires periodic administration of booster doses. Inactivated vaccines may not elicit the range of immunologic response provided by live-attenuated agents. For example, an injected, inactivated viral vaccine may evoke sufficient serum antibody or cell-mediated immunity but fail to evoke local antibody in the form of secretory immunoglobulin A (IgA). Thus, mucosal protection after administration of inactivated vaccines is generally inferior to the mucosal immunity induced by live vaccines, and local infection or colonization with the agent can occur, although systemic infection is prevented or ameliorated by the presence of serum and cellular factors. However, inactivated vaccines cannot replicate or be excreted as infectious agents by the vaccinee and thereby adversely affect immunosuppressed hosts or their contacts.

Recommendations for dose, route, technique of administration, and schedules should be followed for predictable, effective immunization. Related recommendations are critical to the success of immunization practices.

Immunizing Antigens

Physicians should be familiar with the major constituents of the products they use. These are listed in the package inserts. If a vaccine is produced by different manufacturers, some differences may exist in the active and inert ingredients contained in the various products. The major constituents of vaccines include the following:

1. *Active immunizing antigens.* Some vaccines consist of a single antigen that is a highly defined constituent (eg, pneumococcal polysaccharide, or tetanus or diphtheria toxoid); in other vaccines, the antigens are complex and/or less well defined (eg, live viruses or killed bacteria).

Table 1.1. Vaccines Licensed in the United States and Their Routes of Administration

Vaccine*	Type	Route†
Adenovirus‡	Live virus	Oral
Anthrax§	Inactivated bacteria	SC
BCG	Live bacteria	ID (preferred) or SC
Cholera	Inactivated bacteria	SC, IM, or ID
DTP	Toxoids and inactivated bacteria	IM
DTaP	Toxoids and inactivated bacterial components	IM
Hepatitis A	Inactivated virus	IM
Hepatitis B	Inactivated viral antigen	IM
Hib conjugates‖	Polysaccharide-protein conjugate	IM
Hib conjugate-DTP (HbOC‖-DTP and PRP-T‖ reconstituted with DTP)	Polysaccharide-protein conjugate with toxoids and inactivated bacteria	IM
Hib conjugate-DTaP (PRP-T‖ reconstituted with DTaP)	Polysaccharide-protein conjugate with toxoids and inactivated bacterial components	IM
Hib conjugate (PRP-OMP‖)-hepatitis B	Polysaccharide-protein conjugate with inactivated virus	IM
Influenza	Inactivated virus (whole-virus), viral components	IM IM
Japanese encephalitis	Inactivated virus	SC
Measles	Live virus	SC
Meningococcal	Polysaccharide	SC
MMR	Live viruses	SC
Measles-rubella	Live viruses	SC
Mumps	Live virus	SC
Pertussis§	Inactivated bacteria	IM
Plague	Inactivated bacteria	IM
Pneumococcal	Polysaccharide	IM or SC
Poliovirus: OPV	Live virus	Oral
IPV	Inactivated virus	SC
Rabies	Inactivated virus	IM or ID¶
Rubella	Live virus	SC
Tetanus	Toxoid	IM
Tetanus-diphtheria (Td, DT)	Toxoids	IM
Typhoid Parenteral	Inactivated bacteria	SC
Parenteral	Capsular polysaccharide	SC (boosters may be ID)
Oral	Live bacteria	Oral
Varicella	Live virus	SC
Yellow fever	Live virus	SC

* Vaccine abbreviations: BCG indicates bacillus Calmette-Guerin vaccine; DTP, diphtheria and tetanus toxoids and pertussis vaccine, adsorbed; DTaP, diphtheria and tetanus toxoids and acellular pertussis vaccine, adsorbed; Hib, *Haemophilus influenzae* type b vaccine; MMR, live measles-mumps-rubella viruses vaccine; OPV, oral poliovirus vaccine; IPV, inactivated poliovirus vaccine; Td, tetanus and diphtheria toxoid (for children ≥7 years and adults); and DT, diphtheria and tetanus toxoids (for children <7 years).
† Route abbreviations: SC indicates subcutaneous; ID, intradermal; and IM, intramuscular.
‡ Available only to US Armed Forces.
§ Distributed by the Division of Biologic Products, Michigan Department of Public Health, Lansing, Mich.
‖ See Table 3.8, p 225.
¶ Human diploid cell rabies vaccine for intradermal use is different in constitution and potency from the intramuscular vaccine; it should be used for preexposure immunization only. Rabies vaccine adsorbed (RVA) should not be used intradermally.

2. ***Suspending fluid.*** The suspending fluid frequently is as simple as sterile water for injection or saline, but it may be a complex tissue-culture fluid. This fluid may contain proteins or other constituents derived from the medium and biologic system in which the vaccine is produced (eg, egg antigens, gelatin, or tissue-culture-derived antigens).

3. ***Preservatives, stabilizers, and antibiotics.*** Trace amounts of chemicals (eg, mercurials, such as thiomersal, and certain antibiotics, such as neomycin or streptomycin) are frequently necessary to prevent bacterial growth or to stabilize the antigen. Allergic reactions may occur if the recipient is sensitive to one or more of these additives. Whenever feasible, these reactions should be anticipated by identifying known host hypersensitivity to specific vaccine components.

4. ***Adjuvants.*** An aluminum salt is frequently used to increase immunogenicity and to prolong the stimulatory effect, particularly for vaccines containing inactivated microorganisms or their products (eg, hepatitis B, and diphtheria and tetanus toxoids). Investigational adjuvants are under evaluation.

Vaccine Handling and Storage

Inattention to vaccine storage conditions can contribute to vaccine failure. Certain vaccines, such as oral poliovirus vaccine (OPV), measles, varicella, and yellow fever vaccine, are very sensitive to increased temperature. Others are sensitive to freezing; examples are diphtheria and tetanus toxoids and pertussis vaccines (DTaP, DTP, DT, and Td), inactivated poliovirus vaccine (IPV), and *Haemophilus influenzae* conjugate, hepatitis A and B, and influenza vaccines. Some products may show physical evidence of altered integrity (eg, DTP vials containing clumps of antigen that cannot be resuspended by vigorous shaking of the vial), but others may retain their normal appearance despite a loss of potency. Therefore, all personnel responsible for handling vaccines in an office or clinic setting should be familiar with standard procedures designed to minimize the risk of vaccine failure. Recommended storage conditions for commonly used vaccines are listed in Table 1.2 (p 10). New vaccines and new formulations of currently available products may have storage requirements different from those listed in the table. In addition, storage recommendation may be revised by the manufacturer. Revisions require approval by the FDA.

Recommendations for the handling and storage of selected biologicals are summarized in the package insert for each product and in a publication, *Vaccine Management,* available from the CDC.* The most current information concerning recommended vaccine storage conditions and handling instructions can be obtained directly from manufacturers; their phone numbers are listed in the product label (package insert) and in the *Physicians' Desk Reference (PDR),* which is published yearly. The following guidelines are suggested as part of a quality control system for safe handling and storage of vaccines in an office or clinic setting.

---

* Centers for Disease Control and Prevention. *Vaccine Management: Recommendations for Handling and Storage of Selected Biologicals.* Atlanta, Ga: US Department of Health and Human Services, Public Health Service; March 1991.

PERSONNEL

- Designate one person as the vaccine coordinator, and assign to this person responsibility for ensuring that vaccines and other biologic products are carefully handled in a safe, documentable manner.
- Inform all persons who will be handling vaccines about specific storage requirements and stability limitations of the products they will encounter (see Table 1.2, p 10). The details of proper storage conditions should be posted on or near each refrigerator or freezer used for vaccine storage or should be readily available.

EQUIPMENT

- Ascertain that refrigerators and freezers in which vaccines are to be stored are working properly.
- Do not connect refrigerators or freezers to an outlet with a ground-flow interrupter (GFI) or one activated by a wall-switch. Utilize plug guards to prevent accidental dislodging of the wall plug.
- Equip each refrigerator with a thermometer located at the center of the storage compartment. This thermometer should be of the constant recording type with graphed readings or one that indicates the upper and lower extremes of temperature during the observation period ("minimum-maximum" thermometer). These thermometers provide a means of establishing whether vaccines have been exposed to potentially harmful temperatures. Placement of vaccine cold-chain monitor cards* in refrigerators can serve to detect potentially harmful elevations in temperature.
- Keep a log book in which temperature readings are systematically recorded daily and the date and time of any mechanical malfunctions or power outages are noted.
- Place in the refrigerator a tray in which all opened vials of vaccine are kept. To avoid mishaps, do not store other pharmaceuticals in the same tray.
- Equip refrigerators with several bottles of chilled water and freezers with several ice trays or ice packs to fill empty space to minimize temperature fluctuations, should a brief electrical or mechanical failure occur.

PROCEDURES

- Acceptance of vaccine upon receipt of shipment:
  — Check that the delivered product has not expired.
  — Examine the merchandise and its shipping container for any evidence of damage during transport.
  — Consider whether the interval between shipment from the supplier and arrival of the product at its destination is excessive (more than 48 hours), and whether the product has likely been exposed to excessive heat or cold that might alter its integrity. Check vaccine cold chain monitor cards if included in the vaccine shipment.
  — Do not accept the shipment if reasonable suspicion exists that the delivered product may have been damaged by environmental insult or improper handling during transport.

---

* Available from 3M Pharmaceuticals, St Paul, Minn.

- — Contact the vaccine supplier or manufacturer when unusual circumstances raise questions regarding the stability of a delivered vaccine. Store suspect vaccine under proper conditions until its viability is determined.
- Refrigerator inspection:
  - — Measure the temperature of the central part of the storage compartment daily, and record this temperature in a log book. If a "minimum-maximum" thermometer is available, record the extremes in temperature fluctuation and reset to baseline.
  - — Inspect the unit weekly for outdated vaccine and dispose of expired products appropriately.
- Routine procedures:
  - — Store vaccines according to the recommended temperatures in the package insert.
  - — Promptly remove expired (outdated) vaccines from the refrigerator or freezer and dispose of them appropriately at the earliest possible time to avoid accidental use.
  - — Keep opened vials of vaccine in a tray so that they are readily identifiable.
  - — Indicate on the label of each vaccine vial the date and time it was reconstituted or first opened.
  - — Promptly discard opened, multidose vials of vaccines that contain a bacteriostatic agent when outdated or if contaminated.
  - — Discard reconstituted, live-virus and other vaccines, if not used within the interval specified in the package insert. Examples include varicella vaccine after 30 minutes, measles-mumps-rubella (MMR) vaccine after 8 hours, and Pedvax HIB* (PRP-OMP) after 24 hours.
  - — Store vaccines in the refrigerator throughout the office day.
  - — Do not open more than one vial of a particular vaccine at a time.
  - — Store vaccine only in the central storage area, ie, not on the door shelf or in peripheral areas of the unit where temperature fluctuations are greater.
  - — Do not keep food in refrigerators where vaccine is stored, as this practice will lead to more frequent opening of the unit and greater chance for thermal instability.
  - — Do not store radioactive materials in the same refrigerator in which vaccines are stored.
  - — Publicize among all clinic or office personnel any violation of handling protocol or any accidental storage problem (eg, electrical failure), and contact vaccine suppliers regarding the handling of the affected vaccine.

Vaccine Administration

GENERAL INSTRUCTIONS FOR PERSONS ADMINISTERING VACCINES

Personnel administering vaccines should take appropriate precautions to minimize the risk of spread of disease to or from patients. Such personnel should have evidence of immunity or be immunized against measles, mumps, rubella, varicella, hepatitis B,

---

* Merck and Co, West Point, Pa.

and influenza, as well as tetanus and diphtheria. Hands should be washed before and after each new patient contact. Gloves are not required when administering vaccines unless the health care worker has open hand lesions or will come into contact with potentially infectious body fluids. Syringes and needles must be sterile and preferably disposable. After use, the needle should not be recapped, and disposable needles and syringes should be discarded promptly in puncture-proof, labeled containers to prevent accidental needle sticks or reuse. Different vaccines should not be mixed in the same syringe unless specifically licensed and labeled for such use.

Because of possible hypersensitivity to vaccine components, persons administering vaccines or other biologic products should be prepared to recognize and treat allergic reactions, including anaphylaxis (see Hypersensitivity Reactions to Vaccine Constituents, p 32). Facilities and personnel should be available for treating immediate hypersensitivity reactions. This recommendation does not preclude administration of vaccines in school-based or other nonclinic settings. Whenever possible, patients should be observed for an allergic reaction for 15 to 20 minutes after receiving immunization(s).

Syncope may occur after vaccination, particularly in adolescents and young adults. Personnel should be aware of presyncopal manifestations and take appropriate measures to prevent injuries if weakness, dizziness, or loss of consciousness occur. The relatively rapid onset of syncope in most cases suggests that having vaccinees sit or lie down for 15 minutes after immunization could avert many syncopal episodes and secondary injuries. If syncope does develop, patients should be observed until they are asymptomatic.

SITE AND ROUTE OF IMMUNIZATION
(ACTIVE AND PASSIVE)

Oral Vaccines. Breastfeeding does not interfere with successful immunization with oral poliovirus vaccine (OPV). If the patient immediately spits out, fails to swallow, or regurgitates OPV, the dose should be repeated. Vomiting within 10 minutes of receiving also is an indication for repeating the dose. If the second dose is not retained, neither dose should be counted and the vaccine should be readministered.

*Parenteral Vaccines.** Injectable vaccines should be administered in a site as free as possible from the risk of local neural, vascular, or tissue injury. Data in the medical literature do not warrant recommendation of a single preferred site for all injections, and many manufacturers' product recommendations allow some flexibility in the site of injection. Preferred sites include the anterolateral aspect of the upper thigh and the deltoid area of the upper arm for vaccines administered either subcutaneously or intramuscularly.

Recommended routes of administration are included in the package inserts of vaccines and are listed in Table 1.1 (p 5). The recommended route is based on the results of prior clinical use that demonstrated maximum safety and efficacy. To minimize untoward local or systemic effects and ensure optimal efficacy of the immunizing procedure, vaccines should be given according to the recommended route.

For intramuscular (IM) injections, the choice of site is based on the volume of the injected material and the size of the muscle. In children younger than 1 year

---

* For an informative review on intramuscular injections, see Bergeson PS, Singer SA, Kaplan AM. Intramuscular injections in children. *Pediatrics.* 1982;70:944-948.

Table 1.2. Recommended Storage Conditions for Commonly Used Vaccines*

Vaccine	Recommended Temperature	Duration of Stability†	Normal Appearance
Diphtheria and tetanus toxoids and acellular pertussis vaccine, adsorbed (DTaP)	2–8°C. Do not freeze. As little as 24 hours at <2°C or >25°C may cause antigens to fall from suspension and be very difficult to resuspend.	Not more than 18 mo from the time of issue from manufacturer's cold storage.	Markedly turbid and whitish suspension. If product contains clumps of material that cannot be resuspended with vigorous shaking, it should NOT be used.
Diphtheria and tetanus toxoids and whole-cell pertussis vaccine, adsorbed (DTP)	2–8°C. Do not freeze. As little as 24 hours at <2°C or >25°C may cause antigens to fall from suspension and be very difficult to resuspend.	Not more than 18 mo from the time of issue from manufacturer's cold storage.	Markedly turbid and whitish suspension. If product contains clumps of material that cannot be resuspended with vigorous shaking, it should NOT be used.
Diphtheria and tetanus toxoids, whole-cell pertussis vaccine adsorbed, and *Haemophilus* b conjugate vaccine (DTP-HbOC)	2–8°C. Do not freeze. As little as 24 hours at <2°C or >25°C may cause antigens to fall from suspension and be very difficult to resuspend.	Not more than 18 mo from the time of issue from manufacturer's cold storage.	Markedly turbid, white suspension. If product contains clumps of material that cannot be resuspended with vigorous shaking, it should NOT be used.
Diphtheria toxoid, adsorbed	2–8°C. Do not freeze.	Not more than 2 y from the time of issue from manufacturer's cold storage.	Turbid and white, slightly gray, or slightly pink suspension.
Haemophilus b conjugate vaccine: HbOC (diphtheria CRM₁₉₇ protein conjugate)	2–8°C. Do not freeze.	Not more than 2 y from date of issue from manufacturer's cold storage.	Clear, colorless liquid.

Vaccine	Storage	Shelf life	Appearance
Haemophilus b conjugate vaccine: PRP-D (diphtheria toxoid conjugate)	2–8°C. Do not freeze.	Not more than 2 y from date of issue from manufacturer's cold storage.	Clear, colorless liquid.
Haemophilus b conjugate vaccine; PRP-OMP (meningococcal protein conjugate)	Lyophilized formulation: 2–8°C. Do not freeze formulation or diluent. Reconstituted formulation: 2–8°C. Do not freeze.	Not more than 2 y from date of issue from manufacturer's cold storage. Discard reconstituted vials if not used within 24 h.	Reconstituted: after agitation, slightly opaque, white suspension,
Haemophilus b conjugate vaccine: PRP-T (tetanus toxoid conjugate)	Lyophilized formulation: 2–8°C. Do not freeze formulation or diluent. May be reconstituted with DTP produced by Connaught Laboratories. Reconstituted formulation: 2–8°C. Do not freeze.	Not more than 2 y from date of issue from manufacturer's cold storage. Vaccine should be used immediately when reconstituted.	Reconstituted: clear and colorless.
Hepatitis A vaccine, inactivated	2–8°C. Do not freeze. Do not use if product has been frozen.	2 y, if kept refrigerated.	Opaque, white suspension.
Hepatitis B virus vaccine inactivated (recombinant)	2–8°C. Storage outside this temperature range may reduce potency. Freezing substantially reduces potency.	2 y from date of issue from manufacturer's cold storage.	After thorough agitation, a slightly opaque, white suspension.
Influenza virus vaccine (subvirion)	2–8°C. Freezing destroys potency.	Vaccine is recommended only during the year for which it is manufactured; antigenic composition differs annually.	Clear, colorless liquid.

Table 1.2. Recommended Storage Conditions for Commonly Used Vaccines,* continued

Vaccine	Recommended Temperature	Duration of Stability†	Normal Appearance
Measles-mumps-rubella virus (MMR) vaccine, live	Lyophilized formulation: 2–8° C, but may be frozen. Protect from light, which may inactivate virus. Diluent: store at room temperature or refrigerated, do not freeze. Reconstituted formulation: 2–8° C. Protect from light, which may inactivate virus.	Discard reconstituted vials if not used within 8 hours.	Reconstituted: clean, yellow solution.
Measles virus vaccine, live	See MMR.	See MMR.	See MMR.
Mumps virus vaccine, live	See MMR.	See MMR.	See MMR.
Rubella virus vaccine, live	See MMR.	See MMR.	See MMR.
Pneumococcal vaccine, polyvalent	2–8°C. Freezing destroys potency.	See expiration date on vial.	Clear, colorless, or slightly opalescent liquid.
Poliovirus vaccine, inactivated (IPV)	2–8°C. Do not freeze.	Not more than 1 y from date of issue from manufacturer's cold storage.	Clear, colorless suspension. Vaccine that contains particulate matter, develops turbidity, or changes in color should NOT be used.

Product	Storage	Expiration	Appearance
Poliovirus vaccine, live, oral (OPV)	Must be stored at <0°C. Because of sorbitol in the vaccine, it will remain fluid at temperatures above −14°C. Refreezing the thawed product is acceptable (maximum of 10 thaw-freeze cycles), if the temperature never exceeds 8°C, and the cumulative thawing time is <24 h.	Not more than 1 y from date of issue from manufacturer's cold storage.	Clear solution, usually red or pink, from the phenol red (pH indicator) it contains; may have a yellow color if shipment was packed with dry ice. Color changes that occur during storage or thawing are unimportant, provided the solution remains clear.
Tetanus and diphtheria toxoids, adsorbed (DT and Td)	2–8° C. Do not freeze.	Not more than 2 y from the time of issue from manufacturer's cold storage.	Markedly turbid and white suspension. If product contains clumps of material that cannot be resuspended with vigorous shaking, it should NOT be used.
Varicella virus vaccine‡	Lyophilized formulation: keep frozen, at temperature of −15°C or colder. Protect from light. Diluent: store at room temperature or refrigerated. Reconstituted formulation: use immediately; do not store. For temporary storage, unreconstituted vaccine may be stored at 2–8°C for a maximum of 72 h.	Lyophilized formulation: 18 mo. Discard reconstituted vials if not used within 30 min. Discard if not used within 72 h (do not refreeze)	Lyophilized formulation: whitish powder. Reconstituted formulation: clear, colorless to pale yellow liquid.

* For recently licensed combination vaccines, see package inserts; instructions may be different from those for products listed in the Table. Also, any changes in the formulation of currently available immunizing agents may alter their appearance, stability, and storage requirements.

† **Questions regarding the stability of biologicals subjected to potentially harmful environmental conditions should be addressed to the manufacturer of the product in question.**

‡ For questions concerning stability, contact the manufacturer by calling 1-800-9-VARIVAX.

(ie, infants), the anterolateral aspect of the thigh provides the largest muscle and is the preferred site. In older children, the deltoid muscle is usually large enough for IM injection. Some physicians prefer to use the anterolateral thigh muscles for toddlers. Parents and children, however, often prefer use of the deltoid muscle for immunization at 18 months of age and older because of less discomfort in the affected extremity and in ambulating.

Ordinarily, the upper, outer aspect of the buttocks should not be used for active immunization because the gluteal region is covered by a significant layer of subcutaneous fat and because of the possibility of damaging the sciatic nerve. However, clinical information on the use of this area is limited. Because of diminished immunogenicity, hepatitis B and rabies vaccines should not be given in the buttock at any age. Persons who were given hepatitis B vaccine in the buttock should be tested for immunity and revaccinated if antibody concentrations are inadequate.

When the upper, outer quadrant of the buttocks is used for large-volume passive immunization, such as intramuscular administration of large volumes of immune globulin, care must be taken to avoid injury to the nerve. The site selected should be well into the upper, outer mass of the gluteus maximus, away from the central region of the buttocks, and the needle should be directed anteriorly—that is, if the patient is lying prone, perpendicular to the table's surface, not perpendicular to the skin plane. The ventrogluteal site may be less hazardous for IM injection because it is free of major nerves and vessels. This site is the center of a triangle whose boundaries are the anterior superior iliac spine, the tubercle of the iliac crest, and the upper border of the greater trochanter.

Vaccines containing adjuvants (eg, aluminum-adsorbed DTaP, DTP, DT, Td, hepatitis B, and hepatitis A) and immune globulin must be injected deep in the muscle mass. They should not be administered subcutaneously or intracutaneously because they can cause local irritation, inflammation, granuloma formation, and necrosis. Immune globulin (IG), rabies immune globulin (human), and other similar products for passive immunoprophylaxis are also injected intramuscularly.

The needles used for IM injections should be long enough to reach the substance of the muscle. For very young, small infants, a ⅝-in long needle may be adequate. Ordinarily, a needle ⅞- to 1-in long is required to ensure penetration of the thigh muscle in normal 4-month-old infants, and in the thigh or deltoid in toddlers and older children. The deltoid is preferred for immunization of adolescents and young adults. The needle length should be from 1 to 2 inches depending on the vaccinee's weight (eg, 1 to 1½ in for males ≤120 kg; 1 in for women <70 kg; and 2 in for men >120 kg and women >100 kg). A 22- to 25-gauge needle is appropriate for most IM vaccines.

Serious complications of IM injections are rare. Reported events include broken needles, muscle contracture, nerve injury, bacterial (staphylococcal, streptococcal, and clostridial) abscesses, sterile abscesses, skin pigmentation, hemorrhage, cellulitis, tissue necrosis, gangrene, local atrophy, periostitis, cyst or scar formation, and inadvertent injection into a joint space. Sterile or bacterial abscesses at the injection site are estimated to occur approximately once per 100 000 to 166 000 doses of DTP. The incidence of other complications is unknown.

Subcutaneous (SC) injections can be given in the anterolateral aspect of the thigh or the upper arm by inserting the needle in a pinched-up fold of skin and subcutaneous tissue. A 23- or 25-gauge needle, ⅝- to ¾-in long, is recommended. Immune responses after SC administration of hepatitis B and recombinant rabies vaccine are reduced compared to those after IM administration, and these vaccines should not be given SC. In patients with a bleeding diathesis, the risk of bleeding after IM injection can be minimized by administration immediately after the patient's receipt of replacement factor, use of a 23-gauge (or smaller) needle, and immediate application of direct pressure to the vaccination site for at least 2 minutes. However, certain vaccines (eg, *Haemophilus influenzae* vaccines, except PRP-OMP [PedVaxHIB])* recommended for IM injection may be given subcutaneously to persons at risk for hemorrhage after IM injection, such as those with hemophilia. For these vaccines, immune responses and clinical reactions after either IM or SC injection have generally been reported to be similar.

Intradermal (ID) injections are generally given on the volar surface of the forearm. Because of the decreased antigenic mass administered with ID injections, attention to technique is essential to ensure that the material is not injected subcutaneously. A 25- or 27-gauge needle, ¼- to ¾-in long, is recommended.

Syringes and needles for vaccine injections must be sterile and preferably disposable to minimize the chances of contamination. Changing needles between drawing the vaccine into the syringe and injecting it into the child is generally not necessary, but is recommended for varicella vaccine by the manufacturer in order to reduce the likelihood of varicelliform rash at the injection site. After use, needles and syringes should not be recapped and should be discarded in specially labeled impermeable containers to prevent accidental inoculation or theft.

The patient should be adequately restrained before any injection. When multiple vaccines are administered, separate sites should ordinarily be used if possible, especially for DTP-containing vaccines. When necessary, two vaccines can be given in the same limb at a single visit. The thigh is the preferred site for two simultaneous IM injections because of its greater muscle mass. The distance separating the two injections is arbitrary but should be sufficient (eg, 1 to 2 in apart) so that local reactions are unlikely to overlap. Multiple vaccines should not be mixed in a single syringe unless specifically licensed and labeled for administering in one syringe. A different needle and syringe should be used for each injection. Before the injection is given, the needle should be inserted in the site and the syringe plunger pulled back to see if blood appears; if so, the needle should be withdrawn and a new site selected. The procedure is repeated until no blood appears.

A brief period of bleeding at the injection site is common and can usually be controlled by gentle pressure for several minutes. Use of adhesive bandages for more than 1 or 2 hours can mask an infection and is discouraged.

Scheduling Immunizations

A vaccine is intended to be administered to a person who is capable of an appropriate immunologic response and who will likely benefit from the protection afforded. However, optimal immunologic response for the person must be balanced against the need to achieve effective protection against disease. For example, pertussis-containing vaccines may be less immunogenic in early infancy than later in infancy, but the

---

* Merck and Co, West Point, Pa.

benefit of conferring early protection in young infants dictates that immunization should be given despite a lessened serum antibody response. In some developing countries, poliovirus vaccine is given at birth, in accordance with recommendations of the World Health Organization, for a similar reason.

With parenterally administered live-virus vaccines, the inhibitory effect of residual specific maternal antibody determines the optimal age of administration. For example, live-virus measles vaccine in use in the United States has suboptimal rates of successful immunization during the first year of life because of transplacentally acquired maternal antibody.

An additional factor in selecting an immunization schedule is the need to achieve a uniform and regular response. With some products, a response is achieved after one dose; for others, it is achieved only after multiple doses. Live-virus rubella vaccine is an example of a vaccine that evokes a regular, predictable response at highly acceptable rates after a single dose. In contrast, some persons respond to only one or two types of poliovirus(es) after a single dose of poliovirus vaccine. Hence, multiple doses are given to produce antibody against all three types, thereby ensuring complete protection for the individual and maximum response rates for the population. A single dose of some vaccines (mostly inactivated or killed antigens) confers less than optimal response in the recipient. As a result, several doses are needed to complete the primary immunization, and periodic booster doses (eg, with tetanus and diphtheria toxoids) are administered to maintain immunologic protection.

Most of the widely used vaccines are considered safe and effective when administered simultaneously, although limited data are available for many products at this time. This information is particularly important in scheduling immunization for children with lapsed or missed immunizations and for persons preparing for foreign travel (see Simultaneous Administration of Multiple Vaccines, p 21). Theoretical concerns exist about impaired immune responses to two live-virus vaccines given nonsimultaneously but within 30 days (4 weeks) of each other, but no evidence substantiates this concern with current vaccines. When feasible and when return of the vaccine recipient is reasonably assured, parenterally administered live-virus vaccines not administered on the same day should be given at least 4 weeks apart. Recent receipt of OPV is **not** a contraindication to MMR, which should be given at the first available opportunity, according to age-specific recommendations.

Figure 1.1 (p 18) and Table 1.3 (p 20), respectively, give the recommended routine immunization schedule in the United States for infants and children, and the schedules for those who were not appropriately immunized in the first year of life. **The schedule in Fig 1.1 represents a consensus of the American Academy of Pediatrics, the Advisory Committee on Immunization Practices (ACIP) of the Centers for Disease Control and Prevention (CDC), and the American Academy of Family Physicians for routine childhood immunization in 1997. This schedule is reviewed regularly and an updated national schedule is issued at least annually, usually in January, in order to incorporate new vaccines and revised recommendations.** This schedule gives routinely recommended ages and ranges of acceptable age, and includes recommendations for "catch-up" vaccination of adolescents. Special attention should be given to the footnotes as they summarize major recommendations for routine childhood immunization. Combination vaccine products may be given, provided they are approved by the Food and Drug Administration for the child's age and the administration of other vaccine components is justified.

For those in whom early or rapid immunization is urgent, or those not immunized on schedule, simultaneous vaccination with multiple products allows for more rapid protection. In addition, in some circumstances, immunization can be initiated earlier than at the usually recommended ages and doses given at shorter intervals than is routinely recommended; for guidelines, see the immunization recommendations in the disease-specific chapters in Section 3.

The immunization schedule in the United States may not be appropriate for developing countries because of different disease risks, age-specific immune responses, and vaccine availability. The schedule recommended by the Expanded Programme on Immunization (EPI) of the World Health Organization should be consulted (see Table 1.4, p 21). Modifications may be made by the ministries of health in individual countries, based on local considerations.

Interchangeability of Vaccine Products

Comparable vaccines made by different manufacturers may differ in their components and formulation, and may elicit different immune responses. Such vaccines have been considered interchangeable when administered according to their licensed indications, although data documenting interchangeability are sometimes limited. Vaccines that can be used interchangeably according to their licensed indication during a vaccine series include diphtheria and tetanus toxoids, whole-cell pertussis vaccines, live and inactivated polio vaccines, hepatitis A and B vaccines, and rabies vaccines. Human diploid cell rabies vaccine (HDCV) and rabies vaccine, adsorbed (RVA), are interchangeable when given intramuscularly for preexposure and postexposure prophylaxis, but RVA should not be used intradermally (see Rabies, p 439).

Currently licensed *Haemophilus influenzae* type b (Hib) conjugate vaccines induce different immunologic responses in infants. Available data suggest that infants given sequential doses of different vaccines have a satisfactory antibody response after a complete primary series. The primary vaccine series should be completed with the same conjugate vaccine, if feasible (*Haemophilus influenzae* Infections, p 220). However, if different Hib vaccines are administered, a total of three doses of conjugate vaccine is considered adequate for the primary series among infants, and any combination of licensed vaccines may be used to complete the primary series. Any of the licensed conjugate vaccines can be used for the recommended booster dose at 12 to 15 months of age.

When feasible, the same DTaP vaccine product should be used for the first three doses of the pertussis immunization series (see Pertussis, p 394). No data exist on the safety, immunogenicity, or efficacy of different DTaP vaccines when administered interchangeably in the primary series. However, in those circumstances in which the type of DTaP product(s) received previously is not known or the previously administered product(s) is not readily available, any of the DTaP vaccines licensed for use in the primary series may be used. These recommendations may change as data become available concerning the response to different DTaP vaccines administered interchangeably in a primary series. For the fourth and fifth dose, any licensed product is acceptable, irrespective of prior vaccines received.

Fig 1.1. Childhood immunization schedule.

Recommended Childhood Immunization Schedule
United States, January - December 1997

Vaccines[1] are listed under the routinely recommended ages. Bars indicate range of acceptable ages for vaccination. Shaded bars indicate catch-up vaccination: at 11-12 years of age, hepatitis B vaccine should be administered to children not previously vaccinated, and Varicella vaccine should be administered to children not previously vaccinated who lack a reliable history of chickenpox.

Age ▸ Vaccine ▾	Birth	1 mo	2 mos	4 mos	6 mos	12 mos	15 mos	18 mos	4-6 yrs	11-12 yrs	14-16 yrs
Hepatitis B[2,3]	Hep B-1	Hep B-2	Hep B-2		Hep B-3					Hep B[3]	
Diphtheria, Tetanus, Pertussis[4]			DTaP or DTP	DTaP or DTP	DTaP or DTP		DTaP or DTP[4]		DTaP or DTP	Td	
H. influenzae type b[5]			Hib	Hib	Hib[5]	Hib[5]					
Polio[6]			Polio[6]	Polio		Polio[6]			Polio		
Measles, Mumps, Rubella[7]						MMR			MMR[7] or MMR[7]	MMR[7]	
Varicella[8]						Var	Var			Var[8]	

Approved by the Advisory Committee on Immunization Practices (ACIP), the American Academy of Pediatrics (AAP), and the American Academy of Family Physicians (AAFP).

IS 5081

[1] This schedule indicates the recommended age for routine administration of currently licensed childhood vaccines. Some combination vaccines are available and may be used whenever administration of all components of the vaccine is indicated. Providers should consult the manufacturers' package inserts for detailed recommendations.

[2] **Infants born to HBsAg-negative mothers** should receive 2.5 µg of Merck vaccine (Recombivax HB) or 10 µg of SmithKline Beecham (SB) vaccine (Engerix-B). The 2nd dose should be administered ≥ 1 mo after the 1st dose.

Infants born to HBsAg-positive mothers should receive 0.5 mL hepatitis B immune globulin (HBIG) within 12 hrs of birth, and either 5 µg of Merck vaccine (Recombivax HB) or 10 µg of SB vaccine (Engerix-B) at a separate site. The 2nd dose is recommended at 1-2 mos of age and the 3rd dose at 6 mos of age.

Infants born to mothers whose HBsAg status is unknown should receive either 5 µg of Merck vaccine (Recombivax HB) or 10 µg of SB vaccine (Engerix-B) within 12 hrs of birth. The 2nd dose of vaccine is recommended at 1 mo of age and the 3rd dose at 6 mos of age. Blood should be drawn at the time of delivery to determine the mother's HBsAg status; if it is positive, the infant should receive HBIG as soon as possible (no later than 1 wk of age). The dosage and timing of subsequent vaccine doses should be based upon the mother's HBsAg status.

[3] Children and adolescents who have not been vaccinated against hepatitis B in infancy may begin the series during any childhood visit. Those who have not previously received 3 doses of hepatitis B vaccine should initiate or complete the series during the 11-12 year-old visit. The 2nd dose should be administered at least 1 mo after the 1st dose, and the 3rd dose should be administered at least 4 mos after the 1st dose and at least 2 mos after the 2nd dose.

[4] DTaP (diphtheria and tetanus toxoids and acellular pertussis vaccine) is the preferred vaccine for all doses in the vaccination series, including completion of the series in children who have received ≥1 dose of whole-cell DTP vaccine. Whole-cell DTP is an acceptable alternative to DTaP. The 4th dose (DTaP or DTP) may be administered as early as 12 months of age, provided 6 months have elapsed since the 3rd dose, and if the child is considered unlikely to return at 15-18 mos of age. Td (tetanus and diphtheria toxoids, absorbed, for adult use) is recommended at 11-12 years of age if at least 5 years have elapsed since the last dose of DTP, DTaP, or DT. Subsequent routine Td boosters are recommended every 10 years.

[5] Three *H. influenzae* type b (Hib) conjugate vaccines are licensed for infant use. If PRP-OMP (PedvaxHIB [Merck]) is administered at 2 and 4 mos of age, a dose at 6 mos is not required. After completing the primary series, any Hib conjugate vaccine may be used as a booster.

[6] Two poliovirus vaccines are currently licensed in the US: inactivated poliovirus vaccine (IPV) and oral poliovirus vaccine (OPV). The following schedules are all acceptable by the ACIP, the AAP, and the AAFP, and parents and providers may choose among them:
1. IPV at 2 and 4 mos; OPV at 12-18 mos and 4-6 yr
2. IPV at 2, 4, 12-18 mos, and 4-6 yr
3. OPV at 2, 4, 6-18 mos, and 4-6 yr
The ACIP routinely recommends schedule 1. IPV is the only poliovirus vaccine recommended for immunocompromised persons and their household contacts.

[7] The 2nd dose of MMR is routinely recommended at 4-6 yrs of age or at 11-12 yrs of age, but may be administered during any visit, provided at least 1 month has elapsed since receipt of the 1st dose and that both doses are administered at or after 12 months of age.

[8] Susceptible children may receive Varicella vaccine (Var) at any visit after the first birthday, and those who lack a reliable history of chickenpox should be immunized during the 11-12 year-old visit. Children ≥ 13 years of age should receive 2 doses, at least 1 mos apart.

Table 1.3. Recommended Immunization Schedules for Children Not Immunized in the First Year of Life*

Recommended Time/Age	Immunization(s)[†‡§]	Comments
Younger Than 7 Years		
First visit	DTaP (or DTP), Hib,[‖] HBV, MMR, OPV[¶]	If indicated, tuberculin testing may be done at same visit.
		If child is 5 y of age or older, Hib is not indicated in most circumstances.
Interval after first visit 1 mo (4 wk)	DTaP (or DTP), HBV, Var[#]	The second dose of OPV may be given if accelerated poliomyelitis vaccination is necessary, such as for travelers to areas where polio is endemic.
2 mo	DTaP (or DTP), Hib,[‖] OPV[¶]	Second dose of Hib is indicated only if the first dose was received when younger than 15 mo.
≥8 mo	DTaP (or DTP), HBV, OPV[¶]	OPV and HBV are not given if the third doses were given earlier.
Age 4–6 y (at or before school entry)	DTaP (or DTP), OPV,[¶] MMR**	DTaP (or DTP) is not necessary if the fourth dose was given after the fourth birthday; OPV is not necessary if the third dose was given after the fourth birthday.
Age 11–12 y	See Fig 1.1	
7–12 Years		
First visit	HBV, MMR, Td, OPV[¶]	
Interval after first visit 2 mo (8 wk)	HBV, MMR,** Var,[#] Td, OPV[¶]	OPV also may be given 1 mo after the first visit if accelerated poliomyelitis vaccination is necessary.
8–14 mo	HBV,[††] Td, OPV[¶]	OPV is not given if the third dose was given earlier.
Age 11–12 y	See Fig 1.1	

* Table is not completely consistent with all package inserts. For products used, also consult manufacturer's package insert for instructions on storage, handling, dosage, and administration. Biologics prepared by different manufacturers may vary, and package inserts of the same manufacturer may change from time to time. Therefore, the physician should be aware of the contents of the current package insert.

    Vaccine abbreviations: HBV indicates hepatitis B virus vaccine; Var, varicella vaccine; DTP, diphtheria and tetanus toxoids and pertussis vaccine; DTaP, diphtheria and tetanus toxoids and acellular pertussis vaccine; Hib, *Haemophilus influenzae* type b conjugate vaccine; OPV, oral poliovirus vaccine; IPV, inactivated poliovirus vaccine; MMR, live measles-mumps-rubella vaccine; Td, adult tetanus toxoid (full dose) and diphtheria toxoid (reduced dose), for children ≥7 years and adults.

† If all needed vaccines cannot be administered simultaneously, priority should be given to protecting the child against those diseases that pose the greatest immediate risk. In the United States, these diseases for children younger than 2 years usually are measles and *Haemophilus influenzae* type b infection; for children older than 7 years, they are measles, mumps, and rubella. Before 13 years of age, immunity against hepatitis B and varicella should be ensured.

‡ DTaP, HBV, Hib, MMR, and Var can be given simultaneously at separate sites if failure of the patient to return for future immunizations is a concern.

§ For further information on pertussis and poliomyelitis immunization, see the respective chapters (Pertussis, p 394, and Poliovirus Infections, p 424).

‖ See *Haemophilus influenzae* Infections, p 220, and Table 3.9 (p 226).

¶ IPV is also acceptable. However, for infants and children starting vaccination late (ie, after 6 months of age), OPV is preferred in order to complete an accelerated schedule with a minimum number of injections (see Poliovirus Infections, p 424).

Varicella vaccine can be administered to susceptible children any time after 12 months of age. Unvaccinated children who lack a reliable history of chicken pox should be vaccinated before their 13th birthday.

** Minimal interval between doses of MMR is 1 month (4 weeks).

†† HBV may be given earlier in a 0-, 2-, and 4-month schedule.

Table 1.4. **Immunization Schedule of the Expanded Programme on Immunization (EPI) of the World Health Organization**

Age*	Vaccines†	Hepatitis B‡ Schedule A	or Schedule B
Birth	BCG, OPV	HBV	...
6 wk	DTP, OPV	HBV	HBV
10 wk	DTP, OPV	...	HBV
14 wk	DTP, OPV	HBV	HBV
9 mo	Measles, yellow fever§	...	...

* In many countries, OPV is administered to all children on the same day in national immunization campaigns. This strategy has been very effective in eliminating transmission of wild-type poliomyelitis virus.
† Vaccine abbreviations: BCG indicates bacillus Calmette-Guerin; OPV, oral poliovirus vaccine; DTP, diphtheria and tetanus toxoids and pertussis vaccine; and HBV, hepatitis B vaccine.
‡ Schedule A is recommended in countries where perinatal transmission of HBV is important (eg, Southeast Asia) and B in countries where perinatal transmission is less important (eg, Sub-Saharan Africa).
§ In countries where yellow fever poses a risk.

Simultaneous Administration of Multiple Vaccines

Most vaccines can be safely and effectively administered simultaneously. No contraindications to the simultaneous administration of multiple vaccines routinely recommended for infants and children are known. Immune responses to one vaccine generally do not interfere with those to other vaccines; exceptions include interference among the three oral poliovirus serotypes in trivalent OPV and concurrent administration of cholera and yellow fever vaccines. Simultaneous administration of MMR, DTP, and OPV has resulted in rates of seroconversion and of side effects similar to those observed when the vaccines are administered at separate times. Because simultaneous administration of common vaccines is not known to affect the efficacy or safety of any of the routinely recommended childhood vaccines, if return of a vaccine recipient for further immunization is doubtful, simultaneous administration of all vaccines (DTaP [or DTP], OPV or IPV, MMR, varicella, hepatitis B, and Hib vaccines) appropriate for the age and previous vaccination status of the recipient is recommended. Simultaneous administration of multiple vaccines can raise immunization rates significantly.

For persons preparing for foreign travel, multiple vaccines can generally be given concurrently. An exception is the simultaneous administration of yellow fever and cholera vaccines. Antibody responses to both cholera and yellow fever vaccines are decreased if given simultaneously or within a short time of each other. If possible, these vaccines should be separated by at least 3 weeks; alternatively, cholera vaccine could be omitted since its effectiveness is limited and few indications for its use exist. If both vaccines are necessary and time constraints exist, these vaccines can be given simultaneously or within a 3-week period with the understanding that antibody responses may not be optimal.

When vaccines commonly associated with local or systemic reactions (eg, cholera, parenteral typhoid vaccines, and plague) are given simultaneously, the reactions can be accentuated. Thus, in most circumstances, if feasible, these vaccines should be given on separate occasions.

Lapsed Immunizations

A lapse in the immunization schedule does not require reinstitution of the entire series. If a dose of DTaP (or DTP), poliovirus vaccine (IPV or OPV), Hib, or hepatitis B vaccine is missed, immunizations should be given at the next visit as if the usual interval had elapsed. The charts of children in whom immunizations have been missed or postponed should be flagged to remind health care providers to complete immunization schedules at the next available opportunity.

Reimmunization

Epidemics of measles involving large numbers of high school and college-age students led to the decision to recommend universal measles reimmunization. Some data suggest that control of mumps may require reimmunization. A second dose of MMR, therefore, is recommended for children at 4 to 6 years of age and no later than at 11 to 12 years of age if not vaccinated at 4 to 6 years of age. Adolescents and young adults enrolled in a college or university and those traveling abroad who have not received the second dose of MMR should be reimmunized.

Unknown or Uncertain Immunization Status

The physician may encounter some children with an uncertain immunization status. Many young adults and some children do not have adequate documentation of immunizations, and recollection by the parent or guardian may be of questionable validity. In general, these individuals should be considered susceptible and appropriate immunizations should be administered. No evidence indicates that administration of MMR, varicella, Hib, hepatitis B, or poliovirus vaccine to already immune recipients is harmful; Td, rather than DTaP (or DTP) should be given to those 7 years or older.

Immunizations Received Outside the United States

Persons vaccinated in other countries including international adoptees, refugees, and exchange students should be immunized according to recommended schedules in the United States for healthy infants, children, and adolescents (see Fig 1.1 and Table 1.3, p 18 and p 20). Although occasional vaccines of inadequate potency have been produced in other countries, the majority of vaccines used worldwide, including those in developing nations, are produced with adequate quality control standards and are reliable. Only written documentation should be accepted as evidence of prior immunization. In general, written immunization records may be considered valid if the vaccine, date of administration, interval between doses, and age of the patient at the time of vaccination would be appropriate for a comparable vaccine produced in the United States. If uncertainty exists, the person should be considered susceptible and given appropriate immunizations. The immunization schedules of other countries are acceptable if they meet the minimum requirements of the World Health Organization schedule (see Table 1.4, p 21).

Vaccine Dose

The recommended doses of vaccines are derived from experimental trials and clinical experience. Reduction in the recommended doses can result in an inadequate response and continuing susceptibility of the recipient. Exceeding the recommended dose also may be hazardous. Excessive local concentrations of injectable, inactivated vaccines might result in enhanced tissue or systemic reactions, whereas administering an increased dose of a live vaccine constitutes a theoretical but unproven risk.

Reducing or dividing doses of DTP or any other vaccine, including those given to premature or low-birth-weight infants is not indicated. The efficacy of this practice in reducing the frequency of adverse events associated with DTP has not been demonstrated. Such a practice also might confer less protection against disease than that which is achieved with the recommended doses. A diminished antibody response in both term and premature infants to reduced doses of DTP has been reported. A previous immunization with a dose that was less than the standard dose or one administered by a nonstandard route should not be counted and the patient should be revaccinated as appropriate for age.

Active Immunization of Persons Who Recently Received Immune Globulin

Live-virus vaccines given parenterally can have diminished immunogenicity when given shortly before or during a period of several months after receipt of immune globulins. High doses of immune globulin have been demonstrated to inhibit the response to measles vaccine for a prolonged period. The duration of inhibition varies directly with the dose of immune globulin administered. Inhibition of immune response to rubella, while of shorter duration, also has been demonstrated. The appropriate suggested interval between immune globulin administration and measles vaccination will vary with the indication (which determines the dose) and specific product (eg, IG vs intravenously administered immune globulin; suggested intervals are given in Table 3.37 (p 353). If immune globulin must be given within 14 days after the administration of measles or measles-containing vaccines, these live-virus vaccines should be administered again after the period specified in Table 3.37 unless serologic testing indicates immunity, ie, adequate serum antibodies were produced.

The effect of administration of immune globulin on the antibody response to varicella vaccine is not known. Because of potential inhibition of the response, however, varicella vaccine should not be administered for at least 5 months after receipt of an immune globulin preparation or a blood product (except washed red blood cells) and for 9 months after administration of prophylactic respiratory syncytial virus immune globulin intravenous (RSV-IGIV*). In addition, immune globulin preparations, if possible, should not be administered for 3 weeks after vaccination.

---

* RespiGam, Medimmune Inc, Gaithersburg, Md.

If an immune globulin is given in this interval, the vaccinee either should be revaccinated 5 months later or tested for varicella immunity at that time and revaccinated if seronegative.

In contrast to live-virus vaccines, administration of immune globulin preparations has not been demonstrated to cause significant inhibition of the immune responses to inactivated vaccines and toxoids. For example, concurrent administration of recommended doses of Hepatitis B Immune Globulin (HBIG), Tetanus Immune Globulin (TIG) or Rabies Immune Globulin (RIG), and the corresponding inactivated vaccine or toxoid in postexposure prophylaxis does not impair the efficacy of vaccine and provides immediate as well as long-term immunity, ie, active and passive immunoprophylaxis. Standard doses of the corresponding vaccines are recommended. Increases in the vaccine dose volume or number of immunizations are not indicated. Vaccines should be administered at sites different from that of the intramuscularly administered immune globulin. For further information, see chapters on specific diseases in Section 3.

Administration of hepatitis A vaccine together with IG has been recommended for situations in which both immediate and prolonged protection against hepatitis A virus (HAV) infection is desired. Although this combined active-passive immunization has been demonstrated to result in significantly lower serum antibody concentrations than those induced by vaccine administration only, these concentrations are still many times higher than those considered protective and seroconversion rates are not affected. The reduced immunogenicity, therefore, is not expected to be of clinical significance.

A possible exception to the lack of inhibition of immune responses to inactivated vaccines may be the effect of RSV-IGIV on antibody responses to some routinely inactivated vaccines. However, the data, as of December 1996, are inconclusive and supplemental doses of these vaccines for RSV-IGIV recipients are not indicated. Other than deferral of MMR and varicella vaccine, as previously discussed, these recipients should be immunized according to the recommended schedule for routine childhood immunization (see Fig 1.1, p 18).

Administration of IG does not interfere with the antibody response to OPV given as a booster dose to young adults who already had received primary immunization or to yellow fever vaccination. Hence, these live-virus vaccines can be administered simultaneously with immune globulin, such as to travelers whose departure is imminent.

Tuberculin Testing

Recommendations for tuberculin testing (see Tuberculosis, p 541) are independent of those for immunization. Tuberculin testing at any age is not a prerequisite before administration of live-virus vaccines such as MMR, varicella, or yellow fever. A tuberculin skin test can be applied at the same visit that these vaccines are administered. Because measles vaccine can temporarily suppress tuberculin activity, if tuberculin testing is indicated and cannot be done at the same time as measles vaccination, tuberculin testing should be postponed for 4 to 6 weeks. The effect of live-virus varicella and yellow-fever vaccines on tuberculin skin test reactivity is not known.

Record Keeping and Immunization Registries

PATIENT'S PERSONAL IMMUNIZATION RECORD

Each state health department has developed an official immunization record. This record should be given to the parents of every newborn infant and should be accorded the status of a birth certificate or passport and retained with vital documents for subsequent referral. Physicians should cooperate with this endeavor by recording immunization data in this record and by encouraging patients not only to preserve the record but also to present it at each visit to a health care provider.

The immunization record is especially important for patients who move frequently. It will facilitate an accurate patient medical record, enable the physician to evaluate the child's immunization status, and fulfill the need for documentation of immunizations for child care and school attendance and admission to other institutions and organizations.

Many states are developing computer-based immunization registries that eventually will help remind parents when immunizations are due or overdue and determine for health providers the immunization needs of their patients at the time of each visit, incorporating the latest recommendations; and serve to measure immunization coverage. The Academy urges physicians to cooperate with states and local health officials in providing needed immunization information.

Until such registries are functioning reliably throughout the United States, parents and physicians must rely on the personal immunization record to document each child's immunization status.

PHYSICIAN'S IMMUNIZATION RECORDS

Every physician should maintain the immunization history of each patient in a permanent office record that can be reviewed easily and updated when subsequent immunizations are administered. The format of the record should facilitate identification and recall of patients in need of immunization.

Records of children whose immunizations have been postponed should be flagged to indicate the need to complete immunizations. For all immunizations, the following data should be entered into the patient's permanent medical record and the patient's personal immunization record: (1) month, day, and year of administration; (2) vaccine or other biologic administered; (3) manufacturer; (4) lot number and its expiration date; (5) site and route of administration; and (6) name, address, and title of the health care provider administering the vaccine.

The National Childhood Vaccine Injury Act of 1986 requires recording this information (with the exception of site and route of administration) in the patient's personal medical record for childhood-mandated vaccines. As of December 1996, those vaccines include diphtheria, tetanus, pertussis, poliovirus, measles, mumps, and rubella vaccines. In addition, reporting of selected events that occur after vaccination is required (see Reporting of Adverse Events, p 27).

Vaccine Safety and Contraindications

RISKS AND ADVERSE EVENTS

All licensed vaccines in the United States are safe and effective, but none is either absolutely safe or completely effective. Some vaccinees will have an untoward reaction, and some will not always be fully protected. The goal in vaccine development is to achieve the highest degree of protection with the lowest rate of untoward effects.

Risks of vaccination vary from trivial and inconvenient to severe and life threatening. In developing immunization recommendations, vaccine benefits and safety are weighed against the risks of natural disease to the person and to the community. Recommendations attempt to maximize disease prevention and to minimize risk by providing specific advice on dose, route, and timing of the vaccine and by delineating persons who should be immunized and circumstances that warrant precaution or contraindicate vaccination.

Common vaccine side effects are usually mild to moderate in severity and without permanent sequelae. Because such reactions are intrinsic to the immunizing antigen or some other component of the vaccine, they occur frequently and are unavoidable. Examples include fever and local irritation after administration of DTP vaccine, and fever and rash 1 to 2 weeks after administration of live-virus measles vaccine.

Sterile abscesses have occurred at the site of injection of a number of killed vaccines. The abscesses presumably result from the irritating nature of the vaccine or its adjuvant; in some instances they may be caused by inadvertent subcutaneous inoculation of a vaccine intended for intramuscular use.

Rarely, serious side effects of vaccination occur that can result in permanent sequelae or be life threatening. These individual events are not predictable (eg, paralytic poliomyelitis after administration of OPV to an apparently healthy child).

The occurrence of an adverse event after immunization does not prove that the vaccine caused the symptoms or signs. Vaccines are administered to infants and children during a period in their lives when certain clinical conditions most often become manifest (eg, seizure disorders). For most live-virus vaccines, definitive etiologic association between the vaccine and a subsequent illness requires isolating the vaccine strain from the patient. However, even this generalization has exceptions. For example, vaccine-type poliovirus is commonly found in the throat of vaccinees for 1 to 2 weeks and in stool of vaccinees for several weeks after immunization. The occurrence of a neurologic syndrome, such as encephalitis, during this period does not prove that the poliovirus vaccine caused the illness. Better evidence can be obtained by isolating the agent from normally sterile tissues or body fluids, such as the brain or the cerebrospinal fluid. Association of an adverse clinical event with a specific vaccine is suggested if the event occurs at a significantly higher rate in recipients than that in nonvaccinated groups of similar age and residence, or the same event occurs following sequential doses of the same vaccine. Unusual temporal clustering of a condition in vaccinees after vaccination also may support a causal association.

Although a specific condition occurring in a single person after immunization does not provide sufficient evidence to establish that the condition was caused by the vaccine, reporting of adverse events following immunization is important because, in conjunction with other reports, it may provide clues to an unanticipated adverse reaction.

REPORTING OF ADVERSE EVENTS

Before administering a subsequent dose of any vaccine, parents and patients should be questioned concerning side effects and possible reactions after previous doses. No recommendations can anticipate all possible contingencies, particularly with newly developed vaccines. Physicians should be alert to possible deviations from the expected outcome. Unexpected events occurring soon after administration of any vaccine, particularly those severe enough to require medical attention, should be described in detail in the patient's medical record and a VAERS (Vaccine Adverse Events Reporting System) report should be made, as subsequently described.

The National Childhood Vaccine Injury Act of 1986 requires physicians and other health care providers who administer vaccines to maintain permanent vaccination records and to report occurrences of certain adverse events stipulated in the Act (see Table 1.5, p 29) to VAERS.* The vaccines to which these requirements, as of December 1996, apply are measles, mumps, rubella, polio, pertussis, diphtheria, and tetanus (see Record Keeping and Immunization Registries, p 25).

Adverse events other than those listed in Table 1.5 (p 29), or those occurring after administration of other vaccines, especially events that are serious or unusual, should also be reported to VAERS. Forms (see Fig 1.2, p 28) can be obtained from VAERS*; instructions also are available in the *Physicians' Desk Reference (PDR)*.

All reports of possible adverse events after administration of any vaccine, irrespective of the age of the recipient, are accepted. Submission of a report does not necessarily denote that the vaccine caused the adverse event. All patient-identifying information is kept confidential. Written notification that the report has been received is provided to the person submitting the form. Staff from VAERS will contact the reporter for follow-up of the patient's condition at 60 days and at 1 year after serious adverse events.

VACCINE INJURY COMPENSATION

The National Vaccine Injury Compensation Program is a no-fault system in which persons thought to have suffered an injury or death as a result of administration of a covered vaccine may seek compensation. The program is intended as an alternative to civil litigation in the traditional tort system in that negligence need not be proven.

Claims arising from covered vaccines currently administered must first be adjudicated through the program before civil litigation can be pursued. Operational since 1988, the program has reduced lawsuits against health care providers and manufacturers while ensuring a stable vaccine supply and marketplace.

The program relies upon a Vaccine Injury Table (see Appendix III, p 681) listing the vaccines covered by the program as well as injuries, disabilities, illnesses, and conditions (including death) for which compensation may be awarded. The Table defines the period of time during which the first symptoms or significant aggravation of an injury must appear after immunization. Successful claimants receive a "legal presumption of causation" if a Table condition is proven, thus avoiding the need to prove actual causation in an individual case. Claimants may also prevail for conditions not listed in the Table if they prove causation.

---

* See Directory of Telephone Numbers, p 667.

Fig 1.2. **VAERS form.**

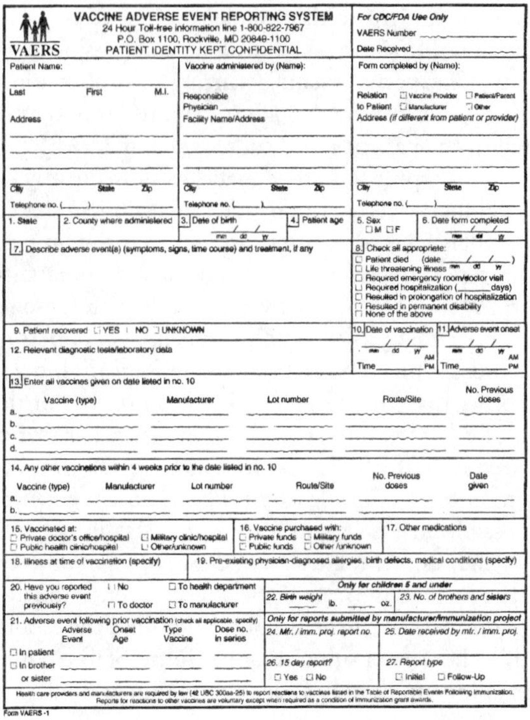

VAERS

VACCINE ADVERSE EVENT REPORTING SYSTEM
24 Hour Toll-free information line 1-800-822-7967
P.O. Box 1100, Rockville, MD 20849-1100
PATIENT IDENTITY KEPT CONFIDENTIAL

For CDC/FDA Use Only
VAERS Number ______
Date Received ______

Patient Name: ______
Last First M.I.
Address ______
City State Zip
Telephone no. (____) ______

Vaccine administered by (Name): ______
Responsible Physician ______
Facility Name/Address ______
City State Zip
Telephone no. (____) ______

Form completed by (Name): ______
Relation to Patient ☐ Vaccine Provider ☐ Patient/Parent ☐ Manufacturer ☐ Other
Address *(if different from patient or provider)* ______
City State Zip
Telephone no. (____) ______

1. State
2. County where administered
3. Date of birth __/__/__ mm dd yy
4. Patient age
5. Sex ☐ M ☐ F
6. Date form completed __/__/__ mm dd yy

7. Describe adverse event(s) (symptoms, signs, time course) and treatment, if any

8. Check all appropriate:
☐ Patient died (date __/__/__ mm dd yy)
☐ Life threatening illness
☐ Required emergency room/doctor visit
☐ Required hospitalization (____days)
☐ Resulted in prolongation of hospitalization
☐ Resulted in permanent disability
☐ None of the above

9. Patient recovered ☐ YES ☐ NO ☐ UNKNOWN

10. Date of vaccination __/__/__ mm dd yy Time ____ AM PM

11. Adverse event onset __/__/__ mm dd yy Time ____ AM PM

12. Relevant diagnostic tests/laboratory data

13. Enter all vaccines given on date listed in no. 10

	Vaccine (type)	Manufacturer	Lot number	Route/Site	No. Previous doses
a.					
b.					
c.					
d.					

14. Any other vaccinations within 4 weeks prior to the date listed in no. 10

	Vaccine (type)	Manufacturer	Lot number	Route/Site	No. Previous doses	Date given
a.						
b.						

15. Vaccinated at:
☐ Private doctor's office/hospital ☐ Military clinic/hospital
☐ Public health clinic/hospital ☐ Other/unknown

16. Vaccine purchased with:
☐ Private funds ☐ Military funds
☐ Public funds ☐ Other /unknown

17. Other medications

18. Illness at time of vaccination (specify)

19. Pre-existing physician-diagnosed allergies, birth defects, medical conditions (specify)

20. Have you reported this adverse event previously? ☐ No ☐ To doctor ☐ To health department ☐ To manufacturer

21. Adverse event following prior vaccination (check all applicable, specify)

	Adverse Event	Onset Age	Type Vaccine	Dose no. in series
☐ In patient				
☐ In brother or sister				

Only for children 5 and under
22. Birth weight ____ lb. ____ oz.
23. No. of brothers and sisters

Only for reports submitted by manufacturer/immunization project
24. Mfr. / imm. proj. report no.
25. Date received by mfr. / imm. proj.
26. 15 day report? ☐ Yes ☐ No
27. Report type ☐ Initial ☐ Follow-Up

Health care providers and manufacturers are required by law (42 USC 300aa-25) to report reactions to vaccines listed in the Table of Reportable Events Following Immunization. Reports for reactions to other vaccines are voluntary except when required as a condition of immunization grant awards.

Form VAERS -1

As of March 10, 1995, the Table was changed for cases filed after this date. The changes include addition of chronic arthritis for rubella-containing vaccines, the removal of residual seizure disorder and hypotonic-hyporesponsive episode (HHE) for pertussis-containing vaccines, and the narrowing of the time interval for anaphylaxis from 24 hours to 4 hours.

Further modifications to the Table were made, effective March 24, 1997. These changes include addition of brachial neuritis and removal of encephalopathy for tetanus-containing vaccines; addition of thrombocytopenia and vaccine-strain measles virus infection, and removal of residual seizure disorder for measles-containing vaccines; and addition of vaccine-strain poliovirus infection for live poliovirus vaccine. The Table also will include hepatitis B, *Haemophilus influenzae* type b and varicella vaccines as well as any future licensed vaccine recommended by the CDC for routine administration to children, but the effective date of their inclusion in the Compensation Program is delayed until Congress enacts an excise tax for these new vaccines.

Additional information about the Program is available from the following:

National Vaccine Injury Compensation Program
Health Resources and Services Administration
Parklawn Building, Room 8A-35
5600 Fishers Ln
Rockville, MD 20857
Telephone: 800-338-2382

Table 1.5. **Reportable Events Following Vaccination***

These events are reportable by law to the Vaccine Adverse Event Reporting System (VAERS). In addition, individuals are encouraged to report any clinically significant or unexpected events (even if uncertain whether the vaccine caused the event) for any vaccine, whether or not it is listed in the table. Manufacturers also are required to report to the VAERS program all adverse events made known to them for any vaccine.

Vaccine/Toxoid	Event	Interval From Vaccination
Tetanus in any combination; DTaP, DTP, DTP-HiB, DT, Td, TT	A. Anaphylaxis or anaphylactic shock B. Brachial neuritis C. Any sequela (including death) of above D. Events described in manufacturer's package events insert as contraindications to additional doses of vaccine	7 d 28 d No limit See package insert
Pertussis in any combination; DTaP, DTP, DTP-HiB, P	A. Anaphylaxis or anaphylactic shock B. Encephalopathy (or encephalitis) C. Any sequela (including death) of above events D. Events described in manufacturer's package insert as contraindications to additional doses of vaccine	7 d 7 d No limit See package insert
Measles, mumps and rubella in any combination; MMR, MR, M, R	A. Anaphylaxis or anaphylactic shock B. Encephalopathy (or encephalitis) C. Any sequela (including death) of above events D. Events described in manufacturer's package insert as contraindications to additional doses of vaccine	7 d 15 d No limit See package insert
Rubella in any combination; MMR, MR, R	A. Chronic arthritis B. Any sequela (including death) of above events C. Events described in manufacturer's package insert as contraindications to additional doses of vaccine	42 d No limit See package insert
Measles in any combination; MMR, MR, M	A. Thrombocytopenic purpura B. Vaccine-strain measles viral infection in an immunodeficient recipient C. Any sequela (including death) of above events D. Events described in manufacturer's package insert as contraindications to additional doses of vaccine	30 days 6 mo No limit See package insert

* Effective March 24, 1997.

Table 1.5. **Reportable Events Following Vaccination, continued**

Vaccine/Toxoid	Event	Interval From Vaccination
Oral polio (OPV)	A. Paralytic polio	
	—in a non-immunodeficient recipient	30 d
	—in an immunodeficient recipient	6 mo
	—in a vaccine-associated community case	No limit
	B. Vaccine-strain polio viral infection	
	—in a non-immunodeficient recipient	30 d
	—in an immunodeficient recipient	6 mo
	—in a vaccine-associated community case	No limit
	C. Any sequela (including death) of above events	No limit
	D. Events described in manufacturer's package insert as contraindications to additional doses of vaccine	See package insert
Inactivated polio (IPV)	A. Anaphylaxis or anaphylactic shock	7 d
	B. Any sequela (including death) of the above events	No limit
	C. Events described in manufacturer's package insert as contraindications to additional doses of vaccine	See package insert
Hepatitis B	A. Anaphylaxis or anaphylactic shock	7 d
	B. Any sequela (including death) of the above events	No limit
	C. Events described in manufacturer's package insert as contraindications to additional doses of vaccine	See package insert
Haemophilus influenzae type b	A. Early onset Hib disease	7 d
	B. Any sequela (including death) of the above events	No limit
	C. Events described in manufacturer's package insert as contraindications to additional doses of vaccine	See package insert

Persons wishing to file a claim for a vaccine injury should call or write to the following:

United States Court of Federal Claims
717 Madison Place, NW
Washington, DC 20005-1011
Telephone: 202-219-9657

PRECAUTIONS AND CONTRAINDICATIONS

Precautions and contraindications to vaccination are described in specific chapters on vaccine-preventable diseases and in the manufacturer's product labeling (ie, package insert). In some of these situations, after careful assessment, vaccine administration may still be indicated because the benefits to the individual child are judged to outweigh the risks.

Minor Illness and Fever. Most vaccines are intended for use in healthy persons or in those whose diseases or conditions are not affected by immunization. For optimal safety, vaccines should not be used if an undesirable side effect or adverse reaction to the vaccine may be seriously accentuated by an underlying illness. A common situation is the child needing immunization who has an acute illness. Minor illnesses with or without fever ($\geq 38°C$) do not contraindicate immunization. No evidence indicates an increased risk of adverse events associated with immunization administered in the course of minor illness. Deferring immunization in such situations constitutes a missed opportunity and frequently results in unimmunized children, some of whom may develop or transmit vaccine-preventable disease.

Fever *per se* **is not a contraindication to immunization.** For the child with an acute, febrile ($\geq 38°C$) illness, guidelines for immunization are based on the physician's assessment of the child's illness and the specific vaccines the child is scheduled to receive. However, if fever or other manifestations suggest a moderate or serious illness, the child should not be vaccinated until recovered. Specific recommendations are as follows:

- *Live-virus vaccines.* Minor respiratory, gastrointestinal, or other illnesses with or without fever do not contraindicate the use of live-virus vaccines such as MMR, varicella, or OPV. Children with febrile upper respiratory tract infections have serologic responses similar to those of well children after vaccination. The potential benefit of immunization at the recommended age, irrespective of the presence of a minor illness, outweighs the possible increased risk of vaccine failure.
- *DTaP and DTP.* Mild illnesses (eg, upper respiratory tract illnesses) do not contraindicate administration of DTaP or DTP. However, a moderate or severe illness with or without fever is a generic contraindication to vaccination, in part because evolving signs and symptoms associated with the illness may be difficult to distinguish from a vaccine reaction.
- *Child with frequent febrile illnesses.* A child who repeatedly has moderate or severe febrile illnesses at the time of scheduled immunizations should be asked to return as soon as the current febrile illness resolves so that immunization can be completed.

- *Immunocompromised children.* Special consideration needs to be given to immunocompromised children, such as those with congenital immunodeficiencies, HIV infection, malignancy, or recipients of immunosuppressive therapy (see Immunodeficient and Immunosuppressed Children, p 50).

A concise summary of contraindications and precautions to immunizations is given in the *Standards for Pediatric Immunization Practices* (see Appendix II, p 668).

HYPERSENSITIVITY REACTIONS TO VACCINE CONSTITUENTS

Hypersensitivity reactions to constituents of vaccines are rare. In some instances, although symptoms appear soon after a vaccine is administered, differentiation between an allergic reaction to the vaccine and a reaction to an environmental allergen is impossible. Facilities and personnel should be available for treating immediate hypersensitivity reactions in all settings where vaccines are administered. This recommendation does not preclude administration of vaccines in school-based or other nonclinic settings. Whenever possible, patients should be observed for an allergic reaction for 15 to 20 minutes after receiving immunization(s).

The four types of hypersensitivity reactions considered related to vaccine constituents are (1) allergic reactions to egg-related antigens, (2) mercury sensitivity in some recipients of immune globulins or vaccines, (3) antibiotic-induced allergic reactions, and (4) hypersensitivity to other vaccine components, including the infectious agent.

Allergic Reactions to Egg-Related Antigens. Current measles and mumps vaccines are derived from chick embryo fibroblast tissue cultures and do not contain significant amounts of egg cross-reacting proteins. Recent studies indicate that children with egg allergy, even those with severe hypersensitivity, are at low risk for anaphylactic reactions to these vaccines, singly or in combination (ie, MMR), and that skin testing with dilute vaccine is not predictive of an allergic reaction to vaccination. Although immediate hypersensitivity reactions occur following MMR, most appear to be due to reactions to other vaccine components such as gelatin or neomycin. Therefore, children with egg allergy routinely may be given MMR, measles, or mumps vaccine without prior skin testing. Vaccine should be given in one injection rather than in a series of gradually increasing concentration doses. Some experts recommend that egg-allergic children given MMR, measles, or mumps vaccine should be observed for 90 minutes with immediate availability of equipment for emergency medical treatment of anaphylaxis.

Current yellow fever and influenza vaccines also contain egg proteins and on rare occasions may induce immediate allergic reactions, including anaphylaxis. Skin testing with yellow fever vaccines is recommended before administration to persons with a history of systemic anaphylactic symptoms (generalized urticaria, hypotension, and/or manifestations of upper or lower airway obstruction) after egg ingestion. Skin testing also has been utilized in children with severe, anaphylactic reactions to eggs who are to receive influenza vaccine, but these children generally should not receive influenza vaccine in view of the risk of reaction, the likely need for yearly vaccination, and the availability of chemoprophylaxis against influenza A infection (see Influenza, p 314). Less severe or localized manifestations of allergy to egg or to feathers are not contraindications to yellow fever or influenza vaccine administration and do not warrant vaccine skin testing.

An egg-sensitive person can be tested with vaccine (eg, yellow fever vaccine) before its use as follows:

- **Scratch, prick, or puncture test.** A drop of 1:10 dilution of the vaccine in physiologic saline is applied at the site of a superficial scratch, prick, or puncture on the volar surface of the forearm. Positive (histamine) and negative (physiologic saline) control tests also should be used. The test is read after 15 to 20 minutes. A positive test is a wheal 3-mm larger than that of the saline control, usually with surrounding erythema. The histamine control must be positive for valid interpretation. If the result of this test is negative, an intradermal (ID) test is performed.
- **Intradermal test.** A dose of 0.02 mL of a 1:100 dilution of the vaccine in physiologic saline is injected; positive and negative control skin tests are performed concurrently. A wheal 5 mm or larger than the negative control with surrounding erythema is considered a positive reaction.

If these tests are negative, the vaccine may be given. If the child's test is positive, the vaccine still may be given using a desensitization procedure if immunization is imperative. A suggested protocol is subcutaneous (SC) administration of the following successive doses of vaccine at 15- to 20-minute intervals as follows:

1. 0.05 mL of 1:10 dilution
2. 0.05 mL of full strength
3. 0.10 mL of full strength
4. 0.15 mL of full strength
5. 0.20 mL of full strength

Scratch, prick, or puncture tests with other allergens have resulted in fatalities in highly allergic persons. **Although such untoward effects have not been reported for vaccine testing, all skin tests and desensitization procedures should be performed by trained personnel experienced in the management of anaphylaxis.** Necessary medications and equipment should be readily available (see Treatment of Anaphylactic Reactions, p 45).

Mercury Sensitivity in Some Recipients of Vaccines or Immune Globulins. Exposure to vaccines containing mercury rarely elicits hypersensitivity, usually manifested as a local, delayed-type hypersensitivity reaction. Even when results of patch or local ID tests indicate hypersensitivity, most patients do not react to thimerosal administered as a vaccine component.

Mercury from the organic mercurial preservatives used in the preparation of IG for intramuscular use can accumulate in persons given repeated injections. Only one case of proven mercury poisoning (acrodynia) has been reported. Intravenous immune globulin does not contain preservatives.

Antibiotic-Induced Allergic Reactions. Antibiotic reactions have been suspected in individuals with known allergies who received vaccines containing trace amounts of antibiotics (see package insert for each product for specific listing). Proof of a causal relationship is difficult and often impossible to confirm.

Poliovirus vaccines (IPV and OPV) may contain trace amounts of streptomycin, neomycin, and polymyxin B. Live-virus measles-mumps-rubella (singly or in combination as MMR), and varicella vaccines have trace quantities of neomycin. Some persons allergic to neomycin may experience a delayed-type, local reaction 48 to 96 hours after administration of MMR, varicella, or IPV. The reaction consists of an erythematous, pruritic papule. This minor reaction is of little importance in comparison to the benefit of immunization and should not be considered a contra-indication. However, if a person has a history of anaphylactic reaction to neomycin, neomycin-containing vaccines should not be used. No currently recommended vaccine contains penicillin or its derivatives.

Hypersensitivity to Other Vaccine Components, Including the Infectious Agent. Some live-virus vaccines such as MMR, varicella, and yellow fever contain gelatin as a stabilizer. Persons with a history of food allergy to gelatin very rarely develop anaphylaxis after receipt of gelatin-containing vaccines. Skin testing is a consideration in these persons before administration of a gelatin-containing vaccine, but no protocol or reported experience is available. Because gelatin used in the United States as a vaccine stabilizer is usually porcine and food gelatins may be derived solely from bovine sources, a negative food history does not exclude the possibility of an immunization reaction.

DTP and, to a lesser extent, plague, cholera, and parenterally administered inactivated whole-cell typhoid vaccines, are associated with local and occasionally systemic reactions, usually of a toxic rather than a hypersensitivity etiology. Such reactions are less frequent with DTaP vaccines, in which the pertussis vaccine is comprised of acellular components. On occasion, urticarial or anaphylactic reactions have occurred in DTP, DT, Td, or tetanus toxoid vaccine recipients. Tetanus and diphtheria antigen-specific antibodies of the IgE type have been identified in some of these patients. Although attributing a specific sensitivity to vaccine components is very difficult, an immediate, severe, or anaphylactic allergic reaction to one of these vaccines is a contraindication to subsequent immunization of the patient with the specific product. A transient urticarial rash, however, is not a contraindication to further doses (see Pertussis, p 394).

Persons who have high serum concentrations of tetanus IgG antibody, usually as the result of frequent booster immunizations, can have an increased incidence and severity of reactions to subsequent vaccine administration (see Tetanus, p 518).

Reactions resembling serum sickness have been reported in approximately 6% of patients after a booster dose of human diploid rabies vaccine, probably due to sensitization to human albumin that had been altered chemically by the virus-inactivating agent.

Japanese encephalitis virus vaccine has been associated with generalized urticaria and angioedema, sometimes with respiratory distress and hypotension occurring within minutes of vaccination to as long as 2 weeks after vaccination. The pathogenesis of such reactions is not understood. Persons with history of urticaria are at increased risk for an adverse reaction. Vaccinees should be observed for 30 minutes after vaccination and warned about the possibility of delayed urticaria and potentially life-threatening angioedema.

Significant hypersensitivity reactions occurring as a result of pneumococcal, Hib, hepatitis B, and oral poliovirus vaccines appear to be extremely rare.

An unusual sensitivity to killed measles virus vaccine (KMV) has been documented. This vaccine has not been available for more than 25 years, but it was received by many patients between 1963 and 1967 in the United States. A moderate-to-severe local reaction, occasionally with systemic symptoms, was observed in KMV recipients when live-virus measles vaccine was administered months or years later. In some KMV recipients, exposure to wild measles virus as many as 16 years later resulted in atypical measles (often a severe illness with fever, pulmonary infiltrates, polyserositis, and a vesicular and/or hemorrhagic rash resembling Rocky Mountain spotted fever). Immunologically, the local reaction and atypical illness represent an Arthus reaction and/or a delayed hypersensitivity (cell-mediated) reaction.

MISCONCEPTIONS CONCERNING VACCINE CONTRAINDICATIONS

Some health care providers inappropriately consider certain conditions or circumstances to be contraindications to vaccination. Common conditions or circumstances that are not appropriate contraindications include the following:

- **Mild acute illness with low-grade fever or mild diarrheal illness in an otherwise well child.**
- **Current antimicrobial therapy or the convalescent phase of illness.**
- **Reaction to a previous DTP dose that involved only soreness, redness, or swelling in the immediate vicinity of the vaccination site or temperature of less than 105°F (40.5°C).**
- **Prematurity.** The appropriate age for initiating most immunizations in the prematurely born infant is the usual recommended chronologic age. Vaccine doses should not be reduced for preterm infants (see Preterm Infants, p 48, and Hepatitis B, p 247).
- **Pregnancy of mother or other household contact.** Vaccine viruses in MMR vaccine are not transmitted by vaccinees. Although varicella vaccine virus has been transmitted by a healthy vaccinee to contacts, the frequency is rare, only mild or symptomatic infection has been reported, and use of this vaccine is not contraindicated by pregnancy of the child's mother or other household contact (see Varicella-Zoster Infections, p 583).
- **Recent exposure to an infectious disease.**
- **Breastfeeding.** The only vaccine virus that has been isolated from breast milk is rubella vaccine virus. No evidence indicates that breast milk from women immunized against rubella is harmful to infants. Breastfeeding does not interfere with immunization with OPV.
- **A history of nonspecific allergies or relatives with allergies.**
- **Allergies to penicillin or any other antibiotic, except anaphylactic reactions to neomycin or streptomycin** (see Hypersensitivity Reactions to Vaccine Constituents, p 32). These reactions occur rarely, if ever. None of the vaccines licensed in the United States contains penicillin.
- **Allergies to duck meat or duck feathers.** No vaccine available in the United States is produced in substrates containing duck antigens.
- **Family history of convulsions in person considered for pertussis or measles vaccination** (see Children With a Personal or Family History of Seizures, p 58).
- **Family history of sudden infant death syndrome in children considered for DTP vaccination.**
- **Family history of an adverse event, unrelated to immunosuppression, after vaccination.**
- **Malnutrition.**

Reporting of Vaccine-Preventable Diseases

Most vaccine-preventable diseases are reportable throughout the United States. Public health officials depend on health care providers to report promptly to state or local health departments suspected cases of vaccine-preventable disease. These reports are transmitted weekly to the CDC and are used to detect outbreaks, monitor disease-control strategies, and evaluate national immunization practices and policies.

Standards for Pediatric Immunization Practices (see Appendix II, p 668)

In 1992, national *Standards for Pediatric Immunization Practices* were recommended by the National Vaccine Advisory Committee, approved by the United States Public Health Service, and endorsed by the Academy. These standards are recommended for use by all health professionals providing care in public or private health care settings who are involved in the administration of vaccines or management of immunization services for children. Their use is intended to improve preschool immunization rates, prevent vaccine-preventable disease outbreaks, and achieve the national objectives for immunization by the year 2000 or before.

PASSIVE IMMUNIZATION

Passive immunization entails administration of preformed antibody to a recipient. It is indicated in the following general circumstances for the prevention or amelioration of infectious diseases:

- When persons are deficient in synthesis of antibody as a result of congenital or acquired B-lymphocyte defects, alone or in combination with other immunodeficiencies.
- When a person susceptible to a disease is exposed, or has a high likelihood of exposure to, that infection, especially when that person has a high risk of complications from the disease (eg, a child with leukemia exposed to varicella or measles), or when time does not permit adequate protection by active immunization alone (eg, some postexposure situations involving measles, rabies, or hepatitis B).
- Therapeutically, when a disease is already present, antibody may ameliorate or aid in suppressing the effects of a toxin (eg, food-borne or wound botulism, diphtheria, or tetanus) or suppress the inflammatory response (eg, Kawasaki disease).

Passive immunization or serotherapy has been accomplished with several different types of products. The choice is dictated by the types of products available, the type of antibody desired, the route of administration, timing, and other considerations. These products include immune globulin (IG) and specific ("hyperimmune") immune globulin preparations given intramuscularly (eg, Hepatitis B Immune Globulin [HBIG]); Immune Globulin Intravenous (IGIV); specific ("hyperimmune") IGs given intravenously (eg, Respiratory Syncytial Virus Immune Globulin Intravenous [RSV-IGIV]); human plasma; and antibodies of animal origin.

Indications for administration of immune globulin preparations other than those relevant to infectious diseases are not reviewed in the *Red Book*. Examples include immune thrombocytopenic purpura and treatment of Guillian-Barré syndrome.

Whole blood and blood components for transfusion (including plasma) from registered blood banks in the United States are tested for blood-borne pathogens, including syphilis, hepatitis B virus (HBV), hepatitis C virus (HCV), HIV infection viruses, and human T-cell leukemia viruses (HTLV-I and II). A similar array of tests is performed by US-licensed establishments that collect plasma used only to manufacture plasma derivatives such as IGIV, IG, and specific immune globulins. US-licensed IG and specific immune globulin preparations have not transmitted any of these diseases. Hepatitis C virus transmission has been associated with administration of IGIV produced by one manufacturer and, as a result of this outbreak, the Food and Drug Administration now requires that IGIV and other immune globulins for intravenous administration undergo additional manufacturing procedures that inactivate and/or remove viruses.

Immune Globulin (IG)

Immune globulin is derived from the pooled plasma of adults by an alcohol-fractionation procedure. It consists primarily of the immunoglobulin fraction (at least 95% IgG and trace amounts of IgA and IgM), is sterile, and is not known to transmit hepatitis, HIV, or any other infectious disease agent. It is a concentrated protein solution (approximately 16.5%; that is, 165 mg/mL), containing specific antibodies in proportion to the infectious and immunization experience of the population from whose plasma it was prepared. Large numbers of donors (from 1000 to 5000 donors per lot of final product) are used to ensure inclusion of a broad spectrum of antibodies.

Immune globulin is recommended for intramuscular (IM) administration. Since some recipients experience local pain and most experience local discomfort, IG should be administered deep and in a large muscle mass, usually in the gluteal region (see Site and Route of Immunization, p 9). The amount of discomfort is lessened if the IG is at room temperature when administered. No more than 5 mL ordinarily should be administered in one site in an adult or large child; lesser amounts (1 to 3 mL) should be given to small children and infants. More than 20 mL at any one time is seldom, if ever, warranted.

Peak serum concentrations of antibodies are usually achieved 48 to 72 hours after IM administration. The serum half-life is generally 3 to 4 weeks. Some investigators have used slow subcutaneous administration in special circumstances, such as immunodeficient patients.

Intravenous use of IG is contraindicated. Intradermal use of IG is not recommended.

INDICATIONS FOR THE USE OF IG

Replacement Therapy in Antibody-Deficiency Disorders. The usual dose is 100 mg/kg (equivalent to 0.66 mL/kg) per month. Customary practice is to administer twice this dose initially and to adjust the interval (2 to 4 weeks) between administration of the doses, based on the trough IgG concentrations and on the clinical response (absence of, or decrease in infections). In most cases, however, IG has been replaced by IGIV. Recent studies in adolescents and adults with antibody deficiencies indicate that subcutaneous administration of IG is safe, less expensive than IGIV, convenient, and suitable for home therapy. Systemic allergic reactions occurred in less than 1% of infusions and local tissue reactions are generally mild.

Hepatitis A Prophylaxis. Immune globulin can prevent clinical disease resulting from hepatitis A virus in exposed susceptible persons when given within 14 days of exposure. Indications include foreign travel in children younger than 2 years and postexposure prophylaxis (see Hepatitis A, p 237).

Measles Prophylaxis. Immune globulin administered to exposed, measles-susceptible persons will prevent or modify infection if given within 6 days of exposure (see Measles, p 344).

ADVERSE REACTIONS TO IG

- The most common problem encountered with the use of IG is discomfort and pain at the site of administration (which is lessened if the preparation is at room temperature at the time of injection). Less common reactions include flushing, headache, chills, and nausea.
- Serious reactions are uncommon; these may involve chest pain or constriction, dyspnea, or anaphylaxis and systemic collapse. An increased risk of systemic reaction results from inadvertent intravenous administration. Persons requiring repeated doses of IG have been reported to experience systemic reactions, such as fever, chills, sweating, uncomfortable sensations, and shock.
- Because IG contains trace amounts of IgA, persons who are selectively serum IgA-deficient in rare cases can develop anti-IgA antibodies and react to a subsequent dose of IG, whole-blood transfusion, or plasma infusion with systemic symptoms, including chills, fever, and shocklike symptoms. In those rare cases in which reactions related to anti-IgA antibodies have occurred, use of IgA-depleted IGIV preparations may reduce the likelihood of further reactions. Because of the rarity of these reactions, routine screening for IgA deficiency is not recommended.
- Healthy persons given IG may develop antibodies against heterologous IgG allotypes. Usually, this phenomenon has no clinical significance; however, on rare occasion, a systemic reaction can result.
- Poisoning caused by the mercury in thimerosal is a rare complication that has been reported in patients receiving prolonged courses of IG for agammaglobulinemia or high-dose HBIG after liver transplantation.

PRECAUTIONS IN THE USE OF IG

- Caution should be used in giving IG to a patient with history of adverse reactions to IG.
- Although systemic reactions to IG are rare (see Adverse Reactions to IG), epinephrine and other means of treating acute reactions should be immediately available.
- Immune globulin is not approved by the FDA for use in patients with severe thrombocytopenia or any coagulation disorder that would preclude IM injection. In such cases, use of IGIV is preferred.
- Screening for IgA-deficiency is not routinely recommended for potential recipients of IG (see Adverse Reactions to IG).

Specific Immune Globulins

Specific immune globulins, termed "hyperimmune globulins," differ from other immune globulin preparations in the selection of donors and the number of donors whose plasma is included in the pool from which the product is prepared. Donors known to have high titers of the desired antibody, either naturally acquired or stimulated by immunization, are selected. These globulins are prepared by the same procedure as other immune globulin preparations and contain 10% to 18% protein. Specific immune globulins for use in infectious diseases include Hepatitis B Immune Globulin (HBIG), Rabies Immune Globulin (RIG), Tetanus Immune Globulin (TIG), Varicella-Zoster Immune Globulin (VZIG), Cytomegalovirus Immune Globulin Intravenous (CMV-IGIV) and Respiratory Syncytial Virus Immune Globulin Intravenous (RSV-IGIV). Recommendations for use of these globulins are given in the discussion of specific diseases in Section 3. The precautions and adverse reactions for IG and IGIV are also applicable to the specific immune globulins.

Immune Globulin Intravenous (IGIV)

Immune Globulin Intravenous (IGIV) is derived from the pooled plasma of adults by an alcohol-fractionation procedure; it is then modified to be suitable for intravenous (IV) use. The donor pool is like that of IG. The FDA specifies that all preparations must have a minimum concentration of measles, diphtheria, polio, and hepatitis B antibodies. Antibody concentrations against common pathogens, such as *Streptococcus pneumoniae*, vary widely between products and even among lots of the same product. Immune Globulin Intravenous consists primarily of the immunoglobulin fraction (more than 95% IgG and trace amounts of IgA and IgM). The protein content varies, depending on the product; both liquid and dried products are available. Immune Globulin Intravenous does not contain thimerosal and can be used in mercury-sensitive persons.

INDICATIONS FOR THE USE OF IGIV

Approval by the FDA of specific indications for a manufacturer's IGIV product is based on the availability of data from one or more clinical trials. Thus, not all licensed products are approved for each of the indications listed here; in some cases only a single product has the indication in its product label. Therapeutic differences between IGIV products of different manufacturers may exist but have not been demonstrated. Recommended and possible indications in children and adolescents include the following:

- *Replacement therapy in antibody deficiency disorders.* The usual dose of IGIV in immunodeficiency syndromes is 300 to 400 mg/kg of body weight administered once a month by IV infusion. Dose or frequency of infusions, however, should be based on the effectiveness in the individual patient. Effective doses have ranged from 200 to 800 mg/kg monthly. Maintenance of a trough IgG concentration of 500 mg/dL has been demonstrated to correlate with clinical response.

- *Parvovirus B19 infection.* Treatment of chronic parvovirus B19 infection in the immunodeficient patient with IGIV appears to be effective and should be considered.
- *Kawasaki disease.* Intravenous immune globin administered within the first 10 days of the illness shortens the duration of fever and decreases the frequency of coronary artery abnormalities (see Kawasaki Disease, p 316).
- *Pediatric HIV infection.* The benefit of IGIV in the prevention of bacterial infections in HIV-infected children has been demonstrated in several trials. Intravenous immune globulin can delay the time to development of bacterial infections and decrease the frequency of hospitalizations in infants and children with CD4+ T-lymphocyte counts of $200/mm^3$ or greater, but it does not affect survival. Accordingly, the Working Group on Antiretroviral Therapy of the National Pediatric Resource Center[*] has recommended IGIV every 4 weeks for children with humoral immunodeficiency, including (1) those with hypogamma-globulinemia (serum IgG concentration less than 250 mg/dL), (2) those with recurrent serious bacterial infections (defined as two or more infections such as bacteremia, meningitis or pneumonia in a 1-year period, (3) those who fail to form antibodies to common antigens, such as measles, pneumococcal and/or *Haemophilus influenzae* type b vaccine, and (4) those living in areas where measles is highly prevalent and who have not developed an antibody response after two doses of MMR (see HIV Infection, p 279).

    Rho IGIV[†] is effective in the treatment of children with thrombocytopenia related to HIV infection.
- *Hypogammaglobulinemia in chronic lymphocytic leukemia.* Intravenous immune globulin in adults with this disease has been demonstrated to reduce the incidence of serious bacterial infections, although its cost-effectiveness has been questioned.
- *Bone marrow transplantation.* Intravenous immune globulin may reduce the incidence of infection and death but not acute graft-versus-host disease (GVHD) in pediatric bone marrow recipients. In adult transplant recipients, IGIV decreases the incidence of interstitial pneumonia (presumably caused by cytomegalovirus), reduces the risk of sepsis and other bacterial infections, decreases the incidence of acute GVHD (but not overall mortality), and, in conjunction with ganciclovir, is effective in the treatment of some patients with cytomegalovirus pneumonia.
- *Low-birth-weight infants.* Results of some clinical trials have indicated that IGIV decreases the incidence of late-onset infections in infants less than 1500 g in birth weight, but other studies have not confirmed these results. Trials have varied in IGIV dose, time of administration, and other aspects of study design. A large multicenter placebo-controlled trial, however, did conclude that IGIV was bene-ficial in very-low-birth-weight infants. At present, IGIV is not recommended for routine use in preterm infants to prevent late-onset infection.

---

[*] Working Group on Antiretroviral Therapy: National Pediatric HIV Resource Center. Antiretroviral therapy and medical management of the human immunodeficiency virus-infected child. *Pediatr Infect Dis J.* 1993;12:513-522.

[†] WinRho SD, distributed by Univax Biologics, Rockville, Md.

In other infections, such as group A streptococcal toxic shock syndrome, the use of IGIV has been proposed and studies are in progress. No indications for its use, as of December 1996, have been recommended.

ADVERSE REACTIONS TO IGIV

The reported incidence of adverse events associated with the administration of IGIV ranges from 1% to 15%, but is usually less than 5%. Most of these reactions are mild and self-limited. Severe reactions occur very infrequently and usually do not contraindicate further IGIV therapy. Adverse events include the following:

- Pyrogenic reactions marked by high fever, chills, and systemic symptoms.
- Minor systemic reactions with headache, myalgia, anxiety, light-headedness, nausea, or vomiting.
- Vasomotor or cardiovascular manifestations, marked by flushing, changes in blood pressure, and tachycardia.
- Aseptic meningitis.
- Hypersensitivity reactions.

Anaphylactic reactions induced by anti-IgA can occur in patients with primary antibody deficiency who have a total absence of circulating IgA and antibodies to IgA. These reactions are extremely rare in panhypogammaglobulinemic persons and potentially more common in patients with selective IgA deficiency and subclass IgG deficiencies. In those rare instances when reactions related to anti-IgA antibodies have occurred, use of IgA-depleted IGIV preparations will reduce the likelihood of further reactions. Avoidance of anaphylactic reactions, however, may require the use of globulin preparations that are completely devoid of IgA. Because of the extreme rarity of these reactions, screening for IgA deficiency is not routinely recommended.

An outbreak of hepatitis C occurred in the United States in 1994 among recipients of IGIV lots from a single domestic manufacturer. Procedures and requirements in the preparation of IGIV have been instituted to prevent transmission of hepatitis C virus by IGIV.

PRECAUTIONS IN THE USE OF IGIV

- Caution should be used in giving IGIV to a patient with a history of adverse reactions to IG.
- Because systemic reactions to IGIV may occur (see Adverse Reactions to IGIV), epinephrine and other means of treating acute reactions should be available immediately.
- Adverse reactions often can be alleviated by reducing either the rate or the volume of infusion. For patients with repeated severe reactions unresponsive to these measures, hydrocortisone, 1 to 2 mg/kg, can be given intravenously 30 minutes before infusion. Utilizing a different IGIV preparation or pretreatment with diphenhydramine, acetaminophen or aspirin also may be helpful.
- Seriously ill patients with compromised cardiac function, who are receiving large volumes of IGIV, may be at increased risk of vasomotor or cardiac complications manifested by elevated blood pressure and/or cardiac failure.
- Screening for IgA deficiency is not routinely recommended for potential recipients of IGIV (see Adverse Reactions to IGIV).

Human Plasma

The use of human plasma in the control of infectious diseases should be limited. Human plasma has been administered to burn patients in an attempt to control *Pseudomonas* infections, but the data are insufficient to substantiate this use. Plasma infusions have been useful in treating infants who have protein-losing enteropathy. Plasma infusions also have been substituted for IG in some patients with IgG antibody deficiency when they develop adverse reactions to IG or fail to respond to treatment with IG; however, these immunodeficient patients can be managed with IGIV (or by slow subcutaneous administration of IG).

Antibodies of Animal Origin (Animal Antisera)

Products of animal origin are derived from the serum of horses. Experimental products prepared in other species also may be available. These products are derived by concentrating the serum globulin fraction with ammonium sulfate. Some, but not all, products are also subjected to an enzyme digestion process in an attempt to decrease reactions to foreign proteins.

The use of the following products is discussed in the disease-specific chapters in Section 3:
- Botulism antitoxin types A, B, E
- Diphtheria antitoxin
- Tetanus antitoxin
- Rabies equine globulin (not available in the United States)

INDICATIONS FOR USE OF ANIMAL ANTISERA

Antibody-containing products prepared from animal sera pose a special risk to the recipient and the use of such products should be strictly limited to certain indications for which specific IGs of human origin are not available (eg, diphtheria and botulism).

REACTIONS TO ANIMAL SERA

Before any animal serum is injected, the patient must be questioned about asthma, allergic rhinitis, urticaria, and previous injections of animal sera. Patients with a history of asthma or allergic symptoms, especially from exposure to horses, can be dangerously sensitive to the animal sera and should be given serum only with the utmost caution. Those who have previously received animal sera are at increased risk of developing allergic reactions and serum sickness after administration of sera from the same animal species.

SENSITIVITY TESTS FOR REACTIONS TO ANIMAL SERA

Each patient who is to be given an animal serum should be skin tested before its administration.

Whereas intradermal (ID) skin tests have resulted in fatalities, the scratch test is usually safe. Therefore, scratch tests always should precede the ID tests. Nevertheless, any sensitivity test always should be performed by trained personnel familiar with the treatment of acute anaphylaxis; necessary medications and equipment should be readily available (see Treatment of Anaphylactic Reactions, p 45).

Scratch, Prick, or Puncture Test. *Apply 1 drop of a 1:100 dilution of the serum in preservative-free normal saline to the site of a superficial scratch, prick, or puncture on the volar aspect of the forearm. Positive (histamine) and negative (physiologic saline) control tests for the scratch test also should be applied. A positive test
is a wheal with surrounding erythema at least 3-mm larger than the negative control test, read at 15 to 20 minutes. The histamine control must be positive for valid interpretation. If the scratch test is negative, an ID test is performed.

Intradermal (ID) Test. *A dose of 0.02 mL of 1:1000 saline-diluted serum (enough to raise a small wheal) is administered. Positive and negative control tests as described for the scratch test also should be applied. If the test is negative, it should be repeated using a 1:100 dilution. In persons with negative history for both animal allergy and prior exposure to animal serum, the 1:100 dilution may be used initially if a scratch, prick, or puncture test with the serum is negative. Interpretation is the same as for the scratch test.

Positive tests not due to an irritant reaction indicate sensitivity, but a negative skin test is not an absolute guarantee of lack of sensitivity. Therefore, animal sera should be administered with caution even in persons whose tests are negative. Immediate hypersensitivity testing is performed to identify IgE-mediated disease and does not predict other immune reactions such as serum sickness.

If the intradermal test is positive or if the history for systemic anaphylaxis after previous administration of serum is highly suggestive in a person for whom the need for the serum is unquestioned, desensitization can be undertaken (see Desensitization to Animal Sera).

If the history and sensitivity tests are negative, the indicated dose of serum can be given intramuscularly. The patient should be observed afterwards for at least 30 minutes. Intravenous administration may be indicated if a high concentration of serum antibody is imperative, such as in the treatment of diphtheria or botulism. In these instances, a preliminary dose of 0.5 mL of serum should be diluted in 10 mL of either physiologic saline or 5% glucose solution. This preparation should be given as slowly as possible, and the patient should be observed for 30 minutes for reactions. If no reaction occurs, the remainder of the serum, diluted 1:20, may be given at a rate not to exceed 1 mL/min.

DESENSITIZATION TO ANIMAL SERA

Tables 1.6 (p 44) and 1.7 (p 45) serve as guides for the desensitization procedures for administration of animal sera. Either the intravenous (IV) (Table 1.6) or the intradermal/subcutaneous/intramuscular (ID/SC/IM)regimens (Table 1.7) may be chosen. The IV route is considered safest because it offers better control. The desensitization procedure should be performed by trained personnel familiar with the treatment of anaphylaxis and with appropriate drugs and equipment available (see Treatment of Anaphylactic Reactions, p 45). Some physicians advocate the concurrent use during the procedure of an oral or parenteral antihistamine (such as diphen-

---

* Antihistamines may inhibit reactions in the scratch, prick, or puncture test, and in the intradermal skin test. Hence, testing should not be performed for at least 24, and, preferably, 48 hours after receipt of these drugs.

Table 1.6. **Desensitization to Serum—Intravenous (IV) Route**

Dose Number*	Dilution of Serum in Normal Saline	Amount of IV Injection, mL
1	1:1000	0.1
2	1:1000	0.3
3	1:1000	0.6
4	1:100	0.1
5	1:100	0.3
6	1:100	0.6
7	1:10	0.1
8	1:10	0.3
9	1:10	0.6
10	Undiluted	0.1
11	Undiluted	0.3
12	Undiluted	0.6
13	Undiluted	1.0

* Administer consistently at 15-minute intervals.

hydramine), with or without IV hydrocortisone or methylprednisolone. If signs of anaphylaxis occur, aqueous epinephrine should be administered immediately (see Treatment of Anaphylactic Reactions, p 45). Administration of sera under the protection of a desensitization procedure must be continuous because after administration is interrupted, protection from desensitization is lost.

TYPES OF REACTIONS TO ANIMAL SERUM

The following reactions can occur as the result of administration of animal sera. Of these, only anaphylaxis is mediated by IgE antibodies and, thus, can be predicted in occurrence by prior skin testing.

Acute Febrile Reactions. These reactions are usually mild and can be treated with antipyretics. Severe febrile reactions should be treated with antipyretics, tepid water sponge baths, or other available methods to reduce the temperature.

Serum Sickness. Manifestations consist of fever, urticaria, or a maculopapular rash (90% of cases); arthritis or arthralgia; and lymphadenopathy, which usually begin 7 to 10 days (occasionally as late as 2 to 3 weeks) after the primary exposure to the foreign protein. Local edema can occur at the serum injection site a few days before the systemic signs and symptoms appear. Angioedema, glomerulonephritis, Guillain-Barré syndrome, peripheral neuritis and myocarditis also can occur. However, serum sickness may be mild and resolve spontaneously within a few days to 2 weeks. Persons who have previously received serum injections are at an increased risk after readministration; manifestations in these patients occur shortly (from hours to 2 to 3 days) after administration of serum. Drugs that can be helpful in the management of serum sickness include antihistamines for alleviation of pruritus, edema

Table 1.7. Desensitization to Serum—Intradermal (ID), Subcutaneous (SC), and Intramuscular (IM) Routes

Dose Number*	Route of Administration	Dilution of Serum in Normal Saline	Amount of Injection, mL
1	ID	1:1000	0.1
2	ID	1:1000	0.3
3	SC	1:1000	0.6
4	SC	1:100	0.1
5	SC	1:100	0.3
6	SC	1:100	0.6
7	SC	1:10	0.1
8	SC	1:10	0.3
9	SC	1:10	0.6
10	SC	Undiluted	0.1
11	SC	Undiluted	0.3
12	IM	Undiluted	0.6
13	IM	Undiluted	1.0

* Administer consistently at 15-minute intervals.

and urticaria. Fever, malaise, arthralgia and arthritis can be controlled in most patients by aspirin or other nonsteroidal anti-inflammatory agents. Corticosteroids may be helpful in controlling serious manifestations that are poorly alleviated by other treatment modalities; prednisone or prednisolone in therapeutic doses (1.5 to 2 mg/kg per day) for 5 to 7 days is an acceptable regimen.

Anaphylaxis. The rapidity of onset and the overall severity of anaphylaxis vary considerably. Anaphylaxis usually begins within minutes of exposure to the etiologic agent, and, in general, the more rapid the onset, the more severe the overall course. Major manifestations are the following: (1) cutaneous, including pruritus, flushing, urticaria, and angioedema; (2) respiratory, with hoarse voice and stridor, wheeze, dyspnea, and cyanosis; and (3) cardiovascular, with a rapid, weak pulse, hypotension, and arrhythmias. Anaphylaxis is a major medical emergency.

Treatment of Anaphylactic Reactions

Personnel administering biologic products or serum should be prepared to recognize and treat anaphylaxis. The necessary medications, equipment, and staff competent to maintain the patency of the airway and to manage cardiovascular collapse must be immediately available.

The emergency treatment of anaphylactic reactions is based on the type of reaction. In all instances, epinephrine is the primary drug. Mild symptoms of pruritus, erythema, urticaria, and angioedema should be treated with epinephrine injected subcutaneously, followed by diphenhydramine, hydroxyzine, or other antihistamine given orally or parenterally (see Tables 1.8 and 1.9). Epinephrine administration may be repeated within 10 or 20 minutes. If the patient improves with this management

Table 1.8. **Epinephrine in the Treatment of Anaphylaxis**
(In addition to epinephrine, maintenance of an airway
and administration of oxygen are critical.)

Subcutaneous or intramuscular administration

Epinephrine 1:1000 (aqueous): 0.01 mL/kg per dose repeated every 10–20 min.* Usual dose:
- Infants—0.05–0.1 mL
- Children—0.1–0.3 mL
- Adolescents—0.3–0.5 mL

Intravenous administration†

Epinephrine 1:1000 (aqueous): 0.1 mL/kg diluted to 1:10 000 with physiologic saline. Dose may be repeated every 10–20 min. A continuous infusion should be started if repeated doses are required. One milligram (1 mL) of 1:1000 dilution of epinephrine added to 250 mL of 5% dextrose in water, resulting in a concentration of 4 μg/mL, is infused initially at a rate of 0.1 μg/kg/min and increased gradually to 1.5 μg/kg/min to maintain blood pressure.

---

* If agent causing anaphylactoid reaction was given by injection, epinephrine can be injected into the same site to slow absorption.
† If intravenous access cannot be obtained, intramuscular dose can be injected into posterior one third of sublingual area.

and remains stable, a long-acting epinephrine injection may be given, and an oral antihistamine prescribed for the next 24 hours.

Treatment of more severe or potentially life-threatening systemic anaphylaxis involving severe bronchospasm, laryngeal edema, shock, and cardiovascular collapse necessitates additional therapy. Maintenance of the airway and oxygen administration should be instituted promptly. Intravenous (IV) epinephrine may be indicated; for this use, it must be diluted from the 1:1000 aqueous base using physiologic saline (see Table 1.8). A slow, continuous infusion is preferable to repeated bolus administration. Nebulized albuterol or IV aminophylline is indicated for bronchospasm (see Table 1.9). Rapid IV infusion of physiologic saline, Ringer lactate, or other isotonic solution adequate to maintain blood pressure must be instituted to compensate for the loss of circulating blood volume that occurs.

In some cases, the use of an inotropic agent such as dopamine (see Table 1.9) titrated to maintain blood pressure may be necessary. The combination of histamine H1- and H2-receptor-blocking agents (see Table 1.9) can be synergistic in their effect and should be used. Corticosteroids should probably be used in all cases of anaphylaxis except those that are mild and have responded promptly to therapy (see Table 1.9). Corticosteroids do not exert an immediate effect, however, and should not be considered primary drugs.

All patients showing signs and symptoms of anaphylaxis, regardless of severity, should be observed for several hours. Biphasic and protracted anaphylaxis (as long as 24 hours or more) may be mitigated with early administration of oral corticosteroids, but has occurred in spite of adequate initial management. Hence, even patients with apparent remissions of immediate symptoms should be observed for 12 hours following the onset of symptoms.

Table 1.9. Dosages of Commonly Used Secondary Drugs in the Treatment of Anaphylaxis

Drug	Dose*
H₁-blocking agents (antihistamines)	
Diphenhydramine	Oral, IM, IV: 1-2 mg/kg every 4-6 h (100 mg, maximum single dose)
Hydroxyzine	Oral, IM: 0.5-1 mg/kg every 4-6 h (100 mg, maximum single dose)
H₂-blocking agents (also antihistamines)	
Cimetidine	IV: 5 mg/kg, slowly during 15 min every 6-8 h (300 mg, maximum single dose)
Ranitidine	IV: 1 mg/kg, slowly during 15 min every 6-8 h (50 mg, maximum single dose)
Corticosteroids	
Hydrocortisone	IV: 100-200 mg every 4-6 h
Methylprednisolone	IV: 1.5-2 mg/kg every 4-6 h (40 mg, maximum single dose)
Prednisone	Oral: 1.5-2 mg/kg, single morning dose, for 5 days (60 mg, maximum single dose)
ß₂-agonist	
Albuterol	Nebulizer solution: 0.5% (5 mg/mL), 0.05-0.15 mg/kg per dose in 2-3 mL normal saline, maximum of 2.5 mg per dose every 20 min for 1–2 h or 0.5 mg/kg/h by continuous nebulization (15 mg/h, maximum dose)
Other	
Dopamine	IV: 5-20 µg/kg/min. Mixing 150 mg of dopamine with 250 mL of saline or 5% dextrose in water will produce a solution which if infused at the rate of 1 mL/kg/h will deliver 10 mg/kg/min. The solution must be free of bicarbonate, which may inactivate dopamine.
Aminophylline	IV: 4-6 mg/kg in 20 mL saline by rapid drip every 6 h or 0.9-1.1 mg/kg/h continuous infusion

* IM indicates intramuscular, and IV, intravenous.

Anaphylaxis occurring in persons already taking ß-adrenergic blocking agents presents a unique situation. In such individuals, the manifestations are likely to be more profound and significantly less responsive to epinephrine and other ß-adrenergic agonist drugs. More aggressive therapy with epinephrine may be adequate to override the receptor blockade in some patients. The use of intravenous glucagon for cardiovascular manifestations and inhaled atropine for management of bradycardia or bronchospasm also has been recommended in this situation.

IMMUNIZATION IN SPECIAL CLINICAL CIRCUMSTANCES

Preterm Infants

Prematurely born infants, including those of low birth weight, should be immunized at the usual chronologic age in most cases. Some studies suggest a reduced immune response in very-low-birth-weight infants ($\leq$1500 g) vaccinated by the usual schedule. Additional data are required to define the optimal vaccination schedule better for these infants. Vaccine doses should not be reduced for preterm infants. If an infant is still in the hospital at 2 months of age, the immunizations routinely scheduled at that age should be given, including DTaP (or DTP), *Haemophilus influenzae* conjugate, and poliovirus vaccines (see Fig 1.1, p 18). To avoid nosocomial transmission of poliovirus vaccine strains in the nursery, IPV should be given.

The optimal time to initiate hepatitis B vaccination in preterm infants with birth weights less than 2 kg whose mothers are HBsAg-negative has not been determined. Seroconversion rates in low-birth-weight infants in whom vaccination was initiated shortly after birth have been reported in some studies to be lower than in those in preterm infants vaccinated at a later age, and in term infants vaccinated shortly after birth. Hence, initiation of vaccination in preterm infants with a birth weight of less than 2 kg whose mothers are HBsAg-negative should be delayed until just before hospital discharge if the infant weighs 2 kg or more, or until approximately 2 months of age when other immunizations are given (see Fig 1.1, p 18, and Hepatitis B, p 250).

Preterm infants with birth weights less than 2 kg whose mothers are HBsAg-positive should receive HBIG within 12 hours of birth and concurrent hepatitis B vaccine (at a different site) in the appropriate dose (see Hepatitis B, p 254). If the maternal HBsAg status is not known, vaccine also should be given in accordance with recommendations for the infant of an HBsAg-positive mother (see Hepatitis B, p 254). The maternal status should be determined and HBIG should be given to the infant if she is HBsAg-positive. If the birth weight is less than 2 kg and her status cannot be determined within the initial 12 hours of life, HBIG should be given. The maternal HBsAg status will determine the subsequent doses and schedule for completion of hepatitis B vaccination (see Hepatitis B, p 256).

Preterm infants who develop chronic respiratory disease should be given influenza immunization annually in the fall once they reach 6 months of age. To protect these infants and those with other chronic conditions before this age, the family and other caregivers, including hospital personnel, also should be immunized against influenza (see Influenza, p 307).

Pregnancy

Vaccination during pregnancy poses theoretical risks to the developing fetus. Although no evidence indicates that vaccines in use today have ill effects on the fetus, pregnant women should receive vaccines only when the vaccine is unlikely to cause harm, the risk for disease exposure is high, and the infection would pose a significant risk to the mother or fetus. When a vaccine or toxoid is to be given during pregnancy, delaying until the second or third trimester, when possible, is a reasonable precaution to minimize concern about possible teratogenicity. Influenza vaccine is considered safe at any stage of pregnancy.

The only vaccines routinely recommended for administration during pregnancy in the United States, provided they are otherwise indicated (either for primary or booster immunization), are those for tetanus and diphtheria. In developing countries with a high incidence of neonatal tetanus, immunization is routinely administered in pregnancy without evidence of adverse effects and with striking reductions in the occurrence of neonatal tetanus.

Influenza vaccine is recommended for pregnant women with medical conditions that increase the risk of complications from influenza. In addition, because recent studies indicate that women in the third trimester of pregnancy and early puerperium, even in the absence of underlying risk factors, are at increased risk of complications and hospitalization from influenza, the Advisory Committee on Immunization Practices (ACIP) of the Centers for Disease Control and Prevention (CDC) recommends influenza vaccination of all women who will be beyond 14 weeks of pregnancy during the influenza season.

Pneumococcal immunization can be given if the pregnant woman is at high risk for serious or complicated illness from these infections. Hepatitis A or B vaccination, if indicated, should be given to pregnant women. Although data on the safety of these vaccines for the developing fetus are not available, no risk would be expected because the vaccines contain either formalin-inactivated virus (hepatitis A) or noninfectious surface antigen (hepatitis B). In contrast, infection with either agent in a pregnant woman can result in severe disease in the mother and, in the case of hepatitis B, chronic infection in the newborn.

Pregnancy is a contraindication to administration of all live-virus vaccines, except when susceptibility and exposure are highly probable and the disease to be prevented poses a greater threat to the woman or fetus than does the vaccine. Although no evidence for the theoretical risk to the fetus of a live-virus vaccine exists, the background rate of anomalies in uncomplicated pregnancies may result in a defect that could be attributed to a vaccine; therefore, live vaccines should be avoided. However, both yellow fever vaccine and live oral poliovirus vaccine (OPV) may be given to pregnant women who are at substantial risk of imminent exposure to infection, such as in some circumstances of international travel. Alternatively, inactivated poliovirus vaccine (IPV) should be given if immunization can be completed before anticipated exposure.

Because measles, mumps, rubella, and varicella vaccines are contraindicated in pregnant women, efforts should be made to immunize susceptible women against these illnesses before they become pregnant. Although of theoretical concern, no case of embryopathy caused by rubella vaccine has been reported. Accumulated evidence demonstrates that inadvertent administration of rubella vaccine to susceptible pregnant women very rarely, if at all, causes congenital defects. The effect of varicella vaccine on the fetus, if any, is unknown. The manufacturer, in collaboration with CDC, has established the VARIVAX Pregnancy Registry to monitor the maternal and fetal outcomes of women who inadvertently are given varicella vaccine 3 months before or at any time during pregnancy. Reporting of cases is encouraged and may be done by telephone (800-986-8999).

Immunodeficient and Immunosuppressed Children*

Indications for active immunization of the altered host are an important considera-tion. Experience with vaccine administration in immunodeficient or immunosup-pressed children is limited. For many persons and with most vaccines, theoretical considerations are the only guide because experience with the vaccine in patients with a specific disorder is lacking or because adverse consequences have not been reported. However, considerable data acquired in HIV-infected infants provide reassurance about the lack of adverse events in these patients when vaccinated. Although the contraindications and suboptimal efficacy of immunizations in immunodeficient and immunosuppressed patients are emphasized in these guide-lines, some immunosuppressed children benefit from immunization with vaccines such as *Haemophilus influenzae* type b, pneumococcal, and influenza.

Live-bacterial and live-virus vaccines are contraindicated in patients with congenital disorders of immune function. Fatal poliomyelitis and measles virus infections have occurred in children with these disorders after administration of live-virus vaccines. If an inactivated vaccine is available for a given disease (eg, IPV for protection against poliomyelitis), it should be administered. Since children with deficiency in antibody-synthesizing capacity will be incapable of responding to vac-cines, these children should receive regular doses of immune globulin (usually IGIV) that provide passive protection against many infectious diseases. Specific immune globulins (eg, Varicella-Zoster Immune Globulin [VZIG]) are available for postexpo-sure prophylaxis for some infections.

Immunologically normal siblings and other household contacts of persons with an immunologic deficiency should not receive oral poliovirus vaccine (OPV) because the vaccine strains are transmissible, and, thus, may be acquired by the immuno-compromised contact. However, these siblings and household contacts can receive live measles-mumps-rubella (MMR) vaccine because transmission of the vaccine viruses does not occur. Varicella vaccine is recommended for susceptible contacts of immunocompromised children (see Varicella-Zoster Infections, p 583). Transmission of varicella vaccine virus from healthy persons is rare, and disease, if it develops, is mild, and no precautions need be taken after immunization. However, vaccinees who develop a rash should avoid direct contact with immunocompromised suscep-tible hosts for the duration of the rash. If contact inadvertently occurs, administra-tion of VZIG is not indicated.

---

* For further information, see Centers for Disease Control and Prevention. Recommendations of the Advisory Committee on Immunization Practices (ACIP): use of the vaccines and immune globulins for persons with altered immunocompetence. *MMWR.* 1993;43(No. RR-4):1-18.

For the child receiving immunosuppressive therapy, several factors are considered in immunization, including the underlying disease, the specific immunosuppressive regimen (dose and schedule), and the infectious disease and immunization history of the patient. Live-bacterial and live-virus vaccines generally are contraindicated because of the risk of serious adverse effects. An exception appears to be the judicious use of live-virus varicella vaccine in children with acute lymphocytic leukemia in remission, in whom the risk of natural varicella outweighs the risk from the attenuated vaccine virus (see Varicella-Zoster Infections, p 584). This vaccine may be obtained from the manufacturer on a compassionate-use protocol for patients 12 months to 17 years of age who have acute lymphocytic leukemia in remission for at least 1 year.*

After cessation of immunosuppressive therapy, live-virus vaccine in most circumstances is withheld for an interval of no less than 3 months after immunosuppressive therapy has been discontinued. The exception is corticosteroid therapy (see Corticosteroids). This interval is based on the assumption that immunologic responsiveness will have been restored in 3 months and that the underlying disease for which the immunosuppressive therapy was given is in remission or under control. However, because the interval may vary with the intensity and type of immunosuppressive therapy, radiation therapy, underlying disease, and other factors, a definitive recommendation for an interval after cessation of immunosuppressive therapy when live-virus vaccines can be safely and effectively administered is often not possible.

Patients with leukemia in remission, whose chemotherapy has been terminated for at least 3 months, may receive live-virus vaccines for infections to which they are still susceptible (ie, those diseases that the child neither had nor was vaccinated against, before developing leukemia).

Inactivated vaccines and immune globulin preparations should be used when appropriate, since they are not a risk to immunocompromised persons. The immune responses of immunocompromised children to some inactivated vaccines (eg, DTaP, DTP, hepatitis B, inactivated poliovirus, pneumococcal, and influenza) can be inadequate, and the vaccine's efficacy may be substantially reduced. The ability to develop a quantitatively normal immunologic response usually develops between 3 months and 1 year after discontinuing immunosuppressive therapy. If possible, influenza vaccine should be given to children with malignancy prior to influenza season, no less than 3 to 4 weeks after chemotherapy is discontinued and when they have peripheral granulocyte and lymphocyte counts greater than 1000/mm^3.

Because patients with congenital or acquired immunodeficiencies may not have an adequate response to immunizing agents, they may remain susceptible despite having received an appropriate vaccine. If feasible, specific serum antibody titers or other immunologic responses should be determined after immunization to assess immunity and guide management of future exposures and further immunization.

CORTICOSTEROIDS

Children can become immunocompromised because of corticosteroid therapy. The minimal amount of systemic steroids and duration of administration sufficient to

---

* Available from Varivax Coordinating Center, Bio-Pharm Clinical Services, Inc, 4 Valley Square, Bluebell, PA 19422 (215-283-0897).

cause immunosuppression in an otherwise healthy child are not well defined. The frequency and route of administration of corticosteroids, the underlying disease and concurrent other therapy also are factors affecting immunosuppression. Despite these uncertainties, however, sufficient experience exists to recommend empiric guidelines for live-virus vaccination of previously healthy children receiving corticosteroid therapy for non-immunocompromising conditions. Many clinicians consider a dose equivalent to 2 mg/kg per day or greater of prednisone or equivalent to a total of 20 mg/d or greater for children who weigh more than 10 kg, particularly when given for more than 14 days, sufficient to raise concern about the safety of immunization with live-virus vaccines. Accordingly, guidelines for live-virus vaccination of corticosteroid recipients are as follows:

- *Topical therapy or local injections of corticosteroids.* Administration of topical corticosteroids, either on the skin or in the respiratory system (ie, by aerosol) or eyes, and intra-articular, bursal, or tendon injections of corticosteroids, usually do not result in immunosuppression that would contraindicate administration of live-virus vaccines. However, live-virus vaccines should not be given if clinical or laboratory evidence of systemic immunosuppression results from prolonged application until corticosteroid therapy has been discontinued for at least one month.
- *Physiologic maintenance doses of corticosteroids.* Children who are receiving only maintenance physiologic doses of corticosteroids can receive live-virus vaccines while on treatment.
- *Low or moderate doses of systemic corticosteroids given daily or on alternate days.* Children receiving less than 2 mg/kg per day of prednisone or its equivalent, or less than 20 mg/d if they weigh more than 10 kg, can receive live-virus vaccines while on treatment.
- *High doses of systemic corticosteroids given daily or on alternative days for less than 14 days.* Children receiving 2 mg/kg per day or more of prednisone or its equivalent, or 20 mg or more daily if they weigh more than 10 kg, can receive live-virus vaccines immediately after discontinuation of treatment. Some experts, however, would delay immunization until 2 weeks after corticosteroid therapy has been discontinued, if possible (ie, if the patient's condition allows temporary cessation).
- *High doses of systemic corticosteroids given daily or on alternate days for 14 days or more.* Children receiving 2 mg/kg per day or more of prednisone or its equivalent, or 20 mg or more daily if they weigh more than 10 kg, should not receive live-virus vaccines until steroid therapy has been discontinued for at least 1 month.
- *Children with a disease which, in itself, is considered to suppress the immune response and who are receiving either systemic or locally administered corticosteroids.* These children should not be given live-virus vaccines except in special circumstances.

These guidelines are based on concerns about vaccine safety in recipient of high doses of corticosteroids. In addition, in deciding whether to administer live-virus vaccines, the potential benefits and risks of vaccination in the individual patient and specific circumstances should be considered. For example, some experts will recommend immunization of a patient at increased risk of a vaccine-preventable infection (and its complications) if, despite corticosteroid therapy, the patient does not have clinical evidence of immunosuppression.

The guidelines are based on considerations of safety concerning live-virus vaccines and do not necessarily correlate with those for optimal vaccine immunogenicity. For example, some children receiving moderate doses of prednisone, such as 1.5 mg/kg per day, for several weeks or longer may have a less than optimal serum antibody response to some vaccine antigens. Nevertheless, unless vaccination can be temporarily deferred until corticosteroids are discontinued without compromising the likelihood of immunization, they should be immunized in order to enhance the likelihood of protection in the case of exposure to disease. In contrast, some children receiving relatively high doses of corticosteroids (eg, 30 mg/d of prednisone) may respond adequately to vaccination.

HODGKIN'S DISEASE

Patients who are 24 months or older, including adults, should be immunized with pneumococcal vaccine (see Pneumococcal Infections, p 417); they also should receive *Haemophilus influenzae* type b (Hib) conjugate vaccine, according to age-specific recommendations (see *Haemophilus influenzae* Infections, p 220). These patients are at increased risk for invasive pneumococcal infection; most experts believe that they are also at increased risk for invasive Hib infection. The antibody response is likely to be best when patients are immunized at least 10 to 14 days before initiation of therapy for Hodgkin's disease. During active chemotherapy and shortly thereafter, the antibody responses to the pneumococcal vaccine are impaired. However, the ability of these patients to respond improves rapidly, and immunization as early as 3 months after the cessation of chemotherapy is reasonable. Patients who received vaccine during chemotherapy or radiation therapy should be re-immunized 3 months after discontinuation of the therapy.

TRANSPLANT RECIPIENTS

A special situation is a child recovering from successful bone marrow transplantation. Many factors can affect the child's immunity to vaccine-preventable diseases, including the donor's immunity, type of transplant (ie, autologous or allogeneic), interval since the transplant, receipt of immunosuppressive medications, and graft-versus-host disease (GVHD). Although many children who are transplant recipients acquire the immunity of the donor, some will lose serologic evidence of immunity. Retention of donor immune memory can be facilitated if recalled by antigenic stimulation soon after transplantation. Clinical studies of recipients of bone marrow transplants indicate that pre-transplant administration of diphtheria and tetanus toxoids to the bone-marrow donor and immediate posttransplant administration to the recipient can facilitate response to these antigens. In these studies, serum antibody titers did not increase when immunization of the recipient was delayed until 5 weeks after transplantation. In theory, these results could be expected with other inactivated vaccine antigens, including pertussis, Hib, hepatitis B, pneumococcal, and inactivated poliovirus vaccines.

The risk of acquiring diphtheria or tetanus in the year following bone marrow transplantation is very low. Some experts elect to reimmunize all children without serologic evaluation, while others base the decision to reimmunize against diphtheria and tetanus on the adequacy of serologic titers obtained 1 year after transplantation. Adequate immune responses can be obtained with three doses of diphtheria and tetanus toxoids at 2-month intervals, beginning 1 year after transplantation. Persons with tetanus-prone wounds sustained during the first year after transplantation should be given Tetanus Immune Globulin (TIG), regardless of their tetanus immunization status.

Data on which to base recommendations for reimmunization against *Streptococcus pneumoniae* or Hib are limited. A single dose of either vaccine appears to provide some protection if given at 12 months or more following transplantation. Protection is enhanced by immunization at both 12 and 24 months. Some experts recommend a multiple-dose schedule initiated before 12 months after transplantation, because a regimen in which children were immunized 3, 6, and 12 months after transplantation elicited acceptable immunogenicity; a booster dose at 24 months also is recommended.

Two years after bone marrow transplantation, MMR is often given because recent data indicate that healthy survivors at that time can receive these live-virus vaccines without untoward effects. A second dose of MMR should be given 1 month (4 weeks) or more after the first dose unless serologic response to measles is demonstrated after the first dose. Patients with chronic GVHD should not receive MMR vaccine because of concern about resulting latent virus infection and its sequelae. Susceptible persons who are exposed to measles should receive passive immunoprophylaxis (see Measles, p 346). Varicella vaccine is not recommended for bone marrow transplant recipients because of the lack of data on use of this vaccine in these patients. Passive immunization with VZIG is recommended for susceptible persons with known exposure to chickenpox (see Varicella-Zoster Infections, p 578).

Only inactivated poliovirus vaccine (IPV) should be given to transplant recipients and their household contacts. Bone marrow transplant recipients are at risk of exposure to live poliovirus vaccine (OPV) from contact with vaccinees in the community and, thus, should be immunized with IPV. Although three doses of IPV induced an antibody response in only half of the recipients who were immunized 1 year after transplantation, the effectiveness of giving additional doses is not known. Alternatively, recipients can be tested for immunity, but serologic tests for antibody titers against polioviruses are not readily available in commercial or state laboratories.

Influenza immunization is not effective when given within the initial 6 months after bone marrow transplantation but vaccination may provide protection when given at 1 year. Because the risk of disease is substantial, influenza vaccine should be administered annually in the early fall (see Influenza, p 310) to persons who received a transplant more than 6 months before, even if the interval is less than 12 months.

The immunogenicity of hepatitis B vaccine in transplant recipients has not been adequately assessed. Based on the response of these patients to other protein antigens, initiation of a three-dose series 12 months after transplantation followed by postvaccination serological testing for anti-HBs is reasonable. Additional doses (maximum of three) are given to vaccine nonresponders.

Children who are scheduled to have a solid-organ transplantation and who are older than 12 months, if previously vaccinated, should have serologic antibody titers for measles, mumps, rubella, and varicella. Those who are susceptible should be given MMR and/or varicella vaccine before transplantation. The preferred time to give these vaccines is at least 1 month before transplantation. Serum and varicella antibody titers should be measured in all patients 1 or more years after transplantation. Information about the use of live-virus vaccines in patients after solid-organ transplantation is limited. Annual influenza immunization is indicated, as recommended for bone marrow transplant recipients. The use of passive immunization (ie, immune globulin administration) should be based on serological evidence of susceptibility and exposure to disease.

Because of the limited data on immunizations of transplant recipients, immunization schedules vary in different centers. Physicians managing these patients are encouraged to develop immunization protocols and schedules in conjunction with experts in infectious diseases and immunology.

HIV INFECTION (SEE ALSO HIV INFECTION, P 279)

Data on the use of currently available live-virus and bacterial vaccines in HIV-infected children are limited but complications, until recently, have been reported only after BCG vaccination. In 1996, however, a case of vaccine-related measles pneumonitis was reported in a severely immunocompromised patient 1 year after measles immunization.

Because of reports of severe measles in symptomatic HIV-infected children, including fatalities in as many as 40% of cases, measles vaccination (given as MMR) is recommended for HIV-infected children in most circumstances, including those who are symptomatic but are not severely immunocompromised as well as those who are asymptomatic. Vaccine should be given at 12 months of age in order to enhance the likelihood of an appropriate immune response. In a measles epidemic, vaccine should be given at an earlier age, such as at 6 to 9 months followed by the routinely recommended dose at 12 months (or 1 month [4 weeks] after this initial dose) (see Measles, p 355). The second dose after the 12 month vaccination may be administered as soon as 1 month (4 weeks) later in an attempt to induce seroconversion as early as possible. However, severely immunocompromised patients with HIV infection, as defined by low CD4+ T-lymphocyte counts or percentage of total circulating lymphocytes, should not receive measles vaccine (see HIV Infection, p 293, and Table 3.22 in that chapter).

Varicella vaccine should not be given to known HIV-infected patients, irrespective of their degree of immunosuppression. However, studies are currently in progress to evaluate the benefit and safety of this vaccine in HIV-infected children and may lead to a change in this recommendation.

Children with either asymptomatic or symptomatic HIV infection should receive other routinely recommended childhood vaccines, including DTaP (or DTP), hepatitis B, and Hib conjugate vaccines according to the recommended schedule (see Fig 1.1, p 18). **Oral poliovirus vaccine (OPV) is contraindicated and IPV should be given.** Annual influenza immunization of HIV-infected persons is recommended (see Influenza, p 310). Pneumococcal vaccination is indicated for children 2 years of age and older.

In the United States, BCG is contraindicated in HIV-infected patients. In areas with high incidence of tuberculosis, however, the World Health Organization recommends giving BCG to HIV-infected children who are asymptomatic.

Routine or widespread screening to detect asymptomatic HIV-infected children before routine immunization is not recommended. Children without clinical or epidemiologic manifestations of HIV infection should be immunized in accordance with the recommendations for routine childhood immunization.

Since the ability of HIV-infected children to respond to vaccine antigens is likely related to the degree of immunosuppression at the time of vaccination and may be inadequate, these children should be considered potentially susceptible to vaccine-preventable diseases, even after appropriate immunization, unless a recent serologic test demonstrates adequate antibody concentrations. Hence, passive immunoprophylaxis or chemoprophylaxis after exposure to these diseases should be considered even if the child has previously received the recommended vaccines.

Household contacts of an adult or child with proven or suspected HIV infection also should not receive OPV because the vaccine virus can spread from person to person, particularly in households. Although no cases of poliovirus-vaccine-associated poliomyelitis have been reported in HIV-infected persons, only IPV should be used in polio immunization of household contacts.

Although vaccine-type varicella-zoster virus has been transmitted from healthy persons, household contacts of HIV-infected persons can be immunized with live-virus varicella vaccine (see Varicella-Zoster Infections, p 583). No precautions need be taken after immunization of healthy children who do not develop a rash. Vaccinees who develop a rash should avoid direct contact with susceptible immuno-compromised hosts for the duration of the rash. Disease, if it develops, is mild and use of VZIG to prevent transmission is not indicated.

Asplenic Children

The asplenic state results from (1) the surgical removal of the spleen, (2) certain diseases, such as sickle cell disease (functional asplenia), or (3) congenital asplenia. All asplenic infants, children, and adults, regardless of the reason for the asplenic state, have an increased risk for fulminant bacteremia, which is associated with a high mortality rate. Susceptibility to fulminant bacteremia is influenced considerably by the underlying disease. In comparison with healthy children who have not had splenectomy, the incidence of mortality from septicemia is increased 50-fold in children who have had splenectomy after trauma, approximately 350-fold in children with sickle cell disease, and may even be higher in children who have had splenectomy for thalassemia. The risk of bacteremia is higher in younger children than in older children, and it may be greater in the years immediately after splenectomy. Fulminant bacteremia, however, has been reported in adults as many as 25 years after splenectomy.

Streptococcus pneumoniae and *Haemophilus influenzae* type b are the most important pathogens in asplenic children. Less common causes of bacteremia include *Neisseria meningitidis*, other streptococci, *Escherichia coli*, *Staphylococcus aureus*, and Gram-negative bacilli such as *Salmonella* species, *Klebsiella* species, and *Pseudomonas aeruginosa*. Persons who are functionally or anatomically asplenic also are at increased risk for fatal malaria and severe babesiosis.

Pneumococcal vaccine is indicated for all asplenic children 2 years and older (see Pneumococcal Infections, p 410). Revaccination after 3 to 5 years is recommended for children with asplenia who are 10 years of age or younger and for older children and adults who were immunized at least 5 years before. Immunization against *H influenzae* type b infections should be initiated at 2 months of age, as recommended for otherwise healthy young children (see Fig 1.1, p 18) and in all previously unimmunized children with asplenia. Quadrivalent meningococcal polysaccharide vaccine also should be administered to asplenic children 2 years and older (see Meningococcal Infections, p 357). The efficacy of meningococcal vaccine in asplenic children is not certain, although this vaccine is probably as effective as pneumococcal polysaccharide vaccine. No known contraindication exists to giving these vaccines at the same time in separate syringes at different sites. Since the currently licensed pneumococcal and meningococcal vaccines are unconjugated polysaccharide vaccines, they may not be as effective in preventing disease in children younger than 5 years as they are in older persons.

Daily antimicrobial prophylaxis against pneumococcal infections is recommended for many asplenic children, irrespective of vaccination status. For infants with sickle cell anemia, oral penicillin prophylaxis against invasive pneumococcal disease should be initiated as soon as the diagnosis is established and preferably by 2 months of age. Although the efficacy of antimicrobial prophylaxis has been proven only in patients with sickle cell anemia, other asplenic children at particularly high risk, such as those with malignancies and thalassemia, also should receive daily chemoprophylaxis. Less agreement exists about the need in children who have had splenectomy after trauma. In general, antimicrobial prophylaxis (in addition to vaccination) should be strongly considered for all asplenic children younger than 5 years.

The age at which chemoprophylaxis is discontinued in patients is often an empirical decision. Based on a recent multi-center study, prophylactic penicillin can be discontinued at approximately 5 years of age in children with sickle cell anemia who are receiving regular medical attention and who have not had a prior severe pneumococcal infection or a surgical splenectomy. The duration of prophylaxis for children with asplenia due to other causes is unknown. Some experts continue prophylaxis throughout childhood and in adulthood in particularly high-risk patients with asplenia.

For antimicrobial prophylaxis, oral penicillin V (125 mg twice a day for children younger than 5 years and 250 mg twice a day for children 5 years and older) is usually recommended. Some experts recommend amoxicillin (20 mg/kg per day).

When antimicrobial prophylaxis is used, its limitations must be stressed to parents and patients. They should recognize that some bacteria capable of causing fulminant sepsis are not susceptible to the antimicrobials given for prophylaxis. Parents should be aware that all febrile illnesses are potentially serious in asplenic children, and that immediate medical attention should be sought because the initial signs and symptoms of fulminant bacteremia can be subtle. When bacteremia is a possibility, the physician should hospitalize the child, obtain blood and other cultures as indicated, and immediately begin treatment with an antimicrobial regimen or a regimen effective against *S pneumoniae*, *H influenzae*, and *N meningitidis*. In some clinical situations, other antibiotics such as aminoglycosides may be indicated. If an asplenic child travels or resides in an area where medical care is not accessible, an appropriate antibiotic should be readily available and the child's caregiver instructed in its use.

Whenever possible, alternatives to splenectomy should be considered. Management options include postponement of splenectomy for as long as possible in congenital hemolytic anemias, preservation of accessory spleens, performance of partial splenectomy for benign tumors of the spleen, conservative (nonoperative) management of splenic trauma, or, when feasible, repair rather than removal, and, if possible, avoidance of splenectomy when immunodeficiency is present (eg, Wiskott-Aldrich syndrome).

Children With a Personal or Family History of Seizures

Infants and children with a personal and family history of convulsions are at increased risk for having a convulsion after receipt of either pertussis (as DTP) or measles (usually as MMR) vaccine. In most cases, these seizures are brief, self-limited, and generalized, and occur in conjunction with fever. These characteristics indicate that such vaccine-associated seizures are usually febrile convulsions. No evidence indicates that these seizures (1) cause permanent brain damage or epilepsy, (2) aggravate neurologic disorders, or (3) affect the prognosis in children with underlying disorders.

In the case of pertussis immunization during infancy, however, administration of DTP may coincide with or hasten the inevitable recognition of a disorder associated with seizures, such as infantile spasms or epilepsy, and cause confusion about the role of pertussis vaccination. Hence, pertussis immunization in infants with recent seizures should be deferred until a progressive neurologic disorder is excluded or the cause of the earlier seizure has been diagnosed. In contrast, measles immunization is given at an age when the cause and nature of the recent convulsion and the child's neurologic status are more likely to have been established. This difference provides the basis for the recommendation that measles immunization should not be deferred in children with a personal history of one or more convulsions.

A family history of convulsive disorders is not a contraindication to pertussis or measles vaccination, or a reason to defer immunization. Postvaccination seizures in these children are usually febrile in origin, have a generally benign outcome, and are not likely to be confused with manifestations of a previously unrecognized neurologic disorder. In addition, many children have a family history of convulsion and would remain susceptible to pertussis and measles if family history were a contraindication to immunization.

Specific recommendations for pertussis and measles immunization of children with a personal or family history of convulsions are given in the respective disease-specific chapters (see Pertussis, p 394, and Measles, p 344); detailed discussion and recommendations concerning pertussis immunization of children with neurologic disorders also are given.

Children With Chronic Diseases

Some chronic diseases render children more susceptible to the severe manifestations and complications of common infections. In general, immunizations recommended for healthy children should be given to children with these disorders. However, for children with immunologic disorders, live-virus vaccines are usually contraindicated; the major exception is MMR for HIV-infected children who are not severely immunocompromised (see Immunodeficient and Immunosuppressed Children, p 50). Children with certain chronic diseases (eg, cardiorespiratory, allergic, hematologic, metabolic, and renal disorders, and cystic fibrosis) are at increased risk for complications of influenza and/or pneumococcal infection and should receive influenza and/or pneumococcal vaccine (see Influenza, p 307, and Pneumococcal Infections, p 410).

The appropriateness of administering a live-virus vaccine to a specific child with a rare disorder (eg, galactosemia or renal tubular acidosis) is problematic, particularly if the disease may impair the immune response to the vaccine. The experience in some of these disorders is minimal or nonexistent, and the physician should seek guidance from a specialist before administering the vaccine(s).

Active Immunization After Exposure to Disease

Since not all susceptible persons receive vaccines before exposure, active immunization in a person who has been exposed to a specific disease may be considered. The following situations are most commonly encountered (see the disease-specific chapters in Section 3 for detailed recommendations).

MEASLES

Live-virus measles vaccine given within 72 hours of exposure will provide protection against measles in some cases because immunity induced by parenterally administered, live-virus vaccine appears more rapidly than that induced by natural measles. Infected persons can spread measles virus for 3 to 5 days before the appearance of a rash (and for 1 to 2 days before the onset of symptoms). Thus, those in continuous contact with such persons, as in households, child care, and school settings, would have been exposed before the appearance of clinical manifestations.

Immune globulin (IG) intramuscularly in a dose of 0.25 mL/kg (maximum dose, 15 mL), given within 6 days of exposure, also can prevent or modify measles in a healthy susceptible person. Since measles morbidity is high in children younger than 1 year, IG is recommended for infants exposed to measles as well as for immunocompromised and pregnant persons. Exposed immunodeficient or immunocompromised persons should receive 0.5 mL/kg of IG (maximal dose, 15 mL).

VARICELLA

Live-virus vaccine may be effective in preventing varicella when given within 3 days of exposure to a child with chickenpox. Because studies demonstrating the possible effectiveness of vaccination have not been performed with the current formulation of varicella vaccine, postexposure vaccine prophylaxis is not recommended at this time. However, its use in healthy, susceptible persons following exposure is potentially advantageous and confers little risk.

Susceptible immunocompromised children should be given passive protection as soon as possible with Varicella-Zoster Immune Globulin (VZIG) following contact with an infected person.

HEPATITIS B

Postexposure vaccination is highly effective if combined with passive antibody. Administration of Hepatitis B Immune Globulin (HBIG) does not inhibit active immunization with the hepatitis B vaccine. For postexposure prophylaxis in a newborn whose mother is a hepatitis B surface antigen (HBsAg) carrier, hepatitis B vaccination is essential. For percutaneous or mucosal exposure to HBsAg, combined active and passive immunization is recommended for susceptible persons. Persons with continuing household or sexual contact with an HBsAg carrier also should be vaccinated.

TETANUS

In wound management, unimmunized or incompletely immunized individuals should be given tetanus toxoid immediately in addition to Tetanus Immune Globulin (TIG), depending on the nature of the wound and the immunization history of the person (see Table 3.58, p 520).

RABIES

Postexposure active and passive immunization is an essential aspect of the immunoprophylaxis of rabies.

MUMPS

Exposed susceptible persons are not necessarily protected by postexposure live-virus vaccine administration. However, a common practice in mumps exposure is to administer vaccine to presumed susceptible persons so that if mumps does not result from the current exposure, permanent immunity will be afforded by the immunization. Administration of live-virus vaccine is recommended for exposed adults born after 1956 who have not previously had mumps or mumps vaccination.

RUBELLA

Whether postexposure rubella vaccination is effective is not known and it is not recommended.

Children in Residential Institutions

Children housed together in institutions pose special problems for control of certain infectious diseases. Ensuring appropriate immunization of these children is important because of the risk of transmission within the facility and because the conditions that led to institutionalization may increase the risk of complications from the disease. All children entering a residential institution should have received appropriate routine immunizations for their age (see Fig 1.1 and Table 1.3, p 18 and p 20). If they have not, arrangements should be made to complete these immunizations as rapidly as possible. Employees should be familiar with standard precautions and procedures for handling contaminated blood and body fluids and for accidental trauma involving these fluids. They should be aware of children infected with hepatitis B virus in order to ensure prompt and appropriate management in these circumstances. Specific diseases of concern include the following (see the disease-specific chapters in Section 3 for detailed recommendations).

MEASLES

Epidemics can occur among susceptible children in institutional settings. Recommendations for managing children in an institutional setting when a case of measles is recognized are as follows: (1) administer live measles virus vaccine (as MMR) within 72 hours of exposure to all susceptible children 1 year or older for whom vaccination is not contraindicated, and (2) administer immune globulin (IG) in a dosage of 0.25 mL/kg, or 0.5 mL/kg to immunocompromised children (15 mL, maximum) as soon as possible and within 6 days of exposure to all exposed, susceptible children younger than 1 year. These IG recipients will still require live-virus vaccine (as MMR) at 12 months of age or thereafter, depending on the age and dose of IG administration (see Table 3.37, p 353, for the appropriate interval between IG administration and vaccination).

MUMPS

Epidemics may occur among susceptible, nonimmunized children in institutions. The major hazards are disruption of activities, the need for acute nursing care in difficult settings, and occasional serious complications (eg, in the susceptible adult attendants).

If mumps is introduced into a setting where susceptible persons reside, no prophylaxis is available to limit the spread or modify the disease in a person. Immune globulin is not effective. Although mumps virus vaccine may not be effective after exposure, the vaccine should be administered to susceptible persons to protect against future exposures.

INFLUENZA

This illness can be devastating in a residential or custodial institutional setting. Rapid spread, intensive exposure, and underlying disease can result in a high risk of severe illness that may affect many residents simultaneously or in close sequence. Current measures for control of influenza in institutions include (1) a program of annual influenza immunization, and (2) appropriate use of chemoprophylaxis during influenza A epidemics. In considering the use of chemoprophylaxis, the physician often can obtain information on which strains of influenza are prevalent in the community from local and state health departments.

PERTUSSIS

Since progressive developmental delay is an indication for deferral of pertussis immunization, some children in an institutional setting may not be immunized against pertussis. If pertussis is recognized, these patients as well as close contacts of infected patients should receive chemoprophylaxis.

HEPATITIS A

Outbreaks of hepatitis A can occur in institutions for custodial care from fecal-oral transmission, affecting residents and staff. Infection is usually mild or asymptomatic in young children but can be severe in adults. Although an effective hepatitis A vaccine is available for children 2 years of age and older, its role in helping to control or prevent outbreaks in these settings has not been determined. If an outbreak occurs, residents and staff members in close personal contact with patients should receive IG (0.02 mL/kg intramuscularly).

HEPATITIS B

Children living in residential institutions for the developmentally disabled and their caregivers are assumed to be at increased risk for acquiring hepatitis B infection. The high prevalence of hepatitis B virus (HBV) markers among children living in these facilities indicates that HBV infections have the propensity for spread in an institutional setting, presumably by exposure to blood and body fluids containing HBV. Factors that can be associated with high prevalence of HBV markers include crowding, high client-staff ratios, and lack of in-service educational programs for the staff. In the presence of such factors, the prevalence of HBV increases with the duration of time spent at the institution. Thus, persons entering or already residing in residential institutions for the developmentally disabled should be vaccinated against HBV; preimmunization serological screening for HBV markers is probably not cost-effective because the prevalence of markers will be low.

After parenteral or sexual exposure to an institutionalized patient recognized to be a hepatitis B surface antigen (HBsAg) carrier, unimmunized, susceptible attendees and/or staff should receive active and passive immunoprophylaxis.

PNEUMOCOCCAL INFECTIONS

Children with severe physical or mental disabilities, particularly those who are bedridden, suffer from a compromised respiratory status, or are capable of only very limited physical activity, may benefit from pneumococcal vaccination at 24 months of age or older.

VARICELLA

This infection is very contagious and can occur in a high percentage of susceptible children in an institutional setting. All healthy children, 1 year of age or older, who lack a reliable history of varicella should be immunized. Prophylactic measures during outbreaks are currently recommended only for immunocompromised, susceptible children at risk for serious complications or death from varicella, for whom VZIG is indicated (see Table 3.67, p 578).

OTHER INFECTIONS

Other infections that spread in institutions, for which no immunization is currently available, include *Shigella, Streptococcus pyogenes, Staphylococcus aureus,* respiratory viruses, rotaviruses, cytomegalovirus, *Giardia lamblia,* scabies, and lice.

Children in Military Populations

In general, children of active-duty military personnel require the same immunizations as their civilian counterparts. If delay in pertussis immunization is recommended for any reason, parents should be warned that the risk of contracting the disease in countries where pertussis immunization is not routinely given is significantly higher than that in countries where effective vaccine is used. For military dependents going overseas, the risk of exposure to hepatitis A and B, measles, pertussis, diphtheria, polio, yellow fever, Japanese encephalitis, and other infections may be increased and necessitate additional immunizations (see Foreign Travel, p 68). In these instances, the choice of immunizations will be dictated by the country of proposed residence, expected travel and residence, and the age and health of the child. Information on the risk of specific diseases in different countries and preventive measures is provided in the yearly publication *Health Information for International Travel* (see p 2) and by the Centers for Disease Control and Prevention Information Service on International Travelers Hotline (see Directory of Telephone Numbers, p 667).

Adolescent* and College Populations

Adolescents and young adults may not be protected against vaccine-preventable diseases. This age group can include persons who escaped natural infection and who (1) were not immunized with all recommended vaccines, (2) received appropriate vaccines but at too young an age (eg, measles vaccine before 12 months), (3) received incomplete vaccination regimens (eg, only one or two doses of hepatitis B vaccine), or (4) failed to respond to vaccines administered at the appropriate ages.

To assure age-appropriate immunization, all children should have a routine early adolescent visit at 11 to 12 years of age to (1) vaccinate those who have not previously received two doses of MMR and give varicella and/or hepatitis B vaccine as indicated, (2) provide a booster dose of tetanus and diphtheria (Td) toxoids, and (3) provide other immunization and preventive services that are indicated.* Additional vaccines that may be indicated at the immunization visit include influenza, pneumococcal, and hepatitis A. Specific indications for each of these vaccines are given in the respective disease-specific chapter in Section 3.

Appointments for needed doses of vaccine that are not administered during the visit should be scheduled. During all subsequent adolescent visits, the child's immunization status should be reviewed and deficiencies should be corrected, including completion of the three-dose hepatitis B vaccine series.

School immunization laws encourage "catch-up" programs for older adolescents. Accordingly, school and college health services should establish a system to ensure that all students are protected against vaccine-preventable diseases. Many colleges are implementing the American College Health Association (ACHA) recommendations for prematriculation immunization requirements, mandating protection from measles, mumps, rubella, tetanus, diphtheria, and polio.

MEASLES

Many colleges and universities have experienced measles outbreaks in the past decade, delaying earlier efforts to eliminate this disease from the United States. To prevent measles outbreaks and ensure high levels of immunity among young adults on college and university campuses, the ACHA has recommended that colleges and universities require two doses of measles vaccine as a condition for matriculation. In

---

* See also Centers for Disease Control and Prevention. Immunization of adolescents: recommendations of the Advisory Committee on Immunization Practices, the American Academy of Pediatrics, the American Academy of Family Physicians, and the American Medical Association. *MMWR.* 1996;45 (No. RR-13):1-16.

addition, the Academy recommends a two-dose measles vaccination schedule, given as MMR vaccine, for persons born after 1956 in post-high school educational settings.

RUBELLA

Adolescents and adults should be considered susceptible to rubella if documentation of immunity is lacking. Vaccinating adolescents and adults in college reduces the chance of outbreaks and helps to prevent the congenital rubella syndrome.

VARICELLA

Healthy adolescents past their 13th birthday who have not been immunized previously and have no history of varicella infection should be immunized against varicella by administration of two doses of vaccine 4 to 8 weeks apart. Longer intervals between doses do not necessitate a third dose, but may leave the person unprotected for the intervening months. Varicella immunity also is desirable in adults, especially adults in colleges and universities and nonpregnant women of childbearing age.*

HEPATITIS B

Hepatitis B vaccination is recommended for all adolescents. In addition to assessment of immunization status at 11 to 12 years of age and vaccination of susceptible persons, special efforts should be made to vaccinate any adolescent, especially those who have one or more risk factors for hepatitis B. Risk factors include multiple sexual partners (defined as more than one partner within the previous 6 months), a sexually transmitted disease, sexually active homosexual or bisexual behavior, injection drug use, and occupation or training involving contact with blood or body fluids.

TETANUS/DIPHTHERIA

Td (adult-type tetanus and diphtheria toxoid) should be given at 11 to 12 years of age and no later than 16 years of age. Thereafter, booster vaccination with Td is given every 10 years.

INFLUENZA

Epidemic influenza can affect any closed population. Physicians responsible for health care in schools and colleges should consider annual influenza vaccination of students, particularly those residing in dormitories or who are members of athletic teams, to minimize disruption of routine activities during epidemics.

OTHER RECOMMENDATIONS

Because adolescents and young adults frequently undertake international travel, their immunization status and travel plans should be reviewed 2 or more months before departure to allow time to administer any needed vaccines (see Foreign Travel, p 68).

Some physicians are unaware of the risks of vaccine-preventable diseases to adolescents and young adults, and do not give priority to immunization. Pediatricians should assist in providing information on immunization and vaccine-preventable

---

* Centers for Disease Control and Prevention. Prevention of varicella: recommendations of the Advisory Committee on Immunization Practices (ACIP). *MMWR.* 1996;45(No. RR-11):1-36

disease to others who care for adolescents in their communities and should work to heighten awareness of the importance of immunizing adolescents and young adults.

The possible occurrence of diseases such as measles, mumps, rubella, hepatitis B, pertussis, and influenza in a school or college should be reported promptly to local health officials.

Health Care Personnel

Adults whose occupations place them in contact with patients with contagious diseases are at increased risk for contracting vaccine-preventable diseases and, if infected, for transmitting them to their patients. Health care personnel, including physicians, nurses, students, and auxiliary personnel, should protect themselves and susceptible patients by receiving appropriate immunizations. Physicians, hospitals, and schools for health professionals should play a major role in implementing these policies. Vaccine-preventable infections of special concern to those involved in the health care of children are as follows (see the disease-specific chapters in Section 3 for further recommendations):

- *Rubella.* Outbreaks of rubella among health care workers have been reported. Although the disease is mild in adults, the risk to the fetus necessitates documentation of rubella immunity in hospital personnel of both sexes. Persons for whom the risk of rubella infection is increased include hospital workers in pediatrics, physicians and nurses working in pediatric and obstetric ambulatory care (including emergency departments), and all those working in health care areas in which pregnant women are encountered. Persons should be considered immune only on the basis of serologic tests or documented proof of rubella immunization on or after 12 months of age; a history of rubella is unreliable and should not be used in judging immune status. All susceptible persons should be immunized (with MMR or monocomponent rubella vaccine) before initial or continuing contact with pregnant patients.
- *Measles.* Because measles in health care workers has contributed to the spread of the disease during outbreaks, evidence of immunity to measles should be required for health care personnel born after 1956 who will have direct patient contact. Proof is established by a physician-documented illness, a positive serologic test for antibody, or documented receipt of two doses of live-virus measles vaccine on or after the first birthday. Workers born before 1957 generally have been considered immune to measles. However, since measles cases have occurred in health care workers in this age group, health facilities should consider offering at least one dose of measles-containing vaccine to such workers who lack proof of immunity to measles, particularly in communities with ongoing measles transmission.
- *Mumps.* Transmission of mumps in health care facilities can be disruptive and costly. Adults born before 1957 have generally been considered immune to mumps; those born in 1957 or later are considered immune if they have documentation of a single dose of mumps vaccine received after their first birthday, or laboratory evidence of immunity.
- *Hepatitis B.* Vaccine is recommended for all health care personnel, including physicians, who are likely to be exposed to blood or body fluids. The Occupational Safety and Health Administration (OSHA) of the US Department of Labor has

issued a regulation requiring employers of workers at risk for occupational exposure to hepatitis B to offer vaccines to these employees at the employer's expense.

- **Influenza.** Certain groups of patients, such as those with chronic cardiovascular or pulmonary disease, are at high risk for serious or complicated influenza infection. Because medical personnel can transmit influenza to their patients and because nosocomial outbreaks can occur, influenza immunization programs for hospital workers and other health care professionals should be organized each fall. Since infants younger than 6 months cannot be protected by immunization, vaccination of personnel working in nurseries and infant wards is highly advised.
- **Varicella.** Assurance of varicella immunity is recommended for all susceptible health care personnel. In health-care institutions, serological screening of personnel who have a negative or uncertain history of varicella is likely to be cost-effective. Varicella vaccination is recommended for susceptible persons by the Advisory Committee on Immunization Practices (ACIP) of the Centers for Disease Control and Prevention (CDC).*
- On occasion, susceptible health care workers adequately immunized with measles, mumps, rubella, varicella, or hepatitis B vaccines fail to develop serologic evidence of immunity against one or more of these antigens. In those instances, one additional immunization can be given 4 to 6 weeks later, followed by serologic testing. Failure to develop immunity thereafter suggests that further immunization is unlikely to induce seroconversion.
- **Tuberculosis.** Comprehensive infection control measures, regular tuberculin skin testing, and, if indicated, anti-tuberculous therapy are the recommended strategies for the prevention and control of tuberculosis among health-care personnel. Vaccination with BCG is not recommended in most circumstances for personnel. According to current recommendations of the CDC, BCG vaccination should be considered on an individual basis in settings with a high prevalence of multi-drug resistant *Mycobacterium tuberculosis* infection, situations in which transmission of resistant organisms are likely, and facilities in which comprehensive infection control precautions against *M tuberculosis* transmission have been implemented and have failed.[†]

Refugees

Prevention of infectious diseases in refugee children presents special problems because of the diseases to which these children have been exposed and the immunization practices unique to their native countries. Whereas most of these children will be free of contagious diseases, certain infections are more common in refugees than in residents of the United States (see Table 2.10, p 117).

Children who come from refugee camps may not have been completely immunized before arrival. Refugee children from eastern Europe and countries of the former Soviet Union are less likely to be fully immunized than those arriving from

---

* Centers for Disease Control and Prevention. Prevention of varicella: recommendations of the Advisory Committee on Immunization Practices (ACIP). *MMWR.* 1996;45(No. RR-11):1-36

† Centers for Disease Control and Prevention. The role of BCG vaccine in the prevention and control of tuberculosis in the US: a joint statement by the Advisory Council for the Elimination of Tuberculosis and the Advisory Committee on Immunization Practices. *MMWR.* 1996;45 (No. RR-4):1-18.

southeast Asian refugee camps. For refugee children whose immunizations are not up-to-date for age, as documented by a written immunization record (see Immunizations Received Outside the United States, p 22), required vaccines as indicated for their age should be administered simultaneously (see Fig 1.1 and Table 1.3, p 18 and p 20).

Tuberculosis is the most important public health problem of refugees, particularly those from Southeast Asia and other developing areas. Refugees and immigrants have accounted for a substantial and increasing proportion of new cases of tuberculosis in the United States in the past decade (see Tuberculosis, p 542). Some refugees will have active disease and as many as one-half have positive tuberculin skin tests. All refugee children should be skin tested with Mantoux tuberculin test at the time of the first visit and 3 months later to identify recently acquired infection (see Tuberculosis, p 544). Previous BCG vaccination, which is the case with many of these children, is not a contraindication to skin testing. Although a vaccinated person may have a positive tuberculin skin test, tuberculin hypersensitivity resulting from a single BCG immunization is often minimal or modest and is not persistent, and, thus, a positive skin test should not be attributed to BCG (see Tuberculosis, p 546). A chest roentgenogram is indicated if the skin test is positive in BCG-vaccinated infants or children.

The physician should be aware that refugees are required by US immigration law to be screened for tuberculosis, and, if found to have tuberculosis disease, they must receive treatment until they are no longer infectious before they may enter the country. Some refugees will arrive before treatment is completed; those persons will have been given enough medication to last until they are evaluated by the local health department. All refugees with active or suspected active tuberculosis are provided with copies of medical records that summarize roentgenographic findings, laboratory studies and treatment, and the local health department is notified at the time of the refugee's arrival in the United States. Some refugees will develop active tuberculosis after arrival. Evaluation of these patients must include efforts to obtain the organism for culture and antibiotic susceptibility testing. Initial therapy should be with a regimen recommended for possible drug-resistant bacteria (see Tuberculosis, p 547).

The prevalence of hepatitis B surface antigen (HBsAg) carriers in eastern Asian refugees is estimated to be 10% to 15%. Most of these persons are asymptomatic, and transmission can be limited by universal infant hepatitis B immunization and administration of hepatitis B vaccine to susceptible household contacts. Serologic screening of pregnant refugee women for HBsAg is necessary to identify women whose infants need active and passive immunoprophylaxis (see Hepatitis B, p 248).

All children younger than 11 years residing in households of first-generation refugees from countries in which hepatitis B infection is of intermediate or high endemicity should be vaccinated (see Hepatitis B, p 254). Refugees from endemic areas, particularly eastern Asia and Africa, also should be serologically screened for HBsAg. If a carrier is found, susceptible household contacts of all ages should be vaccinated. Person-to-person (horizontal) transmission of this infection has been documented in immigrant populations from endemic areas among preschool and early school-age children without a known carrier in the family.

Table 1.10. **Recommended Immunizations for Travelers to Developing Countries***

| Immunizations | Length of Travel[†] | | |
	Brief, <2 wk	Intermediate, 2 wk to 3 mo	Long-term Residential, >3 mo
Review and complete age-appropriate childhood schedule (see text for details) — DTaP (or DTP) may be given at 4-wk intervals[‡] — Poliovirus vaccine may be given at 4- to 8-wk intervals[‡] — Measles: extra dose given if 6–11 mo old at 1st dose — Varicella — Hepatitis B[§]	+	+	+
Yellow fever[‖]	+	+	+
Typhoid fever[¶]	±	+	+
Meningococcal meningitis[#]	±	±	±
Rabies[**]	+	+	+
Japanese encephalitis[‖]	–	±	+

* See disease-specific chapters in Section 3 for details. For further sources of information, see text.
† + indicates recommended; ±, consider; and –, not recommended.
‡ If necessary to complete the recommended schedule before departure.
§ If insufficient time to complete 6-month primary series, accelerated series can be given (see text for details).
‖ For endemic regions (see *Health Information for International Travel*, p 2).
¶ Indicated for travelers who will consume food at nontourist facilities.
# For endemic regions of central Africa and during local epidemics.
** Indicated for persons with high risk of wild animal exposure and for spelunkers.

Foreign Travel

Foreign travel requires consideration of additional vaccines depending on circumstances of the visit or new residence, such as hepatitis A, as well as administration of those vaccines routinely recommended for children (see Table 1.10). Other immunizations may be required by local authorities. In addition, travelers to some tropical and subtropical areas often risk exposure to malaria, dengue fever, and other viral diseases for which vaccines are not available. For travelers at risk, malaria chemoprophylaxis and insect precautions are important preventive behaviors (see Malaria, p 335).

An excellent source of comprehensive information is the annually revised publication *Health Information for International Travel* (see p 2). The Centers for Disease Control and Prevention (CDC) also publishes the biweekly *Summary of Health Information* (known as the "Blue Sheet"), which lists areas infected with yellow fever and cholera, and gives changes reported by the World Health Organization (WHO) in the official recommendations for entry to certain countries. Local and state health departments can be consulted for updated information before travel. Information is also available from the CDC Information Service or International Travelers Hotline, which is accessible by telephone 24 hours a day, 7 days a week and provides information by fax as well (see Directory of Telephone Numbers, p 667). This information also can be obtained on the Internet.

Special attention should be given to ensure that infants and children embarking on international travel receive routine immunizations appropriate for their ages, including DTaP (or DTP), poliovirus, *Haemophilus influenzae* type b, MMR, varicella, and hepatitis B vaccines (see Fig 1.1, p 18). To ensure immunity, some vaccines may have to be given at an accelerated rate before departure (see Table 1.10, p 68).

Infants 6 to 12 months of age traveling to geographic areas where poliovirus is still endemic should have received two doses of vaccine before departure. Oral poliovirus vaccine (OPV) is preferred. For older children, the sequential IPV-OPV or OPV-only regimen is preferred in order to achieve optimal intestinal immunity (see Poliovirus Infections, p 430).

Since some cases of measles in the United States result from exposure in foreign countries, persons traveling abroad should be immune to measles (see Measles, p 344). Unless a contraindication exists, a single dose of a measles-containing vaccine (ie, MMR) should be given to all persons born after 1956 traveling abroad who have not already received two doses of measles vaccine or do not have other proof of immunity. For children traveling to areas in which measles is occurring, the age for initiation of measles vaccination should be lowered. Infants 6 to 11 months of age should receive a dose of monovalent measles vaccine or MMR. They should be given two additional doses of MMR, starting at 12 months of age. Children 12 months of age or older should receive MMR before departure. Those who have not yet received their routine second dose of MMR should be vaccinated, provided that at least 1 month (4 weeks) has elapsed since the first dose. Since immune globulin (IG) can interfere with the immunologic response to measles and rubella vaccines and may interfere with mumps and varicella vaccines, the need for IG for hepatitis A prophylaxis should be considered in scheduling these immunizations (see Table 3.37, p 353).

Immunoprophylaxis against hepatitis A is indicated for susceptible persons traveling to countries with intermediate or high rates of hepatitis A infection. Such countries include those other than Australia, Canada, Japan, New Zealand, and Western Europe. Both vaccine and IG are effective. For persons 2 years of age and older, vaccine is preferred but IG is an acceptable alternative. To ensure immediate protection for those whose departure is imminent, both may be given concurrently in some cases (see Hepatitis A, p 242). For children younger than 2 years, IG is indicated since hepatitis A vaccine is not approved in the United States for use in young children.

Hepatitis B vaccine is recommended for travelers of all ages going to areas where the infection is highly endemic, such as countries in Asia and Africa (see Hepatitis B, p 247), and who will have close contact with the local population or are likely to have blood or sexual contact with residents of these areas. An accelerated dosing schedule is approved for one hepatitis B vaccine (Engerix-B*), by which the first three doses

---

* SmithKline Beecham, Philadelphia, Pa.

are given at 0, 1, and 2 months. This schedule may benefit travelers who have insufficient time (ie, less than 4 months) before departure to complete the standard three-dose schedule. If this accelerated schedule is used, a fourth dose should be given at 12 months.

Depending on the destination, planned activity, and length of stay, additional required or recommended travel immunizations can include vaccines against yellow fever, typhoid fever, meningococcal disease, rabies, and Japanese encephalitis. Health authorities at the destination should be consulted if a prolonged stay is contemplated. Recommendations for vaccine-preventable diseases for international travelers are listed in Table 1.10, p 68 (see also disease-specific chapters in Section 3).

Yellow fever vaccine is required by some countries as a condition of entry from infected areas for travelers as young as 6 months of age. Whenever possible, immunization with this live-virus vaccine should be delayed until age 9 months or older to avoid the risk of vaccine-associated encephalitis. Infants between 4 and 9 months of age should be considered for immunization if travel to an endemic area cannot be avoided; most experts believe that the risk of immunization is outweighed by the risk of yellow fever infection. Since infants younger than 4 months are highly susceptible to the vaccine-associated encephalitis, yellow fever vaccine should not be given to infants of this age (see Arboviruses, p 137).

The currently available cholera vaccine has limited efficacy and is no longer required by any country. Despite World Health Organization recommendations to the contrary, some physicians suggest a single dose of vaccine for travel to countries known to have unofficial requirements in order to facilitate entry into the country. If cholera vaccine is given, it should be administered, if possible, at least 3 weeks apart from yellow fever vaccine. If this schedule is not possible, the yellow fever vaccine should be given first (see Simultaneous Administration of Multiple Vaccines, p 21).

Typhoid vaccine is recommended for those who expect to consume food and water at nontourist facilities and to children who will reside in endemic areas. Three typhoid vaccines are available for civilian use in the United States, including an oral vaccine containing live-attenuated *Salmonella typhi* (Ty21a strain), and a Vi capsular polysaccharide (ViCPS) vaccine for parenteral administration (see *Salmonella* Infections, p 462). Of the three vaccines, the choice generally will be between oral and the ViCPS vaccine. For recommendations for use of these vaccines, see *Salmonella* Infections (p 466). The oral vaccine capsules need to be refrigerated, and antibiotic use should be avoided 1 week before, during, and 1 week after vaccine administration. Since the antimalarial mefloquine (but not chloroquine) can affect the immune response, for persons taking this drug, oral typhoid vaccine should be given at least 24 hours before or after a dose. Travelers always should be advised that typhoid vaccination is not a substitute for cautious and careful selection of food and drink.

Meningococcal polysaccharide vaccine (quadrivalent groups A/C/Y/W-135) should be offered for travelers to endemic areas in central Africa and to countries with current meningococcal A or C epidemics. The duration of protection is not established; it is likely to be more than 5 years in adults but less than 3 years in children immunized when younger than 4 years of age (see Meningococcal Infections, p 357). Revaccination, thus, in some circumstances, is warranted.

Rabies immunization should be offered if children will be living for more than 1 month (4 weeks) in areas where they may encounter rabid animals or if they engage in activities entailing increased risk of rabies transmission (eg, spelunking). The three-dose series may be given as an intradermal or intramuscular injection, depending on the vaccine product given (see Rabies, p 435). Since administration of chloroquine for malaria chemoprophylaxis may decrease the efficacy of intradermal rabies immunization, rabies vaccine by this route is not indicated when the person is taking chloroquine or a related antimalarial, such as mefloquine.

Japanese encephalitis virus, which is spread by mosquitoes, is a potential risk in Asia, adjacent countries of the former Soviet Union, and the Indian subcontinent. It should be offered to persons who will be spending a month or longer in endemic areas during the transmission season, especially if travel will include rural farming areas. However, the rate of allergic reactions to Japanese encephalitis vaccine is high and its use is not recommended for most travelers to these areas. No data are available on vaccine safety and efficacy in infants younger than 1 year. Immunization requires three doses administered subcutaneously on days 0, 7, and 30. The last dose should be administered at least 10 days before travel to an endemic area. If time constraints necessitate an abbreviated schedule, vaccine can be given at 0, 7, and 14 days (see Arboviruses, p 140).

Influenza vaccination may be warranted for foreign travelers, depending on the destination, duration of travel, risk of acquisition (based, in part, on the season of the year), and possible consequences to the traveler (see Influenza, p 307).

Skin testing for tuberculosis before departure is recommended for intermediate and long-term travelers who will reside and work in developing countries. Some countries may require BCG vaccine for issuance of work and residency permits for expatriate workers and their families.

Of all the diseases faced by international travelers going to the tropics, malaria is probably the greatest threat. For recommendations on appropriate use of chemoprophylaxis including pregnant women, infants, and breastfeeding mothers, see Malaria (p 335).

Prevention of mosquito bites is important in minimizing the risk of malaria, dengue fever, and other arbovirus diseases endemic in high-risk areas. Appropriate personal protective measures, particularly during the mosquito-biting period from dusk to dawn, can be highly effective. These include wearing long-sleeved cotton shirts and long trousers; sparing application to exposed skin of long-acting insect repellent such as DEET*; use of window screens and bednets; and use of insect sprays containing permethrin on clothing and bednets. Long-acting permethrin sprays are available that provide residual protection for as long as 2 weeks when applied to materials and allowed to dry.

Travelers' diarrhea is a significant problem that may be mitigated by attention to the foods and beverages ingested. Chemoprophylaxis is not recommended for general use, but provision of an antibiotic for the treatment of travelers' diarrhea is a useful precaution (see *Escherichia coli* Diarrhea, p 204). Giardiasis and, less commonly, amebiasis and cryptosporidiosis are transmitted in some areas by contaminated water supplies.

---

* Diethyltoluamide.

Recommendations for Care of Children in Special Circumstances

•••••••••••••••••••••••••••••••

HUMAN MILK

Breastfeeding provides numerous health benefits to young infants, including protection against morbidity and mortality from infectious diseases of bacterial, viral, and parasitic origin. While providing an ideal source of infant nutrition, largely uncontaminated by environmental pathogens, human milk contains protective factors, including cells, specific secretory antibodies, and nonimmune factors such as glycoconjugates, for infants. Breastfed infants have stools with high concentrations of protective bifidobacteria and lactobacillus, which increase resistance to pathogenic organisms. Increasing evidence indicates that human milk may modulate development of the infant's immune system. Protection by human milk is established most clearly for pathogens causing gastrointestinal tract infection. In addition, human milk appears to provide protection against otitis media, *Haemophilus influenzae* type b, respiratory syncytial virus, and other causes of lower respiratory tract infections.

The American Academy of Pediatrics (AAP) Committee on Nutrition issues statements and publishes a manual on infant feeding that provides further information about the benefits of breastfeeding and recommended feeding practices.* In the *Pediatric Nutrition Handbook*, questions about immunization of lactating mothers and nursing infants, transmission of infectious agents via human milk, and potential effects on nursing infants of antimicrobial agents administered to lactating mothers also are addressed.

Immunization of Mothers and Infants

EFFECT OF MATERNAL IMMUNIZATION

Women who have not received the recommended immunizations before or during pregnancy may be immunized postpartum regardless of lactation status. No evidence exists for concern about the potential presence in maternal milk of live virus from vaccines if the mother is immunized during lactation. Lactating women may be immunized, as recommended for other adults, to protect against measles, mumps, rubella, tetanus, diphtheria, influenza, and hepatitis B. If previously unvaccinated or if traveling to a highly endemic area, a lactating mother may be given inactivated poliovirus vaccine (IPV). Although rubella vaccine virus has been detected in milk after maternal immunization, no evidence indicates that administration of rubella vaccine to the postpartum mother has any potential for harm to the term or preterm infant. Rubella seronegative mothers who could not be immunized during pregnancy

---

* American Academy of Pediatrics, Committee on Nutrition. *Pediatric Nutrition Handbook*. 3rd ed. Elk Grove Village, Ill: American Academy of Pediatrics; 1993.

should be immunized postpartum. Whether varicella vaccine is secreted in human milk, and if so whether it would infect the infant, is not known. Therefore, varicella vaccine may be considered for a susceptible nursing mother if the risk of exposure to varicella-zoster virus is high.

EFFICACY OF IMMUNIZATION IN BREASTFED INFANTS

The immunogenicity of some currently recommended vaccines is enhanced by breastfeeding, but the importance of these observations in their efficacy is unknown. Although high concentrations of anti-poliovirus antibody in milk of some mothers theoretically could interfere with the immunogenicity of oral polio vaccine (OPV), no such association has been demonstrated. Infants should be immunized according to the recommended schedule regardless of the infant's mode of feeding.

Transmission of Infectious Agents Via Human Milk

BACTERIA

Mastitis and breast abscesses have been associated with the presence of bacterial pathogens in human milk. In general, infectious mastitis resolves with continued lactation during antibiotic therapy, and does not pose a significant risk for the healthy term infant. Breast abscesses occur rarely and have the potential to rupture into the ductal system, releasing large numbers of organisms, such as *Staphylococcus aureus*, into milk. In general, feeding an infant using a breast affected by an abscess is not recommended. However, some experts recommend that infant feeding using the affected breast may resume once the mother is treated adequately with an appropriate antimicrobial and the abscess is drained surgically. Even when nursing is interrupted on the affected breast, nursing may continue on the opposite (unaffected) breast.

Women with tuberculosis who have been treated appropriately for 2 or more weeks and who are otherwise considered to be noncontagious may breastfeed. Women with active tuberculosis suspected of being contagious should refrain from breastfeeding or any other close contact with the infant, due to potential transmission through respiratory droplets (see Tuberculosis, p 541). *Mycobacterium tuberculosis* rarely causes mastitis or a breast abscess, but if a breast abscess caused by *M tuberculosis* is present, breastfeeding should be discontinued until the mother is no longer contagious.

Expressed human milk can become contaminated with a variety of bacterial pathogens including *Staphylococcus* species and Gram-negative enteric bacilli. Outbreaks of Gram-negative bacterial infections in neonatal intensive care units occasionally have been attributed to contaminated human milk specimens that have been collected or stored improperly. Human milk fed to infants from women other than the biologic mother should be treated according to the guidelines of the Human Milk Banking Association of North America. However, routine culturing or heat treatment of mother's milk fed to her infant has not been demonstrated to be necessary or cost-effective (see Human Milk Banks, p 76).

VIRUSES

Cytomegalovirus (CMV). Cytomegalovirus may be shed intermittently in human milk. Although transmission of CMV through human milk has occurred, disease in the neonate usually does not result, presumably because of passively transferred maternal antibody. Preterm infants, however, are at greater potential risk of symptomatic disease and sequelae than term infants. Infants born to CMV-seronegative women who seroconvert during lactation and premature infants with low concentrations of transplacentally acquired maternal antibodies to CMV can develop symptomatic disease with sequelae from acquiring CMV through breastfeeding. Decisions regarding breastfeeding of premature infants by mothers known to be CMV-seropositive should consider both the potential benefits of human milk and the risk of CMV transmission. Pasteurization of milk appears to inactivate CMV; freezing milk at −20°C (−4°F) will decrease viral titers but does not reliably eliminate CMV.

Hepatitis B. Hepatitis B surface antigen (HBsAg) has been detected in milk from HBsAg-positive women. However, studies from Taiwan and England have indicated that breastfeeding by HBsAg-positive women does not increase significantly the risk of infection among their infants. In the United States, infants born to known HBsAg-positive women should receive both Hepatitis B Immune Globulin (HBIG) and hepatitis B vaccine, effectively eliminating any theoretical risk of transmission through breastfeeding. Immunoprophylaxis of infants with hepatitis B vaccine alone also provides protection (see Hepatitis B, p 247).

Hepatitis C. Hepatitis C virus (HCV) RNA and antibody to HCV have been detected in milk of mothers infected with HCV. Although published data are limited, HCV transmission via breastfeeding has not been documented in anti-HCV positive, anti-HIV negative mothers. HCV-infected mothers should be counseled that transmission of HCV by breastfeeding theoretically is possible, but has not been documented. According to current guidelines of the US Public Health Service, maternal HCV infection is not a contraindication to breastfeeding. The decision to do so should be based on informed discussion between the mother and the health care provider.

HIV. Human immunodeficiency virus has been isolated from human milk and can be transmitted through breastfeeding. The risk of transmission may be higher for women who acquire HIV infection during lactation (ie, postpartum) than in those with pre-existing infection. In populations such as in the United States where risk of mortality from infectious diseases and malnutrition is low, and where safe and effective alternate sources of feeding are readily available, HIV-infected women should be counseled not to breastfeed their infants or donate milk. All pregnant women in the United States should be counseled and encouraged to be tested for HIV infection. In areas where infectious diseases and malnutrition are important causes of mortality early in life, the World Health Organization recommends that mothers should be advised to breastfeed their infants regardless of the mother's HIV status (see HIV Infection, p 279).

Human T-Cell Leukemia Virus Type 1 (HTLV-1). This retrovirus, which is endemic in Japan, the Caribbean, and parts of South America, is associated with development of malignancies and neurologic disorders among adults. Epidemiologic and laboratory studies suggest that mother-to-infant transmission of HTLV-1 occurs primarily through breastfeeding. Women in the United States who are HTLV-1 seropositive should be advised not to breastfeed.

Human T-Lymphotrophic Virus Type II (HTLV-II). This retrovirus has been detected among American and European injection drug users and some indigenous Native American groups. Although apparent maternal-infant transmission has been reported, the rate and timing of transmission have not been established. Until additional data regarding possible transmission through breastfeeding become available, women in the United States who are seropositive should be advised not to breastfeed.

Herpes Simplex Virus Type 1 (HSV-1). The virus has been isolated from human milk in the absence of vesicular lesions or drainage from the breast, or concurrent positive cultures from the maternal cervix, vagina, or throat. Several cases of HSV-1 transmission after breastfeeding in the presence of maternal breast lesions have been reported. Since development of extragenital lesions appears to occur more often with primary than recurrent HSV infection, some experts have recommended that women with primary mucocutaneous disease should not breastfeed their infants until all lesions have resolved and viral shedding has ceased. However, because identification of primary HSV infection is often difficult, implementation of these recommendations is problematic. Women with herpetic lesions on their breasts should refrain from breastfeeding; active lesions elsewhere should be covered.

Rubella. Both wild and vaccine strains of rubella virus have been isolated from human milk. However, the presence of rubella in human milk has not been associated with significant disease in infants, and transmission is more likely to occur through other routes. Women with rubella or those who have just been immunized with rubella live-attenuated virus vaccine need not refrain from breastfeeding.

HUMAN MILK BANKS

Some conditions, such as premature delivery, may preclude breastfeeding. In these cases, infants may be fed milk collected from their own mothers or from unrelated individual donors. The potential for transmission of infectious agents through human milk requires appropriate selection and screening of donors, and careful collection, processing, and storage of milk. Currently, seven US donor milk banks belonging to the Human Milk Banking Association of North America voluntarily follow guidelines drafted in consultation with the Food and Drug Administration (FDA) and the Centers for Disease Control and Prevention (CDC). These guidelines include screening of all donors for antibodies to HIV-1, HIV-2, HTLV-I, HTLV-II, HBsAg, hepatitis C, and syphilis. Donor milk is dispensed only on prescription after it is heat-treated at 56°C (133°F) or greater for 30 minutes and bacterial cultures reveal no growth.

Heat treatment at 56°C or greater for 30 minutes reliably eliminates bacteria, inactivates HIV, and decreases the titers of other viruses, but heating to 56°C (133°F) in one small study did not completely eliminate CMV. Holder pasteurization (62.5°C [144.5°F] for 30 minutes) reliably inactivates HIV and CMV, and will eliminate or significantly decrease titers of most other viruses.

Freezing at −20°C (−4°F) will eliminate HTLV-1 and will decrease the concentration of CMV, but will not destroy most other viruses or bacteria. Although few data are available regarding appropriate microbiologic quality standards for fresh, unpasteurized, expressed milk, the Human Milk Banking Association of North America recommends use of only specimens with less than 10^4 CFU/mL of non-pathogenic bacteria. The presence of Gram-negative bacteria, *S aureus,* or α- or β-hemolytic streptococci precludes use of milk specimens.

Antimicrobial Agents in Maternal Milk

Antimicrobial agents taken by a lactating mother often can appear in her milk. A general guideline is that an antimicrobial agent is safe to administer to a lactating woman if it is safe to administer to an infant. The AAP Committee on Drugs has reviewed the risks to infants of specific antimicrobial agents taken by lactating mothers.* Recommendations are included in Tables 2.1 (p 78) and 2.2 (p 79). Although important exceptions exist, the majority of antimicrobial agents that might be taken by lactating mothers are compatible with breastfeeding. If metronidazole or chloramphenicol is administered, breastfeeding is precluded during the course of therapy. When treatment with metronidazole is indicated for the lactating mother, the infant's exposure can be minimized by alteration of the dosing schedule and temporary interruption of breastfeeding. For example, for treatment of *Trichomonas vaginalis* infection, a single 2-g dose of metronidazole may be taken by the lactating mother; following which she should pump and discard her milk for 24 hours, then resume nursing. The alternative is a 10-day course with a cessation in breastfeeding during that time. Women receiving chloramphenicol should not breastfeed because of the theoretical risk of idiosyncratic as well as dose-related bone marrow suppression in the nursing infant.

The AAP Committee on Drugs considers maternal use of isoniazid to be compatible with breastfeeding. While potential hepatotoxicity in nursing infants is a concern, no adverse effects have been demonstrated. The infant should receive pyridoxine (see Tuberculosis, p 557). Although not evaluated by the Committee on Drugs, maternal use of the fluoroquinolones, such as ciprofloxacin, norfloxacin, and ofloxacin, is not recommended during breastfeeding by many experts because these compounds are excreted in human milk in high concentrations and, based on experimental data in immature animals, might affect cartilage development of weight-bearing joints of infants. In addition, a case has been reported of pseudomembranous colitis in a 2-month-old breastfed infant associated with ciprofloxacin self-administered by the mother. In one study, norfloxacin was found not to be excreted in detectable concentrations in human milk. Therefore, some experts consider the use of norfloxacin to be compatible with breastfeeding.

Maternal use of tetracycline usually is compatible with breastfeeding, since absorption of the drugs by the nursing infant is negligible. However, some experts recommend that use of tetracycline by a lactating mother should be avoided, if possible, because of the potential for dental staining in the infant's unerupted teeth.

The amount of drug an infant receives from a lactating mother depends on a number of factors, including maternal dose, frequency and duration of administration, absorption, and distribution characteristics of the drug. When a lactating woman receives appropriate doses of an antimicrobial agent, the concentration of

---

* American Academy of Pediatrics, Committee on Drugs. The transfer of drugs and other chemicals into human milk. *Pediatrics.* 1994;93:137-150.

Table 2.1. Antimicrobial Agents Taken by Mothers That Are Not Compatible With Breastfeeding or Are Cause for Concern

Maternal Antimicrobial Agent	Reported Sign or Symptom in Infant or Possible Cause for Concern	Committee on Drugs Evaluation
Chloramphenicol	Possible idiosyncratic bone marrow suppression.	Unknown effect on nursing infant but may be of concern.
Metronidazole	In vitro mutagen; may discontinue breastfeeding 12–24 h to allow excretion of dose when single-dose therapy is given to mother.	Unknown effect on nursing infant but may be of concern.
Ciprofloxacin	Theoretically may affect cartilage development of weight-bearing joints; case report of pseudo-membranous colitis in a 20-mo-old nursing infant.	Not evaluated.
Norfloxacin, ofloxacin, lomefloxacin, cinoxacin, enoxacin	Theoretically may affect cartilage development of weight-bearing joints.	Not evaluated.
Isoniazid	None; acetyl metabolite also secreted; may be hepatotoxic.	Usually compatible with breastfeeding.
Nalidixic acid	Hemolysis in infant with G6PD* deficiency.	Usually compatible with breastfeeding.
Nitrofurantoin	Hemolysis in infant with G6PD* deficiency.	Usually compatible with breastfeeding.
Sulfapyridine	Caution in infant with jaundice or G6PD* deficiency, and in ill, stressed, or premature infant.	Usually compatible with breastfeeding.
Sulfisoxazole	Caution in infant with jaundice or G6PD* deficiency, and in ill, stressed, or premature infant.	Usually compatible with breastfeeding.

* Glucose-6-phosphate dehydrogenase.

the compound in her milk usually is less than the equivalent of a therapeutic dose for the infant. A breastfed infant who requires antimicrobial therapy should receive recommended doses directly, even if the same agent is administered to the mother. In theory, an infant could develop bacterial resistance to an antimicrobial agent by receiving subtherapeutic doses in maternal milk, but in practice no known cases of therapeutic failure caused by lactational exposure have occurred.

The characteristics of the recipient infant should be considered when assessing the potential effect of specific antimicrobial agents taken by the mother. The maturity of the infant at birth, the chronologic postpartum age, the infant's clinical prob-

Table 2.2. Antimicrobial Agents Listed by the American Academy of Pediatrics (AAP) Committee on Drugs as Usually Compatible With Breastfeeding*

Acyclovir	Dapsone[†‡]
Amoxicillin	Erythromycin[§]
Aztreonam	Kanamycin
Cefadroxil	Moxalactam
Cefazolin	Pyrimethamine
Cefotaxime	Quinine
Cefoxitin	Rifampin
Cefprozil	Streptomycin
Ceftazidime	Sulbactam
Ceftriaxone	Tetracycline[‡‖]
Chloroquine	Ticarcillin
Clindamycin	Trimethoprim-sulfamethoxazole[‡]

* American Academy of Pediatrics, Committee on Drugs. The transfer of drugs and other chemicals into human milk. *Pediatrics.* 1994;93:137-150.
† Sulfonamide detected in infant's urine.
‡ While not listed as such by the Committee on Drugs, some experts recommend that the drug should be avoided in lactating women.
§ Concentrated in human milk.
‖ Negligible absorption by infant.

lems, and the pattern of breastfeeding will alter the possible risk. If an infant has a glucose-6-phosphate dehydrogenase deficiency, maternal use of nalidixic acid, nitrofurantoin, or sulfonamides should be avoided (see Table 2.1). With premature, stressed, or ill infants, maternal use of sulfonamide compounds should be avoided. In addition, pharmacokinetic properties of the antimicrobial agent may be helpful in deciding about the safety of a new agent whose appearance in milk is not known. If the drug is not orally bioavailable (ie, it must be given parenterally), it will not be absorbed from milk by the infant.

Another consideration is the potential for interaction of the drug the mother is receiving and that which an infant is receiving. Hence, physicians caring for infants who are breastfeeding should be aware of the medications the mother is taking and their potential for adverse interaction with drugs that might be prescribed for the infant.

In making the decision about use of appropriate antimicrobial agents for a lactating woman, the physician should weigh the benefits of breastfeeding against the potential risk to the nursing infant of exposure to a drug. In most cases, the benefits exceed the risks. The circumstance would be rare in which the only effective medication for treatment of maternal infection would be contraindicated because of risks to the infant.

CHILDREN IN OUT-OF-HOME CHILD CARE*

Infants and young children who are cared for in groups have an increased rate of certain infectious diseases, greater severity of illness, and an increased risk for acquiring resistant organisms. Prevention and control of infection in out-of-home child care (day care) settings is influenced by (1) the caregivers' practice of personal hygiene and immunization status, (2) environmental sanitation, (3) food handling procedures, (4) the ages and immunization status of the children, (5) the ratio of children to caregivers, (6) the physical space and quality of the facilities, and (7) frequency of antimicrobial therapy in children in child care. Adequately addressing problems of infection control in child care settings requires collaborative efforts of public health officials, licensing agencies, child care providers, physicians, nurses, parents, employers, and the community.

Child care programs should require that all children and staff receive age-appropriate immunizations and routine health care. In addition, these programs have the opportunity to provide young, inexperienced parents with day-to-day instruction in child development, hygiene, appropriate nutrition, and management of minor illnesses.

Classification of Care Service

Child care services commonly are classified by the type of setting, the number of children in care, ages of the children, and their health status. **Small-family child care** is defined as out-of-home care provided in a private residence where a provider cares for fewer than six unrelated children. **Large-family child care** is defined as out-of-home care provided in a private residence for seven to 12 children. **Center child care** is provided in a nonresidential facility and usually serves 13 or more children in a part-day or full-day program. **Sick-child care** describes specialized programs designed to provide care for mildly ill children who are excluded from regular child care programs. All 50 states license out-of-home child care; however, licensing is directed toward center-based child care; few states or municipalities license small- or large-family or sick-child care programs.

Grouping of children by age varies in different programs but in child care centers often consists of **infants** (birth to 12 months), **toddlers** (13 to 35 months), **preschoolers** (36 to 59 months), and **school-age** children (5 to 12 years).

Infants and toddlers require diapering or assistance in using a toilet, explore the environment with their mouths, are careless about their secretions, have immature immune systems, and require hands-on contact with care providers. In addition, toddlers have frequent direct contact with other toddlers. Therefore, child care programs that provide infant and toddler care need to give special attention to infection control measures.

---

* This chapter is modified from the recommendations originally formulated by a joint committee of the American Academy of Pediatrics and the American Public Health Association (*Caring for Our Children. National Health and Safety Performance Standards: Guidelines for Out-of-Home Child Care Programs*. Washington, DC: American Public Health Association; 1992.

Management and Prevention of Illness

The modes of transmission of bacteria, viruses, parasites, and fungi within child care settings are listed in Table 2.3. In most instances, the risk of introducing an infectious agent into a child care group is related directly to its prevalence in the population and to the number of susceptible children in that group. Transmission of the agent within the group depends on (1) characteristics such as mode of spread, infective dose, and survival in the environment; (2) frequency of asymptomatic infection or carrier state; and (3) immunity to the respective pathogen. Transmission also can be affected by characteristics of the child care providers, particularly hygienic aspects of child handling, and by environmental practices and ages and immunization status of the children enrolled. Appropriate and thorough hand washing is the most important factor for reducing transmission of disease in child care settings. Children infected in a child care group subsequently can transmit infection not only within the group, but also within their households and the community.

The major options for management of ill or infected children in child care and for controlling spread of infection include (1) antimicrobial treatment, prophylaxis, or immunization when appropriate, (2) exclusion of ill or infected children from the facility, (3) provision of alternative care at a separate site, (4) cohorting to provide care (ie, inclusion of infected children in a group with separate staff and facilities), and (5) closing the facility (a rarely exercised option). Specific recommendations for controlling the spread of specific infectious agents differ according to the epidemiology of the pathogen (see disease-specific chapters in Section 3).

Table 2.3. Modes of Transmission of Microorganisms in Child Care Settings

Mode of Transmission	Bacteria	Viruses	Parasites and Fungi
Fecal-oral	*Campylobacter, Clostridium difficile, Escherichia coli 0157:H7, Salmonella, Shigella*	Astrovirus, calicivirus, enteric adenovirus, enteroviruses, hepatitis A, rotaviruses	*Cryptosporidium, Enterobius vermicularis, Giardia lamblia*
Respiratory	*Bordetella pertussis, Haemophilus influenzae* type b, *Mycobacterium tuberculosis, Neisseria meningitidis, Streptococcus pneumoniae,* group A streptococcus	Adenovirus, influenza, measles, parainfluenza, parvovirus B19, respiratory syncytial virus, rhinovirus, rubella, varicella-zoster	...
Person-to-person via skin contact	Group A streptococcus, *Staphylococcus aureus*	Herpes simplex, varicella-zoster	Pediculosis, scabies, tinea capitis, tinea corporis
Contact with blood, urine, and/or saliva	...	Cytomegalovirus, hepatitis B, herpes simplex	...

Certain general and disease-specific infection control procedures in child care programs reduce the acquisition and transmission of communicable diseases within and outside the programs. Among these procedures are the following: (1) acquisition and review of child and employee illness records and current immunization records for children and staff; (2) hygienic and sanitary procedures for toilet use and toilet training; (3) hand washing procedures (the single most important measure for preventing infection) and enforcement of these procedures; (4) environmental sanitation; (5) personal hygiene for children and staff; (6) sanitary handling of food; (7) communicable disease surveillance and reporting; and (8) management of pets. Specific staff policies that include training procedures for full- and part-time employees and staff illness exclusion policies also aid in the control of infectious diseases. Health departments should have plans for responding to reportable and nonreportable communicable diseases in child care programs and should provide training, written information, and technical consultation to child care programs when requested. Evaluation of the health status of each child should be performed by a qualified staff member each day, on entry of the child at the site and during the day. Parents should be encouraged to share information with child care staff about their child's acute and chronic illnesses, medication use, and current immunization status.

Recommendations for Inclusion or Exclusion

Mild illness is common among children, and most children will not need to be excluded from their usual source of care for mild respiratory tract illnesses, because transmission is likely to have occurred before symptoms developed in the child or is a result of contact with children with asymptomatic infection. The risk of illness can be reduced by following common-sense hygienic practices.

Exclusion of sick children (and adults) from out-of-home child care settings has been recommended when such exclusion could reduce the likelihood of secondary cases. In many situations, the expertise of the program's medical consultant and the responsible local and state public health authorities is helpful in determining the benefits and risks of excluding children from their usual care program. Most states have laws regarding isolation of persons with communicable diseases. Local or state health departments should be contacted regarding these laws, and authorities in these areas should be notified about cases of reportable communicable diseases and unusual outbreaks of other illnesses involving children or adults in the child care environment.

Children need not be excluded from the child care setting for a minor illness except for the following illnesses:
- Illness that prevents the child from participating comfortably in program activities.
- Illness that results in a greater need for care than the staff can provide without compromising the health and safety of other children.
- The child has any of the following conditions: fever, lethargy, irritability, persistent crying, difficult breathing, and/or other manifestations of possible severe illness.
- Diarrhea or stools that contain blood or mucus.
- E coli 0157:H7, until diarrhea resolves and two stool cultures are negative.
- Vomiting two or more times in the previous 24 hours, unless the vomiting is determined to be caused by a noncommunicable condition and the child is not in danger of dehydration.

- Mouth sores associated with drooling, unless the child's physician or local health department authority states that the child is noninfectious.
- Rash with fever or behavior change, until a physician has determined the illness not to be a communicable disease.
- Purulent conjunctivitis (defined as pink or red conjunctiva with white or yellow eye discharge, often with matted eyelids after sleep and eye pain or redness of the eyelids or skin surrounding the eye), until examined by a physician and approved for readmission, with treatment.
- Tuberculosis, until the child's physician or local health department authority states that the child is noninfectious.
- Impetigo, until 24 hours after treatment has been initiated.
- Streptococcal pharyngitis, until 24 hours after treatment has been initiated, and until the child has been afebrile for 24 hours.
- Head lice (pediculosis), until after the first treatment.
- Scabies, until after treatment has been completed.
- Varicella, until the sixth day after onset of rash or sooner if all lesions have dried and crusted (see Varicella-Zoster Infections, p 573).
- Pertussis, until 5 days of the appropriate antibiotic therapy (which is to be given for a total of 14 days) has been completed (see Pertussis, p 394).
- Mumps, until 9 days after onset of parotid gland swelling.
- Measles, until 6 days after onset of rash.
- Hepatitis A virus infection, until 1 week after onset of illness or jaundice (if symptoms are mild).

Most infections do not constitute a reason for excluding a child from child care. Examples that do not necessitate exclusion include nonpurulent conjunctivitis (defined as pink conjunctiva with a clear, watery eye discharge without fever, eye pain, or eyelid redness); rash without fever and without behavior change; parvovirus B19 infection in an immunocompetent host; cytomegalovirus infection; hepatitis B virus carrier (see p 259 for possible exceptions); and HIV infection (see p 300 for possible exceptions). Asymptomatic children who excrete an enteropathogen usually do not need to be excluded, except when *E coli* 0157:H7 or infection with *Shigella* has occurred in the child care program. Because these infections are transmitted easily and can be severe, exclusion is warranted until two stool cultures are negative for the organism (see *Escherichia coli* Diarrhea, p 204, and *Shigella* Infections, p 472).

During the course of an identified outbreak of any communicable illness in a child care setting, a child determined to be contributing to the transmission of the illness at the program may be excluded. The child may be readmitted when the risk of transmission is determined to be no longer present.

Infectious Diseases—Epidemiology and Control

(See also chapters on the specific diseases in Section 3.)

ENTERIC DISEASES

The close, personal contact and poor hygiene of young children provide ready opportunities for the spread of enteric bacteria, viruses, and parasites in child care groups. Although many enteropathogens can cause diarrhea among children in child care, rotaviruses, *Giardia lamblia,* enteric adenoviruses, astroviruses, *Shigella, E coli* 0157:H7, and *Cryptosporidium* have been the principal organisms implicated in outbreaks; infrequently, *Salmonella, Clostridium difficile,* and *Campylobacter jejuni* have been problems in child care.

The most important aspect of child care that is associated with increased frequency of enteric illness and hepatitis A virus (HAV) infection is the presence of young children who are not toilet trained. Fecal contamination of the environment is frequent in child care programs and is highest in infant and toddler areas where enteric disease and HAV infection occur most often. Enteropathogens can be spread fecally or orally, either directly (by person-to-person transmission) or indirectly (by toys and other objects, environmental surfaces, and food). The risk of food contamination can be increased when staff caring for diapered children also prepare or serve food. Several enteric pathogens, including rotaviruses, HAV, *Giardia* cysts, and *Cryptosporidium* oocysts survive on environmental surfaces for periods ranging from hours to weeks.

Child care programs can be a major source of HAV spread within the community. Hepatitis A differs from most other diseases in child care centers because symptomatic illness occurs primarily among adult contacts of infected, asymptomatic children. To recognize outbreaks and initiate appropriate control measures, health care personnel and staff need to be aware of this epidemiologic characteristic (see Hepatitis A, p 237). Hepatitis A vaccine should be considered for the staff of child care centers with ongoing or recurrent outbreaks and in communities where cases in the center are a major source of hepatitis A virus.

The single most important procedure to minimize fecal or oral transmission is frequent hand washing combined with staff training and monitoring of staff procedures. A child in whom acute diarrhea or jaundice develops while in child care should be moved to a separate area, away from contact with other children, until the child can be removed by a parent or guardian. Exclusion for acute diarrhea should continue until the diarrhea ceases; children with *Shigella* infection also should receive antimicrobial therapy before readmission. The child with symptomatic HAV infection should be excluded until 1 week after the onset the illness. Specialized child care facilities, which care for mildly ill children, could be provided for children with enteric illness and hepatitis A virus infection. Asymptomatic children without diarrhea who excrete enteropathogens other than *E coli* 0157:H7 or *Shigella* do not require treatment or exclusion from child care in the absence of specific public health indications. Asymptomatic excretion illustrates the need for frequent hand washing and environmental cleaning in out-of-home child care facilities.

RESPIRATORY DISEASES

Diseases spread by the respiratory route include those causing acute upper respiratory tract infections or invasive diseases caused by pathogens, such as *Haemophilus influenzae* type b, *Streptococcus pneumoniae, Neisseria meningitidis, Bordetella pertussis,* and *Mycobacterium tuberculosis.* Possible modes of spread of respiratory tract viruses include aerosols, respiratory droplets, and direct hand contact with contaminated secretions, toys, and other objects. The viral pathogens responsible for respiratory tract disease in child care settings are those that cause disease in the community, including respiratory syncytial virus, parainfluenza virus, influenza virus, adenovirus, and rhinovirus. The incidence of viral infections of the respiratory tract is increased in child care settings, and outbreaks can occur.

Hand washing may decrease the incidence of acute respiratory tract disease among children in child care. However, exclusion from child care of children with respiratory tract symptoms associated with the common cold, croup, bronchitis, pneumonia, sinusitis, and/or otitis media probably will not decrease the spread of infection. Children with such conditions should be separated from other children in the program if their illness is characterized by one or more of the following conditions: (1) it has a specified etiology, which requires exclusion, (2) it limits the child's comfortable participation in child care activities, or (3) it results in a greater need for care than can be provided by the staff without compromising the health and safety of other children.

Transmission of *H influenzae* type b is likely among unimmunized young children in group child care, especially those younger than 24 months. Transmission can originate from an asymptomatic carrier or a carrier with a respiratory tract infection. Immunization of children with an *H influenzae* conjugate vaccine, according to current recommendations, prevents the occurrence of disease and decreases the rate of carriage, thereby decreasing the risk of transmission to others. In an outbreak of invasive *H influenzae* type b disease in attendees, defined as two or more cases within 60 days, rifampin prophylaxis is indicated for all children and personnel exposed to unvaccinated or incompletely vaccinated children attending child care; after a single case of *H influenzae* type b, the need for rifampin is controversial (see *Haemophilus influenzae* Infections, p 220).

Infections caused by *N meningitidis* occur in all age groups. The highest attack rates occur in children younger than 1 year. Close contact for an extended time of children and staff exposed to an index case of meningococcal disease predisposes to secondary transmission, and outbreaks have occurred in child care settings. Thus, chemoprophylaxis is indicated for child care contacts among children in child care settings is increased (see Meningococcal Infections, p 357).

The risk of primary invasive disease among children in child care settings is increased and secondary spread of *S pneumoniae* in child care centers has been reported, but the degree of risk of secondary spread in child care facilities is unknown. Prophylaxis of contacts after the occurrence of a single case of invasive *S pneumoniae* disease is not recommended at this time.

Group A streptococcal infection among children in child care generally has not been a common problem. A child with proven group A streptococcal infection should be excluded from classroom contact until 24 hours after initiation of antibiotic therapy. While outbreaks of streptococcal pharyngitis in these settings have occurred, the risk of secondary transmission following a single case of severe invasive group A streptococcal infection remains very low. Therefore, no recommendation for prophylaxis of contacts following a single case of severe invasive group A streptococcal infection can be made at this time.

Infants and young children with tuberculosis are not as infectious as adults with *M tuberculosis* disease, because children are less likely to have cavitary pulmonary lesions and are unable to forcefully expel large numbers of organisms into the air. If approved by health officials, children may attend a child care group after chemotherapy is begun and when they are considered noninfectious to others. Infants and young children who have both HIV and *M tuberculosis* infection may need to be excluded from group child care. Because an adult with tuberculosis poses a hazard to children in a child care group, tuberculin screening with a Mantoux skin test of all adults who have contact with children in a child care setting is recommended before the contact is initiated. The need for periodic, subsequent tuberculin testing of persons without clinically important reactions should be based on their risk of acquiring new infection and local or state health department recommendations. If found to have active tuberculosis, care providers should not be allowed to care for children until chemotherapy has rendered them noninfectious to others (see Tuberculosis, p 541).

Parvovirus B19. The spectrum of illness produced by parvovirus B19 includes asymptomatic infection in 20% of infected persons; erythema infectiosum, which is the most common manifestation of illness and usually occurs in children; arthritis in adults; chronic anemia in immunocompromised hosts; aplastic crisis; and fetal hydrops. Isolation or exclusion of immunocompetent persons with parvovirus B19 infection in child care settings is unwarranted because little or no virus is present in respiratory tract secretions at the time of occurrence of the rash of erythema infectiosum. In addition, because less than 1% of pregnant teachers during erythema infectiosum outbreaks would be expected to experience an adverse fetal outcome, exclusion of pregnant women from employment in child care or teaching is not recommended (for more information, see Parvovirus B19, p 383).

VARICELLA-ZOSTER VIRUS

Children with varicella who have been excluded from child care may return on the sixth day after onset of rash or sooner if all lesions have dried and crusted. All staff members and parents should be notified when a case of varicella occurs; they should be informed about the greater likelihood of serious infection in susceptible adults and adolescents and of the potential for fetal damage if infection occurs during pregnancy. Approximately 5% to 10% of adults will be susceptible to varicella-zoster virus and should be offered varicella vaccine, unless medically contraindicated. Susceptible child care staff who are pregnant and exposed to children with varicella should be referred to qualified physicians or other professionals for counseling and management within 24 hours of the exposure.

Exclusion of staff members or children with herpes zoster (shingles) whose lesions cannot be covered should be based on similar criteria to those for varicella. Lesions that can be covered pose little risk to susceptible persons because transmission usually occurs from direct contact with fluid from the lesion. Lesions should be covered by clothing or a dressing until they have crusted. Thorough hand washing is warranted whenever contact with fluid from the lesion has occurred.

HERPES SIMPLEX VIRUS (HSV) AND CYTOMEGALOVIRUS (CMV) INFECTION

Children with HSV gingivostomatitis, who do not have control of oral secretions (drooling), should be excluded from child care when active lesions are present. Although HSV can be transmitted from the mother to the fetus or newborn, maternal HSV infections that are a threat to offspring usually are acquired by the infant during birth from genital infections of the mother; therefore, maternal exposure to HSV in a child care setting carries little risk for the fetus. Care providers should be instructed on the importance of hand washing and other measures for limiting transfer of infected material from children with varicella-zoster virus or HSV infection (eg, saliva, tissue fluid, or fluid from a skin lesion).

Spread of CMV from asymptomatic infected children in child care to their mothers or to child care providers is the most important consequence of child care–related CMV infection (see also Cytomegalovirus Infection, p 187). Children enrolled in child care programs are more likely to acquire CMV than those cared for primarily at home. The highest rates (eg, 70%) of viral excretion occur in children between 1 and 3 years of age, and excretion often continues for years. Studies of CMV seroconversion among child care providers have found annualized seroconversion rates of 8% to 20%. Exposure to CMV with the increased rate of acquisition that occurs in child care staff most likely leads to an increased rate of gestational CMV infection in seronegative staff and an increased risk of congenital CMV infection in their offspring. Women who are seropositive before pregnancy are not at risk from exposure to children but seropositive women whose CMV infection reactivates have a small (approximately 1 in 500) risk of having an infant with congenital CMV infection; only about 5% of these infected infants have sequelae, which are mild and consist mostly of moderate hearing loss.

Transmission of CMV appears to require direct contact with virus-containing secretions. Therefore, careful attention to hygiene, specifically hand washing, is critical. Avoiding contact with secretions is recommended to prevent infection in child care providers. However, the effectiveness of these measures in an environment where CMV is ubiquitous has not been determined. Because CMV excretion is so prevalent, attempts at isolation or segregation of children who excrete CMV are impractical and inappropriate. Similarly, testing of children to detect CMV excretion is inappropriate because excretion is often intermittent, and results of testing can be misleading.

In view of the risk of CMV infection in child care staff and the potential consequences of gestational CMV infection, child care staff should be counseled about the risks. This counseling may include testing for serum antibody to CMV to determine the child care provider's immunity against CMV, but routine serologic testing currently is not recommended.

BLOOD-BORNE VIRUS INFECTIONS — HEPATITIS B VIRUS AND HIV

Hepatitis B Virus (HBV). Possible transmission of HBV in the child care setting is a concern to public health authorities. Because of a low risk for transmission, children known to be HBV carriers (hepatitis B surface antigen [HBsAg] positive) may attend child care in most circumstances.

Transmission of HBV in a child care setting is most likely to occur through direct exposure to blood after an injury or from bites or scratches that break the skin and introduce blood or body secretions from an HBV carrier into another person. Indirect transmission through environmental contamination with blood or saliva is possible but has not been documented in the child care setting in the United States. Because saliva contains much less virus than does blood, the potential infectivity of saliva is low. Infectivity of saliva has been demonstrated only when inoculated through the skin of gibbons and chimpanzees.

On the basis of limited data, the risk of disease transmission from a child or staff member who is an HBV carrier but who behaves normally and is without injury, generalized dermatitis, or bleeding problems is minimal. This slight risk usually does not justify exclusion of a child who is an HBV carrier from child care or the necessity of hepatitis B vaccination of the child's contacts at the care program, most of whom already should be already protected by prior HBV immunization as part of their routine immunization schedule.

Routine screening of children for HBV carriage state before admission to child care is not justified. The admission of a child previously identified to be an HBV carrier with one or more risk factors for transmission of blood-borne pathogens (eg, biting, frequent scratching, generalized dermatitis, or bleeding problems) should be assessed by the child's physician, child care provider, or program director. The responsible public health authority should be consulted as appropriate. Regular assessment of behavioral risk factors and medical conditions of enrolled HBV carriers is necessary, and requires that the child care director and primary care providers are informed about enrollment of a known HBV carrier.

Children who bite pose an additional concern. Existing data in humans suggest a small risk of HBV transmission from the bite of an HBV carrier. Several episodes and one outbreak have been reported in which the most likely route of HBV transmission was through bites by HBV carriers. For victims of bites by HBV carriers, prophylaxis with Hepatitis B Immune Globulin (HBIG) and hepatitis B immunization is recommended in susceptible persons (see Hepatitis B, p 247).

The risk of HBV acquisition when a susceptible child bites an HBV carrier is not known. A theoretical risk exists if HBsAg-positive blood enters the oral cavity of the biter, but transmission by this route has not been reported. Although data on risks of transmission are limited, most experts would not give HBIG to the susceptible biting child who does not have oral mucosal disease when the amount of blood transferred is small.

In the common circumstance in which the HBsAg status of both the biting child and the victim is unknown, the risk of HBV transmission is extremely low because of the expected low seroprevalence of HBsAg in most groups of preschool-age children, the low efficiency of disease transmission from bites, and routine hepatitis B immunization of preschool children. Because all preschool children attending child care settings should be immunized, concern about bites and HBV transmission associated with breaks in the skin should be lessening. Serologic testing generally is not warranted for the biting child or the recipient of the bite, but each situation should be evaluated individually. Bites and other possible percutaneous exposures should serve to remind all parents of the need for routine HBV immunization.

Efforts to reduce the risk of disease transmission in child care through hygienic and environmental standards in general, and particularly when a known HBV carrier is enrolled, should focus primarily on precautions in blood exposures and limiting potential saliva contamination in the environment. Toothbrushes should not be shared among children. Accidents that lead to bleeding or contamination with blood-containing body fluids by any child should be handled as follows: (1) disposable gloves should be used when cleaning or removing all blood or blood-containing body fluid spills; (2) the area should be disinfected with a freshly prepared solution of 1:64 household bleach (¼ cup diluted in 1 gallon of water) applied for 2 minutes, rinsed, and dried; (3) persons involved in cleaning contaminated surfaces should avoid exposure of open skin lesions or mucous membranes to blood or blood-containing body fluids and to wound or tissue exudates; (4) hands should be washed thoroughly after exposure to blood or blood-containing body fluids; (5) optimally, disposable towels or tissues should be used and properly discarded, and mops should be rinsed in the disinfectant; and (6) blood-contaminated material and diapers should be placed in a plastic bag with a secure tie for disposal.

HIV Infection (see also HIV Infection, p 279). The risk of transmission of HIV infection to children in the child care setting appears to be negligible. No need exists to restrict the placement of HIV-infected children without risk factors for transmission of blood-borne pathogens in child care facilities to protect other children or personnel in these settings. Because HIV-infected children whose status is unknown may attend child care, routine procedures should be adopted for handling spills of blood and blood-containing body fluids and wound exudates of all children, as previously described.

The decision to admit HIV-infected children to child care is best made on an individual basis by qualified persons, including the child's physician, who are able to evaluate whether the child will receive optimal care in the program and whether an HIV-infected child poses a significant risk to others. Specifically, admission of each HIV-infected child with one or more potential risk factors for transmission of blood-borne pathogens (eg, biting, frequent scratching, generalized dermatitis, or bleeding problems) should be assessed by the child's physician and the program director. A responsible public health authority should be consulted as appropriate. Information about a child who has immunodeficiency, irrespective of cause, should be available to the caretakers who need to know how to help protect the child against other infections. For example, immunodeficient children exposed to measles or varicella should immediately receive postexposure immunoprophylaxis (see Measles, p 344, and Varicella-Zoster Infections, p 573).

Available data provide no reason to believe that HIV-infected adults will transmit HIV to children in the course of their normal duties. Therefore, HIV-infected adults who do not have open and uncoverable skin lesions, other conditions that would allow contact with their body fluids, or a transmissible infectious disease, may care for children in child care programs. However, immunosuppressed adults with HIV infection may be at increased risk to acquire infectious agents from children and should consult with their physicians about the safety of their continuing child care work.

IMMUNIZATIONS

Routine immunization at the appropriate age is important for children in child care because preschool-aged children can have high age-specific incidence rates of measles, rubella, *H influenzae* type b disease, and pertussis. Outbreaks of mumps in child care settings have not been reported but any cluster of susceptible persons can sustain transmission.

Written documentation of immunizations appropriate for age should be provided by parents or guardians of all children enrolling in child care. Unless contraindications exist, immunization records should demonstrate the following:

- One dose of DTaP (or DTP) vaccine by 3 months, two doses by 5 months, three doses by 7 months, and four doses by 19 months of age
- One dose of poliomyelitis vaccine (either OPV or IPV) by 3 months, two doses by 5 months, and three doses by 19 months of age
- One dose of MMR vaccine by 16 months of age
- One or more doses of *Haemophilus influenzae* type b conjugate vaccine by 16 months of age; for younger children, see the age-appropriate recommendations (see *Haemophilus influenzae* Infections, p 220)
- Two doses of hepatitis B vaccine by 7 months and three doses by 19 months of age
- One dose of varicella vaccine by 19 months of age

Children who have not received recommended age-appropriate immunizations before enrollment should have their immunization series initiated as soon as possible—no later than within 1 month of enrollment—and completed according to Fig 1.1 (p 18) and Table 1.3 (p 20). In the interim, unimmunized or inadequately immunized children should be allowed to attend child care unless a vaccine-preventable disease to which they are susceptible occurs in the child care program. In such a situation, all underimmunized children should be excluded for the duration of possible exposure or until they have completed their immunizations.

Child care providers should have received all immunizations routinely recommended for adults. All staff should have completed a primary series for tetanus and diphtheria, and should receive a booster every 10 years, and they should have been immunized against measles, mumps, rubella, varicella and poliomyelitis according to guidelines for adult immunization of the Advisory Committee on Immunization Practices of the Centers for Disease Control and Prevention and the American College of Physicians. Consideration should be given to annual immunization of child care providers against influenza. Hepatitis B vaccination also should be considered, especially for providers who may manage blood spills.

Because hepatitis A virus (HAV) can cause symptomatic illness in adult contacts and child care programs have been a source of infection in the community, HAV vaccine in some current circumstances may be justified (see Hepatitis A, p 237). However, since the prevalence of HAV infection does not appear to be significantly increased in staff members of child care centers in comparison to that in the general population, routine immunization of staff members is not recommended. During HAV outbreaks, vaccination should be considered (see p 84).

Child care providers should be asked about a history of varicella disease. These child care providers with a negative or uncertain history of varicella either should be vaccinated or serologically tested for susceptibility; those who are nonimmune should be offered varicella vaccine, unless it is medically contraindicated.

Because the incidence of rubella has been high in preschoolers, children and staff members in child care programs are probably at higher risk of exposure than is the general population. Of particular concern are susceptible women of childbearing age (staff members and mothers of young children) who might deliver an infant with congenital rubella if they are infected during pregnancy. Child care providers who have not been immunized against poliomyelitis and who will be caring for infants and children who are receiving OPV may become infected and have a small risk of vaccine-associated paralytic poliomyelitis, since children excrete the virus in their stools for several weeks after OPV immunization. Transmission can be prevented by appropriate hand washing, especially after diaper changing, and by immunization of child care providers.

General Practices

The following practices are recommended to reduce the transmission of infectious agents in a child care setting without losing the developmentally desirable features of child care:

- Each child care facility should have **written policies** for managing child and employee illness in child care.
- **Toilet areas and toilet training equipment** should be maintained in sanitary condition.
- **Diaper changing surfaces** should be nonporous and sanitized between uses. Alternatively, the diaper changing surface should be covered with a paper pad, which is discarded after each use. If the surface becomes wet or soiled, it should be cleaned and sanitized.
- **Diaper changing procedures** should be posted at the changing area. Soiled disposable diapers or soiled disposable wiping cloths should be discarded in a secure, foot-activated, plastic-lined container. Diapers should be able to contain urine and stool and minimize fecal contamination of children, providers, and environmental surfaces and objects in the child care program. The diaper should have an absorbent inner lining completely contained within an outer covering made of waterproof material that prevents escape of feces and urine. The outer covering and inner lining must be changed as a unit and not reused unless both are cleaned and disinfected. The two types of diapers that meet these requirements are modern disposable paper diapers with absorbent gelling material or carboxymethyl cellulose, and single-unit reusable systems with an inner cotton lining attached to an outer waterproof covering. Reusable cloth diapers worn with a modern front-closure waterproof cover are acceptable only if the diaper and cover are removed simultaneously and not in two separate pieces, each of which must not be reused until cleaned and disinfected. If these reusable diaper products are used in child care, the user should determine the waterproof characteristics of the covering material at frequent intervals. Reusable cloth diapers worn either without a covering or with pull-on pants made of waterproof material are not acceptable. Clothes should be worn over diapers while the child is in the child care facility. Fecal contents may be placed in a toilet but diapers should not be rinsed.
- **Diaper changing areas should never be located in food preparation areas, and should never be used for temporary placement of food.**
- The use of **child-sized toilets** or access to steps and modified toilet seats that provide for easier maintenance should be encouraged in child care programs; the use of potty chairs should be discouraged. If potty chairs are used, they should be emptied into a toilet, cleaned in a utility sink, and disinfected after each use. Staff should sanitize potty chairs, flush toilets, and diaper changing areas with a freshly prepared solution of 1:64 household bleach (¼ cup diluted in one gallon of water) applied for 2 minutes, rinsed, and dried.

- **Written procedures for hand washing,** which is the single most important measure for preventing infection, should be established and enforced. Hand washing sinks should be adjacent to each diaper changing and toilet area. These sinks should be washed and disinfected at least daily and, when soiled, should not be used for food preparation. These sinks should not be used for rinsing soiled clothing or for cleaning potty chairs. Children should have access to height-appropriate sinks, soap dispensers, and disposable paper towels.
- Written **personal hygiene policies** for staff and children are necessary.
- Written **environmental sanitation policies and procedures** should include cleaning and disinfecting floors, covering sandboxes, cleaning and sanitizing play tables, and cleaning and disinfecting spills of blood or body fluids and wound or tissue exudates. In general, routine housekeeping procedures using a freshly prepared solution of commercially available cleaner (eg, detergents, disinfectant-detergents, or chemical germicides) compatible with most surfaces are satisfactory for cleaning spills of vomitus, urine, and feces. For spills of blood or blood-containing body fluids and of wound and tissue exudates, the previously described procedures using a freshly prepared solution of 1:64 household bleach (¼ cup diluted in one gallon of water) applied for 2 minutes, rinsed, and dried should be used.
- Each item of **sleep equipment** should be used only by a single child while enrolled in the program, and it should be cleaned and sanitized before assigning to another child. Crib mattresses should be cleaned and sanitized when soiled or wet. Sleeping mats should be stored so contact with the sleeping surface of another mat does not occur. Bedding (sheets and blankets) should be assigned to each child and cleaned when soiled or wet.
- Optimally, **toys** that are placed in children's mouths or otherwise contaminated by body secretions should be cleaned with water and detergent, disinfected, and rinsed before handling by another child. All frequently touched toys in rooms that house infants and toddlers should be cleaned and disinfected daily. Toys in rooms for older children (nondiapered) should be cleaned weekly and when soiled. The use of soft, nonwashable toys in infant/toddler areas of child care programs should be discouraged.
- **Food** should be handled safely and carefully to prevent the growth of bacteria, viruses, fungi, and parasites and to prevent contamination by insects or rodents. Tables and countertops used for food preparation and food service should be cleaned and sanitized between uses and before and after eating. No one who has signs or symptoms of illness, including vomiting, diarrhea, or infectious skin lesions that cannot be covered, or who is infected with potential food-borne pathogens, should be responsible for food handling. Hands should be washed using soap and water before handling food. Because of their frequent exposure to feces and children with enteric diseases, staff who work with diapered children, whenever possible, should not prepare food for others. Caregivers who prepare food for infants should be especially aware of the importance of careful hand washing. No unpasteurized milk or milk products should be served.
- The living quarters of **pets** should be enclosed and kept clean of waste to reduce the risk of human contact with the waste. Hands should be washed after handling all animals or animal wastes. Dogs and cats should be kept away from child play

areas, handled only with staff supervision, and be in good health and immunized appropriately for age.

- Written policies, which comply with local and state regulations, for filing and regularly updating each child's **immunization record** should be maintained.
- Each child care program should use the services of a **health consultant** to assist in the development and implementation of written policies for the prevention and control of communicable diseases and the provision of related health education to children, staff, and parents.
- The child care provider should, on registering each child, **inform parents of the need to share information about illness** that could be communicable, in the child or in any member of the immediate household, to facilitate prompt reporting of disease and institution of any measures necessary to prevent transmission to others. The child care provider or program director, after consulting with the program's health consultant or the responsible public health authority, should follow the recommendations of the consultant or authority for **notification of parents** of children who attend the program about exposure of their child to a communicable disease.
- Local and/or state **public health authorities should be notified** about cases of communicable diseases involving children or care providers in the child care setting.

SCHOOL HEALTH

Clustering of children together in the school setting provides opportunities for the spread of infection. Determining the likelihood that infection in one or more children will pose a risk for schoolmates depends upon an understanding of (1) the mechanism by which the infection is spread, (2) the ease with which the infection is spread (contagion), and (3) the likelihood that classmates are immune either because of immunization or prior infection. Decisions to intervene to prevent the spread of infection within a school should be made through collaboration between school officials and health care providers, considering (1) the availability and effectiveness of specific prevention methods and (2) the risk of serious complications from infection.

Infectious agents are spread through one or more of the following four routes of transmission: fecal-oral, respiratory, contact with infected skin, and contact with blood, urine, or body secretions. In the care of preschool children in out-of-home child care (see Children in Out-of-Home Child Care, p 80) and older children with health problems or developmental disabilities, transmission via the fecal-oral route and through contact with urine are important considerations. In the school setting, respiratory and skin contact provide the most frequent means of transmission of infection. Specific circumstances, such as care of bleeding injuries or intimate contact between classmates, provide an opportunity for spread via blood and body fluids.

Generic methods for control and/or prevention of spread of infection in the school setting include the following:

- For vaccine-preventable diseases, documentation regarding immunization status of enrolled children should be reviewed. Schools have a legal responsibility to ensure that students have been immunized against poliomyelitis, pertussis, diphtheria, measles, mumps, and rubella at the time of enrollment in accordance with state requirements. Hepatitis B immunization is now mandatory in many states. Immunization against varicella, however, is not yet mandatory, although many children will have had the disease or have been vaccinated. Policies established by the state health department regarding exclusions of unimmunized children and exemptions for families with religious objection to immunization should be followed.

- Infected children can be excluded from school until they are no longer considered contagious (for recommendations on specific diseases, see relevant disease-specific chapters in Section 3).
- In many instances, administration of appropriate antimicrobial therapy will limit further spread of infection (eg, streptococcal pharyngitis and *Bordetella pertussis*).
- Antimicrobial prophylaxis given to close contacts of infected children may be warranted in some circumstances.
- Temporary school closing can be used to prevent the spread of infection or in the event of an infection expected to affect a large number of susceptible students when available control measures are considered inadequate (eg, outbreak of influenza) or is expected to have a high rate of morbidity and/or mortality.

Physicians involved with school health should be aware of current public health guidelines to prevent and control infectious diseases. In all circumstances requiring intervention to prevent spread of infection within the school setting, the privacy of children infected should be protected.

Diseases Preventable by Routine Childhood Immunization

Students who have received one dose of varicella (two doses for children immunized after 13 years of age), mumps and rubella vaccines, and two doses of measles vaccine should be considered immune to these infections. Those with a history of physician-documented infection also are considered immune.

Measles vaccine has been demonstrated to provide protection in some exposed persons if administered within 72 hours following exposure. Vaccine should be recommended immediately for all nonimmune persons during an outbreak, except for those with a contraindication to measles vaccination. Students immunized for the first time under these circumstances should be allowed to return to school immediately.

Mumps vaccine given after exposure has not been demonstrated to prevent infection among susceptible contacts, but immunization should be recommended for unimmunized students in order to protect them from infection after possible subsequent exposure.

Although rubella infection usually does not pose a major risk to preadolescent school-age children, the immunization status of contacts should be reviewed and documentation of rubella immunization should be required for previously unimmunized students. Pregnant contacts whose immunity against rubella has been confirmed by serologic testing early in pregnancy should be reassured. Physician consultation should be recommended for susceptible pregnant women who are exposed (see Rubella, p 456).

Other Infections Spread by the Respiratory Route

Some pathogens that cause severe, lower respiratory tract disease in infants and toddlers, such as respiratory syncytial virus, are of less concern in healthy school-age children. Respiratory viruses, however, are associated with exacerbation of reactive airway disease and can cause significant complications for the child with chronic respiratory disease, such as cystic fibrosis, or for the child who is immunocompromised.

Although influenza virus infection is a frequent cause of febrile respiratory disease and school absenteeism during outbreaks, routine, annual immunization of children with influenza vaccine or mandatory exclusion of children with suspected influenza infection from school is not warranted. However, children with chronic cardiac or pulmonary disease, including asthma, as well as children receiving immunosuppressive therapy, those with sickle cell disease or other hemoglobinopathies, and those with HIV infection, should receive influenza vaccine annually (see Influenza Vaccine, p 310). Influenza immunization also may be indicated for students to prevent disruption of academic or athletic activities, especially those residing in dormitories or other circumstances of particularly close contact.

Mycoplasma pneumoniae causes both upper and lower respiratory tract infection in school-age children, and outbreaks of *M pneumoniae* infection occur in communities and schools. The nonspecific symptoms and signs of this infection and the lack of a rapid diagnostic test make distinguishing *M pneumoniae* infection from other causes of respiratory illness difficult. Antibiotic therapy does not eradicate the organism or necessarily prevent spread. Thus, intervention to prevent secondary infection in the school setting is difficult.

Symptomatic contacts of students with group A streptococcal pharyngitis should be evaluated and treated if streptococcal infection is demonstrated. Infected students may return to school 24 hours after the initiation of antimicrobial therapy, if afebrile. Asymptomatic contacts usually require neither evaluation nor therapy.

Bacterial meningitis in school-age children usually is caused by *Neisseria meningitidis*. Infected persons are considered no longer contagious after 24 hours of antibiotic therapy. After hospitalization, they pose no risk to classmates and may return to school. Prophylactic antibiotic therapy is not recommended for school contacts in most circumstances. Close observation for these students is recommended, however, and they should be evaluated promptly if a febrile illness develops. Students who have been exposed to oral secretions of the infected student, such as would occur during kissing or sharing of food and drink, should receive chemoprophylaxis (see Meningococcal Infections, p 357). Immunization of school contacts with meningococcal vaccine, which contains polysaccharide antigens only for serogroups A, C, Y, and W-135, should be considered, in consultation with local public health authorities, if evidence suggests an outbreak within the school of meningococcal infection due to one of the serogroups contained in the vaccine.

Students and staff with pertussis, if their medical condition allows, should be excluded until they have received 5 days of erythromycin. In some circumstances, chemoprophylaxis is recommended for their school contacts (see Pertussis, p 397).

Children with tuberculosis disease generally are not contagious, but students who are in close contact with an infected child, teacher, or other adult should be evaluated for infection, including skin testing (see Tuberculosis, p 560). If an adult source is found outside the school (eg, parent or grandparent of a student), efforts should be made to determine if other students have been exposed to the same source and if they warrant evaluation for infection.

Children with erythema infectiosum should be allowed to attend school, since the period of contagion occurs before a rash is evident. Parvovirus B19 infection poses no risk of significant illness for healthy classmates, although infected children with sickle cell disease and other hemoglobinopathies can develop aplastic crisis. The relatively low risk of fetal damage should be explained to pregnant students and/or teachers exposed to children in the early stages of parvovirus B19 infection, 5 to 10 days before appearance of the rash. All such women should be referred to their physician for possible serologic testing.

Infections Spread by Direct Contact

Infection and infestation of skin, eyes, and hair can spread through direct contact with the infected area or through contaminated hands or fomites, such as brushes, hats, and clothing. *Staphylococcus aureus* and group A streptococcus may colonize the skin or the oropharynx of asymptomatic persons. Lesions may develop when these organisms are passed from a carrier or a person with infected skin to another child. Organisms also can be transmitted to open skin lesions in the same child or to other children. Although most skin infections due to *S aureus* and group A streptococci are minor and require only topical or oral antibiotic therapy, person-to-person spread should be interrupted by appropriate treatment whenever lesions are recognized. Exclusion of affected children prior to the initiation of therapy is not necessary. Severe and disseminated disease (eg, toxic shock syndrome) occur rarely.

Herpes simplex virus (HSV) infection of the mouth and skin is common among school-age children. It is spread usually through direct contact with virus from infected saliva. Asymptomatic shedding of virus from oral secretions is common. Infection of the fingers (herpetic whitlow) can occur following direct contact with oral or genital secretions. Cutaneous infection can occur following direct contact with infected lesions or following contact of abraded skin with a contaminated surface, as occurs among wrestlers (herpes gladiatorum) and rugby players (scrum pox). Although asymptomatic shedding of virus from the throat and oral secretions is common, spread of infection requires direct contact with these secretions, and, thus, is unlikely to occur during normal school activities. "Cold sore" lesions of herpes labialis identify persons with active and probably recurrent infection, but no evidence suggests that these students pose any greater risk to their classmates than the unidentified asymptomatic shedders. Herpes simples virus, type 1, the usual cause of oropharyngeal and cutaneous lesions, will infect virtually all persons by adulthood. Most of these infections are entirely asymptomatic and, although sometimes painful, even symptomatic infection poses virtually no risk of serious disease to the healthy school-age child. Symptomatic children should be advised to avoid direct or indirect (eg, sharing cups and bottles) oral contact with other children and to wash their hands, but excluding them from normal school activities is not justified. Exclusion of students with obvious skin or oral lesions from wrestling or rugby, and careful cleaning of wrestling mats after use with a freshly prepared solution of household bleach (¼ cup of bleach diluted in 1 gallon of water) is reasonable.

For immunocompromised children and for children with open skin lesions (eg, severe eczema), herpes simplex infection may pose significant risk. Because of the frequency of both symptomatic and asymptomatic shedding of HSV among classmates and teachers and staff, careful hygienic practices are the best means of preventing infection.

Infectious conjunctivitis can be caused by bacterial (eg, *Haemophilus influenzae* and *Streptococcus pneumoniae*) or viral (eg, adenovirus, enteroviruses, HSV) pathogens. Bacterial conjunctivitis is uncommon in children older than 5 years. Infection occurs through direct contact or through contamination of the hands followed by auto-inoculation. Respiratory spread from large droplets also may occur. Topical antibiotic therapy is indicated for bacterial conjunctivitis, which is usually distinguished by a purulent exudate. Herpes simplex virus conjunctivitis is usually unilateral and may be accompanied by vesicles on the nearby skin. Evaluation by an ophthalmologist and specific antiviral therapy are indicated. Conjunctivitis due to adenovirus or enteroviruses is self-limited and requires no specific antiviral therapy. Spread of infection is minimized by careful hand washing, and infected persons should be presumed to be contagious until symptoms have resolved. Except when viral or bacterial conjunctivitis is accompanied by systemic signs of illness, infected children should be allowed to remain in school once any indicated therapy is implemented unless their behavior is such that close contact with other students cannot be controlled.

Fungal infections of the skin and hair are spread both by direct person-to-person contact and through contact with contaminated surfaces or objects. *Trichophyton tonsurans*, the predominant cause of tinea capitis, remains viable for long periods of time on combs, brushes, furniture, and fabric. The fungi that cause tinea corporis (ringworm) are transmissible by direct contact. Tinea cruris (jock itch) and tinea pedis (athlete's foot) occur in adolescents and young adults. The fungi that cause these infections have a predilection for moist areas and are spread both through direct contact and through contact with contaminated surfaces. Students with fungal infections of the skin or scalp should be treated, both for their benefit and to prevent spread of the infection. Spread of infection by students with tinea capitis may be decreased by the use of selenium sulfide shampoos, but treatment requires oral griseofulum (see Tinea Capitis, p 523). Students with tinea capitis receiving treatment may attend school and participate in their usual activities. Students with tinea cruris, tinea corporis, or tinea pedis should not be excluded from school even prior to the initiation of therapy. Students with tinea capitis should be instructed not to share combs, brushes, or hair ornaments with classmates until they have been treated. Students with tinea pedis should be excluded from swimming pools and from walking barefoot on locker room and shower floors until treatment has been initiated.

Sarcoptes scabiei (scabies) and *Pediculosis capitis* (head lice) are both transmitted primarily through person-to-person contact. Combs, brushes, hats, and hair ornaments can transmit head lice but away from the scalp they do not remain viable. Shampooing with an appropriate pediculocide is usually effective in eradicating viable lice. Lice within nits adherent to the hair shaft should be killed by the same treatment, and removal of nits after treatment is not necessary to prevent spread. However, removal of nits for cosmetic purposes serves to alleviate concern of school officials and parents (see Pediculosis, p 387).

Scabies can be transmitted via clothing and bedding to household contacts, but direct skin contact is the predominant means of transmission in the school setting. The parasite survives on clothing for several days only without skin contact. Caregivers who have prolonged skin-to-skin contact with infested students during the school day, because of physical or mental disabilities, may benefit from prophylactic treatment (see Scabies p 468).

Children identified as having scabies or head lice should be excluded from school only until they are treated. School contacts should generally not be treated prophylactically.

Infections Spread by the Fecal-Oral Route

For developmentally normal school-age children, pathogens spread through the fecal-oral route constitute a risk only if the infected person fails to maintain good hygiene, ie, hand washing after toileting, or if contaminated food is shared between or among schoolmates.

Hepatitis A infection outbreaks in schools can occur, but are usually associated with community outbreaks. Schoolroom exposure generally does not pose an appreciable risk of infection, and immune globulin (IG) administration is not indicated. However, if transmission within a school is documented, IG could be used to limit further spread (see Hepatitis A, p 237). Alternatively, vaccine should be considered as a means of prophylaxis and has the advantage of resulting sustained prevention. If an outbreak occurs, consultation with the local health authorities is indicated before initiating interventions.

Enteroviral infections are probably spread by the oral-oral as well as by the fecal-oral route, and the attack rate is so high during yearly summer and fall epidemics that control measures specifically aimed at the school classroom likely would be futile. Person-to-person spread of *Salmonella* and *Shigella* infections within school settings are infrequent, but food-borne outbreaks of *Salmonella* and other enteric pathogens can occur. Symptomatic persons with bacterial gastroenteritis should be excluded.

Children in diapers at any age and in any setting constitute a far greater risk for the spread of gastrointestinal infection due to enteric pathogens. Guidelines for control of these infections in child care settings should be applied for developmentally disabled school-age students in diapers (see Children in Out-of-Home Child Care, p 80).

Infections Spread by Blood and Body Fluids

Contact with blood and body fluids of another person requires more intimate exposure than normally occurs in the school setting. The care required for the developmentally disabled child, however, may result in exposure of caregivers to urine, saliva, and, in some cases, blood. The application of routine precautions for prevention of transmission of blood-borne pathogens, as recommended in out-of-home child care, prevents spread of infection from these exposures (see Children in Out-of-Home Child Care, p 80). School staff who provide acute care for children with epistaxis or bleeding from injury should wear gloves to protect themselves from blood-borne pathogens. Routine use of these precautions avoids the necessity of identifying children known to be infected with HIV, hepatitis B, or hepatitis C viruses, and acknowledges that unrecognized infection poses at least as much risk as the identified child.

During adolescence, the likelihood of infection due to hepatitis B, HIV, and other sexually transmitted diseases (STDs) increases in proportion to sexual activity. All children should be immunized against hepatitis B before age 13 years and adolescents should be instructed in appropriate methods of prevention of sexually transmitted diseases.

Students infected with HIV, hepatitis B, or hepatitis C viruses do not need to be identified to school personnel. Therefore, policies and procedures to manage potential exposures to blood should be established and implemented. Parents and students should be educated about the types of exposure that present a risk for school contacts. Although the student's right to privacy should be maintained, decisions concerning activities at school should be made by parents or guardians together with a physician on a case-by-case basis, keeping the health needs of both the infected student and his or her classmates in mind.

Prospective studies to aid in determining the risk of transmission of HIV, hepatitis B virus (HBV), or hepatitis C (HCV) virus during contact sports among high school students have not been performed, but the available evidence indicates that the risk is extremely small.

Guidelines for management of bleeding injuries have been developed for college and professional athletes in recognition of the possibility of unidentified HIV or HBV infection in any competitor. Application of these same guidelines for all adolescent athletes is appropriate. Precautions recommended by the Academy for the prevention of transmission of HIV and other blood-borne pathogens in the athletic setting were issued in 1991* and are expected to be updated in the near future.

Athletes infected with HIV, HBV, or HCV should be allowed to participate in all competitive sports, and their condition should be kept confidential by coaches and teachers. Routine testing of athletes for HIV infection is not indicated. Physicians counseling a known HIV-, HBV-, or HCV-infected athlete in a sport, such as wrestling or football, should inform the student of the theoretical risk of contagion to others, including from potential blood exposure. All athletes should be informed that the policy of their athletic program is to allow participation of students with HIV infection without disclosure of the persons' status of infection to its participants or staff.

---

* American Academy of Pediatrics, Committee on Sports Medicine and Fitness. Human immunodeficiency virus (acquired immunodeficiency syndrome [AIDS] virus) in the athletic setting. *Pediatrics.* 1991;88:640-641.

INFECTION CONTROL FOR HOSPITALIZED CHILDREN

Isolation Precautions

Hospital-acquired infections are a major cause of morbidity and mortality in hospitalized children, particularly those in intensive care units. Procedures and policies for prevention of these infections include routine hygienic practices used in the care of all patients, such as hand washing and isolation precautions for patients suspected to be potential sources of transmission of infection. **Hand washing before and after each patient contact remains the single most important routine practice in the control of nosocomial infections.**

The Hospital Infection Control Practices Advisory Committee of the Centers for Disease Control and Prevention (CDC) in 1996 issued new isolation guidelines for the care of hospitalized patients.* These new guidelines are simpler than previous CDC recommendations and rely on very consistent strategies to prevent the spread of infection between infected and uninfected hospitalized patients. These recommendations state that "no guideline can address all of the needs of the more than 6000 US hospitals, which range in size from five beds to more than 1500 beds and serve very different patient populations. Hospitals are encouraged to review the recommendations and to modify them according to what is possible, practical, and prudent." Therefore, with the new recommendations as a guide, each institution must create its own specific isolation policies. These isolation policies, supplemented by hospital policies and procedures for other aspects of infection and environmental control and occupational health, should result in policies that are "possible, practical, and prudent" for each hospital.

These new guidelines rely on the routine and optimal performance of an expanded set of universal practices, designated **Standard Precautions**, designed for the care of all patients regardless of their diagnosis or presumed infection status; and pathogen- and syndrome-based precautions, designated **Transmission-Based Precautions,** to be utilized in caring for patients who are infected or colonized with pathogens spread by the airborne, droplet, and/or contact routes.

STANDARD PRECAUTIONS

Since medical history and examination cannot reliably identify all patients infected with the human immunodeficiency virus (HIV) or other blood-borne pathogens, the CDC recommends **Standard Precautions** for all patients to protect health care workers from infectious body fluids. These new, expanded precautions apply to blood, all body fluids, secretions, and excretions (regardless of whether they contain visible blood), nonintact skin, and mucous membranes. These general methods of infection prevention are designed to reduce the risk of transmission of microorganisms

---

* Garner JS. Hospital Infection Control Practices Advisory Committee. Guidelines for isolation precautions in hospitals. *Infect Control Hosp Epidemiol.* 1996;17:53-80.

from both recognized and unrecognized sources of infection in hospitals. **Standard Precautions** include the following techniques:

- **Hand washing** is necessary after touching blood, body fluids, secretions, excretions, and contaminated items, whether or not gloves are worn. Hands should be washed immediately after removing gloves, between patient contacts, and when otherwise indicated to avoid transfer of microorganisms to other patients or environments.
- **Gloves** should be worn when touching blood, body fluids, secretions, excretions, and items contaminated with these fluids. Clean gloves should be used before touching mucous membranes and nonintact skin. Gloves should be promptly removed after use, before touching noncontaminated items and environmental surfaces, and before going to another patient.
- **Masks, eye protection, and face shields** should be worn to protect mucous membranes of the eyes, nose, and mouth during procedures and patient care activities likely to generate splashes or sprays of blood, body fluids, secretions, or excretions.
- **Nonsterile gowns** will protect skin and prevent the soiling of clothing during procedures and patient care activities likely to generate splashes or sprays of blood, body fluids, secretions, or excretions. Soiled gowns should be promptly removed.
- **Patient care equipment** that has been used should be handled in a manner that prevents skin and mucous membrane exposures and contamination of clothing.
- **Linen** soiled with blood and body fluids, secretions, and excretions should be handled, transported, and processed in a manner that prevents skin and mucous membrane exposure and contamination of clothing.
- **Blood-borne pathogen** exposure should be avoided by taking all precautions to prevent injuries when using, cleaning, and disposing of needles, scalpels, and other sharp instruments and devices.
- **Mouthpieces, resuscitation bags, and other ventilation devices** should be readily available in all patient care areas and used instead of mouth-to-mouth resuscitation.

TRANSMISSION-BASED PRECAUTIONS

Transmission-Based Precautions are designed for patients documented or suspected to be infected with pathogens for which additional precautions beyond **Standard Precautions** are necessary to interrupt transmission. The three types of transmission on which these precautions are based are airborne, droplet, and contact.

- **Airborne transmission** occurs by dissemination of either airborne droplet nuclei (small-particle residue [5 μm or less in size] of evaporated droplets containing microorganisms that remain suspended in the air for long periods of time) or dust particles containing the infectious agent. Microorganisms spread by this route can be widely dispersed by air currents and may become inhaled by or deposited on a susceptible host within the same room or a long distance from the source patient, depending on environmental factors. Therefore, special air handling and ventilation are required to prevent airborne transmission. Examples of microorganisms transmitted by airborne transmission are *Mycobacterium tubercuberlosis*, rubeola and varicella viruses. Specific recommendations in **Airborne Precautions** are as follows:

— Private room (preferred)
— Negative air-pressure ventilation (minimum of six air changes per hour) with externally exhausted or HEPA*-filtered air, if recirculated
— Masks at all times
— If infectious pulmonary tuberculosis is suspected or proven, respiratory protective devices (ie personally "fitted" and "sealing" respirator masks) should be worn at all times.

Susceptible health care workers should not enter rooms of patients with measles or disseminated infection with varicella-zoster virus if other immune caregivers are available. Specific infections requiring **Airborne Precautions** include the following:
— Measles
— Varicella (or disseminated zoster)
— Tuberculosis

• **Droplet Transmission** occurs when droplets containing microorganisms generated from the infected person, primarily during coughing, sneezing, and talking and during the performance of certain procedures such as suctioning and bronchoscopy, are propelled a short distance and deposited on the host's conjunctivae, nasal mucosa, and/or mouth. Because droplets do not remain suspended in the air, special air handling and ventilation are not required to prevent droplet transmission; droplet transmission should not be confused with airborne transmission. Specific recommendations in **Droplet Precautions** are as follows:
— Private room (preferred)
— Use of a mask if within 3 ft of patient

Specific illnesses and infections requiring **Droplet Precautions** include the following:
— Invasive *Haemophilus influenzae* infection
— Invasive *Neisseria meningitidis* infection
— Diphtheria (respiratory)
— *Mycoplasma pneumoniae* infection
— Pertussis
— Plague (pneumonic)
— Streptococcal pharyngitis, pneumonia or scarlet fever in infants and young children
— Adenovirus
— Influenza
— Mumps
— Parvovirus B19 (during the initial phase of the illness; see Parvovirus B19, p 383)
— Rubella

• **Contact Transmission,** the most important and frequent route of transmission of nosocomial infections, is divided into two modes; direct and indirect. *Direct-contact* transmission involves a direct body surface-to-body contact and physical transfer of microorganisms between a susceptible host and an infected or colonized person, such as occurs when a person turns a patient, gives a patient a bath, or

---

* High Efficiency Particulate Air.

performs other patient care activities that require direct personal contact. Direct-contact transmission also can occur between two patients in which one serves as the source of the infectious microorganisms and the other as a susceptible host. *Indirect-contact* transmission involves contact of a susceptible host with a contaminated intermediate object, usually inanimate, such as contaminated instruments, needles, or dressings, or contaminated hands that are not washed and gloves that are not changed between patients. Specific recommendations in **Contact Precautions** are as follows:

— Private room (preferred; cohorting permissible)
— Gloves at all times
— Hand washing with an antimicrobial agent after glove removal
— Gowns at all times

Specific illnesses and infections requiring **Contact Precautions** include the following:

— Multidrug-resistant bacteria (eg, vancomycin-resistant enterococci, methicillin-resistant *Staphylococcus aureus*, multiple resistant Gram-negative bacilli) judged by the infection control program, based on current state, regional, or national recommendations to be of special clinical and epidemiological significance
— *Clostridium difficile* infection in diapered and/or incontinent patients
— *Escherichia coli* 0157:H7 infection in diapered and/or incontinent patients
— *Shigella* infection in diapered and/or incontinent patients
— Hepatitis A in diapered and/or incontinent patients
— Rotavirus infection in diapered and/or incontinent patients
— Respiratory syncytial virus infection in infants and young children
— Parainfluenzae virus infection in infants and young children
— Enteroviral infections in infants and young children
— Diphtheria (cutaneous)
— Herpes simplex virus cutaneous infection
— Impetigo
— Major (noncontained) abscesses, cellulitis, or decubitus
— Pediculosis (lice)
— Scabies
— *Staphylococcus aureus* cutaneous infection
— Herpes zoster, disseminated or in immunocompromised patients
— Conjunctivitis, viral and/or hemorrhagic
— Viral hemorrhagic fevers (Ebola, Lassa, or Marburg)

Airborne, Droplet, and **Contact Precautions** may be combined together for diseases that have multiple routes of transmission. When used either singularly or in combination, these transmission-based precautions are always to be used in addition to **Standard Precautions** which are recommended for all patients. The specifications for these categories of isolation precautions are summarized in Table 2.4 (p 104) and Table 2.5 (p 105); the latter lists illnesses that are highly suspicious for infection (eg conjunctivitis, gastroenteritis, and pneumonia) and the CDC-recommended guidelines until a pathogen is identified. When the specific pathogen is known, recommended isolation recommendations are given in the pathogen- or disease-specific chapter in Section 3.

Table 2.4. Transmission-Based Precautions for Hospitalized Patients

These recommendations are in addition to those for
Standard Precautions for all patients.

Category of Precautions	Single Room	Masks	Gowns	Gloves
Airborne	Yes, with negative air-pressure ventilation	Yes	No	No
Droplet	Yes*	Yes for those close to patient	No	No
Contact	Yes*	No	Yes	Yes

* Preferred but not required. Cohorting of children infected with the same pathogen is acceptable.

PEDIATRIC CONSIDERATIONS

The new guidelines are generally easy to understand and apply to the care of hospitalized adults as well as children. However, unique differences in pediatric care from that for adults necessitate possible modifications of these guidelines including (1) diaper changing, (2) the use of single-room isolation, and (3) the use of common areas such as hospital waiting rooms, play rooms, and school rooms.

Since diapering is routine in infants and preschool-age children in the nursery or among uninfected children, gloving for routine diapering is not mandatory. Nevertheless, the routine use of gloves for diapering could minimize the potential transmission of colonizing microbes (eg, cytomegalovirus and *Clostridium difficile*) to another patient in whom infection might result. Hospitals, in developing policies for children requiring diapers, should consider the value of consistency as exceptions to routine glove use can cause confusion and impede implementation of recommended infection control practices.

In the new CDC guidelines, private rooms are recommended for all patients in Transmission-based precautions (ie, **Airborne, Droplet**, and **Contact**). For patients with an infection requiring **Airborne Precautions**, a single room with negative air-pressure is indicated. When a private room is mandated by the possibility of airborne transmission, such as for infants with chickenpox, a forced-air incubator is not a substitute for a private room because such an incubator does not filter the air discharged into the environment. The guidelines for **Standard Precautions** also state that patients who cannot control body excretions should be in single rooms. Since most young children are incontinent, this recommendation is inappropriate for routine care of uninfected children. Even with infection in settings such as nurseries, intensive care units, and infant wards, single room isolation for **Droplet** and **Contact Precautions**, although preferred, is not mandatory given that these infants are confined to a crib. If airborne transmission is not likely, an isolation area can be defined within an intensive care unit by curtains, partitions, or other barriers. For newborn infants, including those in intensive care units, separate isolation rooms are not necessary if the following conditions are met:
- Transmission of the infection is not by the airborne route.
- Sufficient space is available for a 4- to 6-ft aisle or area between newborn infant stations.

Table 2.5. Clinical Syndromes or Conditions Warranting Additional Empiric Precautions to Prevent Transmission of Epidemiologically Important Pathogens Pending Confirmation of Diagnosis*

Clinical Syndrome or Condition[†]	Potential Pathogens[‡]	Empiric Precautions
Diarrhea		
Acute diarrhea with a likely infectious cause in an incontinent or diapered patient	Enteric pathogens[§]	Contact
Diarrhea in an adult with a history of recent antibiotic use	*Clostridium difficile*	Contact
Meningitis	*Neisseria meningitidis*	Droplet
Rash or exanthems, generalized, etiology unknown		
Petechial/ecchymotic with fever	*Neisseria meningitidis*	Droplet
Vesicular	Varicella	Airborne and contact
Maculopapular with coryza and fever	Rubeola (measles)	Airborne
Respiratory infections		
Cough/fever/upper lobe pulmonary infiltrate in an HIV-negative patient or a patient at low risk for HIV infection	*Mycobacterium tuberculosis*	Airborne
Cough/fever/pulmonary infiltrate in any lung location in an HIV-infected patient or a patient at high risk for HIV infection	*Mycobacterium tuberculosis*	Airborne
Paroxysmal or severe persistent cough during periods of pertussis activity in the community	*Bordetella pertussis*	Droplet
Respiratory viral infections, particularly bronchiolitis and croup, in infants and young children	Respiratory syncytial or parainfluenza virus	Contact
Risk of multidrug-resistant microorganisms[‖]		
History of infection or colonization with multidrug-resistant organisms	Resistant bacteria	Contact
Skin, wound, or urinary tract infection in a patient with a recent hospital or nursing home stay in a facility where multidrug-resistant organisms are prevalent	Resistant bacteria	Contact
Skin or wound infection		
Abscess or draining wound that cannot be covered	*Staphylococcus aureus,* group A streptococcus	Contact

* Modified from Garner JS. Hospital Infection Control Practices Advisory Committee. Guidelines for isolation precautions in hospitals. *Infect Control Hosp Epidemiol.* 1996;17:53-80. Infection control professionals are encouraged to modify or adapt this table according to local conditions. To ensure that appropriate empiric precautions are implemented always, hospitals must have systems in place to evaluate patients routinely according to these criteria as part of their preadmission and admission care.

† Patients with the syndromes or conditions listed below may present with atypical signs or symptoms (eg, pertussis in neonates and adults may not have paroxysmal or severe cough). The clinician's index of suspicion should be guided by the prevalence of specific conditions in the community, as well as clinical judgment.

‡ The organisms listed under this column are not intended to represent the complete, or even most likely, diagnoses, but rather possible etiologic agents that require additional precautions beyond **Standard Precautions** until they can be excluded.

§ These pathogens include enterohemorrhagic *Escherichia coli* 0157:H7, *Shigella*, hepatitis A, and rotavirus.

‖ Resistant bacteria judged by the infection control program, based on current state, regional, or national recommendations, to be of special clinical or epidemiological significance.

- An adequate number of sinks for hand washing are available in each nursery room and area.
- Continuing instruction is given to personnel about the mode of transmission of infections.

For children who are not crib-confined, **Droplet** and **Contact Precautions** are extremely important because young children are unable to limit the spread of secretions. Accordingly, single rooms are recommended. The exception to the need for a single room is for children infected with the same documented pathogen (eg, respiratory syncytial virus) who can be cohorted.

The new CDC isolation guidelines specifically are recommended for the care of hospitalized children. Settings such as schools, out-of-home child care centers, and other settings in which children are grouped in environments with sharing of common space are different in that the children are healthy and not defined by illness. These recommendations, therefore, should not be extrapolated to those settings.

Employee Health

Prevention of the transmission of infectious agents between pediatric patients and health care personnel is particularly important in the care of children. Some infections pose increased risks for pregnant health care workers principally because of the possible adverse effect on the fetus (eg, parvovirus B19, cytomegalovirus, rubella, herpes simplex, and varicella) or for workers who are immunocompromised and at increased risk of severe infection (eg, *Mycobacterium tuberculosis*, cytomegalovirus, measles, herpes simplex virus and varicella).

The consequences to pediatric patients of acquiring infections from infected adults are also significant. Since children often lack immunity to many common viruses and bacteria, they are a highly susceptible population. Mild illness in adults, such as viral gastroenteritis, upper respiratory tract viral infection (eg, respiratory syncytial virus), varicella-zoster virus infection, pertussis, herpes simplex infection, and tuberculosis, can cause life-threatening disease in children. Those at greatest risk are premature infants, children who have heart disease or chronic pulmonary disease, and immunocompromised patients.

The transmission of infectious agents within hospitals is facilitated by the inevitable close contact between patients and health care providers. In addition, children do not routinely have good hygienic practices.

To limit the risks of infection to and from children and caregivers, hospitals should have established employee health policies and services, including those for immunization (see Health Care Personnel, p 65). These policies should include measles, rubella, mumps, hepatitis B, varicella, influenza, and tetanus and diphtheria (Td) vaccines.

For non-vaccine-preventable infections, employees should be counseled about exposures and possible need for leave if they are exposed to, ill with, or a carrier of, a specific infectious agent, whether the exposure occurs in the home, community, or the medical setting.

Employees should be screened by Mantoux skin testing for tuberculosis. Those with common infections, such as gastroenteritis, dermatitis, or upper respiratory tract infections, should be evaluated to determine the resulting risk of transmission to their patients or to other health care workers.

Pregnant personnel should be counseled about the risks of caring for children with potentially contagious diseases. Specific concerns include exposure to HIV; hepatitis B, C and E; rubella; varicella; cytomegalovirus; and parvovirus B19 infection.

Employee education is of paramount importance in infection control. Pediatric health care providers should be knowledgeable about the modes of transmission of infectious agents, proper handwashing technique, and the potential serious risks to children of certain mild infections in adults.

Sibling Visits

Sibling visits to birthing centers, postpartum rooms, pediatric wards, and ICUs are encouraged. Newborn intensive care, with its increasing sophistication in medical care, often results in long hospital stays for the sick newborn, making family visits an important part of neonatal care. Sibling visits in newborn intensive care units are favorably received by parents, and bacterial colonization or subsequent infection is not increased in either the sick or well newborn who has been visited by his or her brothers or sisters.

Guidelines for sibling visits should be established to maximize opportunities for visiting and to minimize the risks of nosocomial spread of pathogens brought into the hospital by these young visitors. They may need to be modified by local nursing, pediatric, obstetric, and infectious disease staffs to address specific issues in their hospital settings. Basic guidelines for sibling visits to pediatric patients are as follows:

- Sibling visits should be encouraged in both the healthy infant nursery and the newborn intensive care nursery, for chronically and critically ill children, and for other hospitalized children.
- Before the visit, a nurse or physician should interview the parents at a site outside the unit to assess the current health of each sibling visitor. No child with fever or symptoms of an acute illness, including an upper respiratory tract infection, gastroenteritis, or dermatitis, should be allowed to visit. Siblings who have recently been exposed to a known communicable disease and are susceptible should not be allowed to visit. These interviews should be documented in the patient's record, and approval for each sibling visit should be noted.
- Asymptomatic siblings who have been exposed recently to varicella but have been previously vaccinated should be assumed to be immune.
- Adequate observation and monitoring of all visitors by the medical and nursing staff should occur.
- The visiting sibling should visit only his or her sibling.
- Children should carefully wash their hands before patient contact, especially in the case of neonatal and immunocompromised siblings.

Throughout the visit, sibling activity should be supervised by parents or a responsible adult and limited to the mother's or patient's private room and/or other designated areas.

SEXUALLY TRANSMITTED DISEASES*

The incidence of sexually transmitted diseases (STDs), including HIV infection, is increasing in children, adolescents, and young adults. Among other factors, the increase has been associated with the declining age at first intercourse. Approximately 50% of American adolescents are sexually active by 16 years of age. Sexually experienced adolescents have the highest rates of STDs of any age group; an estimated 25% are estimated to develop an STD before graduating from high school.

Physicians should be aware of the increasing prevalence of STDs, their myriad presentations and microbiologic courses, methods for their diagnosis and prevention, the potential seriousness of their sequelae for adolescents and their offspring, and the implications related to child abuse when the diagnosis of an acquired STD is made in a prepubescent child. In all 50 states, minors can be evaluated and treated for STDs without parental consent or knowledge.

The traditional STDs (eg, syphilis, gonorrhea, chancroid, and lymphogranuloma venereum) account for only a fraction of the recognized sexually transmitted pathogens. For example, hepatitis B, *Chlamydia trachomatis*, papillomavirus as well as HIV infection are now recognized as major STDs, as both heterosexual and homosexual activity are important modes of transmission of these agents.

Management

Physicians need to identify patients at risk for STDs and diagnose and appropriately treat infections caused by sexually transmitted pathogens. Adolescents with STDs, particularly females, are often asymptomatic. Screening by history, physical examination, and appropriate laboratory tests as well as patient education are indicated for high-risk groups, which include the following:
- Adolescents who are heterosexually or homosexually active.
- Pregnant adolescents and their sexual contacts.
- Adolescents undergoing therapeutic abortion.
- Adolescents with symptoms compatible with an STD, such as cervical or urethral discharge, lower abdominal or right upper quadrant pain in a female, testicular tenderness, tenesmus, rectal pain, or rectal discharge.
- Prepubescent children with genital, anal, or perineal ulcers; perineal pruritus; condyloma acuminata; or vaginitis and dysuria.
- Adolescents living in group homes or in detention homes.
- Any child or adolescent suspected of being a victim of sexual abuse, rape, or incest.
- Adolescent prostitutes.
- Street youth.
- Drug and alcohol abusers.

Because more than one STD frequently coexists in the patient, the detection of one infection should lead to a search for others, regardless of the presenting

---

* For further information, see the specific chapters in Section 3 on sexually transmitted diseases and American Academy Pediatrics, Committee on Adolescence. Sexually transmitted diseases. *Pediatrics.* 1994;94:568-572.

symptoms. A careful physical examination, including examination of the oropharynx, rectum, genitalia, and skin, should be performed. Relevant laboratory studies include urinalysis, appropriate serologic tests, Gram stains of cervical or urethral discharge, wet mounts and/or cultures of vaginal secretions, diagnostic tests for *Chlamydia trachomatis* on cervical (vaginal in prepubertal girls) or urethral specimens, and gonococcal cultures of the oropharynx, rectum, and cervix, or penile urethra in individual circumstances. The detection of concurrent HIV infection may alter the management of STDs. For example, follow-up of syphilis may need to be more prolonged in an HIV-infected patient (see Syphilis, p 504).

Recommendations for antimicrobial therapy of specific infection(s) according to microbial etiology and to syndrome, respectively, and given in the disease- or organism-specific chapters in Section 3 and in Table 5.3 (see p 623).

The diagnosis of a primary case of an STD incurs additional major responsibilities for public health reporting, evaluation for possible sexual abuse (see Sexual Abuse, p 112), contact tracing, and patient education. All adolescents should be immunized against hepatitis B. Patients who have an STD or who have multiple sexual partners (defined as two or more in 6 months) are at increased risk for hepatitis B and should initiate or complete hepatitis B immunization, which can be given at the time of treatment for the STD (see Hepatitis B, p 247). The physician should explain to the patient the route of transmission of STDs and the importance of examining partners, and should report diseases to the responsible health department to facilitate partner notification. The potential long-term sequelae of disease(s) should be emphasized. Whereas control through partner notification and identification of secondary spread is frequently best coordinated by public health departments, the patient's physician is responsible for educating and appropriately treating the patient. In general, health departments have been active in partner notification when the index patient has syphilis; however, they have been less so with other STDs, particularly chlamydial infection. Physicians should actively facilitate treatment of their patient's current partners.

The style and content of counseling should be adapted for adolescents, including the need for a nonjudgmental approach and identification of other problem behaviors (eg, drug use, school failure, or depression).

Sequelae

Major sequelae of STDs in adolescents include chronic hepatitis, salpingitis, ectopic pregnancies, infertility, and carcinoma of the cervix. Although approximately 50% of adults with HIV infection acquired this disease during adolescence, manifestations often do not develop for at least 6 or more years. Sexually transmitted diseases also cause fetal and neonatal infections, and the risk of these infections is increased in adolescent pregnancies. Failure to consider the possibility of an STD in the mother can result in delay or omission of neonatal therapy with possibly serious consequences. Hence, screening and treatment in pregnancy and early diagnosis and treatment of the infant are essential. Neonatal consequences of certain maternal STDs are listed in Table 2.6 (p 110).

Table 2.6. **Neonatal Consequences of Certain Maternal Sexually Transmitted Pathogens**

Maternal Infection	Infant Consequences	Prevention	Neonatal Treatment
Candida albicans	Thrush, dermatitis	None	Nystatin, clotrimazole, miconazole
Chlamydia trachomatis	Conjunctivitis, pneumonia	Screen and treat mother and her sexual partner	Erythromycin
Cytomegalovirus	Congenital infection	None	None
Hepatitis B virus	Development of chronic hepatitis	Screen mother	Hepatitis B Immune Globulin (HBIG) and hepatitis B vaccine
Herpes simplex virus	Central nervous system disease, disseminated infection, spontaneous abortion, prematurity	Cesarean section	Acyclovir
HIV	AIDS	Screen mother; if negative, counsel regarding prevention; if positive, consider abortion or zidovudine treatment	Zidovudine
Neisseria gonorrhoeae	Conjunctivitis, arthritis, sepsis, meningitis, premature delivery	Screen and treat mother and her sexual partner; ocular prophylaxis for the infant	Ceftriaxone
Treponema pallidum	Stillbirth, low birth weight, prematurity, congenital infection	Screen and treat mother and her sexual partner	Penicillin G
Papillomavirus	Respiratory tract papillomatosis	None	Mechanical removal

Prevention of STDs

Sexually transmitted diseases are a major and growing source of morbidity in children and adolescents. Active cooperation and involvement of the public and private sectors of medicine are necessary to control this significant problem. **Primary prevention is vastly more effective than treating STDs and their sequelae.**

Adolescents consider health care providers to be accurate and confidential sources of information about STDs, including HIV infection. Physicians caring for adolescents not only need to be knowledgeable about the diagnosis and management of STDs, but also need to educate adolescents about STDs and their prevention. Providing information about STDs, the role of masturbation and abstinence, and the proper use of and education about condoms (see Table 2.7, p 111) can help over-

Table 2.7. **Recommendations for Use of Condoms***

1. Latex condoms should be used because they may offer greater protection against HIV and other viral sexually transmitted diseases (STDs) than natural membrane condoms.

2. Condoms should be stored in a cool, dry place out of direct sunlight.

3. Condoms in damaged packages or those that show obvious signs of age (eg, those that are brittle, sticky, or discolored) should not be used. They cannot be relied on to prevent infection or pregnancy.

4. Condoms should be handled with care to prevent puncture.

5. The condom should be put on before any genital contact to prevent exposure to fluids that may contain infectious agents. Hold the tip of the condom and unroll it onto the erect penis, leaving space at the tip to collect semen, yet ensuring that no air is trapped in the tip of the condom.

6. Only water-based lubricants should be used. Petroleum- or oil-based lubricants (such as petroleum jelly, cooking oils, shortening, and lotions) should not be used because they weaken the latex and may cause breakage.

7. Use of condoms containing spermicides may provide some additional protection against STDs. However, vaginal use of spermicides along with condoms is likely to provide still greater protection.

8. If a condom breaks, it should be replaced immediately. If ejaculation occurs after condom breakage, the immediate use of spermicide has been suggested. However, the protective value of postejaculation application of spermicide in reducing the risk of STD transmission is unknown.

9. After ejaculation, care should be taken so that the condom does not slip off the penis before withdrawal; the base of the condom should be held throughout withdrawal. The penis should be withdrawn while still erect.

10. Condoms should never be reused.

* From Centers for Disease Control and Prevention. 1989 sexually transmitted diseases treatment guidelines. *MMWR.* 1989;38(No. S-8):ix.

come many myths and erroneous beliefs (see Table 2.8, p 112), and can reduce the patient's risk of acquiring a sexually transmitted pathogen. The efficacy of female condoms for protection against HIV or other STDs has not been well evaluated.

Advice to abstain from sexual intercourse or always to use condoms together with a discussion about ways to do so should be given. The fact that no chemical or barrier method can assure protection against STDs (ie, absolutely "safe sex" does not exist) should be emphasized. Counseling about monogamous relationships may convey a false sense of security that works against the use of more reliable preventive strategies. Adolescents often interpret monogamy as having one sexual relationship at a time, which is not as effective a strategy to prevent STDs (including HIV infection) as practicing abstinence or using condoms.

Immunization of adolescents against hepatitis B, with appropriate methods to assure follow-up and completion of the series, should be emphasized by all health care providers.

Table 2.8. **Barriers to Condom Use and Ways to Overcome Them***

Perceived Barrier	Intervention Strategy
Decreases sexual pleasure (sensation)	• Often perceived by those who have never used a condom. Encourage patient to try. • Try a thinner latex condom.
Decreases spontaneity of sexual activity	• Encourage incorporation of use of condom during time before actual intercourse. Peace of mind may actually enhance pleasure. • Demonstrates responsibility and respect.
Embarrassing, juvenile, "unmanly"	• This feeling is not shared by many in the population, especially now.
Poor fit, either too small or too big, slips off, uncomfortable (actually due to constriction of the urethra with subsequent painful ejaculation)	• Smaller and larger condoms are available. • Natural skin condoms are another alternative for "large" patients but are less reliable for prevention of sexually transmitted diseases.
Requires prompt withdrawal after ejaculation	• Reinforce the protective nature.
Fear of breakage may lead to less vigorous sexual activity	• With prolonged intercourse, lubricant wears off and the condom begins to rub. Have a water-soluble lubricant available to reapply.

* From Canadian guidelines for the prevention, diagnosis, management, and treatment of sexually transmitted diseases in neonates, children, adolescents, and adults. *CCDR.* 1992;18S1:8.

Sexual Abuse

Some infections known to be sexually transmitted in adults are similarly spread to children. An estimated 20% of girls and 10% of boys will be sexually abused before they reach adulthood. Child sexual abuse is defined as contact or interaction between a child and an adult when the child is used for the sexual stimulation of the adult or another person. Sexual abuse also may be committed by another minor when that person is significantly older than the victim or in a position of power or control over the child.

Assessment for possible sexual abuse should be considered in infants and pre-pubertal children with any of the following infections:
• Genital or rectal *Chlamydia trachomatis* or herpes simplex virus infection
• Genital or pharyngeal *Neisseria gonorrhoeae* infection
• Anogenital warts in a child older than 2 years
• HIV infection or syphilis in an infant or child whose mother is seronegative for these conditions
• Vaginal *Trichomonas vaginalis* infection
• *Pediculus pthirus* (crab louse) infestation of the eyelashes

The majority of victims of sexual abuse frequently are physically asymptomatic and do not acquire infection; prevalence rates of STDs among such children generally do not exceed 4%. Hence, physicians need to determine which patients warrant laboratory evaluation for STDs. Evaluation should be performed if (1) the suspected offender has an STD or is considered at high risk; (2) the child has a history or physical findings indicative of penetrating trauma; (3) the child has signs or symptoms of an STD; (4) the victim is an adolescent or high-risk sexually active patient; (5) the patient or family is anxious about the possibility of acquiring an STD; and/or (6) follow-up is unlikely. Many experts advise culturing all children examined for sexual abuse for *C trachomatis* and *N gonorrhoeae*, regardless of circumstances.

Initial STD screening should be performed within 72 hours after an acute sexual assault in adolescents, including high-risk sexually active patients, and repeated 2 weeks later or at the onset of symptoms. Among low-risk prepubertal children, however, screening can be deferred until the 2-week follow-up visit (unless an initial decision was made to treat empirically the likely STDs). Serologic testing for HIV, syphilis, and hepatitis B should be performed on all victims who have evidence of contact with the abuser's genital or oral secretions 12 weeks after an acute assault. If sexual abuse is considered to be chronic or to have occurred more than 72 hours before evaluation, specimens can be collected immediately for evaluation of STDs (see Table 2.9, p 115, and subsequent discussion in this chapter).

Antimicrobial prophylaxis following sexual assault should be considered for all adolescents, particularly postpubertal females. An appropriate regimen for chlamydial, gonococcal, and trichomonal infections and for bacterial vaginosis includes the following: (1) ceftriaxone, 125 mg intramuscularly in a single dose; (2) metronidazole, 2 g orally in a single dose; and (3) doxycycline, 100 mg orally twice a day for 7 days. In addition, hepatitis B vaccination is indicated for all nonvaccinated victims of assault, regardless of age (unless otherwise demonstrated to be immune).

Presumptive antibiotic treatment for sexually abused prepubertal children is not widely recommended because girls appear to be at lower risk for ascending infection than adolescent or adult women, and regular follow-up usually can be assured. However, the degree of anxiety among children, their parents, or guardians about possible STD acquisition may be adequate justification for initiating therapy. Patients who develop abdominal pain, dysuria, or vaginal discharge should be reexamined as soon as possible and treated appropriately.

Specimens obtained from a child or adolescent alleged to have suffered sexual abuse or assault must be properly collected, labeled, stored, and evaluated, for both medical and legal reasons, given the implications of a positive test. An unbroken and documented "chain of custody" is important to preserve the admissibility of evidence in later court proceedings.

Techniques for testing for *N gonorrhoeae, C trachomatis,* and syphilis are as follows:

- **Neisseria gonorrhoeae.** Swabs of the throat, rectum, urethra, and vagina (in prepubertal girls) or endocervix (in adolescents) should be obtained and placed immediately into commercially available transport media for *N gonorrhoeae* or plated immediately on a selective medium (eg, Thayer-Martin) and chocolate agar and incubated in a CO_2-enriched atmosphere. For boys, a urethral swab culture should be obtained only if urethral discharge, dysuria, positive urine leukocyte esterase test, and/or erythema are present. Isolates should be confirmed by biochemical and enzyme substrate or serologic techniques, preferably using at least two confirmatory techniques.

Rapid-detection techniques directly applied to patient specimens, such as Gram stain of discharge in a symptomatic child, should be used only to guide initial therapy, pending culture results. They cannot be used as legal evidence of an STD. A positive culture for *N gonorrhoeae* in a child older than 1 month, and particularly after 6 months of age, is most likely due to sexual contact rather than persistence of perinatally acquired infection. (see Gonococcal Infections, p 212).

- **Chlamydia trachomatis.** Specimens should be obtained from the throat, rectum, urethral meatus, and vagina (in prepubertal girls) or endocervix (in adolescents) for culture. For boys, a urethral swab culture should be obtained only if urethral discharge, dysuria, positive urine leukocyte esterase, or erythema is present. Rapid detection techniques, such as enzyme immunoassay and direct fluorescent antibody tests, should not be used, except to guide presumptive therapy, because of the risk of false-positive and false-negative reactions. Genital or rectal chlamydial infection in children older than 1 year of age suggests sexual contact, although perinatally acquired *C trachomatis* can result in colonization and may persist until 3 years of age (see *Chlamydia trachomatis,* p 170).

- **Syphilis.** Darkfield microscopy should be performed on fluid from a genital lesion, if present. Serology for syphilis (ie, VDRL, rapid plasma reagin [RPR], or automated reagin test [ART]) should be obtained at the time of abuse and 6 to 12 weeks later (see Syphilis, p 504). Reactive nontreponemal tests should be confirmed by a treponemal test (eg, fluorescent treponema antibody or microhemagglutination assay–*Treponema pallidum*). If not congenitally acquired, a confirmed reactive serology is highly suggestive of sexual contact.

Other infectious agents with serious health implications can be found in sexually abused children. Knowledge of this fact can be a source of extreme anxiety to both parents and child. Evaluation and management of these infections is indicated as follows:

- **Human immunodeficiency virus.** If feasible, serologic evaluation of the alleged offender should be performed. The child should be tested serologically at the time of abuse and at 6, 12, and 24 weeks after sexual contact with an assailant likely to be HIV infected. Counseling of the child and family should be provided. The risk of transmission of HIV is small.

- **Hepatitis B.** If the victim is incompletely or previously unimmunized, hepatitis B vaccine should be given as soon as possible and the vaccination schedule should be subsequently completed (see Hepatitis B, p 252). If the victim is less than 11 years old, the recommended dose(s) is that for an infant born to an HBsAg-positive mother. For those 11 years and older the dose is that recommended according to the victim's age. If the alleged offender is known to have acute hepatitis B, passive immunoprophylaxis with Hepatitis B Immune Globulin (HBIG) also should be given. If the 3-dose hepatitis B immunization series has been completed, neither vaccine nor HBIG is indicated.

- **Herpes simplex virus (HSV).** Types 1 and 2 of HSV may be spread sexually or nonsexually, but type 2 is usually acquired through sexual transmission. Lesions should be cultured for HSV (see Herpes Simplex, p 266). Routine cultures in the

Table 2.9. **Testing for Sexual Abuse**

	Organism/Syndrome	Specimens
All children	*Neisseria gonorrhoeae*	Rectal, throat, urethral, vaginal, and/or endocervical* culture(s)
	Chlamydia trachomatis	Rectal, urethral discharge, vaginal, and/or endocervical* culture(s)
	Syphilis	Darkfield examination of chancre fluid, if present; blood for serologic tests at time of abuse and 6–12 wk later
Selected cases	HIV	Serology of abuser (if possible), serology of child at time of abuse and 6, 12, and 24 wk later
	Hepatitis B virus (HBV)	Serum HBsAg testing of abuser
	Herpes simplex virus	Culture of lesion
	Bacterial vaginosis	Wet mount and culture of vaginal discharge
	Papillomavirus	Biopsy of lesion
	Trichomonas vaginalis	Wet mount and culture of vaginal discharge

* Postpubertal patients only.

absence of lesions are not recommended. The use of commercially available serologic tests is not of value.

- *Bacterial vaginosis (nonspecific or Gardnerella vaginalis–associated vaginitis).* Bacterial vaginosis is more common in children who have had sexual contact, but is not diagnostic of abuse. "Clue cells" may be seen in a wet preparation obtained from a vaginal discharge or vaginal wash, and a fishy odor develops after 10% potassium hydroxide is added to vaginal fluid (see Bacterial Vaginosis, p 149).
- *Human papillomavirus.* Diagnosis is usually clinical; however, a biopsy may be done for histologic examination of genital or rectal warts (condyloma acuminata) that develop within one month or later after sexual abuse if the diagnosis is uncertain. Perinatally acquired disease can appear as laryngeal, genital, or rectal warts as long as several years after birth (see Papillomaviruses, p 374).
- *Trichomonas vaginalis.* A wet-mount preparation, enzyme immunoassay, or immunofluorescent antibody test of vaginal secretions, or culture can be performed. Although infection has been reported to be spread from mother to infant, most infections in prepubertal girls probably are caused by sexual abuse (see *Trichomonas vaginalis* Infections, p 536).

Several organisms usually thought to be sexually transmitted can be recovered from children where sexual abuse does not appear likely. Although infection with *G vaginalis*, *Mycoplasma hominis*, and *Ureaplasma urealyticum* can occur in sexually abused children, their presence in children who have not been abused suggests that acquisition may occur in other ways.

Sexual abuse of children has been endemic for generations, but recognition of its prevalence and potentially devastating psychological effects has only been recent. In addition to the medical evaluation, appropriate social service and law enforcement agencies must be involved whenever sexual abuse is suspected to ensure the child's protection, and counseling must be provided to the child and family.

MEDICAL EVALUATION OF INTERNATIONALLY ADOPTED CHILDREN

Approximately 10 000 children from abroad are adopted each year by families in the United States. Asian nations (such as Korea, India, and the Philippines) and Central and South American countries account for nearly 90% of international adoptees. However, increasing numbers of adoptees are coming from Eastern Europe and the Caribbean. Africa and the Middle East remain unusual sources for international adoption. The diverse origins of these children, their unknown backgrounds before adoption (including their parents' background and their living circumstances), and the inadequacy of health care in many developing countries make appropriate medical evaluation of internationally adopted children an important task.

Internationally adopted children differ from refugee children in terms of their medical evaluation before arrival in the United States and in the frequency of certain infectious diseases. While refugee children who resided in processing camps for some months may have received extensive medical care and treatment, the medical evaluation of international adoptees is so variable as to be usually unreliable. Although all internationally adopted children are required to have a medical examination performed by a physician designated by the United States Embassy or consulate in the country of origin before an immigrant visa is issued, this examination is limited to screening for certain communicable diseases and for serious physical defects and is not a comprehensive assessment of the child's health status. In addition, falsified health documents, including chest radiographs, are sometimes sold to facilitate adoption. Thus, these children are seldom appropriately screened for illness, regardless of country of origin, and preventive health care such as immunizations, may be delayed or omitted.

In prospective studies of internationally adopted children, infectious diseases have constituted most medical diagnoses (see Table 2.10, p 117) and have been found in as many as 60% of children, depending on their country of origin. Because many of these infections are asymptomatic, the diagnosis must be made by screening tests in addition to history and physical examination. Use of screening tests for certain infections is cost-effective, preventive health care for these children and their adoptive families.

Examination of children need not occur immediately after arrival in the United States, but can generally wait for approximately 2 weeks. Parents, however, should notify their physician when their child arrives so they can review basic medical issues and are alerted to potential infectious diseases, such as scabies or lice, that they may encounter.

Table 2.10. **Infectious Diseases of Importance in International Adoptees and Refugees***

Bacteria	Viruses	Protozoa	Helminths	Arthropoda
Campylobacter	Cytomegalovirus	Amebiasis	Ascariasis	Lice
Melioidosis*	Hepatitis A	Giardiasis	Filariasis*	Scabies
Salmonella	Hepatitis B	Malaria*	Hookworm	
Shigella	Hepatitis C	Toxoplasmosis	Liver flukes*	
Syphilis	HIV		Lung flukes*	
Tuberculosis*			Schistosomiasis*	
Typhoid fever*			Strongyloidiasis	
Leprosy			Tapeworm	
			Trichuriasis	

* More commonly encountered in refugee children than in international adoptees.

Infectious Diseases

Some infectious diseases are of particular importance in the care of internationally adopted children as they occur with sufficient frequency to be reviewed for all international adoptees.

VIRAL HEPATITIS

The prevalence of hepatitis B virus (HBV) markers ranges from 5% to 50% in internationally adopted children. Chronic carriers of hepatitis B surface antigen (HBsAg) vary from 1% to 15% in prevalence; adoptees from Asia, Africa, and certain Eastern European countries (such as Romania) have the highest rates. These children should be tested for serum HBsAg, hepatitis B surface antibody (anti-HBs), and hepatitis B core antibody (anti-HBc). Testing for HBsAg and anti-HBs does not identify children in the "window" period of acute HBV infection. They can be identified by the presence of anti-HBc and the absence of HBsAg. Some international adoption agencies require certification that the child is not an HBsAg carrier, but documents provided from most country institutions have incorrectly "certified" that children were not carriers who were determined subsequently to be carriers upon arrival in the United States.

Chronic hepatitis B carriage is defined by the persistence of HBsAg for more than 6 months. Carriers should be evaluated for evidence of chronic active hepatitis by testing of serum hepatic enzyme concentrations and for infectivity by testing for HBsAg. Whenever possible, susceptible household contacts should be immunized before arrival of the child, but adoption need not be delayed until immunization is completed (see Hepatitis B, p 250).

Children whose initial tests for HBsAg and anti-HBc are negative should receive routine immunization for hepatitis B as soon as possible. Infants brought into the country within the first week of life from high-risk areas and whose mothers were not screened for HBsAg can be given Hepatitis B Immune Globulin (HBIG) with their first immunization against hepatitis B, provided the HBIG is given within 7 days of birth.

Hepatitis D, which occurs only in conjunction with active HBV replication, is unusual, but may be found in adoptees from Eastern Europe, Africa, South America, and the Middle East. Serologic tests for diagnoses are available (see Hepatitis D, p 264), but routine testing for hepatitis D is not recommended.

Routine serologic screening for hepatitis A antibodies is not indicated. Many internationally adopted children acquire hepatitis A early in life; thus, acute infections after adoption are rare. Chronic hepatitis A does not occur.

Serologic screening for hepatitis C is not routinely indicated since effective immunoprophylaxis is not available for household and other contacts.

CYTOMEGALOVIRUS

Cytomegalovirus (CMV) is excreted by approximately half of internationally adopted children, who typically acquired the virus perinatally and suffer no sequelae. Because CMV is readily transmitted to susceptible household members from infected children, instructions on the value of good hand washing after contact with urine, diapers and respiratory secretions should be given to adoptive parents. Routine screening for CMV infection is not recommended because of the high prevalence of CMV infection in children in the United States, particularly those attending day care centers. However, adoptive parents should be counseled about CMV infection, especially if an adoptive mother is not immune and is contemplating pregnancy.

INTESTINAL PATHOGENS

Fecal examinations for ova and parasites by an experienced laboratory identify a pathogen in 15% to 35% of most internationally adopted children; Korean children, however, consistently have a low prevalence of intestinal parasites. The most common pathogens are *Giardia, Ascaris,* and *Trichuris; Strongyloides, Entamoeba histolytica,* and hookworm are less frequent. One stool sample is generally sufficient for initial screening unless gastrointestinal symptoms are present or symptoms persist after treatment. In addition, children with diarrhea should have stools cultured for *Salmonella, Shigella, Yersinia,* and *Campylobacter* organisms with appropriate treatment and follow-up cultures as indicated. Therapy decreases intestinal infection with parasites, but complete eradication may not always occur. Thus, enteric symptoms occurring months or even years after a child's arrival should be evaluated for intestinal parasites.

TUBERCULOSIS

Although less common in international adoptees than in refugee children from Indochina, tuberculosis is still frequently encountered. Rates of infection are 50 to 150 times that in American-born children. Because most tuberculosis disease occurs within the first several years of arrival, screening with the Mantoux test is particularly important (see Tuberculosis, p 541), even if the child has previously received BCG vaccine. Routine chest roentgenograms are not warranted in asymptomatic children in whom the Mantoux test is negative. A positive Mantoux test should not be attributed to BCG without further investigation (see Tuberculosis, p 541). When active tuberculosis is found in refugees and international adoptees, efforts to isolate the test and responsible organism for drug sensitivities are imperative because of the high prevalence of drug susceptibilities in many foreign countries.

SYPHILIS

Congenital syphilis, especially with involvement of the central nervous system, is sometimes undiagnosed and often inadequately treated in many developing nations. Each international adoptee should be screened for syphilis by a reliable serologic test (see Syphilis, p 504). Those found to be reactive should have appropriate supplemental testing, and those infected should be treated (see Syphilis, p 504).

HIV INFECTION

The risk of HIV infection in internationally adopted children depends on the country of origin and on individual risk factors. Because of the rapidly changing epidemiology of HIV infection and because adoptees may come from subgroups at high risk for infection, screening should be considered for all internationally adopted children. Test results for HIV from the adoptee's country of origin should not be considered reliable. Transplacentally acquired maternal antibody in the absence of infection can be present in a child younger than 18 months. Hence, positive serologic tests in asymptomatic children of this age require follow-up testing and clinical evaluation (see HIV Infection, p 279).

OTHER INFECTIOUS DISEASES

Because scabies and pediculosis are common, adoptees should be examined immediately after arrival so family members do not become infected. Diseases such as malaria, leprosy, or melioidosis are infrequently encountered in internationally adopted children, except those of southeast Asian origin. While routine screening for these diseases is not routinely recommended, the findings of fever, splenomegaly, anemia, or eosinophilia should prompt an appropriate evaluation. Malaria can be diagnosed by obtaining Giemsa-stained thick and thin smears of peripheral blood (see Malaria, p 335).

Other Medical Conditions

In addition to screening for infectious diseases, international adoptees should be examined for other medical conditions. All children should undergo vision and hearing testing, developmental testing, and nutritional assessment. Some children who are developmentally delayed at adoption have difficulties with learning and will benefit from a thorough developmental assessment before entering school. A careful physical examination should reveal most congenital anomalies. Each child should have a complete blood count to screen for anemia and hemoglobinopathies. In addition, screening for sickle cell hemoglobinopathies may be appropriate in children from India, Central America, or South America. Hemoglobin E can be found in children from Southeast Asia, and ß-thalassemia occurs in children from the Mediterranean, the Indian subcontinent, and Southeast Asia. The finding of anemia should alert the physician to the possibility of dietary deficiency, intestinal nematodes, particularly hookworm infestation, and other chronic infectious or genetic causes. Screening for glucose-6-phosphate dehydrogenase deficiency should be considered in children of Mediterranean or African origin before administering sulfonamides or primaquine.

Immunizations

International adoptees and refugees frequently are not immunized or are underimmunized. They should receive necessary vaccinations according to recommended schedules in the United States for healthy infants and children (see Fig 1.1 and Table 1.3, p 18 and p 20). Only written documentation should be accepted as evidence of prior immunization. In general, written immunization records may be considered valid if the vaccines, dates of administration, number of doses, intervals between doses, and age of the patient at the time of vaccination is comparable to that of the current US schedule (see Immunizations Received Outside the United States, p 22). Although some vaccines with inadequate potency have been produced in other countries, most vaccines used worldwide, including those in developing nations, are produced with adequate quality control standards and are reliable. The immunization schedules of other countries are acceptable if they meet the minimum requirements of the World Health Organization schedule (see Table 1.4, p 21).

INJURIES FROM DISCARDED NEEDLES IN THE COMMUNITY

Injuries from discarded hypodermic needles and syringes in public places, usually by injection drug users, are perceived by victims as a significant risk for transmitting infection caused by blood-borne pathogens. While these injuries pose less of a risk than that resulting from needle stick injuries in health care settings as the observed risk of transmission is very small, the perception of risk often results in the necessity for evaluation, testing, and counseling of the injured person. Some estimate of the possibility that the discarded syringe contains blood-borne pathogens can be made from the prevalence rates of these infections in a community where the injury occurred, but the need to test the injured person usually is not significantly affected by this assessment.

Management of such injuries involves several aspects, including acute wound care, consideration of the need for possible prophylactic management, and prevention. Wound care is the least complicated. Tetanus toxoids and Tetanus Immune Globulin (TIG) should be administered according to the vaccination status of the victim (see Tetanus, p 518). Such wounds rarely require closure.

Prophylaxis of infection by blood-borne pathogens, which include hepatitis B virus (HBV), HIV, and hepatitis C virus (HCV), is more problematic. Extrapolation from similar injuries in health care settings may be inappropriate. Risk of acquisition of various pathogens depends on their respective abilities to survive on fomites and their prevalence rates among local injection drug users. However, syringes may not have been discarded by local users.

Hepatitis B virus is the hardiest of the major blood-borne pathogens as it survives on fomites for at least several days and the need for immunoprophylaxis should be considered. While immunity may be present even in the absence of serum antibody to hepatitis B surface antigen (anti-HBsAg) in a previously vaccinated person, children who have not completed the hepatitis B series should receive an additional dose of vaccine and, if indicated, scheduled to receive the remaining ones to complete the schedule. Administration of Hepatitis B Immune Globulin (HBIG) is usually not indicated if the child has received the three-dose regimen of hepatitis B vaccine (see Hepatitis B, p 259). However, experts differ about the need for HBIG at the time of an injury of an incompletely immunized child.

Hepatitis A virus (HAV) can also be transmitted by blood. Hepatitis A outbreaks have occurred among drug users, and for some outbreaks, person-to-person, blood-borne transmission has been hypothesized. Administration of immune globulin to persons who sustain needle sticks from discarded syringes and needles is not necessary, however, because HAV transmission is highly unlikely.

Infection with HIV is usually the greatest concern of the family and the victim. The need for initial, baseline serological tests for preexisting HIV infection is controversial. Negative results from these initial tests support the conclusion that subsequent positive tests reflect infection acquired from the needle stick. Since positive baseline tests are rare in this circumstance, a decision needs to be made about whether the expense and discomfort of initial testing is justified. Positive tests require further investigation of their causes, such as perinatal transmission or sexual abuse. An alternative option is to obtain and save a baseline serum specimen for later testing for HIV antibody in the unlikely event that a subsequent test is positive. Counseling is necessary before and after testing (see HIV Infection, p 279).

The risk of HIV transmission from a discarded needle in public places appears to be low and data on the efficacy of postexposure prophylaxis with antiretroviral drugs in children are not available. Prophylaxis is recommended by the US Public Health Service for health care workers after occupational blood exposures to HIV, for which the risk of transmission is higher, and may be reasonable for pediatric injuries (see HIV Infection, p 279). Some experts, however, recommend that antiretroviral chemoprophylaxis should be considered only in the unusual circumstance where the syringe is available and is believed to contain fresh blood from an HIV-infected person. Testing the syringe for HIV usually is not practical or reliable. Consultation with a specialist in HIV infection should be considered in the decision of whether to give postexposure chemoprophylaxis.

While testing the child for serum HIV antibody immediately after exposure is controversial, follow-up should include testing at six months, and perhaps also at 6 and 12 weeks after injury. Testing also is indicated in the event of an illness consistent with an acute HIV-related syndrome (see HIV Infection, p 279).

No immune globulins or drugs have been demonstrated to protect against hepatitis C infection. Although transmission by sharing the syringes among injection drug users is efficient, the risk of transmission from a discarded syringe is low. In addition, the viability of this virus on fomites is probably poor. The need for testing for hepatitis C virus is uncertain. If done, it should be done at the time of injury and 6 months later. Positive tests should be confirmed by supplemental confirmatory tests (see Hepatitis C, p 260).

Needlestick injuries of children can be prevented by public health programs for exchange of injection drug users' used syringes and needles for sterile ones. Needle/syringe exchanges reduce improper disposal and the spread of bloodborne pathogens without increasing injection drug use. The American Academy of Pediatrics supports needle exchange programs in conjunction with drug treatment and within the context of continuing research to document their effectiveness and clarify those factors contributing to desired outcomes.

BITE WOUNDS

As many as 1% of all visits to pediatric emergency centers during the summer months are for the treatment of human or animal bite wounds. An estimated 4.7 million dog bites, 400 000 cat bites, 45 000 snake bites, and 250 000 human bites occur annually in the United States. The incidence of infection following cat bites can be more than 50%, and that following dog or human bite wounds can be 15% to 20%. Wild animal bites also are a potential source of serious infection. Parents should be informed about the importance of children avoiding contact with wild animals and of securing garbage containers so that raccoons and other animals will not be attracted to the home and places where children may play. Dead animals should be avoided because they may harbor rabies viruses in their blood and secretions, and be infested with infected arthropods (fleas or ticks).

Generic recommendations for bite wound management are given in Table 2.11 (p 123). Sufficient prospective, controlled studies upon which to base recommendations concerning the closure of bite wounds are lacking; and, thus, these recommendations should be considered guidelines. In general, recent, noninfected, low-risk lesions may be sutured after thorough wound cleansing, irrigation, and debridement. Use of local anesthesia can facilitate these procedures. Because suturing can enhance the risk of wound infection, some clinicians prefer for small wounds approximation of the wound edges with adhesive strips to suturing. Bite wounds on the face, which have important cosmetic considerations, seldom become infected and should be sutured, whenever possible. Hand and foot wounds, however, have a high risk of infection and should be managed in consultation with an appropriate surgical specialist. Elevation of injured areas to minimize swelling is important.

Limited data currently exist concerning the initiation of antimicrobial therapy in patients with wounds that are not overtly infected. The use of antimicrobials within 8 hours of injury, using a suggested guideline for a 2- to 3-day course of therapy, may decrease the rate of infection. Patients with mild injuries in which the skin only is abraded do not need to be treated with antimicrobial agents.

The guidelines for choice of antimicrobial therapy of human and animal bites, given in Table 2.12 (p 125), reflect the organisms likely to cause infection for each biting species. Empiric therapy may be modified based upon culture results.

Prophylaxis or treatment for the penicillin-allergic child with a human or animal bite wound is problematic. Activity of erythromycin and tetracyclines against *Staphylococcus aureus* and anaerobes is unpredictable and use of tetracycline, which does have activity against *Pasteurella multocida,* in children younger than 8 years

Table 2.11. **Prophylactic Management of Human or Animal Bite Wounds to Prevent Infection**

Category of Management	Time From Injury	
	< 8 h	≥ 8 h
Method of cleansing	Sponge away visible dirt. Irrigate with a copious volume of sterile saline by high-pressure syringe irrigation.* Do not irrigate puncture wounds.	Same as that for wounds of less than 8 h duration
Wound culture	No, unless signs of infection exist.	Yes, except in wounds more than 24 h after injury and without signs of infection
Debridement	Remove devitalized tissue	Same as that for wounds of less than 8 h duration
Operative debridement and exploration	Yes, if one of the following: — Extensive wounds (devitalized tissue) — Involvement of the metacarpophalangeal joint (closed fist injury) — Cranial bites by large animal[†]	Same as that for wounds of less than 8 h duration
Wound closure	Yes for nonpuncture bite wounds	No
Assess tetanus immunization status[‡]	Yes	Yes
Assess risk of rabies from animal bites[§]	Yes	Yes
Assess risk of hepatitis B from human bites[‖]	Yes	Yes
Assess HIV risk from human bites[¶]	Yes	Yes

Table 2.11. Prophylactic Management of Human or Animal Bite Wounds to Prevent Infection, continued

Category of Management	Time From Injury	
	< 8 h	≥ 8 h
Initiate antimicrobial therapy[#]	Yes for: — Moderate or severe bite wounds, especially if edema or crush injury is present — Puncture wounds, especially if bone, tendon sheath, or joint penetration may have occurred — Facial bites — Hand and foot bites — Genital area bites — Wounds in immunocompromised and in asplenic persons	Same as that for wounds of less than 8 h duration and for bite wounds with signs of infection
Follow-up	Inspect wound for signs of infection within 48 h	Same as that for wounds of less than 8 h duration

* Use of an 18-gauge needle with a large-volume syringe is effective. Antibiotic or anti-infective solutions offer no advantage and may increase tissue irritation.
† Radiographic studies in facial injuries are indicated if penetrating central nervous system injury is suspected.
‡ See Tetanus, p 519.
§ See Rabies, p 439.
‖ See Hepatitis B, p 259.
¶ See HIV Infection, p 303.
# See Table 2.12 (p 125) for suggested drug choices.

Table 2.12. Antimicrobials for Human or Animal Bite Wounds

Source of Bite	Organism(s) Likely To Cause Infection	Antimicrobial Agent			
		Oral Route	Oral Alternatives for Penicillin-Allergic Patients*	Intravenous Route	Intravenous Alternatives for Penicillin-Allergic Patients*
Dog/cat	*Staphylococcus aureus*, streptococci, *Pasteurella multocida*, *Capnocytophaga canimorsus*, anaerobes	Amoxicillin-clavulanate	Extended spectrum cephalosporin or trimethoprim-sulfamethoxazole **PLUS** clindamycin	Ampicillin-sulbactam	Extended spectrum cephalosporin or trimethoprim-sulfamethoxazole **PLUS** clindamycin
Reptile	Enteric Gram-negative bacteria, anaerobes	Amoxicillin-clavulanate	Extended spectrum cephalosporin or trimethoprim-sulfamethoxazole, **PLUS** clindamycin	Ampicillin-sulbactam **PLUS** gentamicin **OR** ticarcillin-clavulanate	Clindamycin **PLUS** gentamicin
Human	Streptococci, *S aureus*, *Eikenella corrodens*, anaerobes	Amoxicillin-clavulanate	Trimethoprim-sulfamethoxazole **PLUS** clindamycin	Ampicillin-sulbactam	Extended spectrum cephalosporin or trimethoprim-sulfamethoxazole **PLUS** clindamycin

* In patients with history of allergy to penicillin or one of its many congeners, alternative drugs are recommended. In some circumstances, a cephalosporin or other ß-lactam class drug may be acceptable. However, these drugs should not be used in patients with an immediate hypersensitivity (anaphylaxis) to penicillin because approximately 5% to 15% of penicillin-allergic patients also will be allergic to the cephalosporins.

must be weighed against the risk of dental staining. Oral or parenteral treatment with trimethoprim-sulfamethoxazole, which is effective against *S aureus, P multocida,* and *Eikenella corrodens,* in conjunction with clindamycin, which is active in vitro against anaerobic bacteria, streptococci, and *S aureus,* may be effective in preventing bite wound infections. Cefotaxime or ceftriaxone can be used as alternative parenteral therapy for penicillin-allergic patients who can tolerate cephalosporins; clindamycin is the alternative for those who also are cephalosporin-allergic. Metronidazole has an excellent anaerobic spectrum of antibacterial activity and has been used, instead of clindamycin, for that purpose.

CONTROL MEASURES FOR PREVENTION OF TICK-BORNE INFECTIONS

Tick-borne infectious pediatric diseases that can occur in the United States include diseases caused by spirochetes (eg, Lyme disease), rickettsia (eg, Rocky Mountain spotted fever and ehrlichiosis), bacteria (tularemia), viruses (Colorado tick fever), and protozoa (babesiosis). Control of these and other tick-borne diseases requires preventing infected ticks from biting and engorging on humans, or at least minimizing opportunities for them to do so. Physicians should be aware of the epidemiology of tick-borne infections in their local area. Control of the tick population in the field is not always a practical public health measure. Specific control measures for prevention are as follows:

• Physicians, parents, and children, whenever possible, should be aware of the possibility of acquisition of disease from ticks.
• Tick-infested areas should be avoided whenever possible.
• If a tick-infested area is entered, protective clothing that covers the arms, legs, and other exposed areas should be worn. Other measures include tucking pants into boots or socks and buttoning long-sleeved shirts at the cuff. In addition, permethrin (a synthetic pyrethyroid) is effective in decreasing tick attachment and can be sprayed onto clothes. Permethrin toxicity includes itching, edema, erythema, temporary burning, stinging, numbness, and tingling of exposed skin. No systemic reactions have been reported.
• Tick and insect repellents* containing DEET† applied to the skin provide additional protection but require reapplication every 1 to 2 hours for effectiveness. While seizures in young children have been reported coincident with application of DEET-containing insect repellents, the risk is very low when it is used according to product label directions. Accordingly, DEET should be applied sparingly and according to product label duration and only to exposed skin, not to a child's face, hands, or irritated or abraded skin. These preparations should be removed by washing after the child comes indoors.

Persons should be taught to inspect themselves and their children's bodies and clothing daily after possible tick exposure. Special attention should be given to the

---

* For further information, see Insect repellents. *Med Letter.* 1989;31:45-47.
† Diethyltoluamide.

exposed hairy regions of the body, including the head and neck in children, where ticks often attach.

Ticks should be removed promptly. Care should be taken to avoid squeezing the body of the tick. It should be grasped with a fine tweezer close to the skin and removed by gently pulling the tick straight out without twisting motions. If fingers are used to remove ticks, they should be protected with facial tissue and washed after removal of the tick.

Daily inspection of pets and removal of ticks are indicated.

Summaries of Infectious Diseases

Actinomycosis

CLINICAL MANIFESTATIONS: The three major types of disease are cervicofacial, thoracic, and abdominal. Cervicofacial lesions frequently occur after tooth extraction or facial trauma, or are associated with carious teeth. Localized pain and induration progress to "woody hard," nodular lesions that can be complicated by draining sinus tracts. The infection usually spreads by direct invasion of adjacent tissues. It may also contribute to chronic obstructive tonsillitis. Thoracic disease is most commonly secondary to aspiration of oropharyngeal secretions; it rarely occurs after esophageal disruption secondary to surgery or nonpenetrating trauma. Disease manifests as pneumonia, which can be complicated by the development of abscesses, empyema, and, rarely, pleurodermal sinuses. In abdominal infection, the appendix and cecum are the most frequent sites, and symptoms simulate those of appendicitis. Intra-abdominal abscesses and peritoneal-dermal draining sinuses eventually develop.

ETIOLOGY: *Actinomyces israelii* is the usual cause. *Actinomyces israelii*, other *Actinomyces*, and *Arachnia* (a related genus) species are slow-growing, Gram-positive, anaerobic bacteria that can be part of the normal oral flora.

EPIDEMIOLOGY: *Actinomyces* species are worldwide in distribution. Infection is rare in infants and children, and occurs sporadically. The organisms are components of the endogenous gastrointestinal tract flora. Disease results from penetrating trauma (including human bite wounds) and from nonpenetrating trauma. Actinomycosis is not contagious.

The **incubation period** is variable and probably is many years, following oral colonization and days to months after trauma.

DIAGNOSTIC TESTS: A microscopic demonstration of beaded, branched, Gram-positive bacilli in pus suggests the diagnosis. Sulfur granules in drainage or loculations of pus, which are usually yellow and may be visualized microscopically or macroscopically, indicate the diagnosis, when present. A Gram stain of sulfur granules discloses a dense reticulum of filaments; the ends of individual filaments may project around the periphery of the granule, with or without radially arranged hyaline clubs. For recovery of the organism, specimens must be cultured anaerobically on semiselective media in a carbon dioxide-enriched environment.

TREATMENT: Initial therapy should include intravenous penicillin G or ampicillin for 4 to 6 weeks, and is followed by high doses of oral penicillin, amoxicillin, erythromycin, clindamycin, minocycline, or tetracycline for a total of 6 to 12 months of therapy. Minocycline and tetracycline are not recommended for children younger than 8 years. Surgical drainage may be necessary.

ISOLATION OF THE HOSPITALIZED PATIENT: Standard precautions are recommended.

CONTROL MEASURES: Good oral hygiene, adequate regular dental care, and careful cleansing of wounds (including human bite wounds) can prevent infection.

Adenovirus Infections

CLINICAL MANIFESTATIONS: The major clinical syndromes caused by adenoviruses involve upper respiratory tract symptoms accompanied by moderate systemic manifestations in children and adolescents. Severe pneumonia, which is occasionally fatal, can occur in younger infants and, less commonly, in older children and adolescents. Disease is often more severe in immunocompromised patients. Conjunctivitis is common, either alone or in combination with pharyngitis and other respiratory symptoms, and in young children may mimic preseptal cellulitis. They can cause gastroenteritis. The illness is similar to, although less common than, that caused by rotavirus. Adenoviruses are infrequent causes of a pertussis-like syndrome, croup, bronchiolitis, and hemorrhagic cystitis.

ETIOLOGY: Adenoviruses are DNA viruses; 47 distinct serotypes cause human infections. Types 31, 40, and 41 are causes of gastroenteritis.

EPIDEMIOLOGY: Infection in infants and children occurs at any age. Adenoviruses causing respiratory infection are transmitted usually through respiratory secretions by person-to-person contact, fomites, and aerosols. Respiratory adenoviruses also are found in feces. Because adenoviruses are stable in the environment, fomites may be important in transmission. Enteric strains of adenoviruses are transmitted by the fecal-oral route. Other routes have not been clearly defined and may vary with age, type of infection, and environmental or other factors. The eyes can provide a portal of entry; eg, infections have resulted from direct introduction of virus by the use of contaminated ophthalmologic instruments. Epidemics attributed to contaminated swimming pools have occurred. Shared towels and direct inoculation by fingers are involved in epidemic keratoconjunctivitis. Epidemics in military and educational institutions and those resulting from a common source have occurred. Nosocomial outbreaks of adenoviral respiratory and gastrointestinal infections have been documented. The incidence of adenovirus-induced respiratory disease is slightly increased in late winter, spring, and early summer. Enteric disease occurs during most of the year and primarily affects children younger than 4 years. Adenovirus infections are most communicable during the first few days of an acute illness, but persistent and intermittent shedding during longer periods, even months, is frequent. Asymptomatic infections are common.

The incubation period for respiratory infection varies from 2 to 14 days; for gastroenteritis, it is 3 to 10 days.

DIAGNOSTIC TESTS: Adenoviruses can be isolated from pharyngeal secretions, eye swabs, and feces by inoculation of specimens into a variety of cell cultures. A pharyngeal isolate is more suggestive of recent infection than is a fecal isolate, which may indicate prolonged carriage or recent infection. Adenovirus antigen has been detected in body fluids of infected patients by immunoassay techniques. These techniques are especially useful in the diagnosis of diarrheal disease, because the enteric adenovirus types 40 and 41 usually cannot be isolated in standard cell cultures. Enteric adenoviruses also can be identified by electron microscopy of stool specimens. Multiple serologic tests, including fluorescent antibody and enzyme immunoassay (EIA), are now commercially available for antigen and antibody testing. By complement fixation and EIA tests that detect antibody to the common adenovirus antigen (hexon), a fourfold or greater rise in antibody titer in paired acute and convalescent sera is diagnostic of recent infection. Adenoviruses can be serotyped by hemagglutination inhibition or neutralization assays, and by EIA for types 40 and 41. Type-specific antibodies are detectable by hemagglutination inhibition or neutralization techniques.

TREATMENT: Supportive.

ISOLATION OF THE HOSPITALIZED PATIENT*: For young children with respiratory infection, contact and droplet precautions are indicated for the duration of hospitalization. For patients with conjunctivitis, contact precautions are recommended. For diapered and/or incontinent children with adenoviral gastroenteritis contact precautions are indicated for the duration of the illness.

CONTROL MEASURES: Children who participate in group child care, particularly those between the ages of 6 months and 2 years, are at increased risk of adenoviral respiratory infection and gastroenteritis. Measures for preventing spread of adenovirus infection in this setting have not been determined, but frequent hand washing is recommended.

Adequate chlorination of swimming pools is recommended to prevent pharyngoconjunctival fever. Epidemic keratoconjunctivitis associated with ophthalmologic practice can be difficult to control and requires use of single-dose medication dispensing, strict attention to hand washing and instrument sterilization procedures, and cohorting of patients and staff based on infection status.

Health care personnel with known or suspected adenoviral conjunctivitis should avoid direct patient contact, but meticulous hand washing and wearing gloves are recommended in all circumstances. Because adenoviruses are particularly difficult to eliminate from the skin, fomites, and environmental surfaces, assiduous adherence to hand washing and other infection control procedures is required.

Live enteric-coated adenovirus vaccines containing types 4, 7, and 21 have been used successfully to reduce acute respiratory disease among military personnel, but these vaccines are not available for civilian use.

---

* In addition to standard precautions.

Amebiasis

CLINICAL MANIFESTATIONS: The clinical syndromes associated with *Entamoeba histolytica* infection are multiple and varied. They include intestinal disease, which may be asymptomatic or have nonspecific or mild symptoms such as abdominal distention, flatulence, constipation, and, occasionally, loose stools. Other persons may have nondysenteric colitis, with intermittent diarrhea and abdominal pain, or acute amebic colitis (dysentery) associated with abdominal cramps, tenesmus, and diarrhea containing blood and mucus. Progressive involvement of the colon may produce toxic megacolon, fulminant colitis, ulceration of the colon and perianal area, and rarely perforation. An ameboma may present as an annular lesion of the colon that can be mistaken for colonic carcinoma or as a tender extrahepatic mass mimicking a pyogenic abscess.

Extraintestinal disease, found in a small percentage of patients, may occur in a number of organs, including the lung, pericardium, brain, and genitourinary tract, but the liver is the most common site. Liver abscess may present acutely with fever and abdominal pain, tachypnea, and liver tenderness, or subacutely with weight loss, vague abdominal symptoms, and irritability. Rupture of abscesses into the abdomen or chest can lead to death. Pericardial abscesses with tamponade can occur. Evidence of recent intestinal infection is frequently absent. Diarrhea occurs concurrently in 30% to 40% of patients, and the abdominal pain, usually most prominent in the right upper quadrant, may be accompanied by a nonproductive cough and right shoulder pain from diaphragmatic involvement. The liver usually is tender, and most patients have hepatomegaly; jaundice and impaired liver function occur occasionally.

ETIOLOGY: *Entamoeba histolytica* is a protozoan that is excreted as cysts or trophozoites in the stool of infected patients.

EPIDEMIOLOGY: *Entamoeba histolytica* and *E dispar*, which is morphologically indistinguishable from *E histolytica* but nonpathogenic, cause infection worldwide, which is estimated to involve 10% or more of the world's population. Infection rates in tropical areas can be as high as 20% to 50% and in those living in temperate climates as high as 5%, with an estimated 4% prevalence in the United States. Infection with *E histolytica* is transmitted via amebic cysts by the fecal-oral route. Ingested cysts, which are unaffected by gastric acid and dissolve in the alkaline small intestine, produce trophozoites that infect the colon. Cysts that subsequently develop are the source of transmission, especially from asymptomatic cyst excretors. Infected patients excrete cysts intermittently and sometimes for years if untreated. Transmission occasionally has been associated with contaminated food, water, and enema equipment. Risk factors for acquisition of *E histolytica* infection include lower socioeconomic areas with crowding, poor sanitation, and lack of proper indoor plumbing and promiscuity among homosexual males. More severe disease is associated with immunosuppression, malnutrition, young age, and residence in tropical countries.

The **incubation period** is variable, ranging from a few days to months or years, but commonly is 1 to 4 weeks.

DIAGNOSTIC TESTS: Intestinal infection depends on identifying trophozoites or cysts in the stool. Examination of serial samples may be necessary. Specimens, which include liquid stool obtained within 1 to 2 hours of passage, endoscopy scrapings, and biopsies, should be examined by wet mount and fixed in formalin and polyvinyl alcohol (available in kits) for concentration and permanent staining. *Entamoeba histolytica* can be differentiated from nonpathogenic species, such as *E hartmanni*, and *E coli*, by morphology.

Serum anti-amebic antibody tests may be helpful, primarily in the diagnosis of extraintestinal amebiasis with liver involvement. Patients with amebic dysentery or who are asymptomatic cyst excretors are much less likely to demonstrate diagnostic serologic responses. Results of the standard serologic tests are negative in those infected with *E dispar.*

Ultrasound and computed tomography can be effective in identifying liver abscesses and other extraintestinal sites of infection. Aspirates from a liver abscess may be examined for trophozoites, but organisms are often not found.

TREATMENT*: Treatment involves the elimination of the tissue-invading trophozoites as well as the cysts in the intestinal lumen. The following regimens are recommended:

- **Asymptomatic cyst excretors (intraluminal infections):** iodoquinol; alternatively paromomycin or diloxanide furoate[†] which are luminal amebicides.
- **Patients with mild to moderate intestinal symptoms with no dysentery:** metronidazole (or tinidazole[‡]) followed by a therapeutic course of a luminal amebicide.
- **Patients with dysentery or extraintestinal disease (including liver abscess):** metronidazole (or tinidazole[‡]) followed by a therapeutic course of a luminal amebicide.

Dehydroemetine[†] followed by a therapeutic course of a luminal amebicide should be considered for patients for whom treatment of invasive disease has failed. Liver abscess alternatively may be treated with chloroquine phosphate concomitantly with dehydroemetine,[†] followed by metronidazole (or tinidazole[‡]).

To prevent spontaneous rupture of the abscess, patients with large liver abscesses may benefit from percutaneous or surgical aspiration.

ISOLATION OF THE HOSPITALIZED PATIENT: Standard precautions are recommended for both symptomatic and asymptomatic patients.

CONTROL MEASURES: Careful hand washing after defecation, sanitary disposal of fecal material, and treatment of drinking water will control the spread of infection. Sexual transmission may be controlled by using condoms.

---

* For further information, see also Drugs for Parasitic Infections, p 637.

† Available from the Centers for Disease Control and Prevention Drug Service (see Directory of Telephone Numbers, p 667).

‡ Tinidazole is a nitro-imidazole similar to metronidazole, which is not available in the United States, that appears at least as effective as metronidazole and to be better tolerated.

Amebic Meningoencephalitis and Keratitis
(*Naegleria fowleri, Acanthamoeba* and *Balamuthia* Species)

CLINICAL MANIFESTATIONS: *Naegleria fowleri* can cause a rapidly progressive, almost always fatal, primary amebic meningoencephalitis. Early symptoms include fever, headache, and sometimes disturbances of smell and/or taste. The illness rapidly progresses to signs of meningoencephalitis, including nuchal rigidity, lethargy, confusion, and altered level of consciousness. Seizures are common. Death may occur soon after the onset of symptoms. No distinct clinical features differentiate this disease from fulminant bacterial meningitis (except possibly the history of recent swimming in warm water).

Granulomatous amebic encephalitis caused by *Acanthamoeba* species and *Balamuthia* species has a more insidious onset and progression of manifestations occurring weeks to months after exposure and is more common in immunocompromised persons. Signs and symptoms may include personality changes, seizures, headaches, nuchal rigidity, ataxia, cranial nerve palsies, hemiparesis, and other focal deficits. Fever is often low-grade and intermittent. Skin ulcers may be present. The course may resemble that of a bacterial brain abscess or a brain tumor.

Amebic keratitis occurs primarily in those who wear contact lenses and resembles keratitis caused by herpes simplex, bacteria, or fungi, except for a usually more indolent course. Corneal inflammation, photophobia, and secondary uveitis are the predominant features.

ETIOLOGY: *Naegleria fowleri, Acanthamoeba,* and *Balamuthia* species are small, free-living amebae.

EPIDEMIOLOGY: *Naegleria fowleri* is found in warm, fresh water and moist soil. Most infections with *N fowleri* have been associated with swimming in warm, natural bodies of water, but other sources have included tap water, contaminated swimming pools, and baths. Small outbreaks associated with swimming in a warm lake or swimming pool have been reported. A few cases with no history of contact with water, however, have occurred. Disease has been reported worldwide, but is uncommon. In the United States, infection occurs primarily in the summer and usually affects children and young adults. The trophozoites of the parasite directly invade the brain from the nose along the olfactory nerves via the cribriform plate.

The incubation period of *N fowleri* infection is several days to 1 week.

The causative organisms, especially *Acanthamoeba* species, of granulomatous amebic encephalitis are distributed worldwide and are found in soil, fresh and brackish water, dust, hot tubs, and sewage. Infection occurs primarily in debilitated and immunocompromised persons. However, some patients have had no demonstrable underlying disease or defect. Acquisition probably occurs by inhalation or direct contact with contaminated soil or water. The primary focus of infection is most likely the skin or respiratory tract, and spread to the brain is hematogenous.

Acanthamoeba organisms also cause dendritic keratitis mimicking herpes keratitis in persons who wear contact lenses using contaminated saline solutions or tap water rinses for lens care.

The **incubation period** of these infections are unknown.

DIAGNOSTIC TESTS: *Naegleria fowleri* infection can be documented by microscopic demonstration of the motile trophozoites on a wet mount of centrifuged cerebrospinal fluid (CSF). The organism also can be cultured on 1.5% nonnutrient agar layered with enteric bacteria or in Page saline. Immunofluorescent tests to determine the species of the organism are available through the Centers for Disease Control and Prevention.

In infection with *Acanthamoeba* species, cysts can be visualized in sections of brain or corneal tissue and may be present in brain biopsy specimens, but they are seldom seen in CSF examination. The organism also can be cultured by the same method as that for *N fowleri*.

TREATMENT: If meningoencephalitis caused by *N fowleri* is suspected because of the presence of organisms in the CSF, therapy should not be withheld while waiting for the results of confirmatory diagnostic tests. Treatment, however, is often unsuccessful. Amphotericin B is the drug of choice, although only a few cases of survival with complete recovery have been documented. Recovery has occurred with therapy with amphotericin B only or combined with other agents, such as miconazole and rifampin. Early diagnosis and the institution of high-dose drug therapy is probably important in achieving a satisfactory outcome.

Effective treatment for central nervous system infections caused by *Acanthamoeba* species has not been established. Only one case of partial recovery, an adult treated with sulfamethazine, has been reported. Experimental infections can be prevented or cured by sulfadiazine. Strains of *Acanthamoeba* isolated from patients with fatal encephalitis are usually sensitive in vitro to pentamidine, ketoconazole, flucytosine, clotrimazole, and, to a lesser degree, amphotericin B.

Some patients with keratitis due to *Acanthamoeba* organisms have been treated successfully with combinations of topical propamidine, neomycin, polyhexamethylene biguanide, and various azoles (eg, miconazole, clotrimazole, fluconazole, or itraconazole), as well as topical corticosteroids.

ISOLATION OF THE HOSPITALIZED PATIENT: Standard precautions are recommended.

CONTROL MEASURES: People should avoid swimming in hot springs and other bodies of warm, polluted fresh water. *Acanthamoeba* organisms are resistant to freezing, drying, and the usual concentrations of chlorine found in drinking water and swimming pools.

Only sterile saline solutions should be used to clean contact lenses.

Anthrax

CLINICAL MANIFESTATIONS: The spectrum of illness includes cutaneous (malignant pustule), inhalational (woolsorter's disease), oropharyngeal, gastrointestinal, septicemic, and meningeal anthrax. Cutaneous anthrax, which accounts for 95% of the cases in the United States, is characterized by a painless lesion that progresses from a papule to a vesicle to necrosis and, eventually, to eschar formation. In inhalational anthrax, mild upper respiratory tract symptoms occur initially; severe dyspnea, cyanosis, tachycardia, tachypnea, diaphoresis, fever, rales, and, usually, death occur approximately 2 to 5 days later. Gastrointestinal disease is characterized by abdominal pain and distention, vomiting, bloody diarrhea, and, frequently, toxemia and shock. Pharyngeal anthrax with profound submental swelling has also been reported. Septicemia and hemorrhagic meningitis are secondary manifestations of cutaneous, inhalational, or gastrointestinal anthrax. Disease manifestations are similar in adults and children.

ETIOLOGY: *Bacillus anthracis* is a Gram-positive, encapsulated, spore-forming, nonmotile rod.

EPIDEMIOLOGY: Anthrax is a zoonotic disease endemic in many rural regions of the world. It is common in developing countries but is rarely reported in the United States. Human disease occurs after contact with infected animals or their contaminated products. Spores of *B anthracis* are found on hides, carcasses, hair, wool, bone meal, and other by-products of domesticated and wild animals, such as goats, sheep, cattle, swine, horses, buffalo, and deer. Imported dolls and toys decorated with infected hair or hides have been a source of infection. The spore form of the organism has been found in soil in rural farming regions in several areas of the United States. Spores can remain viable for 40 years or more.

Cutaneous anthrax, which occurs principally in agricultural and industrial employees, results from contact with infected animals, carcasses, hair (especially goat hair), wool, or hides. Inhalation anthrax is extremely rare, and has resulted from inhalation of spores aerosolized during industrial processing of animal by-products or laboratory work with *B anthracis*. In gastrointestinal anthrax, ingestion of contaminated, undercooked meat is the mode of acquisition. Biting flies and other insects also may serve as mechanical vectors. Discharges from cutaneous lesions are potentially infectious; accidental infections have occurred in laboratory workers. *Bacillus anthracis* is not known to be transmitted from person to person.

The **incubation period** is 1 to 7 days; most cases occur within 2 to 5 days of exposure.

DIAGNOSTIC TESTS: The following procedures can be used for diagnosis: (1) microscopic visualization of *B anthracis* on direct Gram-stained smears and/or cultures on blood agar of lesions or discharges; (2) fluorescent antibody identification of the organisms in vesicle fluid, cultures, or tissue sections; and (3) detection of antibody to *B anthracis* toxin by enzyme immunoassay and/or immunoblot.

TREATMENT: Penicillin is the antimicrobial of choice and is given for 5 to 7 days. Erythromycin, tetracycline, chloramphenicol, and ciprofloxacin are also effective. High-dose penicillin combined with streptomycin, or possibly parenteral ciprofloxacin, should be used for treating meningitis or inhalational anthrax. Ciprofloxacin should not be used in patients younger than 18 years unless the possible benefits are considered to be greater than the potential risks, and tetracyclines usually should not be given to children younger than 8 years (see Antimicrobials and Related Therapy, p 605).

ISOLATION OF THE HOSPITALIZED PATIENT: Standard precautions are recommended. Contaminated dressings and bedclothes should be burned or steam sterilized to destroy spores.

CONTROL MEASURES: A cell-free vaccine has been developed for persons at significant, continuing risk of acquiring anthrax. The vaccine is effective in preventing or significantly reducing the occurrence of cutaneous anthrax in adults, and it causes minimal adverse effects. No data on vaccine effectiveness or reactogenicity in children are available, and the vaccine is not currently licensed for use in children or pregnant women.*

Surveillance and control of industrial and agricultural sources of *B anthracis* by public health authorities are important.

Arboviruses
(Including Dengue, Japanese Encephalitis, and Yellow Fever)

CLINICAL MANIFESTATIONS: Some arboviruses cause principally a central nervous system infection. Others produce an undifferentiated febrile illness, fever with rash, hemorrhagic manifestations, hepatitis, myalgia, or polyarthritis. Other organ systems also can be involved.

ETIOLOGY: Approximately 570 arthropod-borne viruses, commonly referred to as arboviruses, have been identified. Although originally classified together because of a common mode of transmission, the viruses belong to a variety of taxonomic groups principally in the families *Bunyaviridae, Togaviridae,* and *Flaviviridae* (Table 3.1, p 138). Of the more than 230 recognized arboviruses in the Western hemisphere, more than 30 have been demonstrated to be human pathogens.

EPIDEMIOLOGY: Most arboviruses are maintained in nature through cycles of transmission among birds or small mammals by arthropod vectors, such as mosquitoes, ticks, and phlebotomine flies. Humans and domestic animals are infected incidentally as "dead-end" hosts. Important exceptions include **dengue, yellow fever, Oropouche,** and **Chikungunya** viruses that infected vectors spread from person to person. Direct person-to-person spread does not occur. **Colorado tick fever** has been transmitted through transfusion. In the United States, mosquito-borne arboviral infections usually occur in late summer and early fall. During epidemics of arboviral encephalitis, persons of all ages may be infected, but most infections are asymptomatic. **St Louis encephalitis** and **Western equine encephalitis** are more likely to produce clinical manifestations in the elderly than in children, whereas **California encephalitis** (eg, **LaCrosse virus** infection) occurs almost exclusively in children younger than 15 years. The prevalence of various arboviral diseases is related to ecologic and climatic conditions that affect the natural transmission cycles.

The **incubation periods** and geographic distributions of the principal arboviral infections of the Western hemisphere are given in Tables 3.2 and 3.3 (p 139 and p 140).

---

* Available from the Michigan Biologic Products Institute, Lansing, Mich (see Directory of Telephone Numbers, p 667).

Table 3.1. **Taxonomy of Major Arboviruses**

Family	Genus	Representative Agents
Bunyaviridae	*Bunyavirus*	California serogroup viruses (North and South America, Europe, Asia)
		Oropouche virus (South America)
	Phlebovirus	Sand fly fever virus (Europe, Africa, Asia)
		Toscana virus (Europe)
Togaviridae	*Alphavirus*	Western equine encephalitis virus (North and South America)
		Eastern equine encephalitis virus (North and South America)
		Venezuelan equine encephalitis virus (North and South America)
		Mayaro virus (South America)
		Chikungunya virus (Africa, Asia)
		Ross River virus (Oceania, Australia)
		O'nyong-nyong virus (Africa)
		Sindbis virus (Africa, Scandinavia, former Soviet Union, Asia, Australia)
Flaviviridae	*Flavivirus*	St Louis encephalitis virus (North and South America)
		Japanese encephalitis virus (Asia)
		Dengue viruses (types 1–4) (tropics, worldwide)
		Yellow fever virus (South America, Africa)
		Murray Valley encephalitis virus (Australia)
		West Nile virus (Europe, Africa, Asia)
		Tick-borne encephalitis complex viruses (Europe and Asia)
		Powassan virus (North America, Asia)
Reoviridae	*Orbivirus*	Colorado tick fever (US, Canada, Asia)
Rhabdoviridae	*Rhabdovirus*	Vesicular stomatitis virus (Western hemisphere)

DIAGNOSTIC TESTS: A definitive diagnosis can be made by serologic testing or by viral isolation, techniques that are only available in a few state, research, and reference laboratories. In **dengue, yellow fever, Colorado tick fever, sand fly fever, Chikungunya, epidemic polyarthritis, Oropouche fever,** and **Venezuelan equine encephalitis** infection, virus can be isolated from blood obtained in the acute phase of illness. In cases of encephalitis, viral isolation in cell culture should be attempted from biopsied or postmortem brain tissue. Serological antibody tests confirm the diagnosis, but detailed knowledge of previous immunizations and travel as well as of the interpretation and specificity of serologic tests are required for correct interpretation. Detection of virus-specific IgM antibody in cerebrospinal fluid is diagnostic.

TREATMENT: Supportive.

Table 3.2. Arboviral Infections of the Central Nervous System Occurring in the Western Hemisphere

Diseases (Causal Agent*)	Geographic Distribution of Virus	Incubation Period, d
California encephalitis (primarily LaCrosse and several other California serogroup viruses)	Widespread in the US and Canada, including the Yukon and Northwest Territories; most prevalent in upper Midwest	5–15
Eastern equine encephalitis (Eastern equine encephalitis virus)	Central and eastern seaboard and Gulf states of the US (isolated inland foci); Canada; South and Central America	3–10
Powassan encephalitis (Powassan virus)	Canada; northeastern, north central, and western US	4–18
St Louis encephalitis (St Louis encephalitis virus)	Widespread: central, southern, northeastern, and western US; Manitoba and southern Ontario; Caribbean area; South America	4–21
Venezuelan equine encephalitis (Venezuelan equine encephalitis virus)	Florida, Mexico; Central and South America	2–4
Western equine encephalitis (Western equine encephalitis virus)	Central and western US; Canada; Argentina, Uruguay, Brazil	5–10

* All are mosquito-borne except Powassan encephalitis, which is tick-borne.

ISOLATION OF THE HOSPITALIZED PATIENT: Standard precautions are recommended for viremic patients with dengue, yellow fever, sand fly fever, Oropouche fever, Venezuelan equine encephalitis, Chikungunya virus infection, epidemic polyarthritis, and Colorado tick fever.

CONTROL MEASURES:

Active Immunization.

Yellow Fever Vaccine. The vaccine is a live attenuated virus (17D strain) available at state-approved vaccination centers. A single vaccination is accepted by international authorities as providing protection for periods of at least 10 years and may well confer life-long immunity.

Immunization is recommended for all individuals 9 months or older living in or traveling to endemic areas and is required by international regulations for travel to and from certain countries. **Infants younger than 4 months should not be immunized,** because they are at increased susceptibility to encephalitis temporally associated with yellow fever vaccination. The decision to immunize infants between 4 and 9 months of age should be based upon estimates of the infant's risk of exposure (eg, infants older than 4 months who must travel to an area of ongoing endemic or epidemic activity may receive the vaccine if a high degree of protection against mosquito exposure is not feasible). If possible, cholera vaccine, when indicated,

Table 3.3. **Acute, Febrile Diseases and Hemorrhagic Fevers Caused By Arboviruses in the Western Hemisphere That Are Not Characterized by Encephalitis**

Agent*/Disease	Geographic Distribution of Virus	Clinical Syndrome	Incubation Period, d
Yellow fever virus/ yellow fever	Tropical areas of South America and Africa	Febrile illness, hepatitis, hemorrhagic fever	3–6
Dengue virus types 1 to 4/dengue fever/dengue hemorrhagic fever	Tropical areas worldwide: Caribbean, Central and South America, Asia, Australia, Oceania, Africa	Febrile illness—may be biphasic with rash; hemorrhagic fever and shock	3–14
Mayaro virus/ Mayaro fever	Central and South America	Febrile illness and polyarthritis	1–12
Chikungunya virus	Africa, Asia	Febrile illness rash and polyarthritis	1–12
O'Nyong-nyong virus	Africa	Febrile illness rash and polyarthritis	1–12
Sindbis virus	Africa, Scandinavia, former Soviet Union countries, Asia, Australia	Febrile illness rash and polyarthritis	1–12
Ross River virus	Australia, Oceania	Febrile illness rash and polyarthritis	1–12
Colorado tick fever (Colorado tick fever virus)	South Dakota, Rocky Mountain and Pacific states; western Canada; Asia	Febrile illness—may be biphasic	3–6
Oropouche fever (Oropouche virus)	Central and South America	Febrile illness	2–6

* All are mosquito-borne except Colorado tick fever, which is tick-borne, and Oropouche fever, which is midge-borne.

should not be given concurrently with yellow fever vaccine; ideally, administration of these vaccinations should be separated by at least 3 weeks.

Yellow fever vaccine is prepared in embryonated eggs and contains egg protein, which may cause allergic reactions. Persons who have experienced signs or symptoms of anaphylactic reaction after eating eggs should be excused from vaccination and issued a medical waiver letter to meet health regulations or they should be skin tested according to the package insert before vaccination (also see Hypersensitivity Reactions to Vaccine Constituents, p 32). Pregnant women should not be vaccinated except in high-risk areas. The decision to immunize immunocompromised patients is based on assessment of the patient's risk of exposure and clinical status.

Japanese Encephalitis (JE) Vaccine. *This vaccine is an inactivated vaccine derived from infected mouse brain and is recommended for expatriates living in Asia and for certain travelers.

* Produced in Japan and distributed in the United States by Connaught Laboratories, Swiftwater, Pa.

Vaccine is recommended for (1) persons who will be residing in areas where JE virus is endemic or epidemic; and for (2) travelers planning prolonged stays (more than 30 days) in endemic areas during the transmission season, especially if travel includes rural areas, and/or their activities or itinerary place them at increased risk of exposure (eg, travel into an epidemic focus, bicycling, camping or other unprotected outdoor activity in rural area). Current information on locations of JE virus transmission and detailed information on vaccine recommendations can be obtained from the Centers for Disease Control and Prevention (see Directory of Telephone Numbers, p 667) and from the recommendations of the Advisory Committee on Immunization Practices.*

The recommended primary immunization series is three doses of 1.0 mL each, administered subcutaneously on days 0, 7, and 30. An abbreviated schedule of 0, 7, and 14 days can be used when the longer schedule is precluded by time constraints. The regimen for children 1 to 3 years of age is identical except that each dose is 0.5 mL. No data are available on vaccine safety and efficacy in infants (younger than 12 months).

Other Arboviral Vaccines. An inactivated vaccine for tick-borne encephalitis is licensed in some countries in Europe where the disease is endemic, but it is not available in the United States.

Protection Against Vectors. Public health measures to control arthropod vectors are important. Individuals can help protect themselves by wearing long-sleeved shirts and trousers, and by using insect repellents. Permethrin applied to clothing kills adherent ticks and mosquitoes. Repellents containing DEET† should be applied to exposed skin only and used sparingly. Travelers to tropical countries should bring mosquito bed nets and aerosol insecticide sprays to reduce the risk of mosquito bites at night. The principal vectors of **dengue** and **yellow fever** bite during daytime hours, but many other vector and pest mosquitoes are most active in twilight hours.

Arcanobacterium haemolyticum Infections

CLINICAL MANIFESTATIONS: *Arcanobacterium haemolyticum* appears to be a cause of both pharyngitis and cutaneous infections, although its pathogenicity has not been clearly defined. Acute pharyngitis due to *A haemolyticum* often is indistinguishable from that caused by group A streptococci. Fever, pharyngeal exudate, lymphadenopathy, rash, and pruritis are common, but palatal petechiae and strawberry tongue are absent. In nearly half of all reported cases, a maculopapular exanthem is present, beginning on the extensor surfaces of the distal extremities, spreading centripetally to the chest and back and sparing the face, palms, and soles.

Skin infections, including chronic ulceration, cellulitis, paronychia, and wound infection have been attributed to *A haemolyticum*. Invasive infections including

---

* Inactivated Japanese encephalitis virus vaccine. Recommendations of the Advisory Committee on Immunization Practices (ACIP). *MMWR.* 1993;42(No. RR-1):1-15.
† Diethyltoluamide.

septicemia, peritonsillar abscess, brain abscess, meningitis, endocarditis, osteomyelitis, and pneumonia also have been reported.

ETIOLOGY: *Arcanobacterium haemolyticum* is a Gram-positive bacillus, formerly classified as *Corynebacterium haemolyticum*.

EPIDEMIOLOGY: Humans are the primary reservoir of *A haemolyticum*. Pharyngitis occurs primarily in adolescents and young adults. Although long-term pharyngeal carriage with *A haemolyticum* has been described following an episode of acute pharyngitis, isolation of the bacterium from the nasopharynx of asymptomatic persons is rare. *Arcanobacterium haemolyticum* may be an important cause of tropical ulcers.

The **incubation period** is unknown.

DIAGNOSTIC TESTS: *Arcanobacterium haemolyticum* can be recovered on blood-enriched agar cultures, but growth may be slow and hemolytic colonies may not be visible for 48 to 72 hours after inoculation. Detection is enhanced by culture on human or rabbit blood agar as both larger colony growth and wider zones of hemolysis than that on sheep blood agar occur. Growth also is enhanced by the addition of 5% CO_2. Serologic tests for antibodies to *A haemolyticum* have been used in epidemiologic investigations, but they have not been standardized and are not available commercially.

TREATMENT: Erythromycin is the drug of choice, but to date no prospective therapeutic trials have been performed. *Arcanobacterium haemolyticum* is susceptible in vitro to erythromycin, clindamycin, chloramphenicol, and tetracycline; susceptibility to penicillin is variable. Resistance to trimethoprim-sulfamethoxazole is common.

ISOLATION OF THE HOSPITALIZED PATIENT: Standard precautions are recommended.

CONTROL MEASURES: None.

Ascaris lumbricoides Infections

CLINICAL MANIFESTATIONS: Nonspecific gastrointestinal symptoms occur in some patients, but the frequency is unknown. During the larval migratory phase, an acute transient pneumonitis (Löffler's syndrome) associated with fever and marked eosinophilia may occur. Acute intestinal obstruction may develop in patients with heavy infections. Children are more prone to this complication because they have smaller diameters of the intestinal lumen and often have large numbers of worms. Worm migration can cause peritonitis, secondary to intestinal wall penetration, and common bile duct obstruction resulting in acute obstructive jaundice. The adult worms can be stimulated to migrate by stressful conditions (eg, fever, illness, or anesthesia) and by some anthelmintic drugs. *Ascaris lumbricoides* has been found in the appendiceal lumen in acute appendicitis, but a causal relationship is uncertain.

ETIOLOGY: *Ascaris lumbricoides* is a large roundworm of humans.

EPIDEMIOLOGY: The adult worms live in the small intestine. Females produce 200 000 eggs per day, which are excreted in the stool and must incubate in soil for 2 to 3 weeks for the embryo to form and to become infectious. Ingestion of infective eggs from contaminated soil results in infection, which often is asymptomatic. Larvae hatch in the small intestine, penetrate the mucosa, and are passively transported by portal blood to the liver and subsequently to the lungs. They then ascend through the tracheobronchial tree to the pharynx, are swallowed, and mature into adults in the small intestine. The interval between ingestion of the egg and the development of egg-laying adults is approximately 8 weeks. Infection with *A lumbricoides* is ubiquitous, but is most common in the tropics, in areas of poor sanitation, and wherever human feces are used as fertilizer. If the infection is untreated, adult worms can live for 12 to 18 months, resulting in daily excretion of large numbers of ova.

The **incubation period** is prolonged, as the life cycle of A lumbricoides is 4 to 8 weeks, and feces contain eggs about 2 months after ingestion of embryonated eggs.

DIAGNOSTIC TESTS: Ova can be detected by microscopic stool examination. Occasionally, patients pass adult worms from the rectum, by vomiting, or migration through the nares in febrile patients.

TREATMENT: Pyrantel pamoate in a single dose or mebendazole for 3 days is recommended for treatment of asymptomatic and symptomatic infections. Albendazole is an alternative drug. In children younger than 2 years, in whom experience with these drugs is limited, the risks and benefits of therapy should be considered before drug administration. Reexamination of the stools 3 weeks after therapy to determine whether the worms have been eliminated is helpful in assessing therapy but is not essential.

In cases of partial or complete intestinal obstruction due to a heavy worm load, piperazine citrate solution (75 mg/kg per day, not to exceed 3.5 g) may be given through a gastrointestinal tube. Piperazine paralyzes the worms, allowing them to be excreted with intestinal peristalsis. Piperazine should not be used with pyrantel pamoate because the two drugs are antagonistic. Surgical intervention is occasionally necessary to relieve intestinal or biliary obstruction, or for volvulus or peritonitis secondary to perforation. If surgery is performed for intestinal obstruction, massaging the worms to eliminate the obstruction is preferable to incision of the intestine.

ISOLATION OF THE HOSPITALIZED PATIENT: Standard precautions are recommended.

CONTROL MEASURES: Sanitary disposal of feces should be undertaken. Children's play areas should be given special attention. Vegetables cultivated in areas where human feces are used as fertilizer must be thoroughly cooked or soaked in a dilute iodine solution before eating. Household bleach is ineffective.

Aspergillosis

CLINICAL MANIFESTATIONS: Aspergillosis is manifested by the following types of disease:

- Allergic bronchopulmonary aspergillosis manifests as episodic wheezing, expectoration of brown mucus plugs, low-grade fever, eosinophilia, and transient pulmonary infiltrates. It occurs most frequently in children with chronic asthma or cystic fibrosis.
- Aspergillomas are fungus balls that grow in preexisting cavities or bronchogenic cysts and do not invade pulmonary tissue.
- Invasive aspergillosis occurs almost exclusively in immunocompromised patients with an underlying disease that causes neutrophil dysfunction (eg, chronic granulomatous disease or acute leukemia) or after cytotoxic chemotherapy or immunosuppressive therapy (eg, in organ transplantation).
- Paranasal sinusitis and otomycosis of the external canal occur as benign conditions in otherwise healthy patients in certain warm regions (eg, the Sudan).
- On rare occasion, endocarditis, osteomyelitis, meningitis, infection of the eye or orbit, and cutaneous aspergillosis occur.

ETIOLOGY: *Aspergillus* species are ubiquitous; they grow on decaying vegetation and in the soil. Most infected patients, other than those in whom otomycosis and allergic bronchopulmonary disease develop, have some impairment in host defenses. Nosocomial outbreaks of invasive pulmonary aspergillosis have occurred in which the probable source of the fungus was a nearby construction site or faulty ventilation system. The principal route of transmission is inhalation of airborne conidiospores. Contact transmission through skin or a wound is less likely. Person-to-person spread does not occur.

The **incubation period** is unknown.

DIAGNOSTIC TESTS: Dichotomously branched and septate hyphae, identified by microscopic examination of 10% potassium hydroxide wet preparations or of Gomori methenamine-silver nitrate stain of tissue specimens, are suggestive of the diagnosis. Isolation of an *Aspergillus* species in culture is required for definitive diagnosis. The organism is readily recovered from biologic specimens other than blood on Sabouraud dextrose or brain-heart infusion media (without cycloheximide). *Aspergillus* species also can be found as laboratory contaminants, but when evaluating culture results from immunocompromised patients, recovery of this organism strongly suggests etiological significance. Biopsy of a lesion is usually required to confirm the diagnosis. Serologic antibody tests have no established value in the diagnosis of invasive aspergillosis, and assays for detecting circulating *Aspergillus* antigens, while promising, are investigational. In allergic aspergillosis, elevated concentrations of serum immunoglobulin E, eosinophilia, and serum antibody to *Aspergillus* species are frequently present.

TREATMENT: Amphotericin B in high dose (1.0 to 1.5 mg/kg per day) is the treatment of choice for invasive infection (see Systemic Treatment With Amphotericin B, p 630). Some experts also recommend concomitant flucytosine or rifampin, but other experts do not believe the additional drugs offer any benefit. Amphotericin B Lipid

Complex (ABLC), although initially only approved for use in adults, also should be considered for children who are refractory or intolerant of conventional amphotericin B therapy. Itraconazole is an alternative drug for nonmeningeal cases and for patients who are intolerant of amphotericin B therapy or in whom treatment with amphotericin B fails. The safety and efficacy of itraconazole, however, in children has not been established. Surgical excision of a localized lesion is sometimes warranted. Allergic bronchopulmonary aspergillosis is usually treated with corticosteroids.

ISOLATION OF THE HOSPITALIZED PATIENT: Standard precautions are recommended.

CONTROL MEASURES: Outbreaks of invasive aspergillosis have occurred among hospitalized, immunosuppressed patients during construction in hospitals or at nearby sites. Environmental measures reported to be effective include erecting barriers between patient care areas and construction sites, cleaning of air handling systems, repair of faulty air flow, and replacement of contaminated air filters. High-efficiency particulate air (HEPA) filters and laminar flow rooms markedly reduce the risk of airborne conidiospores in patient care areas. These latter measures, however, may be extremely expensive and difficult for patients to tolerate. Because immunosuppressed patients may be colonized and invasive disease may recur after therapy, prophylactic use of nasal instillation or inhalation of amphotericin B, and low-dose amphotericin B and/or itraconazole are under study and may be of value.

Astroviruses

CLINICAL MANIFESTATIONS: Illness is characterized by abdominal pain, diarrhea, vomiting, nausea, fever, and malaise. Illness in the normal host is self-limited, lasting a median of 5 to 6 days.

ETIOLOGY: Astroviruses are nonenveloped, single-stranded RNA viruses with a characteristic starlike appearance when visualized by electron microscopy.

EPIDEMIOLOGY: Human astroviruses have a worldwide distribution. Outbreaks of gastroenteritis have been detected in the young and the elderly. Multiple antigenic types cocirculate concurrently in the same region. Astroviruses have been detected in as many as 10% of sporadic cases of nonbacterial gastroenteritis. Most astrovirus infections have been detected in children younger than 4 years. Transmission is usually person to person via the fecal-oral route, although outbreaks associated with contaminated food have been documented. Common-source outbreaks tend to occur in closed populations and have a high attack rate. Outbreaks occur among hospitalized children. Astrovirus infections in child care centers appear to be common. Excretion lasts a median of 5 days after the onset of symptoms, but asymptomatic excretion after illness can last for several weeks in healthy children. Persistent excretion may occur in immunocompromised hosts. Asymptomatic infections are common.

The **incubation period** is 3 to 4 days.

DIAGNOSTIC TESTS: Commercial tests for diagnosis are not available. The following tests are available in some research and reference laboratories: electron microscopy for detection of viral particles in stool, enzyme immunoassay for detection of viral antigen in stool or antibody in serum, and reverse transcriptase-polymerase chain reaction (RT-PCR) for detection of viral RNA in stool. Of these tests, RT-PCR is the most sensitive. The virus can be recovered in cell culture.

TREATMENT: Supportive.

ISOLATION OF THE HOSPITALIZED PATIENT*: Contact precautions are recommended for diapered and/or incontinent children with possible astrovirus infection for the duration of the illness.

CONTROL MEASURES: No specific control measures are available. Transmission of astroviruses can be reduced by general measures used to control infection. These measures include training care providers about infection control procedures, maintaining cleanliness of surfaces and food preparation areas, exclusion of ill child care providers or food handlers, adequate hand washing, and exclusion or cohorting of ill children.

Babesiosis

CLINICAL MANIFESTATIONS: Gradual onset of malaise, anorexia, and fatigue typically occurs, followed by intermittent fever with temperatures as high as 40°C (104°F) and one or more of the following symptoms: chills, sweats, myalgias, arthralgias, nausea, and vomiting. Less common findings are emotional lability and depression, hyperesthesia, headache, sore throat, abdominal pain, conjunctival injection, photophobia, weight loss, and nonproductive cough. Signs on physical examination generally are minimal, often consisting only of fever, although mild splenomegaly, hepatomegaly, or both are noted occasionally. Many clinical features are similar to those of malaria. The illness lasts for a few weeks to several months with a prolonged recovery of as long as 18 months. Severe illness is most likely to occur in persons older than 60 years, those who are asplenic, and those who are immunocompromised (eg, persons with HIV infection). Some persons, especially those who have had a splenectomy, can suffer fulminant illness lasting about a week and resulting in death or prolonged convalescence.

ETIOLOGY: *Babesia* species that cause babesiosis are intraerythrocytic protozoa. *Babesia microti* and one or more closely related but genetically and antigenetically distinct organisms are responsible for disease in the United States.

EPIDEMIOLOGY: In the United States, the primary reservoir for *B microti* is the white-footed mouse (*Peromyscus leucopus*) and the primary vector is the tick, *Ixodes scapularis*. This tick also can transmit *Borrelia burgdorferi*, the etiologic agent of Lyme disease. Humans acquire the infection from bites of infected ticks. The white-tailed

---

* In addition to standard precautions.

deer (*Odocoileus virginianus*) is an important host for the tick but is not a reservoir for *B microti*. An increase in the deer population during the past few decades is thought to be a major factor in the spread of *I scapularis* and in the consequent increase in human cases of babesiosis. Rarely, babesiosis is acquired through blood transfusions. Transplacental/perinatal transmission of babesiosis also has been described. Human cases of babesiosis have been reported in California, Connecticut, Georgia, Massachusetts, New York, Rhode Island, Washington, and Wisconsin. Most human cases of babesiosis occur in the summer or fall. In endemic areas, asymptomatic infections are common.

The **incubation period** ranges from 1 to 9 weeks.

DIAGNOSTIC TESTS: Babesiosis is diagnosed by microscopic identification of the organism on Giemsa or Wright-stained thick or thin blood smears. Multiple thick and thin blood smears should be examined in suspected cases or when the initial examination is negative. Serologic tests for detection of *Babesia* antibodies are available at the Centers for Disease Control and Prevention and at several state reference and research laboratories.

TREATMENT: Since many patients have a mild clinical course and recover without specific antibabesial chemotherapy, therapy is reserved for patients who are moderately or seriously ill. The combination of clindamycin and oral quinine for 7 days is the current therapy of choice. Exchange blood transfusions have been used successfully in splenectomized patients with life-threatening *Babesia* species infections, and should be considered for all severely ill persons with a high level of parasitemia.

ISOLATION OF THE HOSPITALIZED PATIENT: Standard precautions are recommended.

CONTROL MEASURES: Specific recommendations concern prevention of tick bites and are similar to those for Lyme disease and other tick-borne infections (see Control Measures for Prevention of Tick-Borne Infections, p 126).

Bacillus cereus Infections

CLINICAL MANIFESTATIONS: Two clinical syndromes are associated with *Bacillus cereus* food poisoning. The emetic syndrome is a disease with a short incubation period, similar to that of staphylococcal food poisoning, characterized by nausea, vomiting, and abdominal cramps, with diarrhea in approximately one third of patients. The diarrhea syndrome has a longer incubation period, similar to that of *Clostridium perfringens* food poisoning, and is characterized predominantly by abdominal cramps and watery diarrhea, with vomiting in approximately one fourth of patients. In both syndromes, illness is mild, not usually associated with fever, and abates within 24 hours.

Bacillus cereus also can cause local skin and wound infections; ocular infections; and invasive disease, including bacteremia, endocarditis, osteomyelitis, pneumonia, and meningitis. Ocular involvement includes panophthalmitis, endophthalmitis, and keratitis.

ETIOLOGY: *Bacillus cereus* is an aerobic and facultatively anaerobic, spore-forming, Gram-positive bacillus. The emetic syndrome is caused by a preformed, heat-stable toxin. The diarrhea syndrome is caused by the in vivo production of a heat-labile enterotoxin. This exotoxin also has tissue necrosis and cytotoxic properties, and is probably the principal determinant of virulence in nongastrointestinal tract infections.

EPIDEMIOLOGY: *Bacillus cereus* is ubiquitous in the environment. It frequently is present in small numbers in raw, dried, and processed foods, but it is an uncommon cause of food poisoning in the United States. Spores of *B cereus* are heat-resistant, and can survive brief cooking or boiling. Vegetative forms can grow and produce enterotoxins over a wide range of temperatures (25° to 42°C; 77° to 107.6°F). The disease is acquired by eating food containing either preformed toxin or food contaminated with *B cereus* spores, which produces toxin in the gastrointestinal tract. The most common foods associated with illness are cooked rice, causing the emetic, short incubation syndrome, and meat or vegetables, causing the diarrheal, long incubation syndrome. The disease is not transmissible from person to person.

Risk factors for invasive disease due to *B cereus* include history of injection drug use, presence of indwelling intravascular catheters or implanted devices, and immunosuppression. Fulminant *B cereus* endophthalmitis has occurred after penetrating ocular trauma and injection drug use.

The **incubation period** of the emetic syndrome is 1 to 6 hours; for the diarrhea syndrome it is 6 to 24 hours.

DIAGNOSTIC TESTS: For food-borne illness, isolation of *B cereus* in a concentration of 10^5 or more per gram of epidemiologically incriminated food establishes the diagnosis. Since the organism can be recovered from some stool samples from well persons, the presence of *B cereus* in feces or vomitus of ill persons is not definitive evidence for infection unless isolates from ill patients are demonstrated to be the same serotype or stool cultures from a control group are negative. Phage typing, DNA hybridization, plasmid analysis, and enzyme electrophoresis have been used as epidemiologic tools in outbreaks of food poisoning.

In patients with risk factors for serious illness, isolation of *B cereus* from wounds or normally sterile body fluids can be significant and should not be dismissed as a contaminant. Repeat cultures may help to confirm the diagnosis.

TREATMENT: Persons with *B cereus* food poisoning require only supportive treatment. Oral rehydration or, occasionally, intravenous fluid and electrolyte replacement for patients with severe dehydration, is indicated. Antibiotics are not indicated.

In contrast, patients with invasive disease require antibiotic therapy and prompt removal of any potentially infected foreign bodies such as catheters or implants. *B cereus* is usually susceptible in vitro to aminoglycosides, chloramphenicol, clindamycin, ciprofloxacin, erythromycin, imipenem, and vancomycin. Ciprofloxacin is not approved by the Food and Drug Administration for persons younger than 18 years (see Antimicrobials and Related Therapy, p 605).

ISOLATION OF THE HOSPITALIZED PATIENT: Standard precautions are recommended.

CONTROL MEASURES: Proper cooking and storage of foods, particularly rice cooked for later use, will help to prevent food-borne outbreaks. Food should be kept at temperatures higher than 60°C (140°F) or rapidly cooled to less than 10°C (50°F) after cooking.

Hand washing and strict aseptic technique in caring for immunocompromised patients or patients with indwelling intravascular catheters are important to minimize invasive disease.

Bacterial Vaginosis

CLINICAL MANIFESTATIONS: Bacterial vaginosis (BV) is a syndrome primarily occurring in sexually active adolescent and adult women, characterized by a profuse vaginal discharge that adheres to the vaginal wall and is usually malodorous (having a fishy smell), nonviscous, homogenous, and white. Bacterial vaginosis may be asymptomatic and is not associated with abdominal pain, significant pruritus, or dysuria. Concurrent sexually transmitted diseases may occur.

Vaginitis and vulvitis in prepubertal girls usually are nonspecific in etiology and, rarely, manifestations of BV. Occasionally other predisposing causes include foreign bodies and other infections, such as group A streptococci, *Trichomonas vaginalis*, herpes simplex virus, *Neisseria gonorrhoeae*, *Chlamydia trachomatis*, or *Shigella* species.

ETIOLOGY: The microbiologic cause of BV has not been clearly delineated. The microbial flora of the vagina are significantly different from that in noninfected persons, with an overgrowth of anaerobic bacteria, *Gardnerella vaginalis*, and *Mycoplasma hominis* and a marked decrease in the concentration of lactobacilli. Despite these changes, little or no inflammation of the vaginal epithelium occurs.

EPIDEMIOLOGY: Bacterial vaginosis is the most prevalent vaginal infection in sexually active adolescents and adults. It may occur with other conditions associated with vaginal discharge, such as trichomoniasis or cervicitis. The evidence about the sexual transmissibility of BV is conflicting, although the condition is uncommon in sexually inexperienced females. Diagnosing BV in a prepubertal girl raises concern about, but does not prove, sexual abuse. Bacterial vaginosis may be a risk factor for pelvic inflammatory disease. Pregnant women with BV are at increased risk for chorioamnionitis and premature delivery. Sexually active women with BV should be evaluated for the presence of other sexually transmitted diseases, including syphilis, gonorrhea, *Chlamydia trachomatis* infection, hepatitis B, and HIV infection.

The **incubation period** of BV is unknown.

DIAGNOSTIC TESTS: The clinical diagnosis of bacterial vaginosis requires the presence of three of the following four signs:
- Homogenous, white, adherent vaginal discharge
- Vaginal fluid pH >4.5

- A fishy, aminelike odor from vaginal fluid before or after mixing with 10% potassium hydroxide
- Presence of "clue cells" (squamous vaginal epithelial cells covered with bacteria, causing a stippled or granular appearance and ragged, "moth-eaten" borders). In BV, clue cells usually constitute at least 20% of vaginal epithelial cells.

Gram staining of vaginal secretions is sometimes useful in establishing a diagnosis. Numerous mixed bacteria, including small curved rods and cocci and few of the large Gram-positive rods consistent with lactobacilli, are characteristic. Cultures for *G vaginalis* are not helpful because the organism may be found in females without BV, including those who are not sexually active.

TREATMENT: Patients with symptoms should be treated with metronidazole (1.0 g orally in two divided doses) for 7 days. Alternative regimens are metronidazole, 2 g orally in a single dose (with a second dose in 48 hours); metronidazole gel, 0.75%, 5 g (one applicator) intravaginally twice a day for 5 days; clindamycin cream, 2%, one applicator (5 g) intravaginally at bedtime for 7 days; and clindamycin, 600 mg/d orally in two divided doses for 7 days. For pregnant women with symptoms, topical clindamycin therapy is the preferred treatment because of possible teratogenicity of metronidazole.

Routine follow-up visits on completion of therapy for BV are not necessary. Recurrences are common and can be treated with the same regimen given initially. The presence of a vaginal foreign body should be excluded. Routine treatment of male sexual partners is not recommended because it does not influence relapse or recurrence rates.

Clindamycin cream is oil-based and may weaken latex condoms for at least 72 hours after terminating therapy.

Recommendations for treatment of BV in females infected with HIV are the same as these for noninfected patients.

ISOLATION OF THE HOSPITALIZED PATIENT: Standard precautions are recommended.

CONTROL MEASURES: None.

Bacteroides and *Prevotella* Infections

CLINICAL MANIFESTATIONS: *Bacteroides* and *Prevotella* species of the oral cavity can cause chronic sinusitis, chronic otitis media, dental infection, peritonsillar abscess, cervical adenitis, retropharyngeal space infection, aspiration pneumonia, lung abscess, empyema, and necrotizing pneumonia. Species from the gastrointestinal tract flora are recovered in patients with peritonitis, intra-abdominal abscess, pelvic inflammatory disease, postoperative wound infection, and vulvovaginal and perianal infections. Soft-tissue infections include synergistic bacterial gangrene and necrotizing fasciitis. Invasion of the bloodstream from the oral cavity or intestinal tract can lead to brain abscess, meningitis, endocarditis, arthritis, or osteomyelitis. Skin involvement includes omphalitis in newborn infants, cellulitis at the site of fetal monitors, human bite wounds, infection of burns adjacent to the mouth or rectum, and decubitus ulcers. Neonatal infections, such as conjunctivitis, pneumonia, bacteremia, or meningitis, occur rarely. Most *Bacteroides* infections are polymicrobial.

ETIOLOGY: Most *Bacteroides* and *Prevotella* organisms associated with human disease are small, pleomorphic, non-spore-forming, obligately anaerobic, Gram-negative bacilli.

EPIDEMIOLOGY: *Bacteroides* and *Prevotella* infections are caused by endogenous organisms of patients' flora. Members of the *Bacteroides fragilis* group predominate in the gastrointestinal tract flora; members of the *Prevotella melaninogenica* (formerly *Bacteroides melaninogenicus*) and *Prevotella oralis* (formerly *Bacteroides oralis*) groups are more common in the oral cavity. These species cause infection as opportunists, usually in conjunction with other endogenous species. Encapsulation of organisms can enhance abscess formation. Endogenous transmission results from aspiration, spillage from the bowel, or damage to mucosal surfaces from trauma, surgery, or chemotherapy. High concentrations of these species in the vagina have been associated with an increased rate of preterm delivery. Peripartum transmission occurs when an infant is exposed during birth to organisms of the vagina or infected tissues. Mucosal injury and granulocytopenia predispose to infection. Except in infections resulting from human bites, no evidence for person-to-person transmission exists.

The **incubation period** is variable and depends on the concentration of organisms and the site of involvement, but generally is 1 to 5 days.

DIAGNOSTIC TESTS: Anaerobic cultures are necessary for recovery of *Bacteroides* and *Prevotella* species. Since infections usually are polymicrobial, aerobic cultures of infected clinical specimens should be obtained. A putrid odor of pus or other discharges is suggestive evidence of anaerobic infection; the Gram stain will show leukocytes and bacteria of differing morphology, but the morphologic features of *Bacteroides* and *Prevotella* species are not sufficiently distinctive to be diagnostic. Use of anaerobic transport tubes or a sealed syringe is recommended for collection of clinical specimens. Collection of clinical material, especially from the respiratory tract, must be performed to avoid contamination of the specimen with anaerobes normally present on mucosal surfaces. Rapid identification techniques are under development.

TREATMENT: Abscesses should be drained when feasible; those involving brain or liver sometimes resolve without drainage if effective antimicrobial agents are administered. Necrotizing lesions should be debrided surgically; the value of hyperbaric oxygenation is controversial.

The choice of antimicrobial agent(s) is based on anticipated or known in vitro susceptibility test results. *Bacteroides* species that cause infections of the mouth and respiratory tract generally are susceptible to penicillin G, ampicillin, broad-spectrum penicillins such as ticarcillin, piperacillin, and cefuroxime. Some species, including members of the *P melaninogenica* and *P oralis* groups, may produce β-lactamase and are resistant to those drugs. Other penicillins and first- and second-generation cephalosporins are less active in vitro. Clindamycin is active against virtually all mouth and respiratory tract *Bacteroides* and *Prevotella* isolates and is recommended by some experts as the drug of choice for anaerobic infections of the oral cavity and lungs. *Bacteroides* species of the gastrointestinal tract usually are resistant to penicillin

G, but are predictably susceptible to metronidazole, chloramphenicol, and, usually, clindamycin. More than 80% of isolates are susceptible to cefoxitin, ceftizoxime, and imipenem. Cefuroxime, cefotaxime, and ceftriaxone are not reliably effective against *Bacteroides* species of the intestinal tract.

ISOLATION OF THE HOSPITALIZED PATIENT: Standard precautions are recommended.

CONTROL MEASURES: None.

Balantidium coli Infections
(Balantidiasis)

CLINICAL MANIFESTATIONS: Acute infection is characterized by the rapid onset of nausea, vomiting, abdominal discomfort or pain, and bloody mucoid diarrhea. Infected patients can develop chronic, intermittent episodes of diarrhea. Rarely, organisms can spread to mesentenic nodes, pleura, or liver. Inflammation of the gastrointestinal tract and local lymphatics can result in bowel dilation, ulceration, and secondary bacterial invasion. Fulminant disease can occur in malnourished or otherwise debilitated patients.

ETIOLOGY: *Balantidium coli*, a ciliated protozoan, is the largest protozoan known to infect humans.

EPIDEMIOLOGY: Most human infections are asymptomatic. Pigs are believed to be the primary reservoir of *B coli*. Cysts excreted in feces can be transmitted directly from hand to mouth or indirectly through fecally contaminated water or food. The excysted trophozoites infect the colon. The patient is infectious as long as the cysts are excreted. The cysts may remain viable in the environment for months.
The **incubation period** is unknown; but may be only several days.

DIAGNOSTIC TESTS: The best source of organisms for diagnosis is from scraping lesions during sigmoidoscopy. Stool examination is less sensitive and repeated stool examination may be necessary to diagnose infection, as shedding of organisms can be intermittent. The microscopic examination of fresh diarrheal stools must be performed promptly to demonstrate rapidly motile trophozoites because trophozoites quickly degenerate.

TREATMENT: Tetracycline is the drug of choice administered for 10 days in a dose of 40 mg/kg per day up to 2 g, divided into four doses. Tetracycline should not be given to children younger than 8 years unless the benefits of therapy are greater than the risks of dental staining (see Antimicrobials and Related Therapy, p 606). Alternative drugs are iodoquinol and metronidazole.

ISOLATION OF THE HOSPITALIZED PATIENT*: Contact precautions are recommended.

---

* In addition to standard precautions.

CONTROL MEASURES: Control measures include sanitary disposal of human feces and avoidance of contamination of food and water with porcine feces. Despite chlorination of water, water-borne outbreaks of disease have occurred.

Blastocystis hominis Infections

CLINICAL MANIFESTATIONS: *Blastocystis hominis* has been associated with symptoms of bloating, flatulence, mild to moderate diarrhea without fecal leukocytes or blood, abdominal pain, and nausea. However, the importance of *B hominis* as a cause of gastrointestinal pathology is controversial. Hence, when *B hominis* is identified in stool from symptomatic patients, other etiologies of this symptom complex, particularly *Giardia* and *Cryptosporidium* species, should be investigated before assuming that *B hominis* is the cause of the signs and symptoms.

ETIOLOGY: *Blastocystis hominis* is a protozoan parasite.

EPIDEMIOLOGY: *Blastocystis hominis* is recovered from 1% to 20% of stool samples examined for ova and parasites. The asymptomatic carrier state is well documented. Because transmission is believed to be via the fecal-oral route, however, the presence of the organism may be a marker for fecal contamination with other pathogens. Transmission from animals also may occur.

The **incubation period** is unknown.

DIAGNOSTIC TESTS: Stool specimens should be preserved in polyvinyl alcohol and stained with hematoxylin or trichrome for microscopic examination. The parasite occurs in varying numbers and infections may be reported as light to very heavy. The presence of five or more organisms per high-power (400× magnification) field suggests heavy infection.

TREATMENT: Indications for treatment are not established. Some experts recommend that treatment should be reserved for immunocompromised patients who are symptomatic and in whom no other pathogen or process is found to explain the patient's gastrointestinal symptoms. Other experts believe that *B hominis* does not cause symptomatic disease and recommend only a careful search for other causes of the symptoms. In anecdotal reports, metronidazole (20 to 35 mg/kg per day divided into three doses for children and 2.25 g/d divided into three doses for adults) for 10 days has also been associated with improvement in symptoms. Iodoquinol (40 mg/kg per day divided into three doses, maximum 2 g/d) for 20 days has effectively eliminated the organism and ameliorated symptoms in some patients. Controlled treatment trials, however, are lacking.

ISOLATION OF THE HOSPITALIZED PATIENT: Standard precautions are indicated.

CONTROL MEASURES: None.

Blastomycosis

CLINICAL MANIFESTATIONS: Infection may be asymptomatic or associated with acute, chronic, or fulminant disease. Symptomatic infection is uncommon, the major clinical manifestations of which are pulmonary, cutaneous, and disseminated disease. Children commonly have pulmonary disease that can cause a wide variety of symptoms and radiographic appearances, resulting in misdiagnosis of tuberculosis, sarcoidosis, or malignancy. Skin lesions can be nodular, verrucous, or ulcerative, often with little inflammation. Abscesses are generally subcutaneous but may involve any organ. Disseminated blastomycosis usually begins with pulmonary infection and can involve the skin, bones, central nervous system, abdominal viscera, and kidney. Intrauterine or congenital infections occur rarely.

ETIOLOGY: The disease is caused by *Blastomyces dermatitidis*, a dimorphic fungus existing in the yeast form at 37°C and in infected tissues, and in a mycelial form at room temperature and in the soil. Conidia, produced from hyphae of the mycelial form, are infectious for humans.

EPIDEMIOLOGY: Infection is acquired through inhalation of conidia from the soil. Person-to-person transmission does not occur. Infection may be epidemic or sporadic and has been reported in the United States, Canada, Africa, and India. Endemic areas in the United States are the southeastern and central states and the midwestern states bordering the Great Lakes. The incidence of infection among persons residing in endemic regions is unknown. Although blastomycosis may be associated with immunocompromised hosts, the disease has been infrequently reported in HIV-infected persons.

The **incubation period** is approximately 30 to 45 days.

DIAGNOSTIC TESTS: Thick-walled, figure-eight, broad-based, single-budding yeast forms may be seen in preparations of sputum, cerebrospinal fluid, urine, or material from lesions processed with 10% potassium hydroxide or a fungal stain. Children with pneumonia who are unable to produce sputum may require an invasive pulmonary procedure, such as an open biopsy or bronchoalveolar lavage, to establish the diagnosis. Organisms can be cultured on brain-heart infusion and Sabouraud's dextrose agar at room temperature. Chemiluminescent DNA probes are available for identification of *B dermatitidis*. The skin test and serologic assays, such as an enzyme-linked immunosorbent test, are not reliable for diagnosis but have been used for epidemiologic studies. A positive immunodiffusion test on sera is a reliable indicator of infection, but a nonreactive test does not exclude the diagnosis.

TREATMENT: Amphotericin B is the treatment of choice for severe or life-threatening infection (see Systemic Treatment With Amphotericin B, p 630). Oral itraconazole and ketoconazole have been used successfully for mild or moderately severe infections, either alone or sequentially following a short course of amphotericin B. Data on safety and efficacy of these drugs in children are limited. Itraconazole is highly effective in the treatment of nonmeningeal, non–life-threatening infections in adults, but it does not achieve effective concentration in the cerebrospinal fluid. In a recent multicenter trial in adults, itraconazole was more effective and associated with less toxic effects than was ketoconazole. Mild pulmonary cases in otherwise healthy individuals with clinical improvement at the time of diagnosis may not require therapy.

Oral therapy is usually continued for at least 6 months for pulmonary and extrapulmonary disease.

ISOLATION OF THE HOSPITALIZED PATIENT: Standard precautions are recommended.

CONTROL MEASURES: None.

Borrelia
(Relapsing Fever)

CLINICAL MANIFESTATIONS: Relapsing fever is characterized by the sudden onset of high fever, shaking chills, sweats, headache, muscle and joint pains, and progressive weakness. A fleeting, macular rash of the trunk and petechiae of the skin and mucous membranes sometimes occur. Complications include hepatosplenomegaly, jaundice, epistaxis, cough with pleuritic pain, pneumonitis, meningitis, and myocarditis. Untreated, an initial febrile period of 3 to 7 days terminates spontaneously by crisis usually with an accompanying Jarisch-Herxheimer reaction. The initial febrile episode is followed by an afebrile period of several days to weeks, then by one or more relapses. Relapses typically become progressively shorter and milder as the afebrile periods lengthen. Infection during pregnancy is often severe and can result in abortion, stillbirth, or neonatal infection.

ETIOLOGY: Relapsing fever is caused by spirochetes of the genus *Borrelia*. *Borrelia recurrentis* is the only species that causes louse-borne (epidemic) relapsing fever. Worldwide, at least 15 *Borrelia* species cause tick-borne (endemic) relapsing fever, including *B hermsii* and *B turicatae* in North America.

EPIDEMIOLOGY: Transmission is vector-borne, by body lice (*Pediculus humanus*) and by soft-bodied ticks (*Ornithodoros*). Louse-borne relapsing fever has been reported recently only in Ethiopia, Eritrea, Somalia, and the Sudan where it sometimes occurs in epidemics, especially among the homeless and in refugee populations. Tick-borne relapsing fever is widely distributed throughout the world, and usually occurs sporadically and in small, often familial, clusters. Most tick-borne relapsing fever in the United States is caused by *B hermsii*. Infection typically results from tick exposures in rodent-infested cabins in western mountainous areas, including state and national parks. *Borrelia turicatae* infections occur less frequently, the majority of which are recognized in Texas. They are most often associated with tick exposures in rodent-infested caves. Soft-bodied ticks have painless bites, feed briefly (10 to 30 minutes), and usually at night, so that patients are often unaware of bites. Ticks become infected by feeding on rodents and transmit infection via saliva and other tick fluid when they take subsequent blood meals; vertical transmission in ticks results in a reservoir. Lice become infected only by feeding on spirochetemic humans; the infection is transmitted when infected lice are crushed and their body fluids contaminate a bite wound or skin abraded by scratching. Infected lice and ticks remain contagious throughout their lives. Direct human-to-human transmission does not occur.

The **incubation period** is 4 to 18 days with a mean of 7 days.

DIAGNOSTIC TESTS: Spirochetes can be observed by darkfield microscopy, and in Wright- Giemsa- or acridine orange-stained preparations of thin or dehemoglobinized thick smears of peripheral blood or in stained buffy-coat preparations. Organisms are found in blood most frequently during the febrile stage of the illness. Spirochetes are cultured from blood by inoculating Barbour-Stoenner-Kelly (BSK) medium or by intraperitoneal inoculation of immature laboratory mice. Serum agglutinins against *Proteus* Ox-K (Weil-Felix test) in convalescent serum support the diagnosis. Serum antibodies to *Borrelia* can be detected by enzyme immunoassay, but the tests are not standardized and subject to antigenic variations between and within *Borrelia* species and strains. Serologic cross-reactions occur with other spirochetes, including *B burgdorferi*, the agent causing Lyme disease. Biologic specimens for laboratory testing can be sent to the Centers for Disease Control and Prevention branch in Fort Collins, Colo.

TREATMENT: Treatment with penicillin, tetracyclines, erythromycin, and chloramphenicol are each effective in producing prompt clearance of spirochetes and remission of symptoms. For children younger than 8 years and for pregnant women, penicillin or erythromycin are the preferred drugs. The use of penicillin may delay the clearance of spirochetes and attenuate the accompanying Jarisch-Herxheimer reaction. Because this reaction can cause transient hypotension and cardiac failure (especially in louse-borne relapsing fever), patients should be monitored closely during the first 12 hours of treatment. The Jarisch-Herxheimer reaction can usually be treated with intravenous volume expansion and antipyretics.

Procaine penicillin or intravenous penicillin G is recommended as initial therapy for those patients unable to take oral therapy. For oral therapy, patients can be given standard doses of penicillin V, erythromycin, tetracycline (if 8 years of age and older), or chloramphenicol. Although single-dose treatment is highly effective in producing cure of louse-borne relapsing fever, less is known about single dose treatment of tick-borne relapsing fever. Continuing treatment for 5 days will ensure prevention of relapses.

ISOLATION OF THE HOSPITALIZED PATIENT: Standard precautions are recommended. If louse infestation is present, contact precautions also are indicated (see Pediculosis, p 387).

CONTROL MEASURES: Contact with ticks can be limited through use of protective clothing, pediculicides, and insect repellents (see Control Measures for Prevention of Tick-Borne Infections, p 126). Prevention of rodent access to the foundations and attics of homes or vacation cabins also reduces the potential for tick exposure. Dwellings infested with soft ticks should be professionally treated with chemical agents and rodent-proofed. When in a louse-infested environment, body lice can be controlled by bathing and washing of clothing at frequent intervals, and by use of pediculicides (see Pediculosis, p 387). Reporting of suspected cases of relapsing fever to health authorities is important for initiating prompt investigation and institution of control measures.

Brucellosis

CLINICAL MANIFESTATIONS: Brucellosis in children frequently is a mild, self-limited disease, with less chronicity when compared to disease in adults. However, in areas where *Brucella melitensis* is the endemic species, disease can be severe. Onset of illness can be acute or insidious. Manifestations are nonspecific and include fever, sweats, weakness, malaise, anorexia, weight loss, arthralgias, myalgias, abdominal pain, and headache. Abnormal physical findings include lymphadenopathy, hepato-splenomegaly, and, occasionally arthritis, but these findings are often minimal. Serious complications include meningitis, endocarditis, and osteomyelitis.

ETIOLOGY: *Brucella* species are small, nonmotile, Gram-negative coccobacilli. The species that infect humans are *B abortus, B melitensis, B suis,* and, rarely, *B canis.*

EPIDEMIOLOGY: Brucellosis is a zoonotic disease of both wild and domestic animals. Humans are accidental hosts, contracting the disease by direct contact with infected animals and their carcasses and secretions, or by ingesting unpasteurized milk or milk products. Persons in occupations such as farming, ranching, and veterinary medicine, as well as abattoir workers, meat inspectors, and laboratory personnel, are at increased risk. Infection is transmitted by inoculation through cuts and abrasions in the skin, by inhalation of contaminated aerosols, by contact with the conjunctival mucosa, or by oral ingestion. Brucellosis is unusual in children in the United States, with fewer than 10% of reported cases occurring in persons younger than 19 years. Human-to-human transmission rarely has been documented.

The **incubation period** varies from less than 1 week to several months, but most patients become ill within 3 to 4 weeks of exposure.

DIAGNOSTIC TESTS: A definitive diagnosis is made by recovering *Brucella* organisms from blood, bone marrow, or other tissues. A variety of media will support the growth of *Brucella* species, but some require 5% to 10% CO_2 for primary isolation. The laboratory should be alerted to the possibility of brucellosis so that cultures can be incubated for a minimum of 4 weeks, if necessary. Lysis-centrifugation techniques may shorten the time necessary to isolate *Brucella.* A presumptive diagnosis can be made by demonstrating elevated serum titers of specific antibodies. The serum agglutination test (SAT) using killed *B abortus* cells as antigen is the most commonly used serologic test. This test will detect antibodies against *B abortus, B suis,* and *B melitensis.* However, detection of antibodies against *B canis* requires use of *B canis*-specific antigen. Although a single titer is not diagnostic, most patients with active infection will have SAT titers of 1:160 or greater. Since lower titers may be found early in the course of infection, repeat tests are recommended in order to demonstrate a rising titer. Since low titers of IgM agglutinins can persist in the serum for months and even years after infection, the 2-mercaptoethanol agglutination test is useful. Elevated concentrations of IgG agglutinins are found in acute infection, chronic infection, and relapse. In interpreting SAT titers, the possibility of cross-reactions of *Brucella* antibodies with those against other Gram-negative bacteria, such as a *Yersinia enterocolitica* serotype 09, *Francisella tularensis*, and *Vibrio cholerae*, should be considered. In addition, the prozone phenomenon can give false-negative results in the presence of high titers of antibody. To avoid this problem, serum should be diluted routinely to 1:320 or higher. Rarely, agglutination is inhibited by the presence of so-called blocking antibodies. These antibodies can be detected by the Coombs' test or by a blocking antibody test, but they rarely interfere with the diagnosis. Enzyme immunoassay (EIA) is probably the most sensitive method for determining IgG, IgA, and IgM anti-*Brucella* antibodies, but until better standardization is established, EIA should be used primarily in suspected cases with negative titers by SAT or for evaluation of relapse or reinfection.

TREATMENT: Prolonged therapy is imperative in achieving a cure. Relapses generally are not caused by development of resistance but rather from premature discontinuation of oral antibiotics.

Oral doxycycline (2 to 4 mg/kg per day; maximum, 200 mg/d in two divided doses) given orally or, alternatively, tetracycline (30 to 40 mg/kg per day; maximum, 2 g/d in four divided doses) given orally should be administered for 4 to 6 weeks. Tetracyclines, however, usually should not be given to children younger than 8 years or to pregnant women after the sixth month of gestation (see Antimicrobials and Related Therapy, p 606). Hence, in children that are younger than 8 years, oral trimethoprim-sulfamethoxazole (trimethoprim, 10 mg/kg per day; maximum, 480 mg/d and sulfamethoxazole, 50 mg/kg per day; maximum, 2.4 g/d) for 4 to 6 weeks is an appropriate alternative therapy.

To decrease the incidence of relapse, many experts recommend combination therapy, given orally, of a tetracycline (or trimethoprim-sulfamethoxazole if tetracyclines are contraindicated) and rifampin (15 to 20 mg/kg per day in one or two divided doses; maximum, 600 to 900 mg/d). Because of the potential emergence of rifampin resistance, rifampin as monotherapy is not recommended.

For the treatment of serious infection or of complications, including endocarditis, meningitis, and osteomylitis, streptomycin (20 mg/kg per day in two divided doses; maximum, 1 g/d intramuscularly) or gentamicin (5 mg/kg per day in three divided doses) for the first 7 to 14 days of therapy in conjunction with a tetracycline (a trimethoprim-sulfamethoxazole if tetracyclines are contraindicated) is recommended. In addition, rifampin (20 mg/kg per day) can be used with this regimen as adjunctive therapy to reduce the rate of relapse.

For life-threatening complications of brucellosis, such as meningitis or endocarditis, the duration of therapy is often extended for several months. For osteomyelitis, early surgical intervention should be considered.

Prednisone has been given with antibiotics in culture-proven meningitis, but the benefits of corticosteroids in neurobrucellosis are unproven. Occasionally, a Jarisch-Herxheimer-like reaction occurs shortly after beginning antibiotics, but it is rarely severe enough to require corticosteroids.

ISOLATION OF THE HOSPITALIZED PATIENT*: Contact precautions are indicated for patients with draining wounds.

CONTROL MEASURES: The control of human brucellosis depends on eradication of *Brucella* from cattle, goats, swine, and other animals. Pasteurization of milk and milk products for human consumption is especially important to prevent disease in children. The certification of raw milk does not eliminate the risk of *Brucella* transmission. In endemic areas, enforcement of and education about control measures are crucial.

Caliciviruses and Calici-like Viruses Causing Gastroenteritis

CLINICAL MANIFESTATIONS: Diarrhea and vomiting, frequently accompanied by fever, headache, malaise, myalgia, and abdominal cramps, are characteristic. Symptoms last from 1 day to 2 weeks.

ETIOLOGY: Caliciviruses are nonenveloped RNA viruses. The four recognized genogroups that cause disease in humans are Norwalk-like, Snow Mountain-like, Sapporo-like caliciviruses and hepatitis E. Sapporo-like caliciviruses are closer genetically to animal caliciviruses than to other human caliciviruses. Hepatitis E virus may represent a distinct genus of caliciviruses.

EPIDEMIOLOGY: Human caliciviruses have a worldwide distribution. Outbreaks of gastroenteritis have been detected in all age groups. Multiple antigenic types circulate simultaneously in the same region. Caliciviruses cause 0.2% to 6.6% of sporadic cases of gastroenteritis requiring hospitalization. Most calicivirus infections have been detected in children younger than 4 years. The Norwalk-like virus is more likely than other strains to cause disease after the first decade of life in developed countries. Transmission presumably is person to person via the fecal-oral route. Outbreaks tend to occur in closed populations and have a high attack rate. Infections in child care centers have been reported. Common-source outbreaks occur in association with the ingestion of contaminated water and food, particularly shellfish and salads. Airborne transmission has been implicated in one institutional outbreak. Excretion lasts 5 to 7 days after the onset of symptoms in half of the infected persons and can be as long as 13 days. Virus excretion may continue as long as 4 days after symptoms cease. Prolonged excretion can occur in immunocompromised hosts. Asymptomatic, persistent virus excretion has been detected for months after primary calicivirus infections in animals.

The **incubation period** is 12 hours to 4 days.

DIAGNOSTIC TESTS: Commercial tests for diagnosis are not available. The following tests are available in some research and reference laboratories: electron microscopy for detection of viral antigen in stool, enzyme immunoassay for detection of viral antigen in stool or antibody in serum, and reverse transcriptase-polymerase chain

---

* In addition to standard precautions.

reaction (RT-PCR) for detection of viral RNA in stool. The most sensitive assay is RT-PCR; electron microscopy is relatively insensitive.

TREATMENT: Supportive.

ISOLATION OF THE HOSPITALIZED PATIENT*: Contact precautions are recommended for diapered and/or incontinent children for the duration of the illness.

CONTROL MEASURES: No specific control measures are available. The spread of infection can be reduced by generic measures for control of diarrhea, such as training care providers about infection control, cleanliness of surfaces and food preparation areas, exclusion of care providers or food handlers who are ill or are carriers, adequate hand washing, and exclusion or grouping of ill children for care. If a mode of transmission can be identified (eg, contaminated food or water) during an outbreak, then specific interventions to interrupt transmission can be effective.

Campylobacter Infections

CLINICAL MANIFESTATIONS: Predominant symptoms are diarrhea, abdominal pain, malaise, and fever. Stools frequently contain visible or occult blood. In neonates, bloody diarrhea can be the only manifestation. Abdominal pain can mimic that produced by appendicitis. Mild infection can last 1 or 2 days and resembles viral gastroenteritis. Most patients recover in less than 1 week, but 20% have a relapse or a prolonged or severe illness. Severe or persistent infection can mimic acute inflammatory bowel disease. Convulsions develop in some young children in association with high fever. Bacteremia is uncommon, but neonatal septicemia occasionally occurs. Immunocompromised hosts may have prolonged, relapsing, or extraintestinal infections. Immunoreactive complications such as reactive arthritis, Guillain-Barré syndrome, Reiter syndrome, and erythema nodosum can occur during convalescence.

ETIOLOGY: *Campylobacter jejuni* are motile, comma-shaped, Gram-negative bacilli that cause gastroenteritis. *Campylobacter fetus*, a related organism, is an infrequent cause of systemic illness in neonates and debilitated hosts.

EPIDEMIOLOGY: The gastrointestinal tract of domestic and wild birds and animals is the reservoir of infection. *Campylobacter jejuni* has been isolated from feces of 30% to 100% of chickens, turkeys, and water fowl. Poultry carcasses usually are contaminated with the organism. Many farm animals and meat sources can harbor the organism, and pets such as dogs, cats (especially young animals), and birds are potential sources. Transmission of *C jejuni* occurs by ingestion of contaminated food, including unpasteurized milk and untreated water, or by direct contact with fecal material from infected animals or persons. Improperly cooked poultry, untreated water, and unpasteurized milk have been the main vehicles of transmission. Outbreaks in school children have occurred after field trips to dairy farms during which children drank unpasteurized milk. Person-to-person spread occasionally occurs,

---

* In addition to standard precautions.

particularly from young children with fecal incontinence. Outbreaks of diarrhea due to *C jejuni* in child care centers have been reported but appear to be uncommon. Person-to-person transmission also has occurred in neonates of infected mothers and has resulted in nosocomial nursery outbreaks. In perinatal infection, *C jejuni* usually causes neonatal gastroenteritis, whereas *C fetus* often results in neonatal septicemia or meningitis. Enteritis occurs in persons of all ages. Communicability is uncommon but is greatest during the acute phase of illness. Convalescent excretion usually is brief, typically 2 to 3 weeks, and is shortened by treatment to 2 to 3 days. Asymptomatic carriage is uncommon.

The **incubation period** is usually 1 to 7 days but can be longer.

DIAGNOSTIC TESTS: Rapid, presumptive diagnosis is possible in laboratories experienced in examining stool smears by darkfield microscopic or Gram-stain techniques, although the sensitivity of these tests is relatively low. *Campylobacter jejuni* can be cultured from feces and both *C fetus* and *C jejuni* can be cultured from blood. Laboratory identification of *C jejuni* in stool specimens requires special isolation techniques, which may not be a routine procedure in some microbiology laboratories. If so, the laboratory should be notified that *C jejuni* is suspected when sending fecal specimens.

TREATMENT:
- When given early in the course of infection, erythromycin shortens the duration of illness and prevents relapse. Treatment with erythromycin usually eradicates the organism from stool within 2 or 3 days. Ciprofloxacin is an alternative agent that is effective, but it is not approved by the Food and Drug Administration for persons younger than 18 years (see Antimicrobials and Related Therapy, p 605).
- If antimicrobial therapy is given for gastroenteritis, the recommended duration is 5 to 7 days.
- Antimicrobial agents for resistant or bacteremic strains should be selected on the basis of laboratory susceptibility tests. Bacteremic strains are nearly always susceptible to aminoglycosides, cefotaxime, and chloramphenicol.

ISOLATION OF THE HOSPITALIZED PATIENT*: Contact precautions are recommended for diapered and/or incontinent children for the duration of illness.

CONTROL MEASURES:
- Hand washing after handling raw poultry, washing cutting boards and utensils with soap after contact with raw poultry, and thorough cooking of poultry are critical.
- Pasteurization of milk and chlorination of water supplies are important.
- Infected food handlers and hospital employees who are asymptomatic pose no known hazard for disease transmission and need not be excluded from work if proper personal hygiene measures are maintained.
- Outbreaks are uncommon in child care centers, and specific strategies for controlling infection in these settings have not been evaluated. General mea-

---

* In addition to standard precautions.

sures for interrupting enteric transmission in child care centers are recommended (see Children in Out-of-Home Child Care, p 80). Infants and children in diapers with symptomatic *C jejuni* infection should be excluded from child care or cared for in a separate protected area until diarrhea has subsided. Erythromycin treatment may further limit the potential for transmission.

- Stool cultures of asymptomatic exposed children generally are not recommended.

Candidiasis
(Moniliasis, Thrush)

CLINICAL MANIFESTATIONS: Mucocutaneous infection results in oral (thrush) or vaginal candidiasis; intertriginous lesions of the gluteal folds, neck, groin, and axilla; paronychia; and onychia. Chronic mucocutaneous candidiasis can be associated with endocrinologic diseases or progressive immunodeficiency, particularly T-cell lymphocyte deficiency, and can be the presenting symptom of HIV infection. Granulomas of the scalp and face are rare. Disseminated candidiasis occurs in very-low-birth-weight newborns and in immunocompromised or debilitated hosts can involve virtually any organ or anatomic site, and may be rapidly fatal. Transient candidemia can occur with or without systemic disease in patients with indwelling catheters or in those receiving prolonged intravenous infusions.

ETIOLOGY: *Candida albicans* causes most infections. Other species, such as *C tropicalis*, can also cause serious infections in compromised hosts. More than 150 species of *Candida* have been identified.

EPIDEMIOLOGY: *Candida albicans* is ubiquitous. Like other *Candida* species, it is present on the skin and in the mouth, intestinal tract, and vagina of healthy individuals. Person-to-person transmission occurs. Vulvovaginal candidiasis is associated with pregnancy and newborns can acquire the organism in utero, during passage through the vagina, or postnatally. Mild mucocutaneous infection is common in healthy infants. Invasive disease occurs almost exclusively in persons with impaired resistance to infection. Individuals with HIV infection or those who are immunodeficient for other reasons, such as neutropenia, diabetes mellitus, or treatment with corticosteroids or antimetabolites, are unusually susceptible. Patients undergoing intravenous hyperalimentation or receiving broad-spectrum antimicrobials also have increased susceptibility.

The **incubation period** is unknown. Most infections are of endogenous origin.

DIAGNOSTIC TESTS: The presumptive diagnosis of mucocutaneous candidiasis or thrush can usually be made by physical examination, but thrushlike lesions also can be caused by other organisms or trauma to the mucous membranes. Both yeast and pseudohyphae can be found in infected tissue and are identified by microscopic examination of scrapings suspended in 10% potassium hydroxide. Gram stains of smears from lesions on the skin and mucous membrane also can identify yeast and pseudohyphae. Barium studies and endoscopy are useful in the diagnosis of esophagitis.

A definitive diagnosis of invasive candidiasis requires the isolation of the organism from an otherwise sterile body fluid or tissue (eg, blood, cerebrospinal fluid, bone marrow, or biopsy specimen) or the demonstration of organisms in a tissue biopsy specimen. Cultures that are negative for *Candida* species, however, do not necessarily exclude invasive infection. Recovery is facilitated by blood culture biphasic or lysis-centrifugation systems. A presumptive identification of *C albicans* can be made by germ tube formation. Cultures from urine or other potentially contaminated sites that are positive for *Candida* species are more difficult to interpret, but may be helpful in diagnosis.

Tests for serum antibody and *Candida* antigens and metabolites are investigational. None of the current commercially available tests have been accepted as dependable diagnostic aids.

TREATMENT:

Mucous Membrane and Skin Infections. Oral candidiasis in otherwise normal hosts is treated with oral nystatin suspension or clotrimazole troches. However, the safety and effectiveness of clotrimazole have not been established in children younger than 3 years.

In immunocompromised patients with oropharyngeal candidiasis, both ketoconazole and fluconazole have therapeutic benefit but may not eradicate the organism. The safety and efficacy of ketoconazole in children younger than 2 years and of fluconazole in infants younger than 6 months have not been established, although both drugs have been safely used in a limited number of patients of these ages.

Mild esophagitis caused by *Candida* species can be treated with high-dose oral nystatin; more severe disease is treated with ketoconazole or fluconazole for a minimum of 14 days or with low-dose intravenous amphotericin B (0.3 mg/kg per day) for at least 5 to 7 days depending on patient factors such as age, severity of the illness, and degree of immunocompromise. Itraconazole also is effective in mucocutaneous candidiasis but its safety and efficacy in children have not been established.

Skin infections are treated with topical nystatin, miconazole, clotrimazole, amphotericin B, ketoconazole, econazole, or ciclopirox (see Topical Drugs for Superficial Fungal Infections, p 632). Nystatin is usually effective and is the least expensive of these drugs.

Vulvovaginal candidiasis is effectively treated with many topical formulations, including clotrimazole, miconazole, butaconazole, terconazole, and tioconazole. Such topically applied azole drugs are more effective than nystatin. Oral azole agents also are effective and should be considered for recurrent or refractory cases. The recommended oral dose for fluconazole for vaginal candidiasis in adolescents and adults is 150 mg given once.

For chronic mucocutaneous candidiasis, ketoconazole and fluconazole are effective drugs. Amphotericin B, given intravenously, with or without oral flucytosine, is also effective in severe cases. Relapses are common when therapy with any of these agents is terminated, but invasive infection is rare.

Keratomycosis is treated with corneal baths of amphotericin B, 1 mg/mL. Patients with cystitis due to *Candida* cystitis can be treated successfully with short courses (3 to 5 days) of low-dose amphotericin B (0.3 mg/kg per day), fluconazole, or flucytosine.

Suppressive therapy with oral fluconazole or other azoles should be considered for HIV-infected patients, including infants, with severe, recurrent mucocutaneous candidiasis, particularly those with esophageal candidiasis.

Systemic Infections. Amphotericin B is the drug of choice for treating invasive candidiasis (see Systemic Treatment With Amphotericin B, p 630). Duration of therapy will vary with the clinical response and presence or absence of neutropenia. Patients at high risk for morbidity and mortality should be treated for a prolonged period of time, usually 6 weeks or more, and until all signs and symptoms of infection have resolved. Low-risk patients usually can be treated adequately with a 7- to 10-day course of therapy. Short-course therapy also may be successful for catheter-associated infections, provided the catheter is removed.

Flucytosine (150 mg/kg per day in four divided doses, given orally) should be given to supplement amphotericin B if infection is severe or associated with central nervous system involvement, because in vitro and clinical studies suggest synergism of flucytosine and amphotericin B against *C albicans*. Susceptibility testing, if available, should be performed because some strains of *C albicans* and other *Candida* species are resistant to flucytosine. Peak plasma concentrations should be maintained between 40 and 60 mg/mL; higher concentrations predispose to toxic effects. The dose of flucytosine must be decreased in patients with renal insufficiency. Adverse effects include thrombocytopenia, leukopenia, hepatic dysfunction, rash, and diarrhea, especially in azotemic patients.

Fluconazole has been used successfully to treat disseminated candidiasis, but since no controlled study has been performed to compare its efficacy with that of amphotericin B in patients with neutropenia, amphotericin B remains the drug of choice. Patients with disseminated candidiasis in whom treatment with amphotericin B failed have responded to fluconazole.

Chemoprophylaxis of candidal infections in immunocompromised patients with drugs such as oral nystatin, ketoconazole, and fluconazole have been evaluated. Success has been variable. Data from a prospective, controlled trial indicate that fluconazole can reduce the risk of mucosal (eg, oropharyngeal and esophageal) candidiasis in patients with advanced HIV disease. However, an increased incidence of fluconazole-resistant *Candida krusei* infections has been reported in patients receiving prophylactic fluconazole in another study of non-HIV-infected patients. Prophylaxis of candidiasis, as the result of these findings, is not routinely recommended in immunocompromised persons, including those with HIV infection.

ISOLATION OF THE HOSPITALIZED PATIENT: Standard precautions are recommended.

CONTROL MEASURES: Prolonged, broad-spectrum, antimicrobial therapy in susceptible patients predisposes to colonization and infection with *Candida*, and should be avoided whenever possible. Meticulous care of the venous catheter site is recommended for any patient requiring long-term intravenous alimentation; such care should include dry gauze dressing changes every 48 hours and application of a povidone-iodine solution, which is fungistatic and bacteriostatic. Transparent dressings are associated with an increased incidence of catheter-related infections.

Cat Scratch Disease

CLINICAL MANIFESTATIONS: The predominant sign is regional lymphadenopathy in an otherwise healthy person. Fever and mild systemic symptoms occur in 30% of patients. A skin papule is often found at the presumed site of bacterial inoculation and usually precedes development of lymphadenopathy by 1 to 2 weeks. Lymphadenopathy usually involves nodes that drain the site of inoculation and may include cervical, axillary, epitrochlear, or inguinal nodes. The area around affected lymph nodes is typically tender, warm, erythematous, and indurated. In as many as 30% of the cases of cat scratch disease (CSD), the affected node(s) will suppurate spontaneously. Occasionally, infection can produce Parinaud's oculoglandular syndrome involving the conjunctiva and an ipsilateral preauricular lymph node. Rare complications include encephalitis, aseptic meningitis, neuroretinitis, osteolytic lesions, hepatitis, microabscesses in the liver and spleen, pneumonia, thrombocytopenic purpura, erythema nodosum, or chronic, systemic disease.

ETIOLOGY: *Bartonella* (formerly *Rochalimaea*) *henselae* is considered to be responsible for most cases of CSD. This conclusion is based primarily on serologic, epidemiologic, and molecular probe rather than culture data, although *B henselae* has been isolated from a few patients with classic signs of CSD as well as from domestic cats. *Bartonella henselae* is a fastidious, slow-growing, Gram-negative bacteria that also has been identified as the etiologic agent of bacillary angiomatosis and peliosis hepatitis, two infections that have been reported in HIV-infected patients. *Bartonella henselae* is closely related to *Bartonella* (formerly *Rochalimaea*) *quintana*, the agent of trench fever and also a cause of bacillary angiomatosis.

EPIDEMIOLOGY: Cat scratch disease is believed to be a relatively common infection, although its true incidence is not known. Approximately 80% of cases occur in patients younger than 20 years. More than 90% of patients have a history of recent contact with cats, often kittens, which are usually healthy. Bacteremia in cats associated with patients with CSD is common. Other animals, such as dogs and monkeys, and inanimate objects have been implicated in transmission. No evidence for person-to-person transmission exists. However, multiple cases have been observed in families, presumably resulting from contact with the same animal. Infection occurs more frequently in the fall and winter. Fleas from cats or kittens may be involved in the transmission of *B henselae* to humans.

The **incubation period**, from the time of the scratch to the appearance of the primary cutaneous lesion, is 7 to 12 days and 5 to 50 days (median of 12 days) from appearance of the primary lesion to appearance of lymphadenopathy.

DIAGNOSTIC TESTS: The indirect fluorescent antibody test for detection of serum antibody to antigens of *Bartonella* species is useful in the diagnosis of CSD. It is available through the Centers for Disease Control and Prevention and the reagents are available to state health departments. An enzyme immunoassay for detection of antibody to *B henselae* also has been developed, and is sensitive and specific. Polymerase chain reaction assays are available in some commercial laboratories. If lymph node, skin, or conjunctival tissue is available, the putative agent of the disease may be identified by the Warthin-Starry silver impregnation stain. Pathologic and microbiologic examinations also are useful to exclude other diseases. Histologic findings in lymph node sections are characteristic but not pathognomic for CSD. Early histologic changes consist of lymphocytic infiltrates with epithelioid granuloma formation, similar to changes in lymphomas and sarcoidosis. Later changes consist of poly-morphonuclear leukocyte infiltrates with granulomas that become necrotic and resemble those of tularemia, brucellosis, and mycobacterial infections. The cat scratch antigen skin test, which has been used in the past to establish the diagnosis, is an investigational test of unproven efficacy and safety; the antigen is prepared from aspirated pus from suppurative lymph nodes of patients with apparent CSD and is not standardized.

TREATMENT: Management is primarily symptomatic since the disease usually is self-limited, resolving spontaneously in 2 to 4 months. Painful, suppurative nodes can be treated with needle aspiration for relief of symptoms; surgical excision gener-ally is unnecessary.

Antibiotic therapy should be considered for acutely or severely ill patients with systemic symptoms, particularly individuals with hepatosplenomegaly or those with large, painful adenopathy. Recent reports suggest that several oral antibiotics (rifampin, trimethoprim-sulfamethoxazole, and ciprofloxacin) and parenteral gen-tamicin may be effective, but no controlled antimicrobial trials have been performed. Doxycycline and erythromycin are effective for treatment of signs and symptoms associated with bacillary angiomatosis if administered for prolonged periods to immunocompromised persons, but their role in persons with CSD is unknown.

ISOLATION OF THE HOSPITALIZED PATIENT: Standard precautions are recommended.

CONTROL MEASURES: Individuals should avoid playing roughly with cats and kittens to minimize cat-induced scratches and bites. Individuals with immune defi-ciencies should avoid contact with cats that scratch or bite.

Chancroid

CLINICAL MANIFESTATIONS: Chancroid is an acute ulcerative disease that usually involves the genitalia. It is associated in approximately 50% of cases with a painful unilateral inguinal adenitis (bubo) and an ulcer that begins as a tender erythematous papule, becomes pustular and erodes during 1 to 2 days, forming a sharply demar-cated, somewhat superficial lesion with a serpiginous border. Its base is friable and may be covered with a gray or yellow, necrotic, and purulent exudate. Men typically have single ulcers, while women usually have multiple lesions. Unlike a syphilitic chancre, the chancroidal ulcer is painful, tender and nonindurated. Buboes frequently suppurate and become fluctuant.

Males usually present with a complaint directly referable to the genital ulcer or to inguinal tenderness. Most females are asymptomatic but can, depending on the site of the ulcer, present with less obvious symptoms, including dysuria, dyspareunia, vaginal discharge, pain on defecation or rectal bleeding. Mild constitutional symptoms can occur.

ETIOLOGY: Chancroid is caused by a short Gram-negative bacillus, *Haemophilus ducreyi*.

EPIDEMIOLOGY: Chancroid is a sexually transmitted disease that is more common in individuals from lower socioeconomic groups. It is endemic in many areas of the United States and also occurs in discrete outbreaks. Coinfection with syphilis or herpes simplex virus (HSV) occurs in as many as 10% of patients. Chancroid is a well-established cofactor for HIV transmission. Because sexual contact is the only known route of transmission, the diagnosis of chancroid in infants and young children is strong evidence of sexual abuse.

The **incubation period** is 3 to 10 days.

DIAGNOSTIC TESTS: The diagnosis of chancroid is usually made on the basis of clinical findings and the exclusion of other infections associated with genital ulcer disease such as syphilis, HSV, genital infection, and lymphogranuloma venereum. Fluorescent antibody stains provide preliminary identification, but require confirmation by recovery of *H ducreyi* from a genital ulcer or lymph node aspirate. Special culture media are required for isolation; if chancroid is suspected, the laboratory should be informed. Purulent material recovered from intact buboes is almost always sterile. Direct examination of clinical material by Gram stain or electron microscopy is rarely helpful because of the wide variety of organisms present in most genital ulcers.

TREATMENT: Azithromycin (1 g orally in a single dose) or ceftriaxone (250 mg intramuscularly in a single dose) is the preferred therapy. Alternative regimens are erythromycin base (500 mg orally four times a day for 7 days), amoxicillin-clavulanic acid (500 mg–125 mg orally three times a day for 7 days), and ciprofloxacin (500 mg orally twice a day for 3 days). Relapses occur in about 5% of patients; retreatment with the original regimen is usually effective. Patients with HIV infection may need more prolonged therapy. Ciprofloxacin should not be administered to pregnant or lactating women or usually to persons younger than 18 years (see Antimicrobials and Related Therapy, p 605).

Clinical improvement occurs within 7 days of onset of successful therapy, and healing is complete in about 2 weeks. Adenitis is often slow to resolve and may require needle aspiration to effect a cure. Patients should be re-examined 7 to 10 days after starting therapy.

Patients should be evaluated for other sexually transmitted diseases, including syphilis, hepatitis B, *Chlamydia trachomatis*, gonorrhea, and HIV at the time of diagnosis and, if test results are negative, 3 months later. All persons having sexual contact with patients with chancroid within 10 days before onset of the patient's symptoms need to be examined and treated, even if they are asymptomatic.

ISOLATION OF HOSPITALIZED PATIENT: Standard precautions are recommended.

CONTROL MEASURES: Examination and treatment of sexual partners of patients with chancroid is an important control measure. Regular condom use may decrease transmission.

CHLAMYDIAL INFECTIONS

Chlamydia pneumoniae

CLINICAL MANIFESTATIONS: Patients may be asymptomatic or mildly to moderately ill. Severe pharyngitis, hoarseness, fever, productive cough, and cervical adenopathy are common findings. In some patients, a sore throat precedes the onset of cough by a week or more. Non-exudative pharyngitis and frequently bronchospasm, but without rales, are present on physical examination. An infiltrate may be present on chest roentgenogram. Illness is prolonged and can have a biphasic course.

ETIOLOGY: *Chlamydia pneumoniae* (formerly termed the TWAR strain) is a species of *Chlamydia* that is antigenically, genetically, and morphologically distinct from other *Chlamydia* species.

EPIDEMIOLOGY: *Chlamydia pneumoniae* infection is assumed to be transmitted from person to person via infected respiratory secretions. No animal or bird reservoir is known. The disease occurs worldwide, but in tropical and less developed areas occurs earlier in life than in developed countries in temperate climates. In the United States, *C pneumoniae*-specific serum antibody is present in most adults. The peak age of initial infection is between 5 and 15 years. Recurrent infection is common, especially in adults. Clusters of infection have been reported in groups of children and young adults.

The **incubation period** averages about 21 days.

DIAGNOSTIC TESTS: No reliable test is commercially available. The organism can be isolated from nasopharyngeal swabs placed into appropriate transport media and held at 4°C until inoculated into cell culture; prolonged shedding can occur for months after acute disease. Methods for detecting *C pneumoniæ* in clinical specimens that are available in research facilities include a fluorescent antibody test using monoclonal antibody specific for *C pneumoniae* and a polymerase chain-reaction test. Complement-fixing *Chlamydia* antibodies are usually present in children and adolescents with illness but are often absent in adults, but the test does not distinguish between antibodies to *C pneumoniae, C trachomatis,* or *C psittaci.* The micro-immunofluorescent antibody test is the most sensitive and specific serological test for infection. A fourfold serum antibody titer rise, an IgM-specific titer of 1:16 or greater, or an IgG-specific titer of 1:512 or greater is evidence of current infection. An increase in antibody titer may be delayed for several weeks after onset of illness. Early antimicrobial therapy may limit the serological rise in antibody titer.

TREATMENT: Erythromycin or tetracycline is recommended. Tetracycline should not be given routinely to children younger than 8 years of age (see Antimicrobials and Related Therapy, p 606). Adolescents and older patients have been successfully treated with erythromycin for 5 to 10 days, but 14- to 21-day courses of therapy may be needed, as prolonged or recurrent symptoms are common. For adolescents and adults, tetracycline or doxycycline for 14 days is also appropriate. In vitro data suggest that *C pneumoniae* is not susceptible to the sulfonamides. The new macrolide drugs, azithromycin and clarithromycin, and some of the new fluoroquinolones may prove effective.

ISOLATION OF THE HOSPITALIZED PATIENT: Standard precautions are recommended.

CONTROL MEASURES: None.

Chlamydia psittaci
(Psittacosis, Ornithosis)

CLINICAL MANIFESTATIONS: Psittacosis (ornithosis) is an acute febrile respiratory tract infection with systemic symptoms and signs that often include fever, a nonproductive cough, headache, and malaise. Extensive interstitial pneumonia can occur with radiographic changes characteristically more severe than those found on physical examination. Pericarditis, myocarditis, endocarditis, superficial thrombophlebitis, hepatitis, and encephalopathy are rare complications.

ETIOLOGY: *Chlamydia psittaci* is the cause. It is antigenically and genetically distinct from other *Chlamydia* species.

EPIDEMIOLOGY: Birds are the major reservoir of *C psittaci*. A number of mammalian species also may become infected, such as cattle, goats, sheep, and cats. In the United States, psittacine birds (such as parakeets, parrots, and macaws), especially those smuggled into the country, pigeons, and turkeys are important sources of human disease. Both healthy and sick birds harbor and transmit the organism, usually via the airborne route in fecal dust or secretions. Excretion of *C psittaci* can be intermittent or continuous for weeks or months. Persons in the environment of infected birds, such as workers at poultry slaughter plants, poultry farms, and pet shops, or pet owners, are at special risk. Laboratory personnel working with *C psittaci* are also at high risk. Psittacosis is worldwide in distribution and tends to occur sporadically in any season. Infections are rare in children. Person-to-person transmission from acutely ill patients, presumably via the respiratory route, is rare. Severe illness and abortion have been reported in pregnant women after exposure to infected sheep.

The **incubation period** is usually 7 to 14 days but may be longer.

DIAGNOSTIC TESTS: The usual method of diagnosis is serologic, based on a four-fold increase in complement fixation (CF) antibody titer between acute and convalescent specimens collected 2 to 3 weeks apart. In the presence of a compatible clinical illness, a single CF titer of 1:32 is considered presumptive evidence of infection. Treatment may suppress the antibody response. The CF test, however, does not distinguish between infection caused by *C psittaci*, *C pneumoniae*, or *C trachomatis*. A microimmunofluorescence assay that is more specific for *C psittaci* has been developed but is not yet widely available. Isolation of the agent from the respiratory tract should be attempted only by experienced personnel in laboratories in which strict measures to prevent spread of the organism are used during the collection and handling of specimens for all cultures.

TREATMENT: A tetracycline is the preferred therapy, except in children younger than 8 years of age. Erythromycin is an alternative drug and is recommended for younger children. The new macrolide drugs, azithromycin and clarithromycin, may also prove effective. Therapy should be administered for at least 10 to 14 days after defervescence.

ISOLATION OF THE HOSPITALIZED PATIENT: Standard precautions are recommended.

CONTROL MEASURES: Reporting cases of human psittacosis to health authorities is mandated in most states. All birds suspected to be the source of human infection should be examined by a veterinarian for evaluation and management. Birds with *C psittaci* infection should be isolated and treated with chlortetracycline for at least 45 days. Birds with suspected infection that have died or have been sacrificed should be sealed in an impermeable container and transported on dry ice to a veterinary laboratory for testing. All potentially contaminated caging and housing areas should be thoroughly disinfected and aired before reuse because these areas contain infectious organisms. *Chlamydia psittaci* is susceptible to most household disinfectants and detergents, including 70% alcohol, 1% Lysol and a 1:100 dilution of household bleach. When cleaning cages and other bird housing areas, care should be taken to avoid scattering the contents. Persons exposed to common sources of infection should be observed for development of fever or respiratory symptoms; early diagnostic tests should be performed and therapy given if symptoms appear.

Chlamydia trachomatis

CLINICAL MANIFESTATIONS: Neonatal chlamydial conjunctivitis is characterized by ocular congestion, edema, and discharge developing a few days to several weeks after birth and lasting for 1 to 2 weeks, occasionally much longer. In contrast to trachoma, scars and pannus formation are rare.

Trachoma is a chronic follicular keratoconjunctivitis with neovascularization of the cornea that results from repeated and chronic infection. Blindness secondary to extensive local scarring and inflammation occurs in 1% to 15% of trachoma patients. Trachoma is very rare in the United States.

Pneumonia in young infants is usually an afebrile illness occurring between 2 and 19 weeks after birth. A repetitive, staccato cough, tachypnea, and rales are characteristic but not always present. Wheezing is uncommon; however, hyperinflation usually accompanies the infiltrates seen on chest roentgenogram. Nasal stuffiness and otitis media may occur. Untreated disease can linger or recur. Severe chlamydial pneumonia has occurred in infants and some immunocompromised adults.

Urethritis, vaginitis in prepubertal females, cervicitis, endometritis, salpingitis, and perihepatitis in postpubertal females; epididymitis in males; and Reiter syndrome in either sex also can occur. Infection can persist for months or years. Reinfection is common. In postpubertal females, chlamydial infection can progress to acute or chronic pelvic inflammatory disease and result in ectopic pregnancy or infertility.

Lymphogranuloma venereum (LGV) is an invasive lymphatic infection with an initial ulcerative lesion on the genitalia accompanied by tender regional lymphadenitis. Anorectal infection has also been described. The disease has a chronic, low-grade course.

ETIOLOGY: *Chlamydia trachomatis* is a bacterial agent with at least 15 serologic variants (serovars) divided between the following two biologic variants (biovars): oculogenital (serovars A–K) and LGV (serovars L1–L3). Trachoma is usually caused by serovars A–C, and genital and perinatal infections are caused by B and D–K.

EPIDEMIOLOGY: *Chlamydia trachomatis* is currently the most common sexually transmitted infection in the United States with high rates among sexually active adolescents and young adults. Prevalence in pregnant women varies between 6% and 12% in most populations, but it can be as low as 2% or as high as 37% in adolescents. Oculogenital serovars of *C trachomatis* can be transmitted from the genital tract of infected mothers to their newborn infants. Acquisition occurs in approximately 50% of infants born vaginally of infected mothers and in some infants delivered by cesarean section with intact membranes. Of infants acquiring *C trachomatis*, the risk of conjunctivitis is 25% to 50% and that of pneumonia is 5% to 20%. The nasopharynx is the most commonly infected anatomic site.

Genital infection in adolescents and adults is sexually transmitted. Prepubertal children beyond infancy who have vaginal, urethral, or rectal chlamydial infection should be suspected of possible sexual abuse, although asymptomatic infection acquired at birth can persist for as long as 3 years. Infection is not known to be communicable among infants and children. The degree of contagiousness of pulmonary disease is unknown but appears to be low.

Lymphogranuloma venereum biovars are worldwide in distribution, but are particularly prevalent in tropical and subtropical areas. Infection is often asymptomatic in women. Perinatal transmission is rare. Lymphogranuloma venereum is infective during active disease, which may last from weeks to many years.

The **incubation period** of chlamydial illness is variable, depending on the type of infection, but is usually at least 1 week.

DIAGNOSTIC TESTS: Definitive diagnosis can be made by isolating the organism in tissue culture. Because chlamydia are obligate intracellular organisms, culture specimens must contain epithelial cells, not just exudate. New nucleic acid amplification methods such as polymerase and ligase chain reactions (PCR and LCR) are more sensitive than cell culture, but are not yet available in many clinical laboratories.

Tests for detection of chlamydial antigen or nucleic acid are useful for evaluating urethral specimens from symptomatic males, cervical specimens from both symptomatic and asymptomatic females, and conjunctival specimens from infants. These tests have not been adequately evaluated for detection of *C trachomatis* in nasopharyngeal specimens. They also should not be used for testing rectal, vaginal, or urethral specimens from infants and children, since fecal bacterial flora cross-react with *C trachomatis* antisera.

Currently available tests for detection of *C trachomatis* infection without cell culture include (1) direct fluorescent antibody (DFA) staining for elementary bodies in clinical specimens using monoclonal antibody, (2) enzyme immunoassay (EIA), (3) DNA probe, and (4) nucleic acid amplification (PCR and LCR). Positive DFA, EIA, or DNA probe test results should be verified if a false-positive test result is likely to have adverse medical, social, or psychological consequences. Confirmation can be accomplished either by culture, with a second nonculture test different from the first, or through use of a blocking antibody (eg, Chlamydiazyme) or competitive probe. When evaluating a child for possible sexual abuse, results of rapid antigen detection or DNA tests are not acceptable and culture of the organism is the only acceptable method of diagnosis at this time.

Serum antibody determinations are difficult to perform and available in only a few clinical laboratories. In children with pneumonia, an acute microimmunofluorescence (MIF) serum titer of *Chlamydia*-specific IgM of 1:32 or greater is diagnostic. A fourfold rise in MIF titer to LGV antigens or a complement fixation titer of 1:32 or greater is suggestive of LGV in the presence of compatible clinical findings.

Indirect laboratory evidence of chlamydial pneumonia includes hyperinflation and bilateral diffuse infiltrates on roentgenograms, eosinophilia of 300 to 400/mm^3 or more in peripheral blood counts, and elevated total serum IgG (500 mg/dL or more) and IgM (110 mg/dL or more) concentrations. However, the absence of these findings does not exclude the diagnosis. Direct antigen tests and culture are now so widely available that a specific diagnosis should be made based on laboratory tests.

Diagnosis of chlamydial disease in an infant, child, or adult should prompt investigation for other sexually transmitted diseases, including syphilis, gonorrhea, hepatitis B, and HIV infection.

TREATMENT:

- **Chlamydial conjunctivitis and pneumonia** in young infants are treated with oral erythromycin (50 mg/kg per day in four divided doses) for 14 days. Oral sulfonamides may be used after the immediate neonatal period for infants who do not tolerate erythromycin. Topical treatment of conjunctivitis is ineffective and unnecessary. Since the efficacy of erythromycin therapy is approximately 80%, a second course is sometimes required. A specific diagnosis of *C trachomatis* infection in an infant should prompt treatment of the mother and her sex partner(s).
- Infants born to mothers known to have untreated chlamydial infection should be evaluated and treated with oral erythromycin for 14 days. Because erythromycin may be poorly tolerated by newborns, an oral sulfonamide is an alternative and therapy (with either drug) may be given after the immediate newborn period.

- Treatment of **trachoma** is more difficult and recommendations for therapy differ. The most widely used therapy is topical treatment with erythromycin, tetracycline, or sulfacetamide ointment twice a day for 2 months or twice a day for the first 5 days of the month for 6 months. Oral erythromycin or doxycycline for 40 days also is given.

- For uncomplicated *C trachomatis* **genital tract infection** in adolescents, oral doxycycline (200 mg/d in two divided doses) for 7 days or azithromycin in a single 1-g oral dose is recommended. Alternatives include oral erythromycin base (2.0 g/d in four divided doses) for 7 days or erythromycin ethylsuccinate (3.2 g/d in four divided doses) for 7 days. Erythromycin or azithromycin is the recommended therapy for children between 6 months and 12 years of age; for infants younger than 6 months, erythromycin is recommended. Erythromycin is recommended for pregnant women. Since the safety of azithromycin in pregnancy has not been completely established, it should only be used if erythromycin cannot be tolerated. Doxycycline during pregnancy is contraindicated. Because the efficacy of erythromycin regimens is approximately 80%, a second course of therapy may be required. If a pregnant woman cannot tolerate erythromycin, half-doses given for 14 days may be given. Alternate but less-effective regimens are oral amoxicillin (1.5 g/d in three divided doses) for 7 to 10 days and sulfisoxazole (2.0 g/d in four divided doses) for 10 days. Sulfisoxazole is contraindicated in pregnant women near term and in nursing mothers.

- For **LGV**, doxycycline (200 mg/d in two divided doses) for 21 days is the preferred treatment for children 8 years of age and older. Erythromycin or sulfisoxazole for 21 days (each at a dose of 2 g/d in four divided doses) are alternative regimens.

Follow-up Testing. Patients do not need to be retested for *Chlamydia* after completing treatment with doxycycline, azithromycin, or ofloxacin unless symptoms persist or reinfection is suspected. Retesting may be considered at 3 or more weeks after completing regimens with erythromycin, sulfisoxazole, or amoxicillin.

ISOLATION OF THE HOSPITALIZED PATIENT: Standard precautions are recommended.

CONTROL MEASURES:

Pregnancy. The identification and treatment of women with *C trachomatis* genital tract infection during pregnancy can prevent disease in the infant. Pregnant women at high risk for *C trachomatis* infection, in particular those younger than 25 years of age and those with new or multiple sex partners, should be targeted for screening. Some experts advocate routine testing of pregnant women in the first trimester and again in the third trimester for high-risk women.

Infants born to mothers with untreated chlamydial infection should be treated with oral erythromycin (see Treatment, p 172). Erythromycin may be poorly tolerated in neonates, in which case therapy with an oral sulfonamide given after the immediate newborn period is an acceptable alternative.

Neonatal Chlamydial Conjunctivitis. The recommended topical prophylaxis with silver nitrate, erythromycin, or tetracycline for all newborns for the prevention of gonococcal ophthalmia will not prevent neonatal chlamydia conjunctivitis or extraocular infection (see Prevention of Neonatal Ophthalmia, p 601).

Contacts of Infants With C trachomatis Conjunctivitis and/or Pneumonia. Mothers (and their sexual partners) of infected infants should also be treated for *C trachomatis*.

Gynecologic Examination. Sexually active adolescents should be routinely tested for *Chlamydia* infection during gynecologic examination even if no symptoms are present. Screening of young adult women aged 20 to 24 years is also desirable, particularly those who do not consistently use barrier contraceptives and who have multiple partners.

Management of Sexual Partners. Sexual contacts of patients with *C trachomatis* infection, nongonococcal urethritis, mucopurulent cervicitis, epididymitis, or pelvic inflammatory disease should be evaluated and treated for *C trachomatis* infection if the last sexual contact was within 30 days of a symptomatic index patient's onset of symptoms or within 60 days of an asymptomatic index patient's diagnosis.

LGV. Nonspecific preventive measures for LGV are those for sexually transmitted diseases in general and include education, case reporting, and avoidance of sexual contact with infected persons.

CLOSTRIDIAL INFECTIONS

Botulism and Infant Botulism
(Clostridium botulinum)

CLINICAL MANIFESTATIONS: Botulism is a neuroparalytic disorder that can be classified into the following categories: food-borne, infant, wound, and undetermined. The latter occurs in persons older than 12 months in whom no food or wound source is implicated. Onset of symptoms either occurs abruptly within a few hours or evolves gradually during several days. Symmetric, descending, flaccid paralysis occurs, typically involving the bulbar musculature initially and later affecting the somatic musculature. Patients with rapidly evolving illness may have generalized weakness and hypotonia initially. Signs and symptoms in older children or adults can include diplopia, blurred vision, dry mouth, dysphagia, dysphonia, and dysarthria. Infant botulism, which occurs predominantly in infants younger than 6 months, usually is preceded by constipation and is accompanied by lethargy, poor feeding, weak cry, diminished gag reflex, subtle ocular palsies, and generalized weakness and hypotonia (eg, "floppy infant").

ETIOLOGY: Seven toxigenic types of *Clostridium botulinum* have been identified. Human botulism is caused by neurotoxins A, B, E, and F (and occasionally by toxins of other *Clostridium* species).

EPIDEMIOLOGY: Food-borne botulism results when a food contaminated with spores of *C botulinum* is preserved or stored improperly under anaerobic conditions that permit germination, multiplication, and toxin production. Recent restaurant-associated outbreaks from foods such as patty-melts and potato salad illustrate that not all food-borne botulism results from ingestion of improperly prepared home-canned foods. Illness occurs when the unheated or incompletely reheated food is eaten and preformed botulinum toxin is ingested. Food-borne botulism rarely occurs in infants or children because they are less likely to be exposed to foods that might contain botulinum toxin. Botulism is not transmitted from person to person.

Infant botulism results after ingested spores of *C botulinum* and related species have germinated, multiplied, and produced botulinum toxin in the intestine. Infant botulism is not transmitted from person to person. In most cases of infant botulism, the source of spores remains unknown, but honey is an identified and preventable source. Light and dark corn syrups are not potential sources.

Wound botulism, the rarest category of botulism, results when *C botulinum* grows in traumatized tissue and produces its toxin. Of the nearly 100 cases of documented wound botulism, approximately half have occurred in children and teenagers.

Immunity to botulinum toxin does not appear to develop, even following severe disease.

The usual **incubation period** for food-borne botulism is 12 to 36 hours (range, 6 hours to 8 days). For wound botulism, it is 4 to 14 days between the time of injury and the onset of symptoms. In infant botulism, the incubation period is estimated at 3 to 30 days from exposure to spore-containing honeys.

DIAGNOSTIC TESTS: A toxin neutralization bioassay in mice is used to identify botulinum toxin in serum, stool, or suspect foods. Enriched and selective media are used to culture *C botulinum* from stool and foods. In infant botulism, the diagnosis is made by demonstrating *C botulinum* organisms or toxin in feces. Toxin has been demonstrated in serum in approximately 1% of infants with botulism. To increase the likelihood of diagnosis, both serum and stool should be obtained from all persons with suspected botulism. Serum specimens collected more than 3 days after ingestion of toxin are usually negative, at which time stool and gastric aspirate cultures are the best diagnostic tests. When obtaining a stool specimen is difficult because of constipation, an enema using sterile, nonbacteriostatic water can be given. Electromyography can be helpful in diagnosis; an incremental response of evoked muscle potentials at high-frequency nerve stimulation (more than 20 cycles per second) can occur, and in infant botulism a characteristic pattern of brief, small, abundant motor action potentials (BSAP) is often found.

TREATMENT:

Meticulous Supportive Care. The most important aspect of therapy in all forms of botulism is meticulous supportive care, particularly respiratory and nutritional.

Antitoxin. For food-borne and wound botulism, botulinum antitoxin should be administered as soon as possible to symptomatic persons after testing for hypersensitivity to equine sera since this antitoxin is of equine origin. Approximately 20% of treated persons experience some degree of hypersensitivity reaction. Trivalent antitoxin (types A, B, and E)* can be obtained from the Centers for Disease Control

---

* Prepared by Connaught Laboratories, Willowdale, Ontario, Canada, and distributed in the United States through the Drug Service of the Centers for Disease Control and Prevention.

and Prevention (CDC) through state health departments. If contact cannot be made with the state health department, the physician should call the CDC Drug Service (see Directory of Telephone Numbers, p 667).

Equine antitoxin rarely has been used in infant botulism because of the risk of inducing lifelong hypersensitivity to equine antigens and lack of evidence of its benefit. However, a human-derived botulism antitoxin, termed "Botulism Immune Globulin," has been prepared, and a clinical trial of its efficacy when given early in the course of the illness is in progress in California.*

Antimicrobial Agents. In infant botulism, antibiotics are used only to treat secondary infections because lysis of intraluminal *C botulinum* may increase the amount of toxin available for absorption. Aminoglycosides may potentiate the effects of the toxin.

ISOLATION OF THE HOSPITALIZED PATIENT: Standard precautions are recommended.

CONTROL MEASURES:
- Prophylactic equine antitoxin for asymptomatic persons who have ingested a food known to contain botulinum toxin is not recommended. Because of the danger of hypersensitivity reactions, the decision to administer antitoxin requires careful consideration. Consultation in this regard may be obtained from the state health department or the CDC (see Treatment, p 175).
- Elimination of ingested toxin may be facilitated by inducing vomiting and/or by gastric lavage, rapid purgation (eg, with magnesium sulfate, 15 to 30 g in children and 30 to 45 g in adults), and high enemas. These measures should not be used in infant botulism. Enemas should not be administered to persons with illness except to obtain a stool specimen for diagnostic purposes. Exposed persons should have close medical observation.

  Although most sources of spores for infant botulism are unavoidable, honey should not be given to children younger than 12 months.

  Contacts of persons with wound or infant botulism are not at an increased risk of acquiring botulism. Botulinum toxoid (types A, B, C, D, and E) is available from the CDC for immunization of laboratory workers whose regular exposure places them at high risk.

  Education to improve home-canning methods should be promoted, but cases also may be restaurant-acquired. Use of a pressure cooker (at 116°C, or 240.8°F) is necessary to kill spores of *C botulinum*. Boiling for 10 minutes will destroy the toxin. Time-temperature-pressure requirements vary with the product being heated. In addition, food containers that appear to bulge may contain gas produced by *C botulinum* and should be discarded. Other foods that appear to be spoiled should not be tasted.

---

* For enrollment of patients (in California), call the Infant Botulism Prevention Program, Health and Human Services (510-540-2646).

Clostridium difficile

CLINICAL MANIFESTATIONS: Infections include pseudomembranous colitis and antimicrobial-associated diarrhea. Pseudomembranous colitis generally is characterized by diarrhea, abdominal cramps, fever, systemic toxicity, abdominal tenderness, and passage of stool with blood, mucus, and pus. The colonic mucosa often contains small (2 to 5 mm), raised, yellowish plaques. Characteristically, the disease begins while the patient is in a hospital receiving antimicrobial therapy, but it may occur weeks after discharge from the hospital or after discontinuation of therapy, or be unassociated with hospitalization or antimicrobial therapy. Severe or fatal disease has been described in severely neutropenic children with leukemia, in infants with Hirschsprung's disease, and in patients with inflammatory bowel disease. Infection also may result only in mild diarrhea or asymptomatic carriage, especially in newborns and in children younger than 1 year.

ETIOLOGY: *Clostridium difficile* is a spore-forming, obligately anaerobic, Gram-positive bacillus. It is the cause of pseudomembranous colitis and of a high percentage of episodes of antimicrobial-associated diarrhea. Disease is related to the action of toxin(s) produced by vegetative organisms. Two toxins, A and B, have been characterized.

EPIDEMIOLOGY: *Clostridium difficile* can be isolated from soil and frequently is present in the hospital environment. Spores of *C difficile* are acquired from the environment or by fecal-oral transmission from colonized persons. Intestinal colonization rates in healthy neonates and young infants can be as high as 50%, but usually are less than 5% in children older than 2 years and in adults. Hospitals are major reservoirs for *C difficile*, and child care facilities may be a source. Risk factors for disease are those that increase exposure to organisms and those that diminish the barrier effect of the normal intestinal flora, allowing *C difficile* to proliferate and elaborate toxin(s) in vivo. Among these factors are repeated enemas, prolonged nasogastric tube insertion, and gastrointestinal tract surgery. Penicillins, clindamycin, and cephalosporins are the antimicrobial drugs most frequently received by patients in whom pseudomembranous colitis subsequently develops, but colitis can be associated with almost any antimicrobial. Although the *C difficile* toxin rarely is recovered from stool specimens from asymptomatic adults, it is recovered frequently from stool specimens from neonates and infants who have no gastrointestinal tract illness. This finding confounds the interpretation of positive toxin assays in patients younger than 12 months. *Clostridium difficile* is a rare cause of diarrhea in children younger than 12 months.

The **incubation period** is unknown.

DIAGNOSTIC TESTS: Endoscopic findings of pseudomembranes and hyperemic, friable rectal mucosa suggest pseudomembranous colitis. To diagnose *C difficile* disease, stool should be tested for the presence of *C difficile* toxins. Since isolation of *C difficile* from stool and testing fecal specimens for *C difficile* by latex agglutination do not distinguish between toxicogenic and nontoxicogenic isolates, testing for toxin either by cell culture or enzyme immunoassay (EIA) should be performed to confirm the presence of toxigenic *C difficile* if these methods are used. Commercially available

EIAs that detect toxin B or both toxins A and B are preferred methods of diagnosis, because most isolates from patients with illness caused by *C difficile* produce toxin B. The EIAs are sensitive and easy to perform. Polymerase chain reaction tests for toxins A and B have been developed but are not commercially available.

TREATMENT:

- Antimicrobial therapy should be discontinued in patients in whom clinically significant diarrhea or colitis develops.
- Antimicrobial therapy is indicated for patients with severe toxicity or in whom diarrhea persists after antimicrobial therapy is discontinued.
- Isolates of *C difficile* are susceptible to metronidazole and vancomycin and both are effective in therapy. To decrease the emergence of vancomycin-resistant enterococci in hospitals, metronidazole (30 mg/kg per day in four divided doses) is the drug of choice in the initial treatment of most patients with colitis; oral vancomycin (40 mg/kg per day in four divided doses) is indicated only for seriously ill patients or those who do not respond to metronidazole. In addition, metronidazole is less expensive than vancomycin. Metronidazole is effective when given either orally or intravenously, but the efficacy of intravenously administered vancomycin is uncertain. Vancomycin is absorbed poorly from the gastrointestinal tract but can accumulate in serum of patients with renal failure. Bacitracin also is active against *C difficile* isolates. It is administered orally and is minimally absorbed by the intestinal tract, but is more costly than metronidazole. Bacitracin, thus, is a second alternative therapeutic choice.
- Antimicrobial agents usually are administered for 7 to 10 days.
- As many as 10% to 20% of patients experience a relapse after discontinuing therapy, but they usually respond to a second course of treatment.
- Cholestyramine resin, which binds toxin, can relieve symptoms. However, its effect has not been evaluated in children with disease caused by *C difficile*. Because cholestyramine also binds vancomycin, the two drugs should not be administered concurrently.
- Intravenous immune globulin has been used successfully in a few patients with chronic relapsing colitis.
- Drugs that decrease intestinal motility should not be given.

ISOLATION OF THE HOSPITALIZED PATIENT*: Contact precautions are recommended for the duration of illness.

CONTROL MEASURES:

- Meticulous hand washing techniques, proper handling of contaminated waste (including diapers) and fomites, and limiting the use of antimicrobial agents are the best available methods for control of *C difficile* disease.
- In child care settings, children with *C difficile* colitis should be in a separate, protected area or excluded from child care for the duration of diarrhea.
- Thorough cleaning of hospital rooms and bathrooms of patients with *C difficile* colitis is essential. Germicide resistance as a cause of survival of *C difficile* in the environment has not been demonstrated.

---

* In addition to standard precautions.

Clostridial Myonecrosis
(Gas Gangrene)

CLINICAL MANIFESTATIONS: The onset is heralded by acute pain at the site of the wound, followed by edema, tenderness, exudate, and progression of pain. Systemic findings, which occur in conjunction with severe local toxicity, initially include tachycardia disproportionate to the degree of fever, pallor, diaphoresis, hypotension, renal failure, and, later, alterations in mental status. Crepitus (which is not always present) is not pathognomonic of *Clostridia* infection. Diagnosis is based on clinical manifestations, including the characteristic appearance of necrotic muscle at surgery. Untreated gas gangrene can lead to death within hours.

ETIOLOGY: Gas gangrene is caused by *Clostridium* species, most commonly *C perfringens,* which are large, Gram-positive, anaerobic bacilli with blunt ends. Mixed infection with other Gram-positive and/or Gram-negative bacteria is frequent.

EPIDEMIOLOGY: Gas gangrene usually results from contamination of traumatic wounds involving muscle injury. The sources of *Clostridia* species are soil, contaminated objects, and human and animal feces. Contamination of wounds can occur as long as open lesions are present. Dirty surgical or traumatic wounds with significant devitalized tissue and foreign bodies predispose to disease. Nontraumatic gas gangrene occurs occasionally from *Clostridia* organisms in a person's gastrointestinal tract.

The **incubation period** is 6 hours to 3 weeks, usually 2 to 4 days.

DIAGNOSTIC TESTS: Anaerobic cultures of wound exudate, involved soft tissue and muscle, and blood should be performed. Because *Clostridia* species are ubiquitous, their recovery from a wound is not diagnostic unless the appropriate clinical manifestations are present. A Gram-stained smear of wound discharge demonstrating characteristic Gram-positive bacilli and absent or sparse polymorphonuclear leukocytes indicates clostridial infection. Tissue samples and aspirates, but not swabs, are appropriate specimens for anaerobic culture; inoculation in the operating room and rapid transport of samples to the laboratory is essential to ensure recovery of anaerobic organisms. A roentgenogram of the affected site may demonstrate gas in the tissue.

TREATMENT:
- Early and complete surgical excision of necrotic infected tissue and removal of foreign material is the most important therapeutic measure.
- Management of shock, fluid and electrolyte imbalance, hemolytic anemia, and other complications is essential.
- High-dose penicillin G (250 000 to 400 000 U/kg per day) should be given intravenously. Chloramphenicol, clindamycin, and metronidazole are alternative drugs for penicillin-sensitive patients.
- Hyperbaric oxygen may be beneficial.
- Treatment with antitoxin is of no value. Equine gas gangrene polyvalent antitoxin is no longer available commercially in the United States.

ISOLATION OF THE HOSPITALIZED PATIENT: Standard precautions are recommended.

CONTROL MEASURES: In wound management, prompt and careful débridement, flushing of contaminated wounds, and removal of foreign material with standard aseptic surgical techniques should be routinely performed.

Penicillin G (50 000 U/kg per day) or clindamycin (20 to 30 mg/kg per day) may be of prophylactic value in patients with grossly contaminated wounds.

Clostridium perfringens Food Poisoning

CLINICAL MANIFESTATIONS: Food poisoning is characterized by sudden onset of watery diarrhea and moderate-to-severe, crampy, midepigastric pain. Vomiting and fever are uncommon. Symptoms usually resolve within 24 hours. The absence of fever in most patients differentiates *Clostridium perfringens* food-borne disease from shigellosis and salmonellosis, and the infrequency of vomiting and longer incubation period contrast with the clinical features of food-borne disease associated with heavy metals, *Staphylococcus aureus* enterotoxins, fish, and shellfish. Diarrheal illness caused by *Bacillus cereus* enterotoxin may be indistinguishable clinically from that caused by *C perfringens*. Enteritis necroticans (known locally as pigbel) is a cause of severe illness and death among children in Papua, New Guinea.

ETIOLOGY: Food poisoning is caused by a heat-labile toxin produced in vivo by *Clostridium perfringens* type A; type C causes enteritis necroticans.

EPIDEMIOLOGY: *Clostridium perfringens* is ubiquitous in the environment and frequently is present in raw meat and poultry. Spores of *C perfringens* survive cooking. The spores germinate and multiply during cooling; once ingested, an enterotoxin produced by the organisms in the lower intestine is responsible for symptoms. Beef, poultry, gravies, and Mexican-style food are common sources. Infection usually is acquired at banquets or institutions (eg, schools and camps) or from food caterers or restaurants where food is prepared in large quantities and kept warm for prolonged periods. Illness is not transmissible from person to person.

The **incubation period** is 6 to 24 hours, usually 8 to 12 hours.

DIAGNOSTIC TESTS: Because the fecal flora of healthy persons frequently includes *C perfringens*, counts of at least 10^6 *C perfringens* spores per gram of feces obtained within 48 hours of onset of illness are required to support the diagnosis in ill persons. The diagnosis can be established by detection of *C perfringens* enterotoxin in stool; kits are available commercially for this purpose. To confirm *C perfringens* as the etiology, the concentration of organisms should be at least 10^5 per gram in the epidemiologically implicated food. Although *C perfringens* is an anaerobe, special transport conditions are not necessary because the spores are durable. Stool rather than rectal swabs should be collected because spores can be enumerated.

TREATMENT: Usually no treatment is required. Oral rehydration or, occasionally, intravenous fluid and electrolyte replacement may be indicated for patients with unusually severe dehydration. Antibiotics are not indicated.

ISOLATION OF THE HOSPITALIZED PATIENT: Standard precautions are recommended.

CONTROL MEASURES: Preventive measures depend on limiting proliferation of *C perfringens* in foods by maintaining food warmer than 60°C (140°F) or cooler than 7°C (45°F). Meat dishes should be served hot shortly after cooking. Foods should never be held at room temperature to cool, but should be refrigerated after removal from warming devices or serving tables. Foods should be reheated to at least 74°C (165.2°F) or higher before serving. Roasts, stews, and similar dishes should be divided into small quantities for cooking and refrigeration to limit the time such foods are at temperatures at which *C perfringens* replicates.

Coccidioidomycosis

CLINICAL MANIFESTATIONS: The primary infection, usually acquired by the respiratory route, is often asymptomatic and inapparent. Symptomatic disease may resemble influenza, with cough, fever, and chest pain. A diffuse erythematous maculopapular rash, erythema multiforme, erythema nodosum, and/or arthralgias frequently occur. Chronic pulmonary lesions are rare in children.

Primary extrapulmonary infection is rare and usually follows trauma. It includes cutaneous lesions and soft-tissue infections with an associated regional lymphadenitis.

Disseminated disease is similar to tuberculosis; the skin, bones and joints, central nervous system, and lungs are frequently affected sites. Limited dissemination to one or more sites is common in children. Meningitis is a serious manifestation of disseminated disease and can be fatal if untreated. Hydrocephalus is a common complication.

Congenital infection is rare.

ETIOLOGY: *Coccidioides immitis* is a dimorphic fungus. In soil, it exists in the hyphal phase. Infectious arthroconidia produced in some of the hyphae subsequently become airborne spores which upon inhalation or inoculation infect the host. In the tissues of the infected host, they enlarge to form spherules. Mature spherules release endospores that develop into new spherules and continue the tissue cycle.

EPIDEMIOLOGY: *Coccidioides immitis* is found extensively in the soil and is endemic in the southwestern United States, northern Mexico, and certain areas of Central and South America. Climatic conditions (ie, hot summers and little winter frost) combine with alkaline, dry soil conditions, and local characteristics of moderate to low rainfall to produce favorable circumstances for propagation of arthroconidia and their dissemination by aerosols. Persons are infected through inhalation of dust-borne arthroconidia. Person-to-person transmission of coccidioidomycosis does not occur. One episode of multiple infections resulting from a contaminated plaster cast with exudate containing arthroconidia has been reported. African-Americans, Asians, pregnant women, and immunocompromised patients have an increased risk of dissemination and fatal outcome.

The **incubation period** is 10 to 16 days; the range is from less than 1 week to approximately 1 month.

DIAGNOSTIC TESTS: Skin tests can be useful in diagnosis. A delayed hypersensitivity reaction to a coccidioidin or spherulin skin test is indicative of past or current infection. The spherule skin test is preferred for general use and its conversion from negative to positive in a patient with a clinically compatible syndrome strongly suggests coccidioidomycosis. A positive skin test can appear from 10 to 45 days after infection, but anergy is common in disseminated disease and overreliance on skin test results can lead to errors in diagnosis.

Serologic tests are useful to confirm diagnoses and provide prognostic information. IgM response can be detected by latex agglutination, enzyme immunoassay, or immunodiffusion. Latex agglutination is a rapid, very sensitive test that lacks specificity; hence, positive results should be confirmed by other tests. An IgM response is detectable 1 to 3 weeks after symptoms appear and lasts 3 to 4 months in most cases.

IgG response can be detected by immunodiffusion or complement fixation (CF). Complement fixation antibodies in serum usually are of low titer and transient if the disease is asymptomatic or mild. High (≥1:32), persistent titers occur in severe disease, and almost always in disseminated infection. Cerebrospinal fluid (CSF) antibodies also are detectable by CF. The concentration and persistence of antibody titers in serum in patients with disseminated, severe disease and in CSF in those with meningitis are useful prognostically and in guiding treatment. Increasing serum and CSF titers indicate progressive disease, while decreasing titers suggest improvement. Low or nondetectable titers in immunocompromised patients should be interpreted with caution.

Spherules as large as 80 μm in diameter, in selected instances, can be visualized in appropriate clinical specimens, such as tracheal aspirates, biopsy specimens of skin lesions or organs, urine, or CSF. A chemiluminescent DNA probe can identify *C immitis* in cultures. The procedure can be applied to nonsporulating cultures, thereby reducing the risk of exposure to infectious fungi. Culture of the organism is possible but is potentially hazardous to laboratory personnel, since spherules can convert to arthroconidial-bearing mycelium on culture plates. Suspect cultures should be sealed at the outset and thereafter handled only by trained persons, using appropriate safety equipment and procedures.

TREATMENT: Antifungal therapy is not indicated in uncomplicated primary infection and is required in less than 5% of cases of coccidioidomycosis.

Amphotericin B is the recommended therapy in severe progressive pulmonary disease, disseminated infection, osteoarticular disease, central nervous system (CNS) infections, and in immunocompromised patients, such as those with HIV infection (see Systemic Treatment With Amphotericin B, p 630). However, because amphotericin B must be administered parenterally and can be toxic, other antifungal azoles recently have been utilized in the treatment of coccidioidomycosis. Specific agents are fluconazole, itraconazole, and ketoconazole (ie, azole drugs). Fluconazole and itraconazole cause fewer side effects than ketoconazole, and are preferred.

Although the efficacy of these azoles has not been directly compared with that of amphotericin B, some experts consider these drugs to be suitable alternatives for the treatment of disseminated disease, particularly in the soft-tissue infections. Their value, however, in treating rapidly progressive or osteoarticular coccidioidomycosis is not established and the required duration of treatment is uncertain, as patients have relapsed after prolonged and seemingly curative courses of therapy.

For CNS infections, intravenous amphotericin B therapy is augmented by repetitive, CSF instillation of this drug. A subcutaneous reservoir can facilitate administration into the cisternal space or lateral ventricle, although technical difficulties are frequent with this route of therapy (see Systemic Treatment With Amphotericin B, p 630). Orally administered fluconazole and itraconazole have suppressed coccidioidal meningitis in many patients, but therapy probably has to be continued for the lifetime of such patients.

In some localized infections with sinuses, fistulae and/or abscesses, amphotericin B has been instilled or utilized for irrigation.

The duration of amphotericin B therapy is variable and depends on the site(s) of involvement, clinical response, and mycologic and immunologic tests. In general, therapy is continued until clinical and laboratory evidence indicates that the active infection has subsided. Minimum treatment for invasive coccidioidomycosis is 1 month, and treatment for several years is frequently necessary for CNS disease. Lifelong, suppressive therapy is indicated for patients with HIV infection.

Surgical debridement or excision of lesions in bone and lung has been advocated for localized, symptomatic, persistent, resistant, or progressive lesions. Shunt procedures are frequently necessary for treatment of hydrocephalus associated with CNS infection.

ISOLATION OF THE HOSPITALIZED PATIENT: Standard precautions are recommended. Care should be exercised in handling, changing, and discarding dressings, casts, and similar materials in which arthroconidial contamination could occur.

CONTROL MEASURES: Measures to control dust are recommended in endemic areas at construction sites, archaeologic projects, or other activities causing excessive soil disturbance.

Coronaviruses

CLINICAL MANIFESTATIONS: Coronaviruses are a common cause of upper respiratory tract infection in adults and children and occasionally have been implicated in lower respiratory tract disease. Coronavirus-like particles, not confirmed as coronavirus, have been associated with several outbreaks of diarrhea in nurseries and, rarely, with neonatal necrotizing enterocolitis in infants.

ETIOLOGY: Coronaviruses are RNA viruses that are large (80 to 160 nm), enveloped with lipid-soluble coats, and pleomorphic (spherical or elliptical). At least two distinct antigenic groups of respiratory coronaviruses have been identified.

EPIDEMIOLOGY: Human coronaviruses most likely are transmitted via respiratory secretions, possibly by small particle and droplet aerosols; transmission is facilitated by close contact. Although several animal coronaviruses have antigens in common with human strains, no evidence implicates animals as reservoirs or vectors for human disease. Coronaviruses are worldwide in distribution. In temperate climates, outbreaks occur in the winter. Young children have the highest infection rate during outbreaks. The period of communicability is unknown but probably persists for the duration of respiratory symptoms.

The **incubation period** is usually 2 to 4 days.

DIAGNOSTIC TESTS: Diagnostic tests, including antibody assays, for human coronavirus infection are not available commercially. Most strains cannot be isolated by the methods commonly used in diagnostic virology laboratories. Viral particles have been visualized by immune electron microscopy and viral antigens detected by immunoassay techniques. Antibody to coronaviruses can be determined by several assay methods, such as neutralization, complement fixation, indirect hemagglutination, hemagglutination-inhibition, fluorescent antibody, enzyme immunoassay, and electron microscopy.

TREATMENT: Supportive.

ISOLATION OF THE HOSPITALIZED PATIENT*: Contact isolation is recommended for the duration of symptoms for diapered and/or incontinent children with possible coronavirus infection.

CONTROL MEASURES: None.

Cryptococcus neoformans Infections

CLINICAL MANIFESTATIONS: Primary pulmonary infection is often inapparent or mild; symptomatic disease may clinically resemble tuberculosis. Dissemination to the central nervous system, bones and joints, heart, skin, and mucous membranes can occur. Usually, several sites are infected, but manifestations of the involvement of one site predominate. Cryptococcal meningitis is the most common and serious form of cryptococcal disease. Cryptococcal fungemia, without apparent organ involvement, occurs in patients with HIV infection.

ETIOLOGY: *Cryptococcus neoformans* is an encapsulated yeast.

EPIDEMIOLOGY: Distribution of *Cryptococcus neoformans* var *neoformans* is worldwide, and is isolated primarily from soil contaminated with bird droppings and causes most human infections. *Cryptococcus neoformans* var *gattii* occurs most commonly in tropical and subtropical regions and causes disease primarily in immunocompetent patients. Acquisition is most likely by inhalation of aerosolized organisms. The fungus is not transmitted from person to person. *Cryptococcus* species infect 5% to 10% of adults with AIDS but is less common in HIV-infected children.

The **incubation period** is not known.

DIAGNOSTIC TESTS: Encapsulated yeast cells can be demonstrated in wet mounts of sputum or pus or in India ink preparations of cerebrospinal fluid (CSF) sediment in some cases. Precise diagnosis depends on the isolation and identification of the organism by culture. The lysis-centrifugation method is the most sensitive and rapid

---

* In addition to standard precautions.

method for blood culture. Media containing cycloheximide, which inhibits growth of *C neoformans*, should not be used as the only fungal isolation medium. Few organisms may be present in the CSF, and large quantities of fluid may need to be cultured to recover the organism. Bronchoalveolar lavage or open lung biopsy may be necessary to establish a diagnosis in children who are unable to produce sputum. The latex agglutination test for detection of cryptococcal antigen in serum or CSF is a useful and rapid diagnostic tool. Cryptococcal skin testing is of no value.

TREATMENT: Amphotericin B (see Systemic Treatment With Amphotericin B, p 630) in combination with oral flucytosine is indicated for meningeal and other serious cryptococcal infections. Combination antifungal therapy is probably superior to amphotericin B alone, but the toxic effects of combined therapy can limit its use. Flucytosine often induces cytopenias, which necessitates discontinuation of the medication, as well as hepatic dysfunction, rash, and diarrhea, especially in azotemic patients. When flucytosine is used, serum concentrations should be monitored. Most patients with meningitis are treated for at least 6 weeks. Fluconazole and itraconazole are possible alternative drugs for the primary treatment of meningeal cryptococcosis in HIV-infected patients as well as in those with less severe disease. Data on the use of these drugs in children with *C neoformans* infection are limited.

Patients infected with HIV who have completed initial therapy for cryptococcosis should receive lifelong maintenance with fluconazole.

ISOLATION OF THE HOSPITALIZED PATIENT: Standard precautions are recommended.

CONTROL MEASURES: None.

Cryptosporidiosis

CLINICAL MANIFESTATIONS: Frequent, watery diarrhea is the most common presenting symptom. Other symptoms include abdominal pain, anorexia, and weight loss. Fever is uncommon in sporadic cases but in outbreaks has occurred in 30% to 60% of patients. In infected immunocompetent individuals, including children, the diarrheal illness is self-limited, usually lasting 1 to 20 days (mean of 10 days). Immunocompromised patients, especially those with HIV infection, can develop chronic, severe diarrhea with malnutrition, dehydration, and death. Although infection usually is limited to the gastrointestinal tract, pulmonary, biliary tract, or disseminated infection has occurred in immunocompromised persons.

ETIOLOGY: *Cryptosporidium parvum* is a coccidian protozoan.

EPIDEMIOLOGY: Cryptosporidia have been found in a variety of hosts, including mammals, birds, and reptiles. Transmission from farm livestock or pets to humans can occur. Person-to-person transmission occurs and can cause outbreaks in child care centers, with high rates (30% to 60%) of infection. Extensive water-borne outbreaks have occurred involving supplies of municipal water contamination and exposure to contaminated swimming pools. *Cryptosporidium* also causes diarrhea of travelers. Infection can be asymptomatic as well as symptomatic. Since the parasite is resistant to chlorine, appropriately functioning water filtration systems are critical for the safety of public water supplies. Most sand filters used for swimming pools are not effective in removing oocysts from contaminated water.

The estimated **incubation period** is 2 to 14 days.

DIAGNOSTIC TESTS: The finding of oocysts on microscopic examination of stool specimens is diagnostic. Either the sucrose flotation method or formalin-K is used to concentrate oocysts in stool prior to staining with a modified Kinyoun acid-fast stain. Monoclonal antibody-based fluorescein-conjugated stain for oocysts in stool and an enzyme immunoassay for detecting antigen in stool are available commercially. Since shedding can be intermittent, at least two stool specimens should be examined before considering the test to be negative. Oocysts are small (4 to 6 μm in diameter) and can be missed in a rapid scan of the slide. Organisms also can be identified on intestinal biopsy tissue.

TREATMENT: Other than rehydration and correction of electrolyte abnormalities, definitive therapy has not been established. Paromomycin or azithromycin may be beneficial in some persons. Nitazoxanide is an investigational agent with potential benefit. In HIV-infected patients with cryptosporidiosis, orally administered hyper-immune immunoglobulin therapy with bovine colostrum or bovine serum has been useful, often in combination with zidovudine therapy. Somatostatin analogues have been used with variable success in controlling secretory diarrhea in patients with AIDS but controlled trials are needed.

ISOLATION OF THE HOSPITALIZED PATIENT*: Contact precautions are recommended for diapered and/or incontinent children.

CONTROL MEASURES: In water-borne outbreaks, advisories to boil water may be issued to prevent cases until proper water treatment is restored.

Cutaneous Larva Migrans

CLINICAL MANIFESTATIONS: Nematode larvae produce itching, reddish papules at the site of skin entry. As the larvae migrate through the skin and advance several millimeters to a few centimeters a day, they leave intensely pruritic, serpiginous tracks. Larval activity can continue for several weeks or months but eventually is self-limiting. An advancing serpiginous tunnel in the skin with an associated intense pruritus is virtually pathognomonic. In infections with a large burden of parasites, pneumonitis (Löeffler's syndrome), which can be severe, and myositis may follow skin lesions. Occasionally the larvae reach the intestine and may cause eosinophilic enteritis.

ETIOLOGY: Infective larvae of cat and dog hookworms, ie, *Ancylostoma braziliense* and *Ancylostoma caninum*, are the usual causes. Other skin-penetrating nematodes are occasional causes.

---

* In addition to standard precautions.

EPIDEMIOLOGY: Cutaneous larva migrans is a disease of children, utility workers, gardeners, sunbathers, and others who come in contact with sandy soil contaminated with cat and dog feces. In the United States, the disease is most prevalent in the Southeast.

DIAGNOSTIC TESTS: Because the diagnosis usually is made clinically, biopsies are not generally indicated. Biopsy specimens typically demonstrate an eosinophilic inflammatory infiltrate, but the migrating parasite is not visualized. Eosinophilia occurs in some cases. Larvae have been detected in sputum and gastric washings in patients with pneumonitis. Serologic testing with an enzyme immunoassay and/or Western blot using antigens of *A caninum* may help detect occult infections. These tests, however, generally are available only in research laboratories.

TREATMENT: The disease is usually self-limited, with spontaneous cure after several weeks or months. Thiabendazole given orally and/or topically relieves cutaneous symptoms. Albendazole has also been reported to be effective.

ISOLATION OF THE HOSPITALIZED PATIENT: Standard precautions are recommended.

CONTROL MEASURES: Skin contact with or ingestion of moist soil contaminated with animal feces should be avoided.

Cytomegalovirus Infection

CLINICAL MANIFESTATIONS: The manifestations of acquired cytomegalovirus (CMV) infection vary with the age and immunocompetence of the host. Asymptomatic infections are the most common, particularly in children. Hepatosplenomegaly is occasionally associated with acquired infection in childhood. An infectious mononucleosis-like syndrome with prolonged fever and mild hepatitis, occurring in the absence of heterophile antibody production, can occur in adults. Pneumonia and retinitis are common in immunocompromised hosts, particularly those receiving treatment for malignancies, those infected with HIV, or those receiving immunosuppressive therapy for organ transplantation.

Congenital infections also have a spectrum of manifestations. Infection usually is asymptomatic, but some congenitally infected infants who appear to be asymptomatic at birth are found in infancy or childhood to have a hearing loss or learning disability. Profound involvement, with intrauterine growth retardation, neonatal jaundice, purpura, hepatosplenomegaly, microcephaly, brain damage, intracerebral calcifications, and chorioretinitis, occurs in approximately 5% of infants with CMV infection. Approximately 15% of infants born after primary infection of mothers will have one or more sequellae of intrauterine infection.

Infection acquired at birth or shortly thereafter from maternal cervical secretions or human milk usually is not associated with clinical illness. Infection resulting from transfusion from CMV seropositive donors to preterm infants has been associated with lower respiratory tract disease.

ETIOLOGY: Human CMV, a DNA virus, is a member of the herpesvirus group.

EPIDEMIOLOGY: Infection in humans is caused almost entirely by human CMV. This virus is ubiquitous and is transmitted both horizontally (by direct person-to-person contact with virus-containing secretions) and vertically (from mother to infant before, during, or after birth). Infections have no seasonal predilection. Cytomegalovirus persists in latent form after a primary infection, and reactivation can occur years later, particularly under conditions of immunosuppression.

Horizontal transmission is probably the result of salivary contamination or sexual transmission, but contact with infected urine also can have a role. Although the virus is not highly contagious, spread of CMV in households and child care centers is well documented. Excretion rates in child care centers can be as high as 70% in children 1 to 3 years of age. Young children can transmit CMV to their parents and other caregivers, such as child care staff (see also Children in Out-of-Home Child Care, p 80). In adolescents and adults, sexual transmission also occurs, as evidenced by virus in seminal and cervical fluids.

Seropositive healthy persons have latent CMV in their leukocytes and tissues; hence, blood transfusions and organ transplantation can result in viral transmission. Severe CMV disease is more likely to occur if the recipient is seronegative or is a premature infant. Latent CMV will frequently reactivate in immunosuppressed individuals, and can result in disease if the immunosuppression is severe (eg, AIDS patients and solid-organ and bone marrow transplant recipients).

Vertical transmission of CMV to the infant occurs (1) in utero by transplacental passage of maternal blood-borne virus, (2) at birth by passage through an infected maternal genital tract, or (3) postnatally by ingestion of CMV-positive human milk. Approximately 1% of all live-born infants are infected in utero and excrete CMV at birth. In utero fetal infection can occur regardless of whether the mother had primary infection or reactivation during pregnancy. Infants, however, infected in utero during maternal reactivation are much less likely to have sequelae than those infected in utero after maternal primary infection, presumably because of immunity in the mother. Of infants whose infection resulted from maternal primary infection, 10% to 20% will have mental retardation or sensorineural deafness. Severe disease with manifestations at birth occurs in approximately 5% of infants infected in utero.

Maternal cervical infection is common, resulting in exposure of many infants to CMV at birth. Cervical excretion rates are highest among young mothers in lower socioeconomic groups. Although interstitial pneumonia caused by CMV can develop in the early months of life, most infected infants remain asymptomatic. Similarly, although symptomatic disease can occur in seronegative infants fed CMV-infected milk from milk banks, most infants infected from human milk do not develop clinical illness, most likely because of the presence of passively transferred maternal antibody. For infants who acquire infection from maternal cervical secretions or human milk, premature infants are at greater risk of symptomatic disease and sequelae than term infants.

The **incubation period** for horizontally transmitted CMV infections in households is unknown. Infection usually manifests 3 to 12 weeks after blood transfusions, and between 4 weeks and 4 months after tissue transplantation.

DIAGNOSTIC TESTS: The diagnosis of CMV is frequently confounded by the ubiquity of the virus, the high rate of asymptomatic excretion, the frequency of reactivated infections, the development of serum IgM CMV-specific antibody in some episodes of reactivation, and the simultaneous presence of other pathogens.

Virus can be isolated in cell culture from urine, pharynx, peripheral blood leukocytes, human milk, semen, cervical secretions, and other tissues and body fluids. Virus present in large quantity also can be identified by electron microscopic examination of urine or tissue. Examination of cells shed in the urine for intranuclear inclusions is an insensitive test.

Only recovery of virus from a target organ provides unequivocal evidence that the disease is caused by CMV infection. However, a presumptive diagnosis can be made on the basis of a fourfold antibody titer rise in paired sera or by virus excretion. Techniques for detection of viral DNA by polymerase chain reaction (PCR) or hybridization are available from specialty laboratories for detection of CMV in tissues and some fluids, especially cerebrospinal fluid.

Complement fixation is the least sensitive serologic method for the diagnosis of CMV infection and should not be used to establish previous infection or passively acquired maternal antibody. Various fluorescence assays, indirect hemagglutination, latex agglutination, and enzyme immunoassays are preferred for this purpose.

Proof of congenital infection requires obtaining specimens within 3 weeks of birth. Viral isolation or a strongly positive test for serum IgM anti-CMV antibody is considered diagnostic. Differentiation between intrauterine and perinatal infection is difficult later in infancy, unless clinical manifestations of the former, such as chorioretinitis or ventriculitis, are present. Special serologic tests that are available only in reference laboratories may help to differentiate between these two possibilities in the first 2 or 3 months of life.

TREATMENT: Ganciclovir (see Antiviral Drugs for Non-HIV Infections, p 634) is beneficial in the treatment of retinitis caused by acquired or recurrent CMV infection in HIV-infected patients. This drug is approved in the United States for the treatment of severe retinitis in immunocompromised adults. Limited data in children suggest that safety and efficacy are similar to those in adults. The drug is often useful in other types of CMV organ involvement. Although ganciclovir has appeared to be beneficial in the treatment of some congenitally infected infants, it is not routinely recommended currently because of insufficient data concerning its efficacy. The combination of cytomegalovirus immune globulin intravenous (CMV-IGIV), given intravenously, and ganciclovir has been reported to be synergistic in the treatment of CMV pneumonia in bone marrow transplant recipients. Foscarnet has also been approved for the treatment of CMV retinitis and is an alternative drug (see Antiviral Drugs for Non-HIV Infections, p 634). This drug is more toxic but may be advantageous for some patients with HIV infection, such as those with disease caused by ganciclovir-resistant virus or those unable to tolerate ganciclovir.

Cytomegalovirus disease in HIV-infected patients is not cured by currently available antiviral agents. Hence, chronic suppressive or maintenance therapy with ganciclovir or foscarnet is indicated.

ISOLATION OF THE HOSPITALIZED PATIENT: Standard precautions are recommended. Since CMV is spread by intimate contact with infectious secretions, hand washing after exposure to secretions is particularly important for pregnant personnel.

CONTROL MEASURES:

Care of Exposed Persons. In caring for all children, hand washing, particularly after changing diapers, is advised to reduce transmission of CMV and other infectious agents. Since asymptomatic infection and excretion of CMV is common in persons of all ages, the child with congenital CMV infection should not be treated differently from other children and should not be excluded from school or institutions. Institution-sponsored screening programs for CMV-excreting children also are not justified. The intermittent and prolonged shedding of CMV in the urine makes screening programs impractical and prohibitively costly.

Although unrecognized exposure to individuals asymptomatically shedding CMV is likely to be frequent, concern arises when immunocompromised or pregnant patients or health care workers are exposed to patients with clinically recognizable CMV infection. Many exposed adults and children are already immune but because most infections are asymptomatic, the history is of no value in assessing susceptibility. Serologic testing can be used to identify nonimmune individuals, although as yet no prophylactic agent is available. Follow-up serologic testing will establish whether infection has occurred. However, routine serologic screening of personnel is not currently recommended.

Prevention of exposure of severely immunocompromised patients to recognized cases of CMV infection is prudent. Since unrecognized exposure may occur, infection control procedures for these patients, such as careful hand washing and other hygienic practices, should be used.

Pregnant personnel who may be in contact with CMV-infected patients should be counseled about the potential risks of acquisition and urged to practice good hygiene, particularly hand washing. Approximately 1% of infants in most newborn nurseries, and a higher percentage of older children, excrete CMV without clinical manifestations. Fetal risks are greatest in the first half of gestation. Amniocentesis has been used in several small series of patients to establish the presence of intrauterine infection.

Child Care (see also Children in Out-of-Home Child Care, p 80). Educational programs about the epidemiology of CMV, its potential risks, and appropriate hygienic measures to minimize occupationally acquired infection should be provided for female workers in child care centers. The prevalence of CMV in urine or saliva of apparently healthy children can be high, and spread to their mothers and child care workers has been documented. Risk appears to be greatest for child care personnel who care for children younger than 2 years. Routine serologic screening for antibody to CMV in staff at child care centers is not currently recommended.

Immunoprophylaxis. Cytomegalovirus Immune Globulin Intravenous (CMV-IGIV) has been developed for prophylaxis of disease in seronegative transplant patients. The initial dose is 150 mg/kg and is followed by doses once every two weeks at a gradually reduced dose for 16 weeks. It appears to be moderately effective in kidney and liver transplant recipients. Results of studies of its use in prevention of CMV transmission to newborn infants, to date, are inconclusive. Evaluation of investigational vaccines in healthy volunteers and renal transplant patients is in progress.

Prevention of Transmission by Blood Transfusion. Transmission of CMV by blood transfusion to preterm infants or others has been virtually eliminated by the use of CMV antibody-negative donors, by freezing blood in glycerol before administration, by removal of the buffy coat, or by filtration to remove the white blood cells.

Prevention of Transmission by Human Milk. Pasteurization or freezing of donated human milk can reduce the likelihood of CMV transmission. If fresh donated milk is needed for infants born to CMV antibody-negative mothers, providing these infants with milk from CMV antibody-negative women only should be considered. For further information on breastfeeding, see Human Milk (p 73).

Prevention of Transmission in Transplant Patients. Cytomegalovirus antibody-negative persons who receive tissue from CMV-seropositive persons are at high risk for CMV disease. If such circumstances cannot be avoided, administration of CMV-IGIV is beneficial in reducing this risk. Treatment with acyclovir or ganciclovir in transplant patients at the onset of CMV viremia may prevent serious CMV disease.

Diphtheria

CLINICAL MANIFESTATIONS: Diphtheria usually occurs as membranous naso-pharyngitis and/or obstructive laryngotracheitis. These local infections are associated with a low-grade fever and the gradual onset of manifestations during 1 to 2 days. Less commonly, the disease presents as cutaneous, vaginal, conjunctival, or otic infections. Cutaneous diphtheria is more common in tropical areas and among the homeless. Life-threatening complications of diphtheria include upper airway obstruction caused by extensive membrane formation, myocarditis, and neurologic problems such as vocal cord paralysis and ascending paralysis similar to that of Guillain-Barré syndrome.

ETIOLOGY: *Corynebacterium diphtheriae* is an irregularly staining, Gram-positive, nonspore-forming, nonmotile, pleomorphic bacillus with three colony types (mitis, intermedius, and gravis). Strains of *C diphtheriae* may be toxicogenic or nontoxico-genic. The ability to produce toxin is mediated by bacteriophage infections of the bacterium and is not related to colony type.

EPIDEMIOLOGY: Humans are the only known reservoir of *C diphtheriae*. Sources of infection include discharges from the nose, throat, eye, and skin lesions of infected persons. Transmission results primarily from intimate contact with a patient or carrier; rarely, fomites and food-borne sources serve as vehicles of transmission. Illness is most common in low socioeconomic groups living in crowded conditions. Infection can occur in immunized and partially immunized persons as well as in persons who are not immunized; disease is most common and most severe in persons who are not immunized or who are inadequately immunized. Since 1990, epidemic diphtheria has occurred throughout the newly independent states of the former Soviet Union, including Russia, the Ukraine, and the central Asian republics, resulting in approximately 48 000 reported cases by 1995. The case-fatality rate has ranged from 3% to

23%. The underlying causes include a highly susceptible adult population lacking routine booster doses of diphtheria toxoid, undervaccination of young children, crowded living conditions, and increased population movement after the dissolution of the Soviet Union.

The incidence of respiratory diphtheria is greatest in the fall and winter, but summer epidemics can occur in warm, moist climates in which skin infections are prevalent. Communicability in untreated persons usually lasts for 2 weeks or less, but occasionally persists for several months. In patients treated with appropriate antibiotics, communicability usually lasts less than 4 days. Occasionally, chronic carriage occurs, even after antimicrobial therapy.

The **incubation period** is usually 2 to 5 days but occasionally longer.

DIAGNOSTIC TESTS: Specimens for culture should be obtained from the nose and throat and from any lesions. Material should be obtained from beneath the membrane, or a portion of the membrane itself should be submitted for culture. Because special media are required, the laboratory should be notified that *C diphtheriae* is suspected. In remote areas, throat swabs can be placed in silica gel packs or tellurite enrichment medium and sent to a reference laboratory for culture. Direct-stained smears and fluorescent antibody-stained smears are unreliable. When *C diphtheriae* is recovered, the strain should be tested for toxicogenicity at a laboratory recommended by state and local authorities. All *C diphtheriae* isolates also should be sent through the state health department to the Diphtheria Reference Laboratory of Centers for Disease Control and Prevention.

TREATMENT:

Antitoxin. Because the condition of patients with diphtheria may deteriorate rapidly, a single dose of equine antitoxin should be administered on the basis of clinical diagnosis, even before culture results are available. The site and size of the diphtheritic membrane, the degree of toxicity, and the duration of the illness are guides for estimating the dose of antitoxin; the presence of soft, diffuse cervical lymphadenitis suggests moderate to severe toxin absorption. Suggested dose ranges are the following: pharyngeal or laryngeal disease of 48 hours' duration, 20 000 to 40 000 U; nasopharyngeal lesions, 40 000 to 60 000 U; extensive disease of 3 or more days' duration or diffuse swelling of the neck, 80 000 to 120 000 U. Antitoxin is probably of no value for cutaneous disease, but some experts, nevertheless, recommend 20 000 to 40 000 U of antitoxin because toxic sequelae have been reported.

To neutralize toxin as rapidly as possible, the preferred route of administration is intravenous. Before intravenous administration, however, tests for sensitivity to horse serum should be performed with a 1:1000 dilution of antitoxin in saline (see Sensitivity Tests for Reactions to Animal Sera, p 42). If the patient is sensitive to equine antitoxin, desensitization is necessary (see Desensitization to Animal Sera, p 43). Although intravenous immunoglobulin preparations contain antibodies to diphtheria toxin, their use for therapy of cutaneous or respiratory diphtheria has not been approved and optimal dosages have not been established.

Antitoxin can be obtained from the National Immunization Program of the Centers for Disease Control and Prevention (see Directory of Telephone Numbers, p 667).

Antimicrobial Therapy. Erythromycin given orally or parenterally (40 to 50 mg/kg per day, maximum 2 g/d) for 14 days; or penicillin G given parenterally (aqueous crystalline, 100 000 to 150 000 U/kg per day, in four divided doses intravenously; or aqueous procaine, 25 000 to 50,000 U/kg per day, maximum 1.2 million units, in two divided doses intramuscularly) for 14 days, constitute acceptable therapy. Antimicrobial therapy is required to eradicate the organism and prevent spread; **it is not a substitute for antitoxin**. Elimination of the organism should be documented by two consecutive negative cultures after completion of treatment.

Cutaneous Diphtheria. Thorough cleansing of the lesion with soap and water and administration of antimicrobials for 10 days are recommended.

Carriers. If not immunized, carriers should receive active immunization promptly, and measures should be taken to ensure completion of the immunization schedule. If a carrier has been previously immunized but has not received a booster within 1 year, a booster dose of a preparation containing diphtheria toxoid (DTaP, DTP, DT, or Td, depending on age) should be given. Carriers should be given antimicrobial therapy, specifically oral erythromycin or penicillin G for 7 days, or a single intramuscular dose of benzathine penicillin G (600 000 U for those weighing less than 30 kg and 1.2 million U for larger children and adults). Follow-up cultures should be obtained at least 2 weeks after the completion of therapy; if they are positive, an additional 10-day course of oral erythromycin should be given. Erythromycin-resistant strains have been identified, but their epidemiologic significance has not been determined.

ISOLATION OF THE HOSPITALIZED PATIENT*: Droplet precautions are recommended for patients and carriers with pharyngeal diphtheria until two cultures from both the nose and the throat are negative for *C diphtheriae*. Contact precautions are recommended for patients with cutaneous diphtheria until two cultures of skin lesions are negative. Material for these cultures should be taken at least 24 hours apart after cessation of antimicrobial therapy.

CONTROL MEASURES:

Care of Exposed Persons. Whenever the diagnosis of diphtheria is strongly suspected or proven, local public health officials should be notified promptly. Management of exposed persons is based on individual circumstances, including immunization status and the likelihood of surveillance and adherence to prophylaxis. The following is recommended:

- Identification of close contacts of a person suspected to have diphtheria should be promptly initiated. Contact tracing should begin in the household and can usually be limited to household members and other persons with a history of habitual, close contact with the person suspected of having the disease.
- Close contacts, *irrespective of their immunization status*, should be (1) kept under surveillance for 7 days for evidence of disease, (2) cultured for *C diphtheria*, and (3) given antimicrobial prophylaxis with oral erythromycin (40 to 50 mg/ kg per day for 7 days, maximum 2 g/d) or a single intramuscular dose of benzathine penicillin G (600 000 U for those weighing less than 30 kg and

---

* In addition to standard precautions.

1.2 million U for larger children and adults). The efficacy of antimicrobial prophylaxis is presumed but not proven. Repeat pharyngeal cultures should be obtained from contacts proven to be carriers at a minimum of 2 weeks after completion of their therapy (see Carriers, p 193).

- Asymptomatic, previously immunized, close contacts should receive a booster dose of a preparation containing diphtheria toxoid (DTaP, DTP, DT, or Td, depending on age) if they have not received a booster dose of diphtheria toxoid within 5 years. Children in need of their fourth dose should be vaccinated.
- For asymptomatic close contacts who are not fully immunized (defined as having had fewer than 3 doses of diphtheria toxoid) or whose immunization status is not known, active immunization should be undertaken with DTaP, DTP, DT, or Td, depending on age.
- Contacts who cannot be kept under surveillance should receive (1) benzathine penicillin G, but not erythromycin because adherence to an oral regimen is less likely; and (2) a dose of DTaP, DTP, DT, or Td, depending on age and the person's immunization history.

The use of equine diphtheria antitoxin in unimmunized close contacts is not recommended because no evidence demonstrates any additional benefit of using diphtheria antitoxin for contacts who have received antimicrobial prophylaxis and because of the 5% to 20% risk of allergic reactions to horse serum.

Immunization. * Universal immunization with diphtheria toxoid is the only effective control measure. Its value is proven by the rarity of the disease in countries in which high rates of immunization with diphtheria toxoid have been achieved. Fewer than five cases have been reported annually in the United States in recent years. As a result of high immunization rates, exposure to persons with diphtheria or to carriers is less frequent now than in the past. However, the decreased frequency of exposure to the organism implies decreased maintenance of immunity secondary to community contact. Therefore, assurance of continuing immunity requires regular booster injections of diphtheria toxoid (as Td) every 10 years after completion of the initial immunization series.

Vaccine is given intramuscularly. *Haemophilus influenzae conjugate* vaccines containing diphtheria toxoid (PRP-D) or CRM197 protein (HbOC), a nontoxic variant of diphtheria toxin, are not substitutes for diphtheria toxoid immunization.

Immunization for children from age 2 months to the seventh birthday (see Fig 1.1 and Table 1.3, p 18 and p 20) should consist of five doses of diphtheria vaccine. The initial three doses are given as DTaP (or DTP), administered at 2-month intervals commencing at approximately 2 months of age. A fourth dose is recommended 6 to 12 months after the third dose, usually at 15 to 18 months of age (see Pertussis, p 397). A fifth dose of DTaP (or DTP) is given before school entry (kindergarten or elementary school) at 4 to 6 years of age, unless the fourth dose was given after the fourth birthday, and it may be given concurrently with other vaccines (see Simultaneous Administration of Multiple Vaccines, p 21).

Immunization against diphtheria for children younger than 7 years in whom pertussis immunization is contraindicated (see Pertussis, p 394) should be accomplished with DT instead of DTP, as follows:

---

* Vaccines containing both tetanus and diphtheria toxoids in use in the United States, including DTaP, DTP, DT, and Td, are absorbed to aluminum salts.

- For children younger than 1 year of age, three doses of DT are given at 2-month intervals; a fourth dose should be given 6 to 12 months after the third dose; and the fifth dose should be given before school entry at 4 to 6 years of age.
- For children aged 1 through 6 years who have not received prior doses of DT, DTaP, or DTP, two doses of DT approximately 2 months apart should be given, followed by a third dose 6 to 12 months later to complete the initial series. DT can be given concurrently with other vaccines. An additional dose is necessary before school entry at 4 to 6 years of age, unless the preceding dose was given after the fourth birthday.
- For children aged 1 through 6 years who have received one or two doses of DTaP, DTP, or DT during the first year of life and for whom further pertussis vaccination is contraindicated, additional doses of DT should be given until a total of five doses of diphtheria and tetanus toxoids are received by the time of school entry. The fourth dose is administered 6 to 12 months after the third dose. The preschool (fifth) dose is omitted if the fourth dose was given after the fourth birthday.

Other recommendations for diphtheria immunization, including those for older children, are as follows:

- For children after their seventh birthday (see Table 1.3, p 20), diphtheria immunization should consist of Td, ie, adult-type tetanus and diphtheria toxoids. The Td preparation contains not more than 2 Lf (limes flocculation) of diphtheria toxoid, as compared to 6.7 to 25 Lf in the DTP, DTaP, and DT preparations for use in infants and younger children. Because of the lower dose of diphtheria toxoid, the Td vaccine is less likely than DTP, DTaP, or DT to produce reactions in older children and adults. Two doses are given 1 to 2 months apart; a third dose should be given 6 to 12 months after the second.
- After the initial immunization series is completed at 4 to 6 years of age, a booster dose of tetanus toxoid (given as Td) is recommended at 11 to 12 years of age and should be given no later than by 16 years of age and every 10 years thereafter. This 10-year period is determined from the time that the last dose was administered, irrespective of whether it was given earlier in routine child-hood immunization or as part of wound management. Since the immunity conferred by absorbed preparations of tetanus toxoid has proved to be of long duration, routine boosters more frequently than every 10 years are not indicated and may be associated with an increased incidence and severity of reactions.
- When children and adults require tetanus toxoid for wound management (see Tetanus, p 518), the use of preparations containing diphtheria toxoid (DTaP, DTP, DT, or Td as appropriate for age or specific contraindication to pertussis immunization) will help ensure continuing diphtheria immunity.
- Active immunization against diphtheria should be undertaken during convalescence from diphtheria in every patient because this exotoxin-mediated disease does not necessarily confer immunity.
- Travelers to countries with endemic or epidemic diphtheria should have their diphtheria immunization status reviewed and updated when necessary.

Precautions and Contraindications. See Pertussis (p 394) and Tetanus (p 518).

Ehrlichiosis
(Human)

CLINICAL MANIFESTATIONS: Human ehrlichiosis in North America consists of at least two distinct diseases that are referred to as human monocytic ehrlichiosis and human granulocytic ehrlichiosis. These two diseases have different etiologies but similar signs, symptoms, and clinical course. Both are acute, systemic febrile illnesses clinically similar to Rocky Mountain spotted fever but with more frequent occurrence of leukopenia and less frequent occurrence of rash. The febrile illness is often accompanied by headache, chills, malaise, myalgia, arthralgia, nausea, vomiting, anorexia, and acute weight loss. Rash is variable in appearance and location, typically develops about 1 week after onset of illness, only occurs in approximately 40% of reported cases of human monocytic ehrlichiosis, and rarely occurs with human granulocytic ehrlichiosis. Diarrhea, abdominal pain, and change in mental status are less frequent in occurrence. Reported complications of either disease include pulmonary infiltrates, bone marrow hypoplasia, respiratory failure, encephalopathy, meningitis, disseminated intravascular coagulation, and renal failure. Anemia, hyponatremia, thrombocytopenia, elevated liver function tests, and cerebrospinal fluid abnormalities (ie, pleocytosis with a predominance of lymphocytes and elevated total protein concentration) are common. Either disease typically lasts 1 to 2 weeks, and recovery generally occurs without sequelae. Fatal as well as asymptomatic infections have been reported. Secondary or opportunistic infections occur in severe illness resulting in possible delayed recognition and appropriate antibiotic treatment.

ETIOLOGY: Human monocytic ehrlichiosis is caused by *Ehrlichia chaffeensis*, a rickettsial species closely related to *Ehrlichia canis*, the causative agent of canine ehrlichiosis. Human granulocytic ehrlichiosis is caused by an as yet unnamed *Ehrlichia* species closely related to *E phagocytophilia* and *E equi*. Sennetsu fever, a self-limited illness diagnosed in the Far East and Southeast Asia, is caused by *E sennetsu*.

EPIDEMIOLOGY: Most human cases of human monocytic ehrlichiosis have been reported from southeastern and south central United States, but cases have been reported in far western states. The disease appears to be transmitted by ticks. *Ehrlichia chaffeensis* has been identified most consistently in the tick vector *Amblyomma americanum* but cases occurring in states out of range of *A americanum* suggest transmission by other tick vectors as well. Most cases of human granulocytic ehrlichiosis have been reported in Wisconsin, Minnesota, and New York, but cases have been acquired in California and other states. Human granulocytic ehrlichiosis has been linked to bites of *Ixodes scapularis*, but definitive identification of the vector is lacking. The natural animal reservoirs for *E chaffeensis* and the agent causing human granulocytic ehrlichiosis are not proven. Compared to those with Rocky Mountain spotted fever (see p 452), patients with ehrlichiosis may be slightly older (particularly patients with human granulocytic ehrlichiosis) but similar regarding gender, race, and recognized tick exposures. Most human infections occur between April and September; peak occurrence is from May through July. The incidence of reported cases appears to be increasing.

The **incubation period** of human monocytic ehrlichiosis and human granulo-cytic ehrlichiosis appears to be 1 to 3 weeks; the median has been 11 to 12 days.

DIAGNOSTIC TESTS: The diagnosis of human ehrlichiosis can be established by demonstrating a fourfold or greater increase or decrease in antibody titer between acute and convalescent sera, obtained 2 to 4 weeks apart, using an indirect fluorescent antibody test with *E chaffeensis* as antigen to diagnose human monocytic ehrlichiosis and *E equi* as antigen to diagnose human granulocytic ehrlichiosis. The tests are available in a limited number of reference laboratories; testing is available through state health departments at the Centers for Disease Control and Prevention. *Ehrlichia chaffeensis* has been isolated from human patients. Examination of peripheral blood smears to detect morulae (inclusions) in peripheral blood monocytes or granulocytes is insensitive and labor intensive; immunocytologic and immuno-histologic testing can be used to determine whether morulalike bodies are *Ehrlichieae*. The use of the polymerase chain reaction test to amplify nucleic acids from peripheral blood of patients with acute phase ehrlichiosis appears sensitive, specific, and most promising for early diagnosis, but currently is available only in research laboratories.

TREATMENT: Doxycycline is the drug of choice for therapy of human ehrlichiosis. The recommended dosage of doxycycline is 3 mg/kg per day in two divided doses. Limited data suggest that chloramphenicol also is effective in treatment of human monocytic ehrlichiosis, but may be less effective and even ineffective in treatment of human granulocytic ehrlichiosis. While tetracycline drugs ordinarily should not be given to children younger than 8 years because of the risk of dental staining (see Antimicrobials and Related Therapy, p 606), comparison of the benefits and risks of a single course of tetracycline with those of chloramphenicol in deciding which anti-microbial agent to give to a child with suspected ehrlichiosis who is younger than 8 years can justify use of doxycycline.

Treatment for a minimum of 5 to 7 days is recommended and should continue for 3 days after defervescence. Staining of teeth by tetracycline drugs is considered to be dose-related, and, thus, minimizing the duration of therapy is prudent. In addition, doxycycline is less likely to stain developing teeth, since it binds less strongly to calcium, than is tetracycline.

The clinical manifestations of ehrlichiosis and Rocky Mountain spotted fever overlap. Because of the importance of initiating appropriate empiric antimicrobial therapy early in the course of either illness and the effectiveness of doxycycline is effective therapy for both infections, and because chloramphenicol may not be effective in human granulocytic ehrlichiosis, doxycycline is recommended as the drug of choice in patients in whom both diseases are possible such as occurs in geo-graphic regions where both diseases are endemic.

ISOLATION OF THE HOSPITALIZED PATIENT: Standard precautions are recommended.

CONTROL MEASURES: Specific measures concern prevention of contact with ticks and are similar to those for Rocky Mountain spotted fever and other tick-borne diseases (see Control Measures for Prevention of Tick-Borne Infections, p 126).

Enterovirus (Nonpolio) Infections
(Coxsackieviruses, Group A and Group B; Echoviruses; and Enteroviruses)

CLINICAL MANIFESTATIONS: Nonpolio enteroviruses are responsible for significant and frequent illnesses in infants and children and result in protean clinical manifestations. The most common presentation is nonspecific febrile illness, which in young infants may appear similar to bacterial sepsis. Manifestations can include the following: (1) respiratory—common cold, pharyngitis, herpangina, stomatitis, pneumonia, and pleurodynia; (2) skin—exanthem; (3) neurologic—aseptic meningitis, encephalitis, and paralysis; (4) gastrointestinal—vomiting, diarrhea, abdominal pain, and hepatitis; (5) eye—acute hemorrhagic conjunctivitis; and (6) heart—myopericarditis. Although each of these findings can be caused by several different enteroviruses, some associations between virus and disease are particularly noteworthy. These associations include coxsackievirus A16 and enterovirus 71 with hand, foot, and mouth syndrome; coxsackievirus A24 and enterovirus 70 with acute hemorrhagic conjunctivitis; enterovirus 71 with encephalitis and poliolike paralysis; echovirus 9 with a petechial exanthem and meningitis; and coxsackieviruses B1-B5 with myopericarditis.

Immunocompromised patients, especially those with humoral deficiencies, can have persistent central nervous system infections lasting for several months or more.

ETIOLOGY: The nonpolio enteroviruses are RNA viruses, which include 23 group A coxsackieviruses (types A1-A24, except type A23), 6 group B coxsackieviruses (types B1-B6), 31 echoviruses (types 1-34, except types 10, 28, and 34), and 4 enteroviruses (types 68-71).

EPIDEMIOLOGY: Humans are the only known natural host for the ubiquitous enteroviruses. They are spread by fecal-oral and respiratory routes, and from mother to infant in the peripartum period. Enteroviruses may survive on environmental surfaces for periods long enough to allow transmission from fomites. Infections and clinical attack rates are typically highest in young children, and infections occur more frequently in lower socioeconomic groups, in tropical areas, and where hygiene is poor. In temperate climates, enteroviral infections are most common in the summer and early fall. In contrast, seasonal patterns can be less evident or absent in the tropics. Fecal viral shedding and transmission can continue for several weeks after the onset of infection, while respiratory shedding is usually limited to a week or less. Viral shedding can occur without signs of clinical illness.

The usual **incubation period** is 3 to 6 days, except for acute hemorrhagic conjunctivitis in which it is 24 to 72 hours.

DIAGNOSTIC TESTS: Specimens providing the highest rate of viral isolation are those obtained from the throat, stool, and rectal swabs. Specimens also should be obtained from any sites of clinical involvement, such as the cerebrospinal fluid (CSF). Enteroviruses also may be recovered from the blood during the acute febrile phase and, rarely, from biopsy material. Specimens should be sent to the laboratory at 4°C. Repeated freezing, thawing, and drying of specimens are detrimental to viral recovery. In patients with serious illnesses, viral isolation as a means of diagnosis is particularly important. Viral isolation from any specimen except feces usually can be considered causally related to the patient's illness. Whether isolation of an enterovirus from the stool alone indicates a causal relationship to the illness has been controversial, as enteroviruses cause a high rate of asymptomatic infections and can persist in the lower gastrointestinal tract for as long as 6 to 12 weeks. However, during some epidemics, depending on the enterovirus serotype, only a small proportion (generally 5% or less) of individuals with fecal shedding of enterovirus are asymptomatic, whereas 60% to 80% have illnesses characteristic of enteroviruses. In less developed countries, however, the fecal rate of shedding in asymptomatic individuals may be as high as 50%. The sensitivity of viral isolation varies by serotype because most viral diagnostic laboratories use only cell culture techniques that are capable of recovering echoviruses, group B coxsackieviruses, and some group A coxsackieviruses. Suckling mouse inoculation, which is not a routine procedure, is required for the recovery of some group A coxsackieviruses. Polymerase chain reaction (PCR) testing for the presence of enterovirus RNA in CSF is available in a few laboratories, and usually, but not always, is more sensitive than viral isolation. Sera for antibody testing can be collected at the onset of illness and 4 weeks later, and stored frozen. The demonstration of a rise in titer of virus-specific neutralizing antibody can be used to confirm infection, particularly when the specific virus has been previously identified during a community outbreak. Serologic screening without a suspected serotype generally is not performed.

TREATMENT: No specific therapy currently exists. Intravenous immune globulin containing high antibody titer to the infecting virus may be beneficial for treatment of immunocompromised patients and has been used in life-threatening neonatal infections.

ISOLATION OF THE HOSPITALIZED PATIENT*: For infants and young children, contact precautions are indicated for the duration of hospitalization.

CONTROL MEASURES: Particular attention should be given to hand washing and personal hygiene, especially after diaper changing.

Epstein-Barr Virus Infections
(Infectious Mononucleosis)

CLINICAL MANIFESTATIONS: Infectious mononucleosis is manifested typically by fever, exudative pharyngitis, lymphadenopathy, hepatosplenomegaly, and atypical lymphocytosis. The spectrum of diseases, however, is extremely variable, ranging from asymptomatic to fatal infection. Infections are frequently unrecognized in infants and young children. Rash, which is more frequent in patients treated with ampicillin, can occur. Central nervous system (CNS) complications include aseptic meningitis, encephalitis, and the Guillain-Barré syndrome. Rare complications include splenic rupture, thrombocytopenia, agranulocytosis, hemolytic anemia, orchitis, and myocarditis. The replication of Epstein-Barr virus (EBV) in B lympho-

---

*In addition to standard precautions.

cytes and the resulting lymphoproliferation usually is inhibited by natural killer and T-cell responses, but in patients who have congenital or acquired cellular immune deficiencies, fatal disseminated infection or B-cell lymphomas can occur.

Epstein-Barr virus causes several other distinct disorders, including the X-linked lymphoproliferative syndrome (also known as Duncan's disease), posttransplantation lymphoproliferation disorders, Burkitt's lymphoma, nasopharyngeal carcinoma, and undifferentiated B-cell lymphomas of the central nervous system. The X-linked lymphoproliferative syndrome occurs in those with an inherited, maternally derived, recessive genetic defect characterized by three phenotypic expressions, the most common of which is the occurrence of infectious mononucleosis early in life among boys. A nodular B-cell lymphoma is the second phenotype and occurs in approximately 25% of recessive carriers, the majority of whom develop disease without antecedent EBV infection and exhibit CNS involvement. Patients with this lymphoproliferative disorder often are profoundly hypogammaglobulinemic.

Posttransplantation EBV-associated lymphoproliferative disorders result in a number of complex syndromes associated with immunosuppression and occur in approximately 2% of graft recipients. The highest incidence occurs after heart transplantation.

Other EBV syndromes are of greater importance outside the United States, including Burkitt B-cell lymphoma, found primarily in Central Africa, and nasopharyngeal carcinoma, found in Southeast Asia.

The chronic fatigue syndrome is not specifically related to EBV infection. However, a small group of patients with recurrent symptoms have abnormal serologic tests for EBV and other viruses.

ETIOLOGY: Epstein-Barr virus, a DNA virus, is a herpesvirus and is the most common cause of infectious mononucleosis.

EPIDEMIOLOGY: Humans are the only source of EBV. Close personal contact is usually required for transmission. Epstein-Barr virus also is occasionally transmitted by blood transfusion. Infection frequently is contracted early in life, particularly among lower socioeconomic groups, in which intrafamilial spread is common. Endemic infectious mononucleosis is common in group settings of adolescents, such as in educational institutions. No seasonal pattern has been documented. Respiratory tract viral excretion can occur for many months after infection, and asymptomatic carriage is common. The period of communicability is indeterminate.

The **incubation period** of infectious mononucleosis is estimated to be 30 to 50 days.

DIAGNOSTIC TESTS: Epstein-Barr virus isolation from oropharyngeal secretions is possible, but techniques for performing this procedure are usually not available in routine diagnostic laboratories, and viral isolation does not necessarily indicate acute infection. Hence, diagnosis depends on serologic testing. Nonspecific tests for heterophile antibody, including the Paul-Bunnell test and slide agglutination reaction, are most commonly available. These tests are often negative in infants and children younger than 4 years with EBV infection, but they identify approximately 90% of cases (proven by EBV-specific serology) in older children and adults.

Multiple specific serologic antibody tests for EBV are available in diagnostic virology laboratories (see Table 3.4). The most commonly performed test is for antibody against the viral capsid antigen (VCA). Since IgG antibody against VCA occurs in high titers early after onset of infection, testing of acute and convalescent sera for anti-VCA may not be useful in establishing infection. Testing for IgM anti-VCA antibody and for antibodies against early antigen (EA) is useful in identifying recent infections. Since serum antibody against EBV nuclear antigens (EBNA) is not present until several weeks to months after onset of the infection, a positive anti-EBNA antibody test excludes acute infection.

Epstein-Barr virus serologic tests are particularly valuable for evaluating patients who have heterophile-negative infectious mononucleosis. Testing for other viral agents, especially cytomegalovirus, is indicated in these patients. In research studies, culture of saliva or peripheral blood mononuclear cells for EBV, in situ DNA hybridization, or the polymerase chain reaction can determine the presence of EBV or EBV DNA, and may implicate EBV with a syndrome, such as lymphoproliferation.

TREATMENT: Corticosteroids have been useful in reducing tonsillar inflammation and preventing airway obstruction. Corticosteroid use otherwise is only considered in cases with complications such as massive splenomegaly, myocarditis, and hemolytic anemia. The dosage of prednisone is usually 1 mg/kg per day orally for 7 days with a subsequent tapering. Although acyclovir has in vitro antiviral activity against EBV, the clinical benefits of treatment have not been demonstrated, with the possible exception of HIV-infected patients with hairy leukoplakia. Reducing immunosuppressive therapy is beneficial in patients with EBV-induced lymphoproliferation, such as the posttransplant lymphoproliferation syndrome.

ISOLATION OF THE HOSPITALIZED PATIENT: Standard precautions are recommended.

CONTROL MEASURES: Patients with a recent history of EBV infection or an illness similar to infectious mononucleosis should not donate blood.

Table 3.4. Serum EBV Antibodies in EBV Infection

Infection	Anti-VCA-IgG*	Anti-VCA-IgM†	Anti-EA (D)‡	Anti-EBNA§
No previous infection	0	0	0	0
Acute infection	+	+	+/0	0
Recent infection	+	+/0	+/0	+/0
Past infection	+	0	0	+

* Anti-VCA-IgG: IgG class antibody to viral capsid antigen.
† Anti-VCA-IgM: IgM class antibody to viral capsid antigen.
‡ EA(D): early antigen diffuse staining.
§ EBNA: Epstein-Barr nuclear antigen. 0 indicates <1:10 or <1:2 for EBNA, and + indicates ≥1:10 or ≥1:2 for EBNA.

Escherichia coli and Other Gram-Negative Bacilli
(Septicemia and Meningitis in Neonates)

CLINICAL MANIFESTATIONS: Neonatal septicemia or meningitis caused by *Escherichia coli* and other Gram-negative bacilli cannot be differentiated clinically from serious infections caused by other infectious agents. The first signs of sepsis may be minimal and similar to those observed in noninfectious processes. Clinical signs of septicemia include fever, temperature instability, apnea, cyanosis, jaundice, hepatomegaly, lethargy, irritability, anorexia, vomiting, abdominal distention, and diarrhea. Meningitis may be concomitant with septicemia without overt signs attributable to the central nervous system.

ETIOLOGY: *Escherichia coli* strains with the K1 capsular polysaccharide antigen cause approximately 40% of cases of septicemia and 75% of cases of meningitis caused by *E coli*. Other important Gram-negative bacilli that can cause neonatal septicemia include non-K1 strains of *E coli*, *Klebsiella*, *Enterobacter*, *Proteus*, *Citrobacter*, *Salmonella*, and *Pseudomonas* species. Anaerobic Gram-negative bacilli are infrequent causes. *Haemophilus influenzae* infection can occur in the newborn period. In contrast to invasive *H influenzae* infections occurring after the newborn period, invasive infections in neonates can be caused by nonencapsulated strains.

EPIDEMIOLOGY: The source of *E coli* and other Gram-negative bacterial pathogens in neonatal infections is usually the maternal gastrointestinal tract. In addition, nosocomial acquisition of Gram-negative flora through person-to-person transmission among nursery personnel and from nursery environmental sites, such as fluid reservoirs of incubators, has been documented, especially in preterm infants requiring prolonged intensive care management. Predisposing host factors in neonatal Gram-negative bacterial infections include maternal perinatal infections, low birth weight, prolonged rupture of membranes, and septic or traumatic delivery. Metabolic abnormalities such as galactosemia, fetal hypoxia, and acidosis also have been implicated as predisposing factors. Neonates with immunologic abnormalities or defects in the integrity of the skin or mucosa (eg, meningomyelocele) or persons with asplenia also are at increased risk for Gram-negative bacterial infections. In intensive care nurseries, sophisticated systems for respiratory and metabolic support, invasive procedures, indwelling vascular lines, and the frequent use of antimicrobial agents enable selection and proliferation of multiply antimicrobial-resistant strains of pathogenic Gram-negative bacilli.

The **incubation period** is highly variable; time of onset of the infection ranges from birth to several weeks of age.

DIAGNOSTIC TESTS: Blood, urine, cerebrospinal fluid, and other body fluids or tissues from a potentially infected neonate should be Gram stained and microscopically examined for bacteria as well as cultured prior to initiation of antimicrobial therapy. Techniques for detection of bacterial antigens, such as latex particle agglutination, are not available commercially for Gram-negative pathogens implicated in neonatal septicemia, with the exception of *H influenzae* type b and *E coli* K1 (whose capsular antigen cross-reacts with that of group B *Neisseria meningitidis*). The value of these tests in patient management, however, is questionable.

TREATMENT:

- Initial empiric treatment of a neonate with suspected bacterial septicemia and/or meningitis entails a combination of ampicillin and an aminoglycoside. An alternative regimen of ampicillin and a cephalosporin (such as cefotaxime or ceftazidime) active against most etiologic Gram-negative bacilli can be used, but rapid emergence of cephalosporin-resistant strains, especially *Enterobacter cloacae, Klebsiella* species, and *Serratia* species, can occur as a result of frequent cephalosporin use in a nursery. Hence, routine use of cephalosporins in newborn units for empiric treatment of infections is not recommended, unless Gram-negative bacterial meningitis is strongly suspected.
- Once the etiologic agent and its in vitro antimicrobial susceptibilities have been determined, bacteremia is treated with an appropriate cephalosporin (such as cefotaxime) and/or an aminoglycoside, or both; meningitis is usually treated with a cephalosporin with or without other drugs.
- Duration of therapy is based on the patient's response; the usual duration of therapy in uncomplicated septicemia is 10 to 14 days and in meningitis the minimum is 21 days.
- Data on the efficacy of granulocyte transfusions or granulocyte stimulating factors in septic, neutrophil-depleted neonates are limited and these therapies remain controversial.
- A therapeutic role for immunoglobulin therapy in septicemia or meningitis caused by *E coli* or other Gram-negative organisms has not been established, although its use may be warranted in low-birth-weight infants of less than 1500 g.
- All infants with meningitis should undergo careful follow-up examinations, including testing for hearing loss, to detect neurologic abnormalities.

ISOLATION OF THE HOSPITALIZED PATIENT: Standard precautions are recommended for the infant with septicemia or meningitis caused by *E coli* or other enteric Gram-negative bacilli. Exceptions include nursery epidemics, infants with *Salmonella* infection, and those with infection caused by multiply antibiotic-resistant Gram-negative bacilli, in which cases contact precautions are indicated.*

CONTROL MEASURES:

The physician in charge of the nursery and all infection control personnel should be aware of pathogens causing infections in the nursery and the nature of infections in personnel, so that clusters of infections are recognized and appropriately investigated. They should be notified by other physicians in the community of serious infections in infants recently discharged from the nursery because nursery-acquired infections can become apparent as late as several weeks to a month after discharge.

Several cases of infection caused by the same genus and species of bacteria occurring in infants in close physical proximity or caused by an unusual pathogen can indicate an epidemic and the need for an epidemiologic investigation. The decision to perform culture surveys of personnel or the environment in an attempt to identify the source should be based on epidemiologic data.

---

*In addition to standard precautions.

The routine performance of ongoing surveillance cultures of the environment or personnel, infants, or families is not cost effective, does not predict infecting pathogens, and is not recommended.

An ongoing, in-service educational program for nursery personnel to review and emphasize concepts of infection control, especially hand washing between all patient contacts, is recommended.

Periodic review of the in vitro antimicrobial susceptibilities of clinically important bacterial isolates from newborns, especially those in the intensive care nursery, can provide useful epidemiologic and therapeutic information.

Escherichia coli Diarrhea
(Including Hemolytic-Uremic Syndrome)

CLINICAL MANIFESTATIONS: At least five different groups of diarrhea-producing *Escherichia coli* strains have been identified. Clinical features of disease caused by each group are summarized as follows (see also Table 3.5, p 205):

- Enterohemorrhagic *E coli* (EHEC) strains are associated with diarrhea, hemorrhagic colitis, hemolytic-uremic syndrome (HUS), and postdiarrheal thrombotic thrombocytopenic purpura. *Escherichia coli* O157:H7 is the prototype for this class of organisms (and is the only one for which extensive epidemiologic and clinical information is available). *Escherichia coli* O157:H7 infections can occur sporadically or in outbreaks (see Epidemiology, p 206). The illness usually begins as nonbloody diarrhea and may progress to grossly bloody diarrhea. Severe abdominal pain is typical; fever occurs in one third of cases.
- Diarrhea caused by enteropathogenic *E coli* (EPEC) typically occurs in neonates and children younger than 2 years in developing countries, either sporadically or in epidemics. Illness is characterized by watery diarrhea that is often severe and can result in dehydration. Enteropathogenic *E coli* is an important cause of chronic diarrhea that can cause failure to thrive.
- Diarrhea caused by enterotoxigenic *E coli* (ETEC) is a self-limited illness of moderate severity with watery stools and abdominal cramps. It occurs in persons of all ages but is an important cause of diarrhea in infants in developing countries. Outbreaks have occurred in adults, usually from ingestion of contaminated food or water. Enterotoxigenic *E coli* is the major cause of travelers' diarrhea.
- Enteroinvasive *E coli* (EIEC) can cause dysentery, similar to that caused by *Shigella*, characterized by fever, diarrhea, vomiting, crampy abdominal pain, and tenesmus. Stools often contain blood and leukocytes. However, most patients experience watery diarrhea without blood or mucus. Outbreaks have occurred, usually secondary to contaminated food.
- Enteroaggregative *E coli* (EAggEC) appear to cause chronic diarrhea in infants and young children.

Late Sequelae of EHEC Infection. Hemolytic-uremic syndrome (HUS) is a sequela of enteric infection with shigalike toxin-producing *E coli* strains, such as *E coli* O157:H7. This syndrome is defined by the triad of microangiopathic hemo-

Table 3.5. Classification of *Escherichia coli* Associated With Diarrhea

Types of E coli	Epidemiology	Type of Diarrhea	Mechanism of Action
Enterohemorrhagic (EHEC)	Hemorrhagic colitis and hemolytic uremic syndrome in all ages and thrombotic thrombocytopenic purpura in adults	Bloody or nonbloody	Cytotoxin production, adherence and effacement
Enteropathogenic (EPEC)	Acute and chronic endemic and epidemic diarrhea in infants	Watery	Adherence, effacement
Enterotoxigenic (ETEC)	Infantile diarrhea in developing countries and travelers' diarrhea	Watery	Adherence, enterotoxin production
Enteroinvasive (EIEC)	Diarrhea with fever in all ages	Bloody or nonbloody	Adherence, invasion of mucosa
Enteroaggregative (EAggEC)	Chronic diarrhea in infants	Watery	Adherence

lytic anemia, thrombocytopenia, and acute renal dysfunction. Many children with hemorrhagic colitis caused by *E coli* O157:H7 develop mild, self-limited, microangiopathic hematologic changes and/or nephropathy in the week after onset of diarrhea. Thrombotic thrombocytopenic purpura (TTP) occurs in adults, may follow EHEC infection and is part of a disease spectrum often designated as TTP-HUS. While the vast majority of cases of childhood HUS are caused by *E coli* O157:H7, most cases of TTP in adults are of unknown etiology.

ETIOLOGY: Each group of *E coli* strains has a distinct group of somatic (O) and flagellar (H) antigens and has specific virulence characteristics that usually are plasmid-mediated. Microbiologic characteristics are as follows:

- Hemorrhagic colitis is caused by *E coli* O157:H7 and, less frequently, by other serotypes of *E coli* that produce cytotoxins resembling those found in *Shigella dysenteriae*, type 1. These toxins are referred to as shigalike toxins or verotoxins.
- The EPEC strains traditionally have been defined as members of specific *E coli* serotypes that have been epidemiologically incriminated as causes of infantile diarrhea and include the following somatic (O) serogroups: O44, O55, O86, O111, O114, O119, O125, O126, O127, O128, O142, and O158. More recently, EPEC has been defined according to specific virulence properties. Enteropathogenic *E coli* strains adhere to intestinal mucosa and produce a characteristic lesion in the gastrointestinal tract termed an "attaching and effacing" lesion. Enteropathogenic *E coli* do not produce enterotoxins and are not invasive.
- The ETEC strains colonize the small intestine without invading and produce either or both heat-labile and/or heat-stable enterotoxins.
- The enteroinvasive *E coli* (EIEC) strains include specific serotypes of *E coli* that are different from EPEC serotypes. The EIEC strains resemble *Shigella* biochemically and can invade intestinal epithelial cells.

- Enteroaggregative *E coli* are defined by their characteristic adherence pattern in tissue-culture-based assays. Unlike EPEC, which demonstrates localized adherence, these strains exhibit a "stacked brick" adherence pattern on HEP-2 or HeLa cells. An additional group of *E coli* that adhere diffusely to these cell lines needs further clarification.

EPIDEMIOLOGY: Transmission of most diarrhea-associated *E coli* strains is from infected symptomatic persons or carriers, or from food or water contaminated with human or animal feces. *E coli* O157:H7 has a bovine reservoir and is transmitted by undercooked ground beef and unpasteurized milk; it also spreads from person to person by fecal-oral transmission. Outbreaks from contaminated apple cider, raw vegetables, salami, yogurt, and water also have occurred. The frequency of HUS as a complication of *E coli* O157:H7 in children has been estimated to be 5% to 10%. Diarrhea caused by *E coli* strains other than O157:H7 is common in areas of the world where food and water supplies are contaminated and facilities for hand washing are suboptimal. Previously, nursery epidemics caused by enteropathogenic *E coli* strains were common in the United States; currently, epidemic diseases in newborn infants from these strains are uncommon. Enteropathogenic *E coli* and *E coli* O157:H7 have caused numerous outbreaks of diarrhea in child care centers. While enteroaggregative *E coli* appear to be associated with persistent diarrhea in infants and young children, their role as a cause of disease needs to be defined more clearly. The period of communicability is for the duration of excretion of the specific pathogen.

The **incubation period** for most *E coli* strains is from 10 hours to 6 days; for *E coli* O157:H7 it is usually 3 to 4 days but can be as long as 8 days.

DIAGNOSTIC TESTS: Diagnosis of infection caused by diarrhea-associated *E coli* usually is difficult, as in most cases clinical laboratories cannot differentiate diarrhea-associated *E coli* from the normal *E coli* stool flora. The exceptions are *E coli* O157:H7 and EIEC, which can be presumptively and/or specifically identified. For definitive identification, isolates suspected to be associated with diarrhea need to be sent to reference or research laboratories.

Stool specimens from all children with bloody diarrhea should be cultured for *E coli* O157:H7. Clinical laboratories can screen for *E coli* O157:H7 by using MacConkey agar base with sorbitol substituted for lactose. Approximately 90% of human intestinal *E coli* strains rapidly ferment sorbitol, whereas *E coli* O157:H7 strains do not. These sorbitol-negative *E coli* can then be serotyped, using commercially available antisera to determine if they are O157:H7.

Serotyping is recommended only for outbreaks when diarrhea-associated *E coli*, such as EPEC, is suspected; for identification of EHEC strains such as O157:H7; and in epidemiologic studies. DNA probes are available in research laboratories for identification of strains in each class of diarrhea-associated *E coli* and are now considered preferable to serotyping in the identification of EPEC.

Suggested indications for EHEC confirmation include the following: bloody diarrhea, hemolytic uremic syndrome (HUS), postdiarrheal thrombotic thrombocytopenic purpura, and any type of diarrhea in contacts of patients with HUS. Persons with presumptive diagnosis of intussusception, inflammatory bowel disease, and ischemic colitis sometimes are found to have disease caused by *E coli* O157:H7. Methods for definitive identification of EHEC that are used in reference or research laboratories include testing strains or stool specimens for shigalike toxin and use of DNA probes, polymerase chain reaction assays, and enzyme immunoassay (EIA). Serologic diagnosis using an EIA to detect serum antibodies to *E coli* O157:H7 lipopolysaccharide is available in reference laboratories.

Hemolytic-Uremic Syndrome (HUS). Patients with HUS should be cultured for enteric pathogens, including *E coli* O157:H7. The absence of EHEC in feces does not preclude the diagnosis of EHEC-associated HUS, since HUS typically is diagnosed a week after onset of diarrhea when the organism no longer may be detectable in stool.

TREATMENT: Dehydration and electrolyte abnormalities should be corrected. Orally administered solutions usually are adequate.* Antimotility agents should not be administered to children or adolescents with inflammatory or bloody diarrhea. Careful follow-up of patients with hemorrhagic colitis is recommended to detect changes suggestive of HUS.

Antimicrobial Therapy. The role of antimicrobial therapy in patients with hemorrhagic colitis caused by EHEC is uncertain. Therapy does not appear to prevent progression to HUS. For infants with mild EPEC diarrhea, nonabsorbable antibiotics such as neomycin or gentamicin, given orally in three to four divided doses for 5 days, can be administered, although resistance may develop. These agents should not be used in infants with inflammatory or bloody diarrhea because of potential toxicity if absorbed. Trimethoprim-sulfamethoxazole should be considered if diarrhea is moderate, severe or intractable, and if the organism is susceptible. If systemic infection is suspected, parenteral antimicrobial therapy should be given. For dysentery caused by EIEC strains and for chronic diarrhea caused by EPEC strains, antimicrobial agents such as trimethoprim-sulfamethoxazole can be given orally. Antimicrobial selection should be based on susceptibility testing of the isolates.

ISOLATION OF THE HOSPITALIZED PATIENT†: Contact precautions are indicated for patients with all types of *E coli* diarrhea for the duration of illness. During outbreaks, contact precautions for infants with diarrhea caused by EPEC strains should be maintained until cultures of stool taken after cessation of antimicrobial therapy are negative for the infecting strain. For patients with HUS, contact precautions should be continued until two consecutive stool cultures are negative for *E coli* O157:H7, or, if these tests are not available, for at least 10 days from onset of diarrhea.

CONTROL MEASURES:

Escherichia coli O157:H7 Infection. In an outbreak of *E coli* O157:H7 diarrhea and HUS in a child care center, immediate involvement of public health authorities is critical. Rapid reporting of cases of *E coli* O157:H7 infection can lead to intervention to prevent further disease. Ill children should not be permitted to reenter their room until diarrhea has stopped and two stool cultures are negative for *E coli* O157:H7.

---

* For further information and detailed recommendations, see Duggan C, Santosham M, Glass RI. The management of acute diarrhea in children: oral rehydration, maintenance, and nutritional therapy. *MMWR.* 1992;41(No. RR-16):1-20.

† In addition to standard precautions.

Strict attention to hand washing and hygiene is important but may not be sufficient to prevent continued transmission. A child care center should be closed to new admissions and care should be exercised to prevent transfer of exposed children to other centers. Because most *E coli* O157:H7 infections are caused by eating contaminated ground beef, it should be thoroughly cooked until no pink meat remains and the juices are clear. Raw milk should not be ingested.

Nursery and Other Institutional Outbreaks. Strict attention to hand washing techniques is essential in limiting spread. Exposed patients should be observed closely and their stools cultured for the causative organism. Unexposed patients should be separated from infants who have been exposed.

In a newborn nursery, management of EPEC infection is based on the number of cases. If a single case occurs, the infant should be isolated in a unit separate from the nursery area. If multiple cases occur, the nursery room should be closed to admissions and not reopened until all infants in the room have been discharged and the room has been cleaned. Infants should be discharged home or, if not possible, transferred to a designated isolation area and not to other infant wards. Personnel caring for infants in the closed nursery cohort should not have duties in other open nursery rooms. If epidemic disease involves more than one room in a nursery, the entire nursery should be closed and not reopened until a strict cohort system has been established in each room of the nursery for the duration of the epidemic. Admissions to a room should be limited to infants born in a 1- to 2-day period. The room should then be closed to admissions until all infants have been discharged and the room has been cleaned. Personnel should be cohorted with the infants.

Travelers' Diarrhea. Travelers' diarrhea has been associated with many enteropathogens, usually is acquired by ingestion of contaminated food or water, and is a significant problem for persons traveling in developing countries. Travelers should be advised to drink only carbonated beverages and boiled or carbonated (bottled) water; they should avoid ice, salads, and fruit they have not peeled themselves. Foods should be eaten hot. Antimicrobial agents usually are not recommended for prevention of travelers' diarrhea in children. Although several antimicrobial agents, such as trimethoprim-sulfamethoxazole, doxycycline, and ciprofloxacin, are effective prophylactically in decreasing the incidence of travelers' diarrhea, the benefit usually is outweighed by the potential risks, including allergic drug reactions, antibiotic-associated colitis, and the selective pressure of widespread use of antimicrobial agents leading to antimicrobial resistance.

If diarrhea does occur, packets of oral rehydration salts can help maintain fluid balance and anti-spasmodic drugs can relieve symptoms. If diarrhea is moderate or severe, or is associated with fever or bloody stool, empirical antimicrobial treatment is indicated. In children, the recommended drug is trimethoprim-sulfamethoxazole; in adults, a fluoroquinolone (eg, ciprofloxacin or ofloxacin) is recommended. Duration of therapy should continue until symptoms resolve, but not for more than 3 days.

Filariasis
(Bancroftian, Malayan, and Timorian)

CLINICAL MANIFESTATIONS: Most filarial infections are asymptomatic. Symptoms are caused by acute inflammation or, most commonly, by inflammation and dysfunction of the lymphatics where the adult worms develop. In the former, fever, headache, myalgia, and lymphadenitis develop in the patient. In lymphatic disease, manifestations usually occur 3 months to 1 year after acquisition. Occasionally, moderate lymphadenopathy, particularly involving the inguinal lymph nodes, occurs. Inflammation of the lymphatics of the extremities and genitalia leads to adenolymphangitis that is characteristically retrograde. Epididymitis, orchitis, and funiculitis also can occur along with fever, chills, and other nonspecific systemic symptoms. Lymphatic dysfunction, with resulting chronically progressive edema of the limbs and genitalia, is relatively infrequent in children. In a few individuals, elephantiasis can result from fibrosis caused by chronic dysfunction of the lymphatic channels. Chyluria can occur as a manifestation of Bancroftian filariasis.

Cough, fever, marked eosinophilia, and high serum IgE concentrations are the manifestations of the tropical pulmonary eosinophilia syndrome.

ETIOLOGY: Filariasis is caused by the following three filarial nematodes: *Wuchereria bancrofti*, *Brugia malayi*, and *B timori*.

EPIDEMIOLOGY: The disease is transmitted by the bite of infected species of various genera of mosquitoes, including *Culex, Aedes, Anopheles*, and *Mansonia*. *Wuchereria bancrofti* is found in many scattered areas of the Caribbean, Venezuela, Columbia, the Guianas, Brazil, Central America, sub-Saharan Africa, North Africa, Turkey, and Asia, extending into a broad zone from Saudi Arabia through the Indonesian archipelago into Southern China and Oceania. *Brugia malayi* is found mostly in India, Southeast Asia, and the Far East. *Brugia timori* is restricted to certain islands at the eastern end of the Indonesian archipelago. Because the adult worms are long-lived, microfilariae infective for mosquitoes are in the patient's blood for decades; individual microfilaria have a life span up to 1.5 years. The adult worm is not transmissible from person to person or by blood transfusion, but microfilariae may be transmitted by transfusion.

The **incubation period** is not well established; the period from acquisition to the appearance of microfilariae in blood can be 3 to 12 months, depending on the nematode.

DIAGNOSTIC TESTS: Microfilariae can be detected microscopically on routine blood smears obtained at night (10 pm to 4 am) after concentration of blood preserved in formalin or by membrane filtration. Adult worms can be identified in tissue specimens obtained at biopsy. Serologic enzyme immunoassay tests are available, but interpretation of results is affected by cross-reactions of filarial antibodies with those against other helminths. Assays for circulating parasite antigen are more specific and are now commercially available. Lymphatic filariasis often must be diagnosed clinically because dependable serologic assays are not available, and in elephantiasis the microfilariae may no longer be present. Eosinophilia of 25% frequently occurs in the early, inflammatory phase of the disease.

TREATMENT: Diethylcarbamazine citrate* is the drug of choice. Because reactions induced by disintegrating microfilariae following treatment occur in heavy infestations, beginning treatment with low doses for the first 4 to 5 days may be advantageous. The late obstructive phase of the disease is not affected by chemotherapy. Ivermectin,† an investigational drug in the United States, is effective against the microfilariae of *W bancrofti,* but is unlikely to become the drug of choice for lymphatic filariasis. Complex, decongestive physiotherapy may be effective in treating elephantiasis. Plastic surgical repair of the genitalia gives variable results. Chyluria originating in the bladder responds to fulguration; chyluria originating in the kidney cannot be corrected. Prompt identification and treatment of superinfections, particularly streptococcal and staphylococcal infections, and careful treatment of intertriginous and ungual infections are important aspects of therapy.

ISOLATION OF THE HOSPITALIZED PATIENT: Standard precautions are recommended.

CONTROL MEASURES: The mosquito population should be controlled. Treatment of those with asymptomatic infection, ie, carriers or an entire community if a substantial percentage are infected, should be considered.

Giardia lamblia Infections
(Giardiasis)

CLINICAL MANIFESTATIONS: Symptomatic infection causes a broad spectrum of clinical manifestations. Acute watery diarrhea with abdominal pain may develop in patients with clinical illness, or they may experience a protracted, intermittent, often debilitating disease, which is characterized by passage of foul-smelling diarrheal or soft stools associated with flatulence, abdominal distention, and anorexia. Anorexia combined with malabsorption can lead to significant weight loss, failure to thrive, and anemia.

ETIOLOGY: *Giardia lamblia* is a flagellate protozoan that exists in trophozoite and cyst forms; the infective form is the cyst. Infection is limited to the small intestine and/or biliary tract.

EPIDEMIOLOGY: Giardiasis has a worldwide distribution. Humans are the principal reservoir of infection, but *Giardia* organisms can infect dogs, cats, beavers, and other animals. These animals can contaminate water with feces containing cysts that are infectious for humans. Persons become infected either directly (by hand-to-mouth transfer of cysts from feces of an infected person) or indirectly (by ingestion of fecally contaminated water or food). Many persons who become infected with *Giardia* remain asymptomatic. Most community-wide epidemics result from contaminated water supplies. Epidemics resulting from person-to-person transmission

---

* Available from Lederle, Pearl River, NY.
† Available from Merck and Co, West Point, Pa.

occur in child care centers, especially those that care for children who are not toilet trained, and in institutions for mentally retarded persons. Staff and family members in contact with persons in these settings occasionally become infected. *Giardia* transmission also has been documented among male homosexuals. Humoral immunodeficiencies predispose to chronic symptomatic *Giardia* infections. Patients with cystic fibrosis have an increased frequency of giardiasis. Surveys conducted in the United States have demonstrated prevalence rates of *Giardia* organisms in stool specimens that range from 1% to 20%, depending on geographic location and age. Duration of cyst excretion is variable and may persist for months. The disease is communicable for as long as the infected person excretes cysts.

The **incubation period** is usually 1 to 4 weeks.

DIAGNOSTIC TESTS: Identification of either trophozoites or cysts on direct smear examination of stool specimens or duodenal fluid, or detection of *G lamblia* antigens in these specimens by enzyme immunoassay (EIA) is diagnostic. Enzyme immunoassay techniques for antigen detection in stool specimens, which are available commercially, have greater sensitivity than microscopy. A single stool microscopic examination detects 50% to 75% of infections; sensitivity is increased to approximately 95% by testing three specimens. Laboratories can reduce reagent and personnel costs by pooling specimens prior to evaluation by microscopy or EIA. Examination of duodenal contents obtained by direct aspiration or by using a commercially available string test (Entero-Test*) is a more sensitive procedure than examination of a single stool specimen. Rarely, duodenal biopsy is performed. To enhance detection, microscopic examination of stool specimens or duodenal fluid should be performed soon after they are obtained, or stool should be mixed, placed in fixative, concentrated, and examined by both wet mount and permanent stain. Commercially available stool collection kits containing a vial of 10% formalin and a vial of polyvinyl alcohol fixative in childproof containers are convenient for preserving stool specimens collected at home.

TREATMENT: Quinacrine hydrochloride is the most effective drug for treatment of symptomatic infections; cure rates range from 85% to 95%. However, because quinacrine hydrochloride is not currently available in the United States, metronidazole and furazolidone are the drugs of choice for treatment of symptomatic infections. Metronidazole is 90% effective in adults, but its safety and effectiveness for children with giardiasis have not been established. Furazolidone is 80% effective, but because it is the only drug available in liquid suspension, it is often more acceptable to children. If therapy fails, a course of any of these drugs can be repeated. Paromomycin, a nonabsorbable aminoglycoside that is 50% to 70% effective, is recommended for treatment of symptomatic infection in pregnant women. Relapse is common in immunocompromised patients and may require continuous therapy for long periods.

Treatment of asymptomatic carriers is not recommended except possibly for prevention of household transmission by toddlers to pregnant women and in patients with hypogammaglobulinemia or cystic fibrosis.

---

* HDC Corp, San Jose, Calif.

ISOLATION OF THE HOSPITALIZED PATIENT*: Contact precautions for the duration of illness are recommended for diapered and/or incontinent children.

CONTROL MEASURES:

- In child care centers, improved sanitation and personal hygiene should be emphasized (see also Children in Out-of-Home Child Care, p 80). Hand washing by staff and children should be stressed, especially after using the toilet or handling soiled diapers. When an outbreak is suspected, an epidemiologic investigation should be undertaken to identify and treat all symptomatic children, child care workers, and family members infected with *Giardia*. Persons with diarrhea should be excluded from the child care center until they become asymptomatic. Treatment of asymptomatic carriers has not been demonstrated to be effective in outbreak control. Exclusion of carriers from child care is not recommended.
- Prevention of water-borne outbreaks requires adequate filtration of municipal water obtained from surface water sources because concentrations of chlorine used to disinfect drinking water are not effective against cysts.
- Backpackers, campers, and persons likely to be exposed to contaminated water should avoid drinking directly from streams. Boiling of water will kill the infective cysts.

Gonococcal Infections

CLINICAL MANIFESTATIONS: Gonococcal infections in children occur in three distinct age groups.

- Infection in the **newborn infant** usually involves the eye. Other types of involvement include scalp abscess (which can be associated with fetal monitoring), vaginitis, and disseminated disease with bacteremia, arthritis, meningitis, or endocarditis.
- In **prepubertal children** beyond the newborn period, gonococcal infection usually occurs in the genital tract and is almost always sexually transmitted. Vaginitis is the most common manifestation; pelvic inflammatory disease (PID) and perihepatitis can occur but are very rare. Gonococcal urethritis in the prepubertal male is uncommon. Anorectal and tonsillopharyngeal infection also can occur in prepubertal children.
- In **sexually active adolescents**, as in adults, gonococcal infection of the genital tract in females is most frequently asymptomatic, and common clinical syndromes are urethritis, endocervicitis, and PID. In males, the infection is usually symptomatic and the primary site is the urethra. Infection of the rectum and pharynx can occur alone or can accompany genitourinary tract infection in either sex. Rectal and pharyngeal infections often are asymptomatic. Extension from primary genital mucosal sites can lead to epididymitis, bartholinitis, PID, and perihepatitis. Even asymptomatic infection can progress to PID with tubal scarring that can result in ectopic pregnancy or infertility. Infection involving

---

* In addition to standard precautions.

other mucous membranes can produce conjunctivitis, pharyngitis, or proctitis. Hematogenous spread can involve skin and joints (arthritis-dermatitis syndrome) causing a maculo-papular rash with petechiae, tenosynovitis and migratory arthritis. Arthritis can occur as a reactive (sterile) or septic arthritis. Meningitis and endocarditis occur rarely.

ETIOLOGY: *Neisseria gonorrhoeae* is a Gram-negative diplococcus.

EPIDEMIOLOGY: Gonococcal infections occur only in humans. The source of the organism is exudate and secretions of infected mucous surfaces; *N gonorrhoeae* is communicable as long as an individual harbors the organism. Transmission results from intimate contact, such as sexual acts, parturition, and, very rarely, household exposure in prepubertal children. Sexual abuse should be strongly considered when genital, rectal, or pharyngeal colonization or infections are diagnosed in children beyond the newborn period and before puberty, and in those who deny that they are sexually active. An estimated 1 million new cases of gonococcal infection occur annually in the United States. Young women 15 to 19 years of age have the highest reported incidence of infection, followed by those 20 to 24 years of age. In males, the highest rates are in young men 20 to 24 years of age, followed by adolescents 15 to 19 years of age. Concurrent infection with *Chlamydia trachomatis* is common.

The **incubation period** is usually 2 to 7 days.

DIAGNOSTIC TESTS: Microscopic examinations of Gram-stained smears of exudate from the eyes, the endocervix of postpubertal females, the vagina of pre-pubertal girls, male urethra, skin lesions, synovial fluid, and, when clinically warranted, cerebrospinal fluid (CSF) are useful in the initial evaluation. Identification of Gram-negative intracellular diplococci in these smears can be helpful, particularly when the organism is not recovered in culture. Gram stains of material obtained from the endocervix of postpubertal females are less sensitive than culture in the detection of infection, but they can be of immediate help in the differential diagnosis of a patient with acute abdominal pain or when immediate therapy is indicated. Other *Neisseria* species and Gram-negative cocci may be present in the female genital tract, but these organisms are seldom observed within polymorphonuclear leukocytes. In prepubertal girls, vaginal specimens are adequate for diagnosis and endocervical specimens are unnecessary.

Culture from normally sterile sites, such as blood, CSF, or synovial fluid, can be accomplished on nonselective chocolate agar with incubation in 5% to 10% CO_2. Selective *N gonorrhoeae* culture media, such as Thayer-Martin (chocolate agar supplemented with antibiotics), inhibit most normal flora and nonpathogenic *Neisseria* found on mucosal surfaces. These selective media are used for culture from nonsterile sites, such as the cervix, vagina, rectum, urethra, and pharynx. Specimens for *N gonorrhoeae* culture from mucosal sites should be inoculated immediately onto the appropriate agar or placed in transport medium because *N gonorrhoeae* is extremely sensitive to drying and temperature changes. Transport systems containing selective medium are available commercially.

Caution should be exercised in interpreting the significance of the isolation of *Neisseria* organisms, as *N gonorrhoeae* can be confused with other *Neisseria* species that colonize the genitourinary tract or pharynx. At least two confirmatory bacteriologic tests involving different principles (eg, biochemical, enzyme substrate or serology) should be performed. Culture results of *N gonorrhoeae* from the pharynx of young children necessitate particular caution because of the high carriage rate of nonpathogenic *Neisseria species.*

Sexual Abuse. In all prepubertal children beyond the newborn period and in non-sexually active adolescents who have gonococcal infection, sexual abuse must be considered to have occurred unless proven otherwise. Genital, rectal, and pharyngeal cultures should be obtained from all patients before antibiotic treatment. All gonococcal isolates from such patients should be preserved. Nonculture gonococcal tests, including Gram stain, DNA probes, or enzyme immunoassay tests of oropharyngeal, rectal, or genital tract specimens in children cannot be relied upon for diagnosis of gonococcal infection for this purpose, since false-positive results can occur. Appropriate cultures should be obtained from persons who have had contact with a child suspected to have been sexually abused. Children in whom sexual abuse is suspected should undergo tests for other sexually transmitted diseases, such as *Chlamydia* infection, syphilis, hepatitis B, and HIV infection (for further information, see Sexual Abuse, p 112).

TREATMENT: Because of the prevalence of penicillin-resistant *N gonorrhoeae*, an extended spectrum (third-generation) cephalosporin (eg, ceftriaxone) is recommended as initial therapy for persons of all ages. High-level resistance to tetracycline is becoming more common. Resistance to spectinomycin is still uncommon.

Parenteral cephalosporins are recommended for use in young children; ceftriaxone is approved for all gonococcal indications in children and cefotaxime is approved only for gonococcal ophthalmia. Antimicrobials administered orally that have been demonstrated to be effective for treating gonococcal urethritis and cervicitis in adults and older adolescents include cefixime, azithromycin, ciprofloxacin, and ofloxacin. While data to support the use of cefixime to treat gonorrhea in young children are not available, experience in adults indicates that this agent may be considered for uncomplicated infections, provided that follow-up is assured. Fluoroquinolones generally are not recommended for persons younger than 18 years of age (see Antimicrobials and Related Therapy, p 605) and are contraindicated in pregnant or nursing women.

All patients with presumed or proven gonorrhea should be evaluated for concurrent syphilis, hepatitis B, HIV and *Chlamydia trachomatis* infection. Patients beyond the neonatal period should be treated presumptively for *C trachomatis* infection (see *Chlamydia trachomatis,* p 170).

Adolescents and adults with uncomplicated gonorrhea who are asymptomatic after treatment with one of the recommended antibiotic regimens need not be cultured for a test of cure. Infected children, however, should have follow-up cultures to ensure that treatment has been effective.

Specific recommendations for management and antimicrobial therapy are as follows:

Neonatal Disease. Infants with clinical evidence of ophthalmia neonatorum, scalp abscess, or disseminated infections should be hospitalized. Appropriate cultures should be obtained from the mother. Cultures of blood, cerebrospinal fluid, eye discharge, or other sites of infection should be obtained from the infant to confirm the diagnosis and determine antimicrobial susceptibility. Tests for concomitant infection with *C trachomatis* should also be performed.

Nondisseminated Infections. Recommended antimicrobial therapy, including for ophthalmia neonatorum, is ceftriaxone (25 to 50 mg/kg per day intravenously or intramuscularly, not to exceed 125 mg) given once. A single dose of cefotaxime (100 mg/kg given intravenously or intramuscularly) is an alternative treatment for ophthalmia neonatorum.

Infants with gonococcal ophthalmia should have their eyes irrigated with saline immediately and at frequent intervals until the discharge is eliminated. Topical antibiotic treatment alone is inadequate, and is unnecessary when recommended systemic antibiotic treatment is given.

Disseminated Infections. Recommended therapy for arthritis and septicemia is ceftriaxone (25 to 50 mg/kg intravenously or intramuscularly, given once a day) for 7 days, or cefotaxime (50 to 100 mg/kg per day given intravenously or intramuscularly, in two divided doses) for 7 days. Cefotaxime is recommended for hyperbilirubinemic infants. If meningitis is documented, treatment should be continued for a total of 10 to 14 days.

Since neonates with gonorrhea acquire the organism from their mothers, both the mother and her sexual partner(s) should be evaluated and treated appropriately.

Gonococcal Infections in Children Beyond the Neonatal Period and in Adolescents. Recommendations for treatment of gonococcal infections, by age and weight, are given in Tables 3.6 and 3.7 (p 216 and p 217).

Presumptive Treatment for Chlamydia Infection. Patients with gonococcal infection also should be treated for presumptive *Chlamydia* infection (see Tables 3.6 and 3.7, p 216 and p 217) and *Chlamydia trachomatis* (p 172). They also should be evaluated for coinfection with syphilis and other sexually transmitted diseases.

Approximately half of recurrent *Chlamydia* infections occurring after treatment with the recommended schedules are caused by reinfection and indicate the need for improved partner notification and patient education.

Special Problems in Treatment of Children (Beyond the Neonatal Period) and Adolescents. Patients with uncomplicated endocervical infection, urethritis, or proctitis who are allergic to cephalosporins should be treated with spectinomycin (40 mg/kg, maximum 2 g, given intramuscularly). Patients for whom doxycycline, tetracycline, and azithromycin are contraindicated or who are unable to tolerate these drugs can be given erythromycin base or stearate (2 g/d orally in four divided doses for adults) or erythromycin ethyl succinate (3.2 g/d orally in four divided doses for adults) for the concurrent treatment of presumptive *Chlamydia* infection.

Patients with uncomplicated pharyngeal gonococcal infection should be treated with ceftriaxone (125 mg, intramuscularly) in a single dose. Those who cannot tolerate ceftriaxone should be treated with ciprofloxacin or ofloxacin (see Antimicrobials and Related Therapy, p 605). Trimethoprim-sulfamethoxazole (720 to 3600 mg) given orally once a day for 5 days may be effective. Spectinomycin is not effective for the treatment of pharyngeal gonorrhea.

Patients who are incubating syphilis (seronegative, without clinical signs) may be cured by regimens that include ceftriaxone, a 7-day course of either doxycycline for those 8 years of age and older, or erythromycin, but few data are available. Fluoroquinolones and spectinomycin are not active against *Treponema pallidum*.

Table 3.6. Uncomplicated Gonococcal Infection: Treatment in Children Beyond the Newborn Period and for Adolescents.*

Disease	Prepubertal Children Who Weigh <100 lb (45 kg)	Disease	Patients Who Weigh ≥100 lb (45 kg) and Are 8 Years or Older
Uncomplicated vulvovaginitis, urethritis, epididymitis, proctitis, or pharyngitis†	Ceftriaxone, 125 mg IM‡ in a single dose *or* Spectinomycin,§ 40 mg/kg (maximum, 2 g) IM in a single dose **PLUS*** Erythromycin, 40 mg/kg/d (maximum, 2 g/d) in 4 divided doses for 7 d *or* Azithromycin, 20 mg/kg (maximum, 1 g) in a single dose	Uncomplicated endocervicitis, urethritis, epididymitis, proctitis, or pharyngitis	Ceftriaxone, 125 mg IM‡ in a single dose *or* Cefixime, 400 mg orally in a single dose *or* Ciprofloxacin,‖ 500 mg orally in a single dose *or* Ofloxacin,‖ 400 mg orally in a single dose *or* Spectinomycin,‡ 2 g IM in a single dose **PLUS¶** Doxycycline or azithromycin

* In addition to the recommended treatment for gonococcal infection, therapy for *C trachomatis* is recommended on the presumption that the patient has concomitant infection.

† Hospitalization should be considered, especially for patients who have been treated as outpatients and have failed to respond, and for those who are unlikely to adhere to treatment regimens.

‡ The discomfort of an intramuscular (IM) injection can be reduced by using 1% lidocaine as a diluent.

§ Spectinomycin is not recommended for treatment of pharyngeal infections; in persons who cannot take a cephalosporin or a quinolone, a 5-day oral regimen of trimethoprim-sulfamethoxazole may be given.

‖ Fluoroquinolones are contraindicated for pregnant women, nursing women, and usually for persons younger than 18 years (see Antimicrobials and Related Therapy, p 605).

¶ In all cases, in addition to the recommended treatment for gonococcal infection, doxycycline (100 mg orally twice a day for 7 days), or tetracycline (500 mg orally 4 times a day for 7 days), or azithromycin (1 g orally in a single dose) is recommended on the presumption that the patient has concomitant infection with *C trachomatis*. Tetracycline (500 mg orally 4 times a day for 7 days) is also acceptable.

Table 3.7. Complicated Gonococcal Infection: Treatment in Children Beyond the Newborn Period and for Adolescents*

Disease[†]	Prepubertal Children Who Weigh <100 lb (45 kg)	Patients Who Weigh ≥100 lb (45 kg) and Are 8 Years or Older
Disseminated gonococcal infection (eg, arthritis-dermatitis syndrome)	Ceftriaxone, 50 mg/kg/d (maximum, 1 g/d) IV or IM[‡] once a day for 7 d Erythromycin, tetracycline, doxycycline, or azithromycin*	See Table 3.44 (p 393)
Pelvic inflammatory disease		
Meningitis or endocarditis	Ceftriaxone, 50 mg/kg/d (maximum, 2 g/d) IV or IM[‡] given every 12 h; for meningitis, duration is 10–14 d; for endocarditis, duration is at least 28 d **PLUS*** Erythromycin, 40 mg/kg/d (maximum, 2 g/d) in 4 divided doses for 7 d	
Disseminated gonococcal infections[‖]		Ceftriaxone, 1 g/d IV or IM[‡] given once a day for 7 d[¶] *or* Cefotaxime, 1 g IV given three times a day for 7 d[¶] *or* Spectinomycin, 2 g IM every 12 h for 7 d for persons allergic to cephalosporin[¶] **PLUS** Doxycycline or azithromycin*
Meningitis or endocarditis[†]		Ceftriaxone, 1-2 g IV given every 12 h; for meningitis, duration is 10–14 d; for endocarditis, duration is at least 28 d
Conjunctivitis[§]	Ceftriaxone, 50 mg/kg (maximum, 1 g) IM[‡] in a single dose	Ceftriaxone, 1 g IM[‡] in a single dose

* In all cases, in addition to the recommended treatment for gonococcal infection, doxycycline (100 mg orally twice a day for 7 days) or azithromycin (1 g orally in a single dose) is recommended on the presumption that the patient has concomitant infection with *Chlamydia trachomatis*. Tetracycline (500 mg orally 4 times daily for 7 days) is also acceptable. For children younger than 8 years and pregnant women, erythromycin is recommended (see p 215). IV indicates intravenously, and IM, intramuscularly.

† Hospitalization is required; follow-up cultures are necessary to ensure that treatment has been effective.

‡ The discomfort of IM injection can be reduced by using 1% lidocaine as a diluent.

§ Eyes should be lavaged with saline to clear accumulated secretions.

‖ Spectinomycin is not recommended for treatment of pharyngeal gonococcal infection.

¶ Alternatively, parenteral therapy can be discontinued 24 to 48 hours after improvement occurs and a 7-day course completed with an appropriate oral antimicrobial such as cefixime, 400 mg orally 2 twice a day, or ciprofloxacin, 500 mg orally twice a day (contraindicated for pregnant women, nursing women, and usually for persons younger than 18 years [see Antimicrobials and Related Therapy, p 605]). Some experts advise a 10- to 14-day course of therapy.

All patients who are treated for gonorrhea should undergo serologic testing for syphilis at the initial visit and 6 to 8 weeks later.

Children or adolescents with HIV infection should receive the same treatment as those without such infection.

Acute Pelvic Inflammatory Disease (PID). *Neisseria gonorrhoeae* and *C trachomatis* are implicated in most cases, and many cases have a polymicrobial etiology. No reliable clinical criteria distinguish gonococcal from nongonococcal PID. Hence, broad-spectrum treatment regimens are recommended (see Pelvic Inflammatory Disease, p 390).

Acute Epididymitis. Sexually transmitted organisms, such as *N gonorrhoeae* or *C trachomatis*, can cause acute epididymitis in sexually active adolescents and young adults. In prepubertal children, *Enterobacteriaceae* and *Pseudomonas* are the most common cause of epididymitis; infection is usually related to predisposing structural anomalies of the genitorurinary tract. *Haemophilus influenzae* type b, group B streptococcus, and meningococci are rare causes in infants and young children.

The recommended regimen is ceftriaxone and erythromycin, azithromycin, or doxycycline, depending on the patient's age (see Table 3.6, p 216).

ISOLATION OF THE HOSPITALIZED PATIENT: Standard precautions are recommended, including for newborn infants with ophthalmia.

CONTROL MEASURES:
Neonatal Ophthalmia. For routine prophylaxis of infants immediately after birth, a 1% solution of silver nitrate, or 1% tetracycline, or 0.5% erythromycin ophthalmic ointment is instilled into each eye; subsequent irrigation should not be performed (see Prevention of Neonatal Ophthalmia, p 601). Prophylaxis may be delayed for as long as 1 hour after birth to facilitate parent-infant bonding.

These prophylactic regimens are ineffective for prevention of chlamydial ophthalmic disease.

Infants Born to Mothers With Gonococcal Infections. When prophylaxis is correctly administered, infants born to mothers with gonococcal infection infrequently develop gonococcal ophthalmia. However, since gonococcal ophthalmia or disseminated infection occasionally can occur in this situation, infants born to mothers with gonorrhea should receive a single dose of ceftriaxone, 125 mg intravenously or intramuscularly; for low-birth-weight infants, the dose is 25 to 50 mg/kg, maximum of 125 mg. Cefotaxime in a single dose (100 mg/kg given intravenously or intramuscularly) is an alternative.

Children and Adolescents With Sexual Exposure to a Patient Known to Have Gonorrhea. Patients should be examined, cultured, and treated the same as those known to have gonorrhea.

Education. Sustained educational efforts are necessary to control sexually transmitted diseases among adolescents (see Sexually Transmitted Diseases, p 108).

Other Infections. Patients with gonococcal infection should be evaluated for other sexually transmitted diseases, including syphilis, *C trachomatis*, and HIV infection. Hepatitis B vaccination is indicated for susceptible persons, ie, those who have not previously been vaccinated (see Hepatitis B, p 247).

Pregnancy. All pregnant females should have an endocervical culture for gonococci as an integral part of their prenatal care at the first visit. A second culture late in the third trimester is recommended for women at high risk of exposure to gonococcal infection. Recommended therapeutic regimens for patients found to be infected are those previously described for uncomplicated gonorrhea, except that a tetracycline or fluoroquinolone should not be used because of the potential toxic effects on the fetus. Women who are allergic to cephalosporins should be treated with spectinomycin.

Case Reporting and Management of Sex Partners. All cases of gonorrhea must be reported. Cases in prepubertal children must be investigated to determine the source of infection. Ensuring that sexual contacts are treated and counseled is essential for community control, prevention of reinfection, and prevention of complications in the contact.

Granuloma Inguinale

CLINICAL MANIFESTATIONS: Initial lesions are single or multiple subcutaneous nodules that progress to form painless, friable, granulomatous ulcers. Lesions usually involve the genitalia. Anal infections occur in 5% to 10% of patients, but lesions at distant sites (eg, face, mouth, or liver) are rare. Subcutaneous extension into the inguinal area results in induration that can mimic inguinal adenopathy, ie, the "pseudobubo" of granuloma inguinale. Fibrosis manifests as sinus tracts, adhesions, and lymphedema, resulting in extreme genital deformity.

ETIOLOGY: The disease is caused by *Calymmatobacterium granulomatis*, a Gram-negative bacillus.

EPIDEMIOLOGY: Granuloma inguinale is extremely rare in the United States and most developed countries, but it is common in New Guinea and parts of India, Africa, and the Caribbean. The highest incidence of disease occurs in tropical and subtropical environments. The incidence of infection appears to correlate strongly with sustained high temperatures and high relative humidity. Infection usually is acquired by sexual intercourse, most commonly with a person with active infection, but possibly also from those with asymptomatic rectal infection. Granuloma inguinale is only mildly contagious and repeated exposure may be necessary for the development of disease. Young children can acquire infection by contact with infected secretions. The period of communicability extends throughout the duration of active lesions or rectal colonization.

The **incubation period** is 8 to 80 days.

DIAGNOSTIC TESTS: The microscopic demonstration of Donovan bodies on Wright or Giemsa staining of a crush preparation from a lesion is diagnostic. The microorganism also can be detected by histologic examination of biopsy specimens. Culture of *C granulomatis* only has been accomplished rarely. Lesions, however, should be cultured for *Haemophilus ducreyi* to exclude chancroid (pseudogranuloma inguinale). Granuloma inguinale is frequently misdiagnosed as carcinoma, which can be excluded by histologic examination of the tissue or by the response of the lesion to antibiotics.

TREATMENT: Tetracycline (which ordinarily should not be given to children younger than 8 years) and trimethoprim-sulfamethoxazole have been reported to be effective. Gentamicin and chloramphenicol are highly effective but reserved for resistant cases. Erythromycin has been used in pregnant patients. Antimicrobial therapy is continued for at least 3 weeks or until the lesions have resolved. If antimicrobial therapy is effective, some healing is usually noted within 7 days.

Patients should be evaluated for other sexually transmitted diseases, such as gonorrhea, syphilis, and infection with *Chlamydia trachomatis*, hepatitis B, and HIV infection.

ISOLATION OF THE HOSPITALIZED PATIENT: Standard precautions are recommended.

CONTROL MEASURES: Sexual partners should be examined, counseled to use condoms, and given prophylactic antimicrobial therapy.

Haemophilus influenzae Infections

CLINICAL MANIFESTATIONS: *Haemophilus influenzae* can cause meningitis, otitis media, sinusitis, epiglottitis, septic arthritis, occult febrile bacteremia, cellulitis, pneumonia, and empyema; occasionally this organism causes neonatal meningitis and septicemia. Other *H influenzae* infections include purulent pericarditis, endocarditis, conjunctivitis, osteomyelitis, peritonitis, epididymo-orchitis, glossitis, uvulitis, and septic thrombophlebitis.

ETIOLOGY: *Haemophilus influenzae* is a small, pleomorphic, Gram-negative coccobacilli. Isolates are classified into six antigenically distinct capsular types (a–f) and nonencapsulated, nontypable strains. Most cases of invasive diseases in children before the introduction of *H influenzae* type b (Hib) conjugate vaccination were caused by type b. Nonencapsulated organisms can cause invasive disease in newborns. Nonencapsulated strains cause upper respiratory tract infection, including otitis media, sinusitis, and bronchitis, and may cause pneumonia.

EPIDEMIOLOGY: The source of the organism is the upper respiratory tract of humans. The mode of transmission is presumably person to person, by direct contact, or through inhalation of droplets of respiratory tract secretions containing the organism. Asymptomatic colonization by nonencapsulated strains is frequent; organisms are recovered from the throat of 60% to 90% of children. Colonization by type b organisms, however, is infrequent, ranging from 2% to 5% of children in the pre-vaccine era, and appears to be even less frequent with widespread Hib conjugate vaccination. The exact period of communicability is unknown but may be for as long as the organism is present in the upper respiratory tract.

Before the introduction of effective vaccines, Hib was the most common cause of bacterial meningitis in children in the United States and in many other countries. Meningitis and other invasive infections were most common in children 3 months to 3 years of age and approximately half of the cases occurred in infants younger than

12 months. The age-specific incidence of invasive type b disease in different populations in countries has varied; the proportion of disease in infants younger than 12 months tends to be greatest in populations with the highest total incidence, resulting in a lower median age of cases. In contrast to meningitis and most other invasive Hib diseases, epiglottitis is rare in infants younger than 12 months; its peak occurrence in the pre-vaccine era was 2 to 4 years of age. Epiglottitis also can occur in older, unvaccinated children and adults.

Invasive disease has been more frequent in boys, African-Americans, Alaskan Eskimos, Apache and Navajo Indians, child care center attendees, children living in overcrowded conditions and children who were not breastfed. Unimmunized children, particularly those younger than 4 years who are in prolonged, close contact (such as in a household) with a child with invasive Hib disease, are at an increased risk for serious infection from this organism. Other factors predisposing to invasive disease include sickle cell disease, asplenia, HIV infection, certain immunodeficiency syndromes, and malignancies. Infants younger than 1 year with documented invasive infection are at an approximate 1% risk of recurrence, if not subsequently vaccinated.

Since 1988 when Hib conjugate vaccines were introduced, the incidence of invasive Hib disease has declined by 95% in infants and young children and the incidence of invasive infections caused by other encapsulated types is now similar to that caused by type b. As a result of this success, the US Public Health Service has targeted Hib disease in children younger than 5 years for elimination in this country. Invasive Hib disease occurs now in this country primarily in undervaccinated children and among infants too young to have completed the primary series of vaccinations.

The **incubation period** is unknown and probably is widely variable.

DIAGNOSTIC TESTS: Cerebrospinal fluid (CSF), blood, synovial fluid, pleural fluid, and middle ear aspirates should be cultured on a medium such as chocolate agar enriched with X and V co-factors. A Gram stain of an infected body fluid can disclose the organism and allows a presumptive diagnosis to be made. Latex particle agglutination for detection of capsular antigen in CSF may be helpful when antimicrobial therapy was initiated before cultures were obtained. However, detection of antigen in serum and in urine can be unreliable for diagnosis since antigen can be detected in these fluids as a result of asymptomatic nasopharyngeal carriage of Hib, recent immunization with an *H influenzae* conjugate vaccine, or contamination of urine specimens by cross-reacting fecal organisms. All *H influenzae* isolates should be serotyped to determine whether the strain is type b. Antimicrobial susceptibility testing should be performed on all clinically important isolates.

Isolates should be serotyped. If testing is not available, isolates should be submitted to a reference laboratory or to the state health department for submission to the Centers for Disease Control and Prevention.

TREATMENT:
- Initial therapy for children with meningitis possibly caused by Hib can be cefotaxime, ceftriaxone, or ampicillin in combination with chloramphenicol. Ampicillin alone should not be used as initial therapy since, depending on the locality, 10% to 40% of Hib isolates produce ß-lactamase and, therefore, are resistant. Chloramphenicol resistance also is common in some countries but has been rare in the United States.

- For patients with uncomplicated meningitis who respond rapidly, therapy for 7 to 10 days with an appropriate antimicrobial agent (ie, to which the organism is susceptible by in vitro testing) administered intravenously in a high dose usually is satisfactory. In selected cases, oral therapy with chloramphenicol has been used, particularly if monitoring of serum chloramphenicol concentrations can be performed. Therapy for more than 10 days may be indicated in complicated cases of meningitis.
- For treatment of other invasive *H influenzae* infections, recommendations are similar but are primarily based on empiric experience.
- Dexamethasone is recommended for infants and children 6 weeks of age and older as adjunctive therapy for Hib meningitis (see Dexamethasone Therapy for Bacterial Meningitis in Infants and Children, p 620).
- **Epiglottitis is a medical emergency. An airway must be established promptly by endotracheal tube or tracheostomy.**
- Infected synovial, pleural, or pericardial fluid should be drained.
- For acute otitis media, most experts recommend treatment with oral amoxicillin (see also Pneumococcal Infections, p 410). Duration of therapy is for 5 to 10 days. In uncomplicated cases, 5 to 7 days is preferred in order to minimize the emergence of resistant bacteria in the community. Effective alternative drugs, especially for ampicillin-resistant strains of *H influenzae* and/or penicillin-resistant strains of *Streptococcus pneumoniae*, include erythromycin-sulfisoxazole, amoxicillin-clavulanic acid, extended-spectrum oral cephalosporins and clarithromycin. Narrow-spectrum drugs, when appropriate, are recommended.

ISOLATION OF THE HOSPITALIZED PATIENT*: Droplet precautions are recommended for 24 hours after initiation of effective antimicrobial therapy.

CONTROL MEASURES (for invasive Hib infections):

Care of Exposed Persons.

Careful observation of exposed household, child care, or nursery contacts is essential. Exposed children in whom a febrile illness develops should receive prompt medical evaluation, irrespective of *Haemophilus* vaccination status. If indicated, antimicrobial therapy appropriate for invasive Hib infection should be administered.

Rifampin Chemoprophylaxis. The risk of invasive Hib disease among unvaccinated household contacts younger than 4 years is increased. Asymptomatic colonization with Hib also is more frequent in household contacts of all ages than in the general population. Rifampin eradicates Hib from the pharynx in approximately 95% of carriers. Limited data indicate that rifampin prophylaxis also decreases the risk of secondary invasive illness in exposed household contacts. Nursery and child care center contacts also may be at increased risk of secondary disease, but experts disagree regarding the magnitude of the risk. The risk of secondary disease in children attending child care centers appears to be lower than that observed for age-susceptible household contacts, and secondary disease in child care contacts is rare

---

* In addition to standard precautions.

when all contacts are older than 2 years. Moreover, the efficacy of rifampin in preventing disease in child care groups is not well established and the difficulties in delivering prophylaxis are considerable.

Indications and guidelines for chemoprophylaxis in different circumstances are as follows:

- **Household.** In those households with at least one contact* younger than 48 months whose immunization status against Hib is incomplete, rifampin prophylaxis is recommended for all household contacts, irrespective of age. Based on the high efficacy of Hib vaccination, prophylaxis is not indicated when all household contacts younger than 48 months have completed their immunization series. Complete immunization is defined as having had at least one dose of conjugate vaccine at 15 months of age or older; two doses between 12 and 14 months; or a two- or three-dose primary series when younger than 12 months with a booster/reinforcing dose at 12 months or older (see Recommendations for Immunization, p 227). Although the risk of secondary disease is low in an infant who has completed the primary two- or three-dose series, all members of a household with a child younger than 12 months (ie, who have not yet received the booster/reinforcing vaccine dose) should receive rifampin prophylaxis.

  The exception to these recommendations is that all members of households with a fully vaccinated but immunocompromised child, regardless of age, should receive rifampin because of concern that the immunization series may not have been effective.

  When indicated, prophylaxis should be initiated as soon as possible since the majority of secondary cases in households occur in the first week after hospitalization of the index patient. The time of occurrence of the remaining secondary cases after the first week suggests that prophylaxis of household contacts initiated 7 days or more after hospitalization of the index patient, although not optimal, may still be of benefit.

- **Child care and nursery school.** When two or more cases of invasive disease have occurred within 60 days and unvaccinated or incompletely vaccinated children attend the child care facility, administration of rifampin to all attendees and supervisory personnel is indicated, as recommended for household contacts. The success of rifampin prophylaxis depends on strict, prompt compliance by attendees and supervisory personnel.

  When a single case has occurred, the advisability of rifampin prophylaxis in exposed child care groups with unvaccinated or incompletely vaccinated children is controversial. In out-of-home child care attended by unvaccinated or incompletely vaccinated children younger than 2 years, and where contact is 25 hours per week or more, rifampin prophylaxis may be given, but where all contacts are older than 2 years, rifampin prophylaxis need not be given, irrespective of vaccination status.

---

* A household contact is defined in these circumstances as an individual residing with the index patient, or a nonresident who spent 4 or more hours with the index patient for at least 5 of the 7 days preceding the day of hospital admission of the index patient.

In addition to these recommendations for chemoprophylaxis, unvaccinated or incompletely vaccinated children should receive a dose of vaccine and should be scheduled for completion of the recommended age-specific immunization schedule (see Immunization).

- ***Index case.*** In families and other groups (eg, out-of-home child care) receiving prophylaxis, the index patient also should receive rifampin prophylaxis, if he or she was treated with ampicillin or chloramphenicol. Prophylaxis of the index case is not indicated for those treated with cefotaxime or ceftriaxone, since these drugs, in contrast to ampicillin and chloramphenicol, eradicate Hib from the nasopharynx. Rifampin, when indicated, should be initiated during hospitalization, usually just before hospitalization.

- ***Dosage.*** Rifampin should be given orally once a day for 4 days (in a dose of 20 mg/kg; maximum dose, 600 mg). The dose for infants younger than 1 month is not established; some experts recommend lowering the dose to 10 mg/kg. For adults, each dose is 600 mg. Rifampin is available in 150- and 300-mg capsules. Patients unable to swallow capsules may be given aliquots of rifampin powder, preweighed by a trained individual. The rifampin dose can then be mixed with a small amount of applesauce immediately before administration. Although rifampin suspension is not available commercially, a liquid suspension (1% in simple syrup) can be prepared (see rifampin package insert). If a suspension is used, it must be prepared freshly for administration to each contact group, shaken vigorously before each administration, and used within 1 week.

- ***Other generic recommendations for contacts in whom prophylaxis may be warranted:***
  — Children who have been immunized with any *H influenzae* vaccine as well as susceptible, unimmunized children should receive prophylaxis.
  — In out-of-home child care, only children who are age-appropriately immunized should be permitted to enter the child care group during the time prophylaxis is given and for 2 months after onset of the cases.
  — Prophylaxis is not recommended for pregnant women who are contacts of cases because the effect of rifampin on the fetus has not been established.

Immunization.

Four Hib conjugate vaccines have been licensed in the United States (see Table 3.8). These vaccines consist of the Hib capsular polysaccharide (ie, polyribosylribotol phosphate [PRP] or PRP oligomers) covalently linked to a carrier protein directly or via an intervening spacer molecule. Protective antibodies are directed against PRP. Conjugate vaccines differ in composition and immunogenicity, and, as a result, recommendations for their use differ. For example, PRP-D is recommended only for children 12 months of age and older, whereas the other three vaccines, HbOC, PRP-T, and PRP-OMP, are recommended for infants beginning at 2 months of age.

A primary series consisting of three doses given at 2, 4, and 6 months of age or two doses given at 2 and 4 months of age, depending on the vaccine product, is recommended (see Recommendations for Immunization, p 227, and Table 3.9). The recommended doses may be given as combination vaccines, provided the product is

Table 3.8. *Haemophilus influenzae* Type b Conjugate Vaccines*†

Manufacturer	Abbreviation	Trade Name	Carrier Protein
Connaught Laboratories	PRP-D	ProHIBit	Diphtheria toxoid
Wyeth-Lederle Laboratories	HbOC	HIBTITER	CRM197 (a nontoxic mutant diphtheria toxin)
Merck and Co	PRP-OMP	PedvaxHIB	OMP (an outer membrane protein complex of *Neisseria meningitidis*)
Pasteur Mérieux Vaccines (Distributed by Connaught Laboratories and by SmithKline Beecham)	PRP-T	ActHIB, OmniHIB	Tetanus toxoid

* HbOC, PRP-OMP, and PRP-T are recommended for infants beginning at approximately 2 months of age. PRP-D is recommended by the Academy only for children 12 months of age or older. The Food and Drug Administration (FDA), however, has approved labeling for PRP-D for booster administration beginning at 12 months of age and for primary administration at 15 months of age.
† These vaccines may be given in combination products or as reconstituted products with DTP or DTaP, provided the combination or reconstituted vaccine is approved by the FDA for the child's age and administration of the other vaccine component(s) also is justified.

approved by the Food and Drug Administration (FDA) for the child's age and administration of the other vaccine component also is justified.

The regimens in Table 3.9 are likely to be equivalent in the protection following completion of the recommended primary series of three or two doses, depending on the vaccine product. All four licensed conjugate vaccines are considered equivalent in the protection achieved in children vaccinated at 12 months of age or older.

In most immunogenicity studies in infants younger than 12 months, the same conjugate vaccine product was given for all doses. However, regimens in which the conjugate vaccine product given at 4 or at 4 and 6 months of age differed from that given at 2 months of age have resulted in mean serum anti-PRP antibody concentrations comparable to those elicited by regimens in which the same conjugate vaccine product was used for all doses. Hence, regimens involving different vaccine products for completion of the primary series are likely to be equivalent in prevention against Hib disease. While all possible regimens have not been evaluated, giving more than a total of three doses of any vaccine to complete the primary series in the first year of life is not necessary. As a result, when the product given at the first or second dose is not known or available, the three-dose primary series can be completed with any of the three products approved for use in children younger than 12 months.

Following administration of the initial two- or three-dose priming regimen (depending on the vaccine product), serum antibody concentrations decline rapidly. Therefore, an additional booster dose of any FDA-licensed conjugate vaccine is recommended at 12 to 15 months of age, regardless of which regimen was used for the primary series. This dose may be given as a combination vaccine, provided the product is FDA-approved for the child's age and administration of the other vaccine component(s) also is justified.

Table 3.9. Currently Recommended Regimens for *Haemophilus influenzae* Type b Conjugate Vaccination for Children Immunized Beginning at 2 to 6 Months of Age*†

Vaccine Product at Initiation	Total No. of Doses To Be Administered	Recommended Regimen
HbOC or PRP-T	4	3 doses at 2-mo intervals initially; when feasible, same vaccine for doses 1–3; fourth dose at 12 to 15 mo of age; any conjugate vaccine for dose 4†‡
PRP-OMP	3	2 doses at 2-mo interval initially; when feasible, same vaccine for doses 1 and 2; third dose at 12–15 mo of age; any conjugate vaccine for dose 3‡

* See text and Table 3.8 for further information concerning specific vaccines.

† These vaccines may be given in combination products or as reconstituted products with DTP or DTaP, provided the combination or reconstituted vaccine is approved by the Food and Drug Administration for the child's age and administration of the other vaccine component(s) also is justified.

‡ The safety and efficacy of PRP-OMP, PRP-D, PRP-T, and HbOC are likely to be equivalent in children 12 months and older.

Dosage and Route of Administration. The dose of each Hib conjugate vaccine is 0.5 mL, given intramuscularly.

Children in Whom DTaP, DTP, or DT Vaccination Is Deferred. The carrier proteins used in PRP-T, PRP-D, and HbOC (but not PRP-OMP) are related chemically and immunologically to toxoids in diphtheria and tetanus vaccine (see Table 3.8). Earlier or simultaneous vaccination with diphtheria or tetanus toxoids may be required to elicit an optimal anti-PRP antibody response to PRP-T, PRP-D, or HbOC. In contrast, the immunogenicity of PRP-OMP is not affected by immunization with DTP. Thus, in infants in whom DTaP, DTP, or DT immunization is deferred (see Pertussis, p 394), PRP-OMP may be advantageous for Hib vaccination.

Children With Immunologic Impairment. Children with chronic illnesses associated with increased risk of Hib disease may have impaired anti-PRP antibody responses to conjugate vaccines. Examples of such children include those with HIV infection, immunoglobulin deficiency, anatomic or functional asplenia, and sickle cell disease, as well as recipients of bone marrow transplants and recipients of chemotherapy for malignancy. Some children with immunologic impairment may benefit from more doses of conjugate vaccine than normally indicated (see Recommendations for Immunization, p 227).

Vaccine Failure. Despite receiving conjugate vaccination, Hib disease can occur. Since serum antibody responses do not occur for 1 to 2 weeks after vaccination, recipients are not expected to be protected during this immediate postvaccination period. The interval after immunization when protection can be anticipated is not known and probably differs depending on the number of previous doses. Providers should be aware of this uncertainty and should not expect protection simultaneously with vaccine administration.

Adverse Reactions. Adverse reactions to the Hib conjugate vaccines are few. Pain, redness, and/or swelling at the injection site occur in approximately 25% of recipients, but these symptoms typically are mild and last less than 24 hours. Systemic reactions such as fever and irritability are infrequent. When conjugate vaccines are administered during the same visit that DTP or DTaP vaccine is given, the rates of systemic reactions do not differ from those observed when only DTP or DTaP, respectively, vaccine is administered. The risk of Hib disease is not increased during the 1 to 2 weeks after administration of a conjugate vaccine.

Recommendations for Immunization.

Indications and Schedule

- All children should be immunized with an Hib conjugate vaccine beginning at approximately 2 months of age or as soon as possible thereafter (see Table 3.9). Only HbOC, PRP-OMP, or PRP-T should be administered to children younger than 12 months. Other generic recommendations are as follows:
  — Immunization can be initiated as early as 6 weeks of age.
  — Vaccine may be given during visits when vaccines for diphtheria, tetanus, pertussis (DTaP or DTP), polio, hepatitis B, MMR, and/or varicella are given (see Simultaneous Administration of Multiple Vaccines, p 21). No known contraindications exist to simultaneous administration of Hib conjugate vaccine with pneumococcal vaccine or meningococcal vaccine when given in separate syringes at different sites.
- For routine immunization of children younger than 7 months; the following guidelines are recommended:
  — *Primary series.* Either a three-dose regimen of HbOC or PRP-T, or a two-dose regimen of PRP-OMP should be administered (see Table 3.9). Doses are given at approximately 2-month intervals. When feasible, the conjugate vaccine product used for the first dose should be used for subsequent doses in children younger than 12 months. When sequential doses of different vaccine products are given or uncertainty exists about which products were previously administered, three doses of any conjugate vaccine are considered sufficient to complete the primary series, irrespective of the regimen employed.
  — *Reinforcing/booster vaccination at 12 to 15 months of age.* For children who have completed a primary series, an additional dose of conjugate vaccine is recommended at 12 to 15 months of age, or as soon as possible thereafter. Any conjugate vaccine (HbOC, PRP-OMP, or PRP-T or PRP-D) is acceptable for this dose regardless of the vaccine previously received by the child.
- Children younger than 5 years who did not receive an Hib conjugate vaccine in the first 6 months of life should be immunized according to the following recommended schedules (see Table 3.10):

Table 3.10. **Recommendations for *Haemophilus influenzae* Type b Conjugate Vaccination in Children in Whom Initial Vaccination Is Delayed Until 7 Months of Age or Older*†**

Age at Initiation of Immunization, mo	Vaccine Product at Initiation	Total No. of Doses To Be Administered	Recommended Vaccine Regimens
7–11	HbOC, PRP-T, or PRP-OMP	3	2 doses at 2-mo intervals‡; when feasible, same vaccine for doses 1 and 2; third dose at 12–18 mo, given at 2 mo after dose 2; any conjugate vaccine for dose 3§
12–14	HbOC, PRP-T, PRP-OMP, or PRP-D	2	2-mo interval between doses‡
15–59	HbOC, PRP-T, PRP-OMP, or PRP-D	1‖	Any conjugate vaccine
60 and older¶	HbOC, PRP-T, PRP-OMP, or PRP-D	1 or 2‖	Any conjugate vaccine

* See text and Table 3.8 for further information concerning specific vaccines.

† These vaccines may be given in combination products or as reconstituted products with DTP or DTaP, provided the combination or reconstituted vaccine is approved by the Food and Drug Administration for the child's age and administration of the other vaccine component(s) also is justified.

‡ For accelerated immunization, a minimum of a 1-month (4-week) interval between doses may be used.

§ The safety and efficacy of PRP-OMP, PRP-T, HbOC or PRP-D are likely to be equivalent for use as a booster dose in children 12 months or older.

‖ Two doses separated by 2 months are recommended by some experts for children with certain underlying diseases associated with increased risk of disease and impaired antibody responses to *H influenzae* type b conjugate vaccination (see text).

¶ Only for children with chronic illness known to be associated with an increased risk for *H influenzae* type b disease (see text).

— For children in whom immunization is initiated at 7 to 11 months of age, the recommended schedules for HbOC, PRP-OMP, and PRP-T are identical and require three doses. The first two doses are given at 2-month intervals using the same vaccine product, when feasible, for both doses. The third (booster) dose should be given at 12 to 18 months of age, preferably 2 months after the second dose. For the third dose, any licensed conjugate vaccine or PRP-D is acceptable.

— For children in whom immunization is initiated at 12 to 14 months of age, the recommended regimens for HbOC, PRP-OMP, PRP-T, and PRP-D are identical and require two doses given at a 2-month interval. However, PRP-D is recommended by the FDA only for primary administration at 15 months of age.

— For children in whom immunization is initiated at 15 months or older, and who have not yet reached their fifth birthday (ie, 59 months or younger), the recommended regimen is a single dose of any licensed conjugate vaccine.

— Circumstances may suggest a need for more rapid "catch-up" immunization, in which case a 1-month (4-week) interval between doses is the minimum.

- Special circumstances are as follows:
  1. *Lapsed immunizations.* Recommendations for children who have had a lapse in the schedule of immunizations are based on limited data. The current recommendations are summarized in Table 3.11.
  2. *Premature infants.* For infants born prematurely, immunization should be based on chronologic age and initiated at 2 months of age according to recommendations in Table 3.9. This recommendation is based on available data suggesting that even very low birthweight (ie, premature) infants have adequate antibody responses to these vaccines, when the recommended number of doses are given, although the serum concentrations of antibody may be decreased in chronically ill infants in comparison to those in full-term infants.
  3. *Deferral and contraindication of pertussis vaccination.* In infants with certain neurologic disorders, DTaP, DTP, or DT vaccination may be deferred until the first birthday (see Pertussis, p 394). Use of PRP-OMP may be advantageous in this circumstance. In infants in whom a decision has been made to use DT vaccine instead of DTaP or DTP, however (ie, pertussis vaccine is contraindicated), any Hib conjugate vaccine may be used. In infants and children in whom pertussis vaccination is contraindicated (see Pertussis, p 394), combination products containing DTaP or DTP should not be used.
  4. *Children who may be at increased risk of invasive Hib disease resulting from immunological or other host defense abnormalities (eg, sickle cell disease and postsplenectomy).* Children with decreased or absent splenic function who have received a primary series of Hib immunizations and a booster dose at 12 months of age or older need not be immunized further. Children who complete a primary series followed by a booster dose who are undergoing scheduled splenectomy (eg, for Hodgkin's disease, spherocytosis, immune thrombocytopenia, or hypersplenism) may benefit from an additional dose of any licensed conjugate vaccine. This dose should be provided at least 7 to 10 days prior to the procedure.

     Patients with HIV infection, IgG_2 subclass deficiency and those receiving chemotherapy for malignancies also are at increased risk for invasive Hib disease. Whether these children will benefit from additional doses after completion of the primary series of immunizations and the booster dose at 12 months of age or later is not known. Every effort should be made to ensure completion of the primary immunization and booster series.

Table 3.11. Recommendations for *Haemophilus influenzae* Type b Conjugate Immunization in Children With a Lapse in Administration*†

Age at Presentation, mo	Previous Vaccination History	Recommended Regimen
7–11	1 dose‡	1 dose of conjugate at 7–11 mo, with a booster dose given at least 2 mo later, at 12–15 mo§
	2 doses of HbOC or PRP-T	Same as above
12–14	2 doses before 12 mo‡	A single dose of any licensed conjugate‖
12–14	1 dose before 12 mo‡	2 additional doses of any licensed conjugate, separated by 2 mo‖
15–59	Any incomplete schedule	A single dose of any licensed conjugate‖

* See text and Table 3.8 for further information concerning specific vaccines.
† These vaccines may be given in combination products or as reconstituted products with DTP or DTaP, provided the combination or reconstituted vaccine is approved by the Food and Drug Administration for the child's age and the administration of the other vaccine component(s) also is justified.
‡ PRP-OMP, PRP-T, or HbOC.
§ For the dose given at 7 to 11 months, when feasible, the same vaccine should be given as was used for the dose given at 2 to 6 months. For the dose given at 12 to 15 months, any licensed conjugate vaccine can be used.
‖ The safety and efficacy of PRP-OMP, PRP-T, or HbOC or PRP-D are likely to be equivalent when used in children 12 months or older.

    For children 12 to 59 months of age with an underlying condition predisposing to Hib disease who are not immunized or have received only one dose of conjugate vaccine before 12 months of age, two doses of any conjugate vaccine, separated by 2 months, are recommended. For those in this age group who received two doses before 12 months of age, one additional dose of conjugate vaccine is recommended.

   5. *Unvaccinated children with an underlying disease possibly predisposing to Hib disease who are older than 59 months of age.* These children should be immunized with any licensed conjugate vaccine. Based on limited data, two doses separated by 1 to 2 months are suggested for children with HIV infection or IgG$_2$ deficiency.

    Some experts believe that a reinforcing dose of an Hib conjugate vaccine should be provided to children undergoing treatment for malignancy. This dose should be provided 3 months after completion of all chemotherapy or thereafter.

   6. *Haemophilus influenzae type b invasive infection.* Children who had invasive disease when younger than 24 months frequently have low anticapsular antibody concentrations in convalescent sera and may remain at risk of developing a second episode of disease. Immunization in these patients should be administered according to the age-appropriate schedule for

unvaccinated children and as if they had reviewed no prior Hib vaccine doses (see Tables 3.9 and 3.11). Immunization should be initiated 1 month after onset of disease or as soon as possible thereafter.

Children whose disease occurred at 24 months of age or older do not need immunization, irrespective of previous immunization status, because the disease most likely induced a protective immune response and second episodes of disease at this age are rare.

Immunized children who experience invasive Hib disease after receiving a dose of a conjugate vaccine at 15 months of age or older have a high incidence of IgG2 deficiency and, therefore, should be considered for immunologic evaluation. Children who completed the recommended immunization schedule before 15 months of age (ie, final dose given at 12 to 14 months of age) and who develop invasive disease also should be considered for immunologic evaluation. Whether immunologic evaluation should be performed for children who experience invasive Hib disease after conjugate immunization given earlier than 12 months of age is uncertain. Nevertheless, evaluation of immunoglobulin concentrations in such children, particularly those with a history of recurrent infection, should be considered.

Reporting. *Haemophilus influenzae* invasive disease, including both type b and non-type b infection and cases in fully or partially immunized children, should be reported to the Centers for Disease Control and Prevention through the local and state public health departments.

Helicobacter pylori Infections

CLINICAL MANIFESTATIONS: Acute infection may be manifest by epigastric pain, nausea, vomiting, hematemesis, and guaiac-positive stools. Symptoms usually resolve within a few days despite the persistence of infection for years or life. Duodenal or gastric ulceration or gastric adenocarcinoma develop in a minority of infected persons. *Helicobacter pylori* infection is not associated with autoimmune or chemical gastritis.

ETIOLOGY: *Helicobacter pylori* are Gram-negative, spirally curved or U-shaped microaerophilic bacilli that have a tuft of flagella at one end.

EPIDEMIOLOGY: *Helicobacter pylori* have been isolated only from humans and other primates. An animal reservoir for human transmission has not been demonstrated. The routes by which organisms are transmitted from the reservoir of infected humans are unknown, but fecal-oral transmission may occur. Infection rates are low in children but rise until age 60 years, at which time 25% to 60% of the population has been infected. Most carriage is asymptomatic, but essentially all infected persons have chronic gastritis. Infection is acquired at a younger age in developing countries and in persons in lower socioeconomic groups.

The **incubation period** is unknown.

DIAGNOSTIC TESTS: *Helicobacter pylori* infection can be diagnosed by culture from gastric biopsy tissue on nonselective media (eg, chocolate agar) or selective media (eg, Skirrow's) at 37°C under microaerobic conditions for 2 to 5 days. Organisms usually can be visualized on histologic sections with Gram, hematoxylin-eosin, silver, Giemsa, or acridine orange staining. Because of the production of urease by the organisms, urease testing of a gastric specimen can give a rapid and specific microbiologic diagnosis. All of these tests require endoscopy and biopsy to obtain tissue. Noninvasive, commercially available tests include detection of labeled CO_2 in expired air after oral administration of isotopically labeled urea, and serology for the presence of antibody to *H pylori*. Each of the diagnostic tests is greater than 95% accurate.

TREATMENT: *Helicobacter pylori* is susceptible to a wide variety of antimicrobial agents including ampicillin, tetracycline, metronidazole, clindamycin, erythromycin, clarithromycin, and bismuth salts, but none have been proved therapeutically effective as single agents. Combination therapy of amoxicillin, metronidazole, and bismuth subsalicylate is often effective in eliminating the organism, healing duodenal ulceration, and avoiding ulcer relapse, but recurrences occur. In adolescents and adults, tetracycline may be substituted for amoxicillin. Alternative therapies include a proton pump inhibitor, such as omeprazole, in combination with amoxicillin or clarithromycin, with or without metronidazole. Therapy results in eradication rates of 70% to 90%, although reinfection is likely.

ISOLATION OF THE HOSPITALIZED PATIENT: Standard precautions are recommended.

CONTROL MEASURES: Disinfection of gastroscopes will prevent transmission of the organism between patients.

Hemorrhagic Fevers Caused By Arenaviruses

CLINICAL MANIFESTATIONS: These diseases range from mild infections to severe acute febrile illnesses in which shock is a prominent feature. Fever, headache, myalgia, conjunctival suffusion, and abdominal pain are common early symptoms in all infections. Axillary petechiae are usual in **Argentine (AHF), Bolivian (BHF),** and **Venezuelan hemorrhagic fevers (VHF),** and exudative pharyngitis often occurs in **Lassa fever.** Mucosal bleeding occurs in severe cases as a consequence of vascular damage, thrombocytopenia, and platelet dysfunction. Proteinuria is common, but renal failure is unusual. Upper and lower respiratory symptoms can develop in **Lassa fever.** Elevated serum concentrations of aspartate aminotransferase can indicate an adverse or fatal outcome of **Lassa fever.** Sensorineural hearing loss is a common sequela of **Lassa fever.** Shock develops 7 to 9 days after onset of the illness in more severely ill patients with these infections. Encephalopathic signs with tremor, alterations in consciousness, and seizures can occur in the South American hemorrhagic fevers as well as in severe cases of **Lassa virus** infections.

ETIOLOGY: Arenaviruses are RNA viruses. The major New World arenavirus hemorrhagic fevers occurring in the Western hemisphere, **AHF, BHF, and VHF,** are caused by **Junin, Machupo,** and **Guanarito viruses,** respectively. A fourth arenavirus associated with hemorrhagic fever, **Sabiá virus,** recently was isolated in Brazil. **Lassa fever,** a disease occurring in West Africa, is caused by Lassa virus, an Old World arenavirus.

EPIDEMIOLOGY: Inhalation or skin contact (eg, through cuts, scratches, or abrasions) with urine and salivary secretions from persistently infected rodents are the principal routes of infection. All arenaviruses are infectious as aerosols; those causing hemorrhagic fever should be considered highly hazardous to laboratory workers. The geographic distribution and habitats of the specific rodents that serve as reservoir hosts largely determine the endemic area and groups of persons at risk. Several hundred cases of **AHF** occur yearly in agricultural workers and inhabitants of the Argentine pampas. Epidemics of **BHF** occurred from 1962 to 1964; sporadic disease activity has continued since then. **Venezuelan hemorrhagic fever** occurs in rural north-central Venezuela. **Lassa fever** is highly endemic in most of West Africa, where its rodent host lives in proximity with humans, causing thousands of infections annually. **Lassa fever virus** (and rarely, **BHF** or **AHF**) can be transmitted from person to person, typically through close contact, including within hospitals. Infection of laboratory workers has been caused by all arenaviruses associated with hemorrhagic fever except **Guanarito virus. Lassa fever** has been imported by travelers from West Africa.

The **incubation periods** are from 6 to 17 days.

DIAGNOSTIC TESTS: Diagnosis is made by demonstrating virus-specific serum IgM, an increase in virus-specific IgG antibody titers in serial serum specimens, viral isolation, or by identifying viral antigen in blood or tissues. Serum antibody detected by immunofluorescence occurs earlier in **Lassa fever** (7 to 10 days) than in the South American diseases (14 to 21 days). Neutralizing serum antibodies occur later and are difficult to detect in **Lassa fever**. These viruses may be recovered from the blood of acutely ill patients, as well as from various tissues obtained postmortem.

TREATMENT: Plasma from convalescent patients has proved effective in reducing the mortality associated with **AHF** from 15% to 30% in untreated patients to less than 1% in those receiving appropriate quantities (based on neutralizing antibody content) within the first 8 days of illness. Intravenous ribavirin reduces mortality significantly in patients with **Lassa fever,** particularly if they are treated during the first week of illness, and it probably is beneficial in treating South American arenavirus infections.

ISOLATION OF THE HOSPITALIZED PATIENT*: Contact precautions, including careful prevention of needle-stick injuries, are recommended for all the hemorrhagic fevers caused by arenaviruses for the duration of the illness. The state health department and the Centers for Disease Control and Prevention should be contacted for specific advice about management of suspected cases.

---

*In addition to standard precautions.

CONTROL MEASURES:

Care of Exposed Persons. No specific measures are warranted for persons exposed to **Lassa fever** unless direct contamination with blood, excretions, or secretions from an infected patient has occurred. If such contamination has occurred, daily temperature recordings for 21 days and prevention of physical contact with other individuals during this interval are recommended. Recommendations are similar for those who have had sexual contact (both immediately before illness and for several weeks afterward).

Rodent Control. In the village-based outbreaks of **BHF,** rodent control has proved successful. Rodent control is not practical for control of **AHF** because the reservoirs are sylvatic and ubiquitous. Rodent control has reduced **Lassa fever** infections but has not eliminated infection in household members because the rodents are also peridomestic and eventually re-invade human dwellings.

Immunoprophylaxis. An investigational live-attenuated **Junin** vaccine developed by the US Army protects against **AHF** and probably against **BHF.** The vaccine is associated with minimal side effects in adults; similar findings have been obtained from limited safety studies in children 4 years of age and older.

Hemorrhagic Fevers and Related Syndromes, Including Hantavirus Pulmonary Syndrome, Caused By Viruses of the Family *Bunyaviridae*

CLINICAL MANIFESTATIONS: These infections are severe, febrile diseases in which shock and bleeding can be significant, and multisystem involvement can occur. Recently in the United States, one of these infections has caused an illness marked by acute respiratory failure (ie, Hantavirus pulmonary syndrome).

Hemorrhagic fever with renal syndrome (HFRS) is a complex, multiphasic disease characterized by vascular instability and varying degrees of renal insufficiency. Fever, flushing, conjunctival injection, abdominal pain, and lumbar pain are followed by hypotension, oliguria, and, subsequently, polyuria. Petechiae and more serious bleeding manifestations are common. Shock and acute renal insufficiency may require intensive care and dialysis. Nephropathia epidemica, the clinical syndrome of **HFRS** in Europe, is a milder disease characterized by a grippelike illness with abdominal pain and proteinuria. Acute renal dysfunction also occurs, which may require hospitalization, but hypotensive shock or a requirement for dialysis is infrequent.

Hantavirus pulmonary syndrome (HPS) is an acute febrile illness with high mortality that progresses to acute respiratory failure and shock. Clinical findings during the prodrome are nonspecific, but usually include fever and marked myalgia, often accompanied by gastrointestinal manifestations and/or dizziness. Hemoconcentration, hypoalbuminemia, thrombocytopenia, arterial oxygen desaturation, and interstitial or alveolar pulmonary edema are often present when patients are admitted to the hospital. Unlike other hantaviral diseases, renal failure has been mild or absent in most recognized cases of **HPS.**

Crimean-Congo hemorrhagic fever (CCHF) is a multisystem disease characterized by hepatitis and, often, profuse bleeding. Fever, headache, and myalgia are followed by signs of a diffuse capillary leak syndrome, such as facial suffusion, conjunctivitis, and proteinuria. Bradycardia is common, and petechiae and purpura frequently appear on the skin and mucous membranes. A hypotensive crisis often occurs after the appearance of frank hemorrhage from the gastrointestinal tract, nose, mouth, or uterus.

Rift Valley fever (RVF), in most cases, is a self-limited, febrile illness. Occasionally, patients develop hepatitis, hemorrhagic fever with shock and bleeding, encephalitis, or retinitis.

ETIOLOGY: Bunyaviridae are RNA viruses with different geographic distributions and vectors. Hantaviruses cause **HFRS** and **HPS**. The prototype Hantaan virus is responsible for severe disease in Asia and the Balkans, and Puumala virus causes the milder disease occurring in Europe. Seoul virus is distributed worldwide and causes **HFRS** of variable severity. Most recognized cases of **HPS** have been caused by Sin Nombre virus from the North American deer mouse, but other viruses in the Americas have been implicated in disease.

EPIDEMIOLOGY: Classic hemorrhagic fever with renal syndrome occurs throughout much of Asia, Eastern and Western Europe, and the Balkans. **Hantaan** and related viruses cause chronic inapparent infections in species of field mice, voles, peridomestic rats, and other small mammals characteristic for each virus. Disease in humans is acquired by contact, most frequently from inhalation of aerosols, infectious secreta and excreta of these animals. The most severe forms of disease are acquired in rural areas of Asia and the Balkan nations; urban-acquired cases that occur in Europe are generally milder. Numerous infections have occurred in the laboratory by contact with chronically infected rodents, either captured wild rodents or colonies of laboratory rats. **Hantaviruses** have been isolated from rodents in the United States but the only association with acute disease is **HPS**. This syndrome was initially identified in the southwestern United States in 1993 but the disease is believed to occur in most areas of Canada and the United States as well as certain regions of South America. **Crimean-Congo hemorrhagic fever (CCHF)** occurs in much of sub-Saharan Africa, the Middle East, areas in West and Central Asia, and Eastern Europe. The **CCHF** virus is transmitted by ticks, and, occasionally, at the slaughter of domestic animals. Nosocomial transmission of **CCHF** is a serious hazard. **Rift Valley fever** (RVF) occurs throughout sub-Saharan Africa and has caused epidemics in Egypt in 1977 and 1993–1995. The virus is arthropod-borne, and is transmitted from domestic livestock to humans by mosquitoes. It can also be transmitted by aerosol, and by direct contact with infected fresh animal carcasses.

The **incubation periods** for **CCHF** and **RVF** range from 2 to 10 days; for **HFRS** they are usually longer, ranging from 9 to 40 days. For **HPS**, the incubation period may be 1 to 3 weeks, but has not been definitively established.

DIAGNOSTIC TESTS: The **CCHF** and **RVF** viruses are readily recovered from blood and tissues of infected patients; recovery of **hantaviruses** is difficult and infrequent. Detection of viral antigen is a useful alternative for the diagnosis of **CCHF** and **RVF**, but it has been unsuccessful for **HFRS**. Serum IgM and IgG virus-specific antibodies typically develop early in convalescence in **CCHF** and **RVF.** In **HFRS** and **HPS,** IgM and IgG antibodies are usually detectable at the time of onset of the illness or within 48 hours. IgM antibodies or rising IgG titers in paired sera, as demonstrated by enzyme immunoassay, are diagnostic. Neutralizing antibody tests provide greater virus-strain specificity. Immunofluorescent and complement-fixing antibody tests also are used for serologic diagnosis. Polymerase chain reaction for viral RNA on fresh or frozen tissue and immunohistochemistry performed on formalin-fixed lung tissue are useful for diagnosis of **HPS.**

TREATMENT: Ribavirin given intravenously to patients with **HFRS** within the first 4 days of illness appears effective in reducing renal dysfunction, vascular instability, and mortality. Supportive therapy for **HFRS** should include (1) avoidance of transporting patients, (2) supportive care for shock, (3) prevention of overhydration (particularly with crystalloid solutions), (4) dialysis for complications of renal failure, and (5) control of hypertension during the oliguric phase.

The treatment of **HPS** is similar to that of **HFRS,** except that the primary consideration is on the prevention of severe hypoxemia and maintenance of adequate tissue perfusion without exacerbation of the pulmonary capillary leak syndrome by excess fluid administration. Ribavirin has been used but controlled trials are lacking.

Ribavirin given to patients with **CCHF** has resulted in clinical responses, although no controlled studies have been performed. Experimental animal data suggest the potential for use of ribavirin in treatment of hemorrhagic **RVF** as well.

ISOLATION OF THE HOSPITALIZED PATIENT*: Contact precautions, with particular attention to the hazards posed by laboratory specimens and needlesticks, are indicated for patients with **CCHF. Rift Valley fever** has not been demonstrated to be contagious, but standard precautions should be scrupulously followed. **Hemorrhagic fever with renal syndrome** and **HPS** are not associated with nosocomial or person-to-person transmission and, therefore, patients with these infections require only standard precautions.

CONTROL MEASURES:

Care of Exposed Persons. Persons having direct contact with blood or other secretions from patients with CCHF should be monitored for fever daily for 14 days and precluded from intimate contact with other persons during this time. For those with parenteral exposure to contaminated objects or extensive blood exposure, close observation and immediate therapy should be instituted with intravenous ribavirin at the first sign of disease in consultation with appropriate experts.

Other Measures.

HFRS. Monitoring of laboratory rat colonies and urban rodent control may be effective for rat-borne disease.

Hantaviruses. Widespread control of sylvatic reservoirs of rurally acquired hantaviruses, including the newly recognized hantaviruses causing HPS, is not practical. However, reduction of human contact with rodents and their excreta through targeted rodent elimination programs is prudent.

---

* In addition to standard precautions.

CCHF. Insecticides for tick control generally have limited benefit, but may be useful in stockyard settings. Personal protective measures (eg, physical tick removal and protective clothing with permethrin sprays) are effective.

RVF. Vaccination of domestic animals is important in limiting or preventing RVF outbreaks and protecting humans. Mosquito control is usually not effective. An investigational vaccine for humans developed by the US Army appears effective in laboratory workers, which suggests it would be useful in other settings, such as for veterinary staff in endemic areas.

Hepatitis A

CLINICAL MANIFESTATIONS: Hepatitis A is characteristically an acute self-limited illness with fever, malaise, jaundice, anorexia, and nausea. In infants and preschool-aged children, symptomatic illness usually causes only mild, nonspecific symptoms without jaundice. Duration of illness is typically several weeks, but prolonged or relapsing disease lasting as long as 6 months can occur. Fulminant hepatitis is rare, and chronic infection does not occur.

ETIOLOGY: Hepatitis A virus (HAV) is an RNA virus classified as a member of the picornavirus (enterovirus) group.

EPIDEMIOLOGY: The most common mode of transmission is person to person, resulting from fecal contamination and oral ingestion, ie, the fecal-oral route. In developing countries, infection is endemic. In the United States, HAV infection is endemic, with periodic outbreaks occurring in selected populations such as Native Americans, Alaskan natives, selected Hispanic communities, and certain Hasidic communities. Among clinical cases of hepatitis A reported to the Centers for Disease Control and Prevention (CDC) from 1990 to 1992, the major identified source was personal contact in 24%, child care center in 15%, international travel in 6%, food- or water-borne outbreaks in 4%, male homosexual contact in 4%, and use of injection drugs in 3%. In 44%, the source was unknown. Fecal-oral spread from asymptomatic infections, particularly young children, likely accounts for most of these cases of unknown source. Infection in households and in child care centers has become an important source for HAV spread in the community and for outbreaks in the United States. In contrast to most other infectious diseases in child care settings, symptomatic (icteric) illness occurs primarily among adult contacts of children in child care and most infected attendees are asymptomatic or have nonspecific manifestations. Hence, spread of HAV infection in and from a child care center frequently occurs before recognition of the index case(s). The risk of spread and of an outbreak occurring in a child care center increases with the number of children enrolled who are younger than 2 years and who wear diapers.

Common-source food- and water-borne epidemics, including several caused by shellfish contaminated by human sewage, have occurred. Nosocomial outbreaks have occurred as the result of shedding of HAV virus from infected, asymptomatic neonates, children, or adults. Transmission by blood transfusion or from mother to newborn infant (ie, vertical transmission) is rare. Infection has been contracted rarely from nonhuman primates.

Age of infection varies with socioeconomic status and associated living conditions. In developing countries, infection in the first decade of life is common; in developed countries, infection occurs at an older age. In the United States, the highest rates for symptomatic HAV infection have occurred in children 5 to 14 years of age and the lowest rates are in children from birth to 4 years and adults older than 40 years. Symptomatic hepatitis occurs in less than 10% of infected children younger than 6 years, 40% to 50% of those from 6 to 14 years, and 70% to 80% of those older than 14 years. No appreciable seasonal variation in the incidence of infection has been noted.

Viral shedding and probably the contagious period last 1 to 3 weeks. The highest titers of HAV in stool of infected patients occur in the 1 to 2 weeks before the onset of illness, during which time patients are most likely to transmit infection. The risk subsequently diminishes and is minimal in the week after the onset of jaundice. No HAV carrier state exists. The presence of serum anti-HAV IgG in unvaccinated persons indicates lifelong immunity to HAV.

The **incubation period** is 15 to 50 days, with an average of 25 to 30 days.

DIAGNOSTIC TESTS: Serologic tests for HAV-specific IgG and IgM are available commercially. Serum IgM is present at the onset of illness and usually disappears within 4 months, thus usually indicating current or recent infection, but may persist for 6 months or longer. Anti-HAV IgG is detectable shortly after the appearance of the IgM-specific titer. The presence of IgG anti-HAV antibodies without virus-specific IgM indicates past infection.

Children who have received HAV vaccine rarely have detectable anti-HAV IgM titers. The relatively low titers of serum antibody resulting from intramuscular immune globulin or HAV vaccine, in comparison to those following infection, may not be detectable by the commercially available antibody assays.

TREATMENT: Supportive.

ISOLATION OF THE HOSPITALIZED PATIENT*: Contact precautions are recommended for diapered and/or incontinent patients, ie, young children, for 1 week after the onset of symptoms.

CONTROL MEASURES:

General Measures. The major methods for prevention of HAV infections are improved sanitation (eg, of water sources and in food preparation) and personal hygiene (eg, hand washing after diaper changes in child care settings).

Schools, Child Care, and Work. Children and adults with acute HAV infection should be excluded for 1 week after onset of the illness.

Immune Globulin. Immune globulin (IG) for intramuscular administration, when given within 2 weeks after HAV exposure, is 80% to 90% effective in preventing symptomatic infection. Peak serum antibody concentrations usually are achieved 48 to 72 hours after IG administration. Indications include pre-exposure and

---

* In addition to standard precautions.

postexposure prophylaxis (see p 242). Recommended pre-exposure and postexposure IG doses and duration of protection are given in Table 3.12 and Table 3.13 (p 240 and p 241).

Intravenous immune globulin (IGIV) is likely to be protective against HAV infection, but protective efficacy, appropriate dose and duration of protection have not been defined. Extrapolation from protective efficacy data on IG and from anti-HAV titers in IG and IGIV suggest that an IGIV dose of 400 mg/kg would be protective for at least 6 months. HAV antibody titers, however, may be variable in lots of IGIV as the result of different manufacturing processes and donors from whom the products were derived, and affect duration of protection.

Hepatitis A Vaccine. Two inactivated HAV vaccines, Havrix[†] and Vaqta,[‡] are currently available in the United States. Both vaccines have pediatric and adult formulations. The vaccines are comprised of viral antigens purified from HAV-infected human diploid fibroblast cell cultures. Antigen content is expressed for Havrix as enzyme-linked immunoassay units (EL.U.) and for Vaqta as units (U).

Administration, Dosages, and Schedules (see Table 3.14, p 242). Both vaccines are approved for children 2 through 18 years of age and for adults. Havrix for children has two licensed formulations, one for a three-dose schedule and the other for a two-dose schedule (see Table 3.14). Vaqta for children is given in a two-dose schedule. The adult formulations of Havrix and Vaqta are recommended for persons 19 years of age and older. All currently licensed vaccines are given intramuscularly. Recommended doses and schedules for these different products and formulations are given in Table 3.14.

Immunogenicity. The different vaccine formulations are similarly immunogenic when given in their respective recommended schedules and doses. Serum antibody titers following vaccination are lower than those resulting from HAV infection and commercially available assays are not always sufficiently sensitive to measure low titers of antibody after administration of vaccine or IG. Postvaccination titers are detectable, however, by immunoassays, the results of which correlate with viral neutralizing antibody assays. Antibody titers in these immunoassays are expressed as milli-international units (mIU) per milliliter; concentrations of 20 mIU/mL or greater are considered to be protective.

One dose of Havrix in adults induces seroconversion by 15 days in 88% and by 1 month in 99%; 1 month after a second dose at 6 months, 100% have serum antibody concentrations and significantly increased titers. Responses in children are similar. Doses of either pediatric formulation of Havrix induce 90% greater seroconversion 1 month after an initial dose and 100% seroconversion after the second dose. Subsequent doses cause a substantial increase in serum antibody titers, indicating an anamnestic response and immunologic memory that may be important for sustained protection against HAV infection.

Limited data on immunogenicity of HAV vaccine in infants indicate high rates of seroconversion, but the geometric mean serum antibody titers are significantly less in those with passively acquired maternal anti-HAV antibody in comparison to recipients lacking anti-HAV antibodies. Further studies of the immunogenicity and safety of HAV vaccine in infants are in progress.

[†] SmithKline Beecham, Philadelphia, Pa.

[‡] Merck and Co, West Point, Pa.

Table 3.12. Recommendations for Pre-exposure Immunoprophylaxis of Hepatitis A Infection for Travelers*

Age, y	Likely Exposure, mo	Recommended Prophylaxis
<2	<3	IG 0.02 mL/kg[†]
	3–5	IG 0.06 mL/kg[†]
	Long term	IG 0.06 mL/kg at departure and every 5 mo thereafter[†]
≥2	<3[‡]	HAV vaccine[§‖]
		or
		IG 0.02 mL/kg[†]
	3–5[‡]	HAV vaccine[§‖]
		or
		IG 0.06 mL/kg[†]
	Long term	HAV vaccine[§‖]

* HAV, hepatitis A virus; IG, immune globulin.
† IG should be administered deep into a large muscle mass. Ordinarily no more than 5 mL should be administered in one site in an adult or large child; lesser amounts (maximum, 3 mL) should be given to small children and infants.
‡ Vaccine is preferable, but IG is an acceptable alternative.
§ To ensure protection in travelers whose departure is imminent, IG also may be given (see text).
‖ Dose and schedule of HAV vaccine as recommended according to age in Table 3.14.

Efficacy. In a large, double-blind, placebo-controlled, randomized efficacy trial of Havrix in Thailand children 1 to 16 years of age living in an endemic region for HAV infection who were given three doses (360 EL.U.) in a schedule of 0, 1, and 12 months, protective efficacy was 94% after two doses and 100% after three doses. A single dose of Havrix in Alaskan natives in villages with endemic HAV disease resulted in a marked decrease in cases within 8 weeks of vaccination. A similar abrupt decrease in HAV cases was observed after two doses of Havrix in two Slovak Republic villages experiencing a large community outbreak. In a trial of Vaqta in a New York community with a high endemic rate of hepatitis A, protective efficacy against clinical hepatitis A, beginning 21 days after vaccination, was 100%. Clinical studies suggest possible herd immunity if more than 80% of the estimated susceptible persons were vaccinated.

Duration of Protection. The need for booster doses cannot be determined because HAV vaccines have been under evaluation for only a short time and long-term efficacy has not been established. Detectable antibody, however, persists for at least 4 years after a three-dose series in adults. While antibody concentrations decline each year in the first year after vaccination, kinetic models suggest that protective concentrations will persist for as long as 20 years. In the New York community trial of Vaqta, protection against HAV disease has persisted thus far for 4 years.

Vaccine in Immunocompromised Patients. The immune response in immunocompromised persons may be suboptimal. In HIV-infected adults, seroconversion rates and geometric mean titers are lower than those in noninfected persons. Data for immunocompromised children are not available.

Table 3.13. **Recommendations for Postexposure Immunoprophylaxis of Hepatitis A Infection**

Time Since Exposure, wk	Future Exposure Likely	Age of Patient, y	Recommended Prophylaxis
≤2	No	All ages	IG (0.02 mL/kg)*
	Yes	≥2	IG (0.02 mL/kg)* **and** HAV vaccine†
>2	No	All ages	No prophylaxis
	Yes	≥2	HAV vaccine†

* Immune globulin (IG) should be administered deep into a large muscle mass. Ordinarily no more than 5 mL should be administered in one site in an adult or large child; lesser amounts (maximum, 3 mL) should be given to small children and infants.
† Dosage and schedule of hepatitis A virus (HAV) vaccine as recommended according to age in Table 3.14.

Effect of Immune Globulin (IG) on Vaccine Immunogenicity. Seroconversion rates are not impaired by simultaneous administration of IG and the first vaccine dose, but lower serum antibody concentrations may be achieved, the significance of which is unclear. Early achievement of protective concentrations of antibody after the first dose of vaccine may require concomitant administration of IG. In a study of travelers receiving HAV immunoprophylaxis, serum antibodies were detectable 5 days later in 92% of subjects receiving IG alone or vaccine and IG, but in only 4% of those receiving vaccine alone

Vaccine Interchangeability. Vaqta and Havrix, when given as recommended, appear to be similarly effective. Since data determining the interchangeability of vaccines from different manufacturers are not available, completion of the immunization regimen with the same product is preferable, but vaccination with either product is acceptable, particularly if the product given for the first dose is not known. Children whose first dose of HAV vaccine either was the Havrix-360 EL.U. (0.5 mL) formulation or is not known should receive two doses of any pediatric vaccine formulation to complete the recommended vaccine schedule.

Administration With Other Vaccines. Hepatitis A virus vaccine may be administered simultaneously with other vaccines, but should be given in a separate syringe and at a separate site (see Simultaneous Administration of Multiple Vaccines, p 21).

Adverse Events. Adverse reactions are mild and similar in frequency to those in hepatitis B vaccine recipients (given as the placebo in vaccine trials). The most common side effect is local pain; induration at the injection site occurs less commonly. No serious adverse events attributed definitively to HAV vaccine have been reported in children or adults.

Precautions and Contraindications. The vaccine should not be administered to persons with a hypersensitivity to any of the vaccine components, such as alum and phenoxyethanol. Safety data in pregnant women are not available, but the risk is considered to be low or nonexistent because the vaccine contains inactivated, purified viral proteins.

Table 3.14. Recommended Doses and Schedules for Hepatitis A Virus (HAV) Inactivated Vaccines

Age, y	Vaccine*	Antigen Dose†	Volume per dose, mL	Number of doses	Schedule
2 through 18	Havrix‡ (SKB)	360 EL.U.	0.5	3	Initial, 1, and 6–12 mo later
	Havrix (SKB)	720 EL.U.	0.5	2	Initial and 6–12 mo later
	Vaqta (Merck)	25 U§	0.5	2	Initial and 6–18 mo later
19 and older	Havrix (SKB)	1440 EL.U.	1.0	2	Initial and 6–12 mo later
	Vaqta (Merck)	50 U§	1.0	2	Initial and 6–12 mo later

* SKB indicates SmithKline Beecham.
† EL.U. indicates enzyme-linked immunoassay units.
‡ Children receiving 360 EL.U. for the first dose should receive two additional doses of either pediatric formulation (360 EL.U. or 720 EL.U.) to complete the schedule.
§ Antigen units (each unit is equivalent to approximately 1 mg of viral protein).

Preimmunization Serologic Testing. Preimmunization testing for HAV antibody generally is not recommended for children. Testing may be cost-effective in individuals who have a high likelihood of immunity from prior infection, such as those whose early childhood was in areas of high endemicity, those with a history of jaundice potentially caused by HAV, and those older than 40 years.

Postimmunization Serologic Testing. Postimmunization testing for HAV antibody titer is not indicated in immunocompetent individuals because of the high seroconversion rates in adults and children. Commercially available anti-HAV tests may not detect low, but protective, concentrations of antibody induced by vaccine. For immunocompromised persons, especially those with liver disease who are at risk of exposure to HAV, postimmunization testing is justified. If no HAV antibody is detected with a sensitive assay, a repeat immunization series should be considered, preferably during periods of least immunosuppression.

RECOMMENDATIONS FOR IMMUNOPROPHYLAXIS

Pre-exposure Prophylaxis (see Table 3.12).

Foreign Travel. For susceptible persons traveling to or working in countries with intermediate or high endemic rates of HAV infection, immunoprophylaxis before departure is indicated. Such countries include those other than Australia, Canada, Japan, and New Zealand, and those in Western Europe and Scandinavia. For persons 2 years of age and older, vaccine is preferable, but IG is an acceptable alternative. Factors to consider in choosing active and/or passive prophylaxis include the interval before departure, the relative costs and availability of IG and HAV vaccine, the duration of the stay, and the likelihood of repeated exposure (see Table 3.12).

Immune globulin is protective against HAV disease immediately after administration, whereas the precise time required from receiving one dose of vaccine to onset of protection has not been established. Since 88% to 96% of children and adults developed detectable antibody within 2 weeks of a single dose, the usual incubation period for HAV disease is 25 to 30 days, and efficacy within 21 days after receipt of a single dose of Vaqta in a community with ongoing endemic HAV disease was 100%, protection is considered likely to occur within a few days after the first dose of vaccine. However, the product label for both vaccines suggests that a 2-week interval is required for protection and the Advisory Committee on Immunization Practices of the Centers for Disease Control and Prevention recommends a 1-month interval. To ensure protection in travelers whose departure is imminent, an alternative option to only vaccination is to administer both IG (see Table 3.12) and the first dose of vaccine (see Effect of Immune Globulin (IG) on Vaccine Immunogenicity, p 241). However, the additional benefit of simultaneous administration of IG and the first dose of vaccine has not been evaluated in field trials and may be marginal.

Whether vaccine alone or vaccine and IG are given for the first dose, the recommended additional dose(s) should be administered in order to produce high antibody titers and ensure likely long-term protection.

Children younger than 2 years should receive only IG because vaccine is not yet approved for this age group (see Table 3.12).

Other Indications for Vaccination. Hepatitis A vaccine is recommended for the following:

- *Children 2 years and older in defined and circumscribed communities with high endemic rates and/or periodic outbreaks of HAV infection (eg, Native Americans or Alaskan Natives).* Immunization is recommended for such children, as vaccine use has markedly diminished the occurrence of HAV cases. Younger children are most apt to be susceptible and should be given priority for immunization. In communities where HAV disease is endemic, children older than 10 to 15 years already may have been infected. Plans for implementation of age-specific immunization in such communities should be based on available seroprevalence and epidemiologic data and should be made in consultation with local public health officials. For control of more widespread community outbreaks, too few data currently exist to recommend routine use of HAV vaccine. In some common-source outbreaks, the source of infection has been removed before recognition of the outbreak and, thus, the subsequent risk to the community is low.

  Widespread prophylactic use of IG during extended community outbreaks for other than contacts of hepatitis A cases has not proved efficacious because protection is of limited duration and spread of the virus may continue through several generations of incubation periods. Although in some community situations IG prophylaxis has been used for control, it cannot be recommended routinely.

- *Patients with chronic liver disease.* These patients have an increased risk for severe hepatitis with HAV infection, which can be prevented by immunization. Although few data currently exist about the immunogenicity and protective efficacy of HAV vaccine in persons with chronic liver disease, no reason exists to suspect that the inactivated HAV vaccine would aggravate the chronic condition.
- *Homosexual and bisexual men.*
- *Users of injection and illicit drugs.*
- *Those at occupational risk of exposure (eg, handlers of nonhuman primates and persons working with HAV in a laboratory setting).*

In addition, any healthy person at least 2 years of age may receive HAV vaccine at the discretion of the physician and the patient or patient's family.

Potential Indications for HAV Vaccination. Other circumstances in which vaccination may be given are as follows:

- *Child care center staff and attendees.* Recent serosurveys have found only a small or no excess of HAV seroprevalence among staff of child care centers compared with that among community control populations. Given the cost of HAV vaccine, routine immunization of staff is not justified. Administration of vaccine, however, should be considered in child care settings with ongoing or recurrent outbreaks and in communities where cases in the child-care centers contribute substantially to the total number of cases of HAV disease.

  The need of HAV vaccine for attendees is more problematic. A national child care survey estimated that 9.5 million children in the United States in 1990 attended child care centers or family child care settings, and 27% were younger than 3 years. Transmission of HAV in centers usually occurs from asymptomatic infection in diapered children less than 2 years of age, the age group for which HAV vaccine is not approved. Immunization of all these children, therefore, is not possible or currently warranted.

- *Custodial care institutions.* Epidemic HAV disease was reported in custodial care institutions in the 1970s and 1980s, but it has not been a problem in recent years. However, HAV vaccine may be considered for staff and residents in institutions where HAV infection is occurring or where HAV seroprevalence data indicate vaccination would be cost-effective.

- *Hospital personnel.* Because hospital personnel generally do not have increased prevalence rates of HAV antibody compared with that in the community, routine pre-exposure use of HAV vaccine in hospital personnel is not recommended. Usually nosocomial HAV disease in hospital personnel has occurred through spread from acutely infected patients in whom the diagnosis of HAV infection was not recognized. If HAV vaccine is demonstrated to be effective in postexposure prophylaxis, immunization in such outbreaks would be indicated. In specific patient care areas with continued occurrence of symptomatic cases or where high seroprevalence of anti-HAV have been found, immunization may be effective.

- *Food handlers.* Food-borne outbreaks usually are associated with contamination of uncooked food during preparation by a food-handler who is infected with HAV. The most effective means to prevent these outbreaks is by careful hygienic practices during food preparation. Little information is available concerning seroprevalence rates of HAV antibody in food handlers compared with that in the general population. Routine HAV vaccination, therefore, in this population is not indicated at this time. However, economic, medicolegal, and public relations implications of a food-borne HAV outbreak from a commercial establishment may indicate that HAV vaccine use should be considered in some circumstances. Factors to consider in this decision include the nature of the food (eg, materials for salads) as well as the demographic characteristics, the average duration of employment, and the number of food handlers.

- *Patients with hemophilia.* Outbreaks of HAV infection in patients with hemophilia receiving solvent-detergent treated factor concentrates have been reported primarily in Europe. However, in the United States, three cases of HAV infection were reported in the mid-1990s in patients with hemophilia who received factor VIII concentrate from a single lot from one manufacturer. Currently available seroprevalence data in the United States from patients with hemophilia do not allow accurate determination of risk. Nevertheless, patients with hemophilia, especially those receiving solvent detergent-treated factor concentrates, may benefit from protection against HAV infection and should be considered for immunization. Preimmunization testing for anti-HAV antibody may be cost-effective because seroprevalence rates among persons with hemophilia may be higher. Studies are planned to determine whether subcutaneous administration of the vaccine in hemophiliac patients would be as immunogenic and safe as the IM route recommended for other individuals.

Postexposure Prophylaxis (see Table 3.13). Use of IG is recommended as follows (see Table 3.13 for dosages):

- *Household and sexual contacts.* All household and sexual contacts of HAV cases should receive IG as soon as possible after exposure. Serologic testing of contacts is not recommended because it adds unnecessary cost and may delay the administration of IG. The use of IG more than 2 weeks after the last exposure is not indicated.

- *Newborn infants of HAV-infected mothers.* Perinatal transmission of HAV is rare in this circumstance. Some experts advise giving IG (0.02 mL/kg) to the infant if the mother's symptoms began between 2 weeks before and 1 week after delivery. Efficacy, however, in this circumstance has not been established. Severe disease in healthy infants appears to be rare.

- *Child care center staff, employees, children, and their household contacts.* Serological testing for HAV IgM antibody to confirm HAV infection in suspected cases is indicated. When an HAV case is identified in an employee or child enrolled in a center in which all children are older than 2 years and all are toilet trained, IG is recommended for employees in contact with the index case and for children in the same room as the index case.

When an HAV infection is identified in an employee or a child or in the household contacts of two of the enrolled children in a child care center where children are not yet toilet trained, IG is recommended for all employees and all enrolled children in the facility. During the 6 weeks after the last case is identified, new employees and children should also receive IG.

The decision to administer IG to household contacts of a case in a child care center is dependent on such factors as whether the child is diapered and the intimacy of contact (eg, primary caregiver).

If recognition of an outbreak of HAV disease in a child care center is delayed by 3 or more weeks from the onset of the index case or if illness has occurred in three or more families, the infection is likely to have already spread widely. Although IG should be considered for use in these situations, it may not prevent additional cases.

Children and adults with acute HAV infection should be excluded from the center until 1 week after onset of the illness, until the IG prophylaxis program has been initiated, or until directed by the responsible health department. Precise data concerning the onset of protection after a dose of IG are not available. Allowing IG recipients, however, to return to the child care center setting immediately following receipt of the IG dose appears reasonable.

Studies are needed to determine the effectiveness of vaccine alone as a means to control such outbreaks. Vaccine alone may be considered an alternative option for prophylaxis of new employees if the risk of exposure is not high during their initial 2 weeks of employment because a single dose induces seroconversion within 15 days in 88% of adults.

- **Schools.** Schoolroom exposure generally does not pose an appreciable risk of infection, and IG administration is not indicated. However, IG could be used if transmission within the school setting is documented. Alternatively, vaccine should be considered as a means of prophylaxis, especially when a longer duration of protection is advisable.

- **Institutions and hospitals.** In institutions for custodial care with an outbreak of HAV infection, residents and staff in close personal contact with infected patients should receive IG. Administration of IG to hospital personnel caring for patients is not indicated routinely, unless an outbreak is occurring.

- **Food- or water-borne outbreaks.** Such outbreaks usually are recognized too late for IG to be effective. Immune globulin may be effective if administered to exposed individuals within 2 weeks of the last exposure to the HAV-contaminated water or food.

- **HAV vaccine for postexposure prophylaxis.** Available data are insufficient to recommend HAV vaccine alone for postexposure prophylaxis. However, several studies and clinical trials suggest that HAV vaccine, with or without concurrent IG administration, may provide effective postexposure prophylaxis by inducing protective serum antibody concentrations before the usual 4-week incubation period for HAV infection.

Hepatitis B

CLINICAL MANIFESTATIONS: Hepatitis B virus (HBV) causes a wide spectrum of manifestations, ranging from asymptomatic seroconversion, subacute illness with nonspecific symptoms (eg, anorexia, nausea, or malaise) or extrahepatic symptoms, and clinical hepatitis with jaundice, to fulminant fatal hepatitis. Anicteric or asymptomatic infection is most common in young children. Arthralgias, arthritis, or macular rashes can occur early in the course of the illness. Chronic HBV infection with persistence of hepatitis B surface antigen (HBsAg) occurs in as many as 90% of infants infected by perinatal transmission, in 30% of children 1 to 5 years old infected after birth, and in 5% to 10% of older children, adolescents, and adults with HBV infection. Chronically infected persons are at increased risk for developing chronic liver disease (eg, cirrhosis, chronic active hepatitis, or chronic persistent hepatitis) or primary hepatocellular carcinoma in later life.

ETIOLOGY: Hepatitis B virus is a DNA-containing, 42-nm hepadenavirus. Important components include HBsAg, hepatitis B core antigen (HBcAg), and hepatitis B e antigen (HBeAg).

EPIDEMIOLOGY: Hepatitis B virus is transmitted through blood or body fluids such as wound exudates, semen, cervical secretions, and saliva that are HBsAg-positive. Blood and serum contain the highest concentrations of virus; saliva contains the lowest. The HBV chronic carrier (defined as a person who is HBsAg-positive for 6 months or who is IgM anti-HBc-negative and HBsAg-positive) is the primary reservoir for infection. Modes of transmission include transfusion of blood or blood products (which is now rare in the United States because of routine screening of blood donors and viral inactivation of certain blood products), sharing or reusing nonsterilized needles or syringes, percutaneous or mucous membrane exposure to blood or body fluids, and homosexual and heterosexual activity. Percutaneous contact with contaminated inanimate objects may transmit infection as HBV can survive for 1 week or longer. Hepatitis B virus is not transmitted by the fecal-oral route.

A substantial proportion of persons with chronic HBV infection ultimately die of chronic liver disease (ie, chronic active hepatitis or cirrhosis) or primary hepatocellular carcinoma (PHC). Persons infected as infants or young children are at higher risk of death due to liver disease than are those infected as adults. The risk of chronic infection with HBV is related inversely to the age at the time infection occurs. Transmission from mother to infant during the perinatal period (ie, vertical transmission) occurs in infants born to HBsAg-positive mothers. Chronic infection develops in 70% to 90% of the infants of mothers who also are HBeAg-positive. If not infected during the perinatal period, infants of HBsAg-positive mothers remain at high risk of acquiring chronic HBV infection by person-to-person (ie, horizontal) transmission during the first 5 years of life. Horizontal transmission during early childhood, which occurs frequently in areas where the prevalence of HBV infection is high, has been documented among infants of Alaskan natives, Pacific Islanders, and first-generation immigrant mothers from geographic areas where HBV infection is highly endemic.

Other young children at risk for infection include (1) residents in institutions for the developmentally disabled, (2) patients with clotting disorders and others receiving blood products, (3) hemodialysis patients, and (4) household contacts of HBV carriers. In child care facilities in the United States, the risk of transmission appears to be small and should become negligible after implementation of universal infant vaccination. However, school contacts of deinstitutionalized, developmentally disabled HBV carriers may be at increased risk for infection.

Most infected persons in the United States acquire the infection as adolescents or adults. Groups at highest risk include users of injection drugs, persons with multiple heterosexual partners, and homosexually active males. Others at increased risk include those with occupational exposure to blood or body fluids, staff of institutions and nonresidential child care programs for the developmentally disabled, patients receiving hemodialysis, and sexual or household contacts of persons with an acute or chronic infection. However, more than one third of infected persons do not have a readily identifiable risk factor. The prevalence of infection among adolescents and adults in the general population is three to four times greater for blacks than for whites. Infection with HBV in adolescents and adults is associated with other sexually transmitted diseases, including syphilis.

The frequency of HBV infection and patterns of transmission vary markedly throughout the world. In most areas of the United States, Canada, Western Europe, Australia, and southern South America, the infection is of low endemicity and occurs primarily in adolescents and adults; 5% to 8% of the total population have been infected, and 0.2% to 0.9% have a chronic infection. Geographic regions of high endemicity, including Alaskan Native and inner city groups, exist within these countries. In contrast, HBV infection is highly endemic in China, Southeast Asia, eastern Europe, the Central Asian republics, most of the Middle East, Africa, the Amazon Basin, some Caribbean islands, and the Pacific Islands. In these areas, most infections occur in infants or children younger than 5 years, 70% to 90% of the adult population has been infected, and 8% to 15% have a chronic infection. In the rest of the world, HBV infection is of intermediate endemicity with chronic HBV carriage occurring in 2% to 7% of the population. Worldwide, HBV is a major cause of chronic liver disease and PHC.

The **incubation period** of acute infection is 45 to 160 days with an average of 120 days.

DIAGNOSTIC TESTS: Commercial serologic antigen tests are available to detect HBsAg and HBeAg. Assays are also available for the detection of antibody to HBsAg (anti-HBs), total antibody to hepatitis B core antigen (anti-HBc), IgM anti-HBc, and antibody to HBeAg (anti-HBe) (see Table 3.15, p 249). Hepatitis B surface antigen is detectable during acute infection. If the infection is self-limited, HBsAg disappears in most patients before serum anti-HBs can be detected (termed the "window phase" of infection). IgM anti-HBc is highly specific in establishing the diagnosis of acute infection as it is present early in the infection as well as during the window phase in older children and adults. However, IgM anti-HBc usually is not present in perinatal HBV infection. Persons with chronic HBV infection have circulating HBsAg and anti-HBc; on rare occasions, anti-HBsAg is present. Both anti-HBs and anti-HBc are detected in persons with resolved infection, whereas anti-HBs alone is

Table 3.15. **Diagnostic Tests for Hepatitis B Virus (HBV) Antigens and Antibodies**

Factor To Be Tested (Abbreviation)	Hepatitis B Virus or Antibody	Use
HBsAg	Surface antigen	Detection of acutely or chronically infected persons
Anti-HBs	Antibody to surface antigen (HBsAg)	Identification of persons who have had infections with HBV; determination of immunity after vaccination
HBeAg	e antigen	Identification of infected persons at increased risk for transmitting HBV
Anti-HBe	Antibody to HBe	Identification of HBsAg carriers with low risk for transmitting HBV
Anti-HBc	Antibody to core antigen (HBcAg)*	Identification of persons with acute or past HBV infection (not present after immunization)
IgM Anti-HBc	IgM antibody to core antigen	Identification of acute or recent HBV infections (including those in HBsAg-negative persons during the "window" phase of infection)

* No test is commercially available to measure core antigen (HbcAg).

present in persons immunized with hepatitis B vaccine. Tests to quantitate HBV-DNA in serum by polymerase chain reaction (PCR) or branched chain DNA methods are now available commercially. These tests have been useful in the selection of candidates to receive interferon therapy and to monitor the response to therapy.

TREATMENT: No specific therapy for acute HBV infection is available. In chronic liver disease in adults, α-interferon has been demonstrated to have approximately 40% efficacy in resolving the chronic infection, but the drug has been less effective for chronic infections acquired during early childhood.

Management of Chronic HBV Infection. Children and adolescents who have chronic HBV infection are at risk for development of serious liver disease, including PHC, with advancing age. While most cases of PHC, however, do not occur until adulthood, with a peak incidence in the fifth decade of life, PHC can occur in children with chronic hepatitis B infection. The primary risk factor for serious liver disease is the acquisition of chronic infection at birth or in early childhood. Children with chronic HBV infection should be screened periodically for hepatic complications. Screening tests such as serum liver function tests, α-fetoprotein concentration, and abdominal ultrasound should be considered, but definitive recommendations on the frequency and the indications for specific tests are precluded by lack of data in children and adults, including that on cost-effectiveness. Patients with persistently elevated serum transaminases concentrations (exceeding twice the upper limits of normal) as well as those with an elevated serum α-fetoprotein concentration or an abnormal abdominal ultrasound should be referred to a gastroenterologist for further management.

ISOLATION OF THE HOSPITALIZED PATIENT: Standard precautions are indicated for patients with acute or chronic HBV infection.

For infants born to HBsAg-positive mothers, no special care other than removal of maternal blood by a gloved attendant and standard precautions is necessary.

CONTROL MEASURES:

Hepatitis B Immunoprophylaxis. Pre-exposure immunization of susceptible persons with hepatitis B vaccine is the most effective means to prevent HBV transmission. To reduce and eventually eliminate transmission of HBV as soon as possible, universal immunization is necessary. Accordingly, hepatitis B vaccination is recommended for all infants as part of the routine childhood immunization schedule and all children who have not received the vaccine previously should be immunized by or before 11 to 12 years of age. Immunization at an earlier age than 11 years (for children not previously immunized) can be advantageous because of more likely compliance with routine medical visits to complete the 3-dose schedule.

Postexposure immunoprophylaxis with hepatitis B vaccine and Hepatitis B Immune Globulin (HBIG) can effectively prevent infection after exposure to HBV. Serologic testing of all pregnant women for HBsAg is essential for identifying infants who require postexposure immunoprophylaxis beginning at birth to prevent perinatal HBV infections (see Care of Exposed Persons, p 256).

Two types of products are available for immunoprophylaxis. Hepatitis B Immune Globulin (HBIG) provides temporary protection and is indicated only in specific postexposure circumstances (see Care of Exposed Persons, p 256). Hepatitis B vaccine is used for both pre-exposure and postexposure protection and provides long-term protection.

Hepatitis B Immune Globulin. * Hepatitis B immune globulin is prepared from hyperimmunized donors whose plasma is known to contain a high titer of anti-HBs and to be negative for antibodies to HIV and hepatitis C virus (HCV). The process used to prepare HBIG inactivates and/or eliminates HIV and HCV from the final product. The concentration of anti-HBs in immune globulin has declined as the result of current blood donor screening practices, and immune globulin is not effective for postexposure prophylaxis against hepatitis B virus infection.

Hepatitis B Vaccine. Two types of hepatitis B vaccine have been licensed in the United States. Both are highly effective and safe. The original vaccine prepared from the plasma of HBsAg carriers is no longer produced in the United States, but plasma-derived vaccines are widely used in other countries. The type of vaccine currently available in this country is produced by recombinant DNA technology, using common bakers' yeast that is genetically modified to synthesize HBsAg. Vaccines contain 2.5 to 40 µg HBsAg protein per milliliter adsorbed to aluminum hydroxide and thimerosal as a preservative. The concentration of HBsAg protein differs in the two recombinant vaccine products currently licensed in the United States. However, equal rates of seroconversion are achieved with both vaccines when given to healthy infants, children, adolescents, or young adults in the doses recommended according to the person's age and other host factors (see Table 3.16, p 252).

---

* Dosages recommended for postexposure prophylaxis are for products licensed in the United States. Because the concentration of anti-HBs in other products may vary, different dosages may be recommended in other countries.

Three doses, given in one of the recommended schedules, induces a protective antibody response (anti-HBs ≥10 mIU*/mL) in more than 90% of healthy adults and in more than 95% of infants, children, and adolescents.

Hepatitis B vaccine can be given concurrently with other vaccines (see Simultaneous Administration of Multiple Vaccines, p 21).

Vaccine Interchangeability. The immune response using one or two doses of a vaccine produced by one manufacturer, followed by one or more subsequent doses from a different manufacturer, has been demonstrated to be comparable to a full course of vaccination with a single product.

Routes of Administration. Vaccine is administered intramuscularly in the anterolateral thigh or deltoid area depending on the age of the recipient (see Vaccine Administration, p 8). Immunogenicity of hepatitis B vaccine in adults is diminished when given in the buttock. In patients with a bleeding diathesis, the risk of bleeding after intramuscular vaccine injection can be minimized by administration immediately after the patient receives replacement factor, use of a 23-gauge needle (or smaller), and application of direct pressure to the vaccination site for at least 2 minutes.

Since low doses of hepatitis B vaccine given by the intradermal route result in lower seroconversion rates and concentrations of anti-HBs, intradermal vaccination should not be used in infants or children and is not recommended for adults.

Efficacy and Duration of Protection. Hepatitis B vaccines licensed in the United States have a 90% to 95% efficacy in preventing HBV infection and clinical hepatitis B among susceptible children and adults. Among young adults, the incidence of loss of detectable serum antibody after 10 years of follow-up has ranged from 13% to 60%. Long-term studies of adults and children indicate that immune memory remains intact for 12 years or more and protects against chronic HBV infection, even though anti-HBs concentrations may become low or undetectable. Follow-up studies of children immunized at birth to prevent perinatal HBV infection have demonstrated continued efficacy for at least 8 years.

Booster Doses. For children and adults with normal immune status, routine booster doses of vaccine are not recommended currently, but their need will continue to be assessed as additional information becomes available. For hemodialysis patients, the need for booster doses should be assessed by annual anti-HBs testing. A booster dose should be given if the anti-HBs concentration is less than 10 mIU/mL.

Adverse Reactions. Pain at the injection site and a temperature greater than 37.7°C are the most frequently reported side effects in adults and children, occurring in 1% to 6% of recipients.

Allergic reactions after hepatitis B vaccination have been reported infrequently. Anaphylaxis appears to be uncommon, occurring in approximately 1 in 600 000 recipients according to passive reporting of vaccine adverse events, and has been rarely reported in children and adolescents.

Postvaccination surveillance for 3 years after licensure of the plasma-derived vaccine suggested an association in adults of borderline significance between Guillain-Barré syndrome and receipt of the first vaccine dose. No association has been demonstrated in postvaccination surveillance for the recombinant hepatitis B vaccines. The Vaccine Safety Committee of the Institute of Medicine in 1993 con-

---

* milli-International Units.

Table 3.16. Recommended Dosages of Hepatitis B Vaccines*

	Vaccine[†]			
	Recombivax HB[‡] Dose, µg (mL)		Engerix-B[§ǁ] Dose, µg (mL)	
Infants of HBsAg-negative mothers and children <11 y	2.5	(0.5)[¶]	10	(0.5)
Infants of HBsAg-positive mothers (HBIG [0.5 mL] also is recommended)	5	(1.0)[¶] (0.5)[#]	10	(0.5)
Children and adolescents 11–19 y	5	(0.5)[#]	10	(0.5)
Adults ≥20 y	10	(1.0)[#]	20	(1.0)
Patients undergoing dialysis and other immunosuppressed adults	40	(1.0)**	40	(2.0)[††]

* Heptavax B (available from Merck and Co), a plasma-derived vaccine, is also licensed but no longer produced in the United States. HBsAg indicates hepatitis B surface antigen; HBIG, hepatitis B immune globulin.
† Vaccines should be stored at 2°C to 8°C. Freezing destroys effectiveness. Both vaccines are administered in a three-dose schedule.
‡ Available from Merck and Co.
§ Available from SmithKline Beecham.
ǁ The Food and Drug Administration has approved this vaccine for use in an optional four-dose schedule at 0, 1, 2, and 12 months.
¶ Pediatric formulation.
# Adult formulation.
** Special formulation for dialysis patients.
†† Two 1.0-mL doses given in one site in a four-dose schedule at 0, 1, 2, and 6 to 12 months.

cluded that the evidence was inadequate to accept or reject a causal relationship between hepatitis B vaccine and Guillain-Barré syndrome.

Vaccination During Pregnancy and Lactation. No adverse effect on the developing fetus has been observed when pregnant women have been vaccinated. Because HBV infection may result in severe disease for the mother and chronic infection in the newborn, pregnancy should not be considered a contraindication to vaccination of women. Lactation also is not a contraindication.

Serologic Testing. Susceptibility testing before vaccination is not routinely indicated for children or adolescents. Because of the higher cost of vaccine, testing for previous infection should be considered for adults in risk groups with high rates of HBV infection, such as users of injection drugs, homosexually or bisexually active men, and household contacts of HBV carriers.

Routine postvaccination testing for anti-HBs is not necessary. However, testing is advised 1 to 2 months after the third vaccine dose for persons whose subsequent management is determined by their anti-HBs status. Such persons include the following: (1) hemodialysis patients, (2) persons with HIV infection, (3) those at occupational risk of exposure from sharp injuries, (4) immunocompromised patients at risk of exposure to HBV, (5) regular sexual contacts of HBV carriers, and (6) infants born to HBsAg-positive mothers. Testing for anti-HBs and HBsAg will identify those few infants who did not respond or who become chronically infected despite immunoprophylaxis, and will aid in their long-term medical management (see Management of Infants Born to HBsAg-Positive Women, p 256).

Management of Nonresponders. Vaccinees who do not develop a serum anti-HBs-antibody response ($\geq$10 mIU*/mL) after a primary vaccine series should be revaccinated (unless they are determined to be HBsAg-positive). Revaccination consists of one to three doses; those who remain anti-HBs-negative after a revaccination series of 3 doses are unlikely to respond to additional doses of vaccine.

Immunocompromised Patients. Larger vaccine doses and/or an increased number of doses may be required to induce protective anti-HBs concentrations in adult hemodialysis patients (Table 3.16). Additional or larger doses also may be necessary for immunocompromised persons, including HIV-seropositive individuals. However, few data in adults and none in children concerning the response to higher doses of vaccine in these patients exist. Specific recommendations, thus, cannot be made.

Pre-exposure Vaccination. Routine pre-exposure immunization is recommended for all infants at or soon after birth (0 to 2 months), for all children by 11 to 12 years of age, and older persons in certain high-risk groups (see Table 3.17, p 254).

High seroconversion rates and protective concentrations of anti-HBs ($\geq$10 mIU/mL) are achieved when hepatitis B vaccine is administered in any of the various three-dose schedules, including those begun soon after birth in term infants. Guidelines for scheduling vaccine doses are as follows: (1) the minimal interval between the first and second doses is 1 month; (2) for the second and third doses, the minimal interval is 2 months; (3) for infants in whom the vaccine series is initiated between birth and 2 months of age, the third vaccine dose should not be given before 6 months of age; and (4) for persons beginning immunization at 2 months and older, the minimal interval between the first and third doses is 4 months. The choice of schedule should be used to facilitate high rates of compliance with the three-dose primary vaccine series. The three-dose schedule for infants should be completed by 18 months of age. For vaccination of older children and adolescents, doses may be given in a schedule of 0, 1, and 6 months or of 0, 2, and 4 months.

The recommended schedule for routine hepatitis B immunization of infants born to HBsAg-negative mothers is given in Fig 1.1 (see p 18). Age-specific vaccine dosages are given in Table 3.16. Combination products containing hepatitis B vaccine may be given, provided they are approved by the Food and Drug Administration for the child's current age and administration of the other vaccine component(s) also is justified.

Lapsed Immunizations. For infants with lapsed immunization (ie, the interval between doses is longer than that in one of the recommended schedules), the three-dose series can be completed, regardless of the interval from the last dose of vaccine (see Lapsed Immunizations, p 22). High seroconversion rates have been demonstrated with intervals as long as 1 year between the second and third doses. Sufficient doses to complete the three-dose series should be administered at appropriate intervals. Routine serologic testing for anti-HBs is not indicated (unless the child's mother is HBsAg-positive).

---

* milli-International Units.

Table 3.17. Persons Who Should Receive Pre-exposure Hepatitis B Immunization*

All infants[†]:

Children at risk of acquisition of HBV by person-to-person (horizontal) transmission should be immunized.

Adolescents[‡]: HBV vaccination should be given by or before 11 to 12 years of age. Special efforts should be made to vaccinate **all** adolescents, not only those at high risk.

Users of intravenous drugs.

Sexually active heterosexual persons with more than one sex partner in the previous 6 months or who have a sexually transmitted disease.

Sexually active homosexual or bisexual males.

Health care workers and others at occupational risk of exposure to blood or blood-contaminated body fluid.

Residents and staff of institutions for developmentally disabled persons.

Staff of nonresidential child care and school programs for developmentally disabled persons if the program is attended by a known HBV carrier.

Patients undergoing hemodialysis.

Patients with bleeding disorders who receive clotting factor concentrates.

Household contacts and sexual partners of HBV carriers.

Members of households with adoptees who are HBsAg-positive.

International travelers to areas in which HBV infection is of high or intermediate endemicity.

Inmates of long-term correctional facilities.

---

* HBsAg indicates hepatitis B surface antigen; HBIG, hepatitis B immune globulin; HBV, hepatitis B virus.
† For those born to HBsAg-positive mothers, HBIG and vaccine is recommended for postexposure immunoprophylaxis (see text for specific recommendations).
‡ Implementation can be initiated before children reach adolescence.

SPECIAL CONSIDERATIONS:

Immunization Between Infancy and Adolescence. Many children and adolescents will remain at risk for HBV infection for several decades after the initiation of routine immunization of infants. For most children in the United States, the risk of HBV infection is low until adolescence and their immunization as, or before, they reach adolescence will provide protection from HBV infection. However, children of certain ethnic groups (eg, Alaskan Natives, Pacific Islanders, and children of immigrants and refugee families from countries with high rates of HBV infection) are at high risk for HBV infection resulting from person-to-person (horizontal) transmission during childhood and should be vaccinated early in childhood. Vaccination of children in these groups is a high priority.

Preterm Infants. The optimal time to initiate hepatitis B immunization in premature infants who weigh less than 2 kg at birth has not been determined. Seroconversion rates in very-low-birth-weight infants in whom vaccination was initiated shortly after birth have been reported in some studies to be lower than those in preterm infants vaccinated at an older age or in term infants vaccinated shortly after birth. Therefore, for preterm infants weighing less than 2 kg at birth and born to HBsAg-negative women, initiation of vaccination should be delayed until just before hospital discharge if the infant weighs 2 kg or more, or until approximately 2 months of age when other routine immunizations are given. These infants do not need to have serologic testing for anti-HBs performed routinely after the third dose if vaccinated according to this recommendation.

All preterm infants born to HBsAg-positive mothers, however, should receive immunoprophylaxis (HBIG and vaccine) beginning as soon as possible after birth, followed by appropriate postvaccination testing (see Prevention of Perinatal HBV Infection, p 256). Preterm infants born to mothers whose HBsAg status is unknown also should receive the first dose of vaccine shortly after birth and HBIG if the maternal HBsAG status cannot be determined within 12 hours of birth (see Prevention of Perinatal HBV Infection).

Immunization of High-Risk Groups (see Table 3.17 for complete listing).
Sexually Active Heterosexual Adolescents and Adults. Those who are diagnosed with a sexually transmitted disease or have had more than one sex partner in the previous 6 months should be vaccinated.

Health Care Workers and Others With Occupational Exposure to Blood. The risk to a health care worker for HBV exposure depends on the tasks the worker performs. Those with contact with blood or blood-contaminated body fluids should be vaccinated. Because the risks for occupational HBV infection are often highest during the training of health care professionals, vaccination should be completed during training and before contact with blood.

Residents and Staff of Institutions for the Developmentally Disabled. Susceptible children in institutions for the developmentally disabled and the staff who work closely with the children should be vaccinated. Susceptible children and staff who live or work in smaller (group) residential settings where other staff members or residents are known to be HBV carriers also should be vaccinated. Children discharged from residential institutions into community programs should be screened for HBsAg to allow appropriate preventive measures for HBV transmission.

Staff of nonresidential child care programs (eg, schools and other group settings) attended by known HBV carriers have a risk of infection comparable to that of health care workers and should be vaccinated. Vaccination of attendees in these programs should be considered, and is strongly encouraged if an attendee who is an HBV carrier behaves aggressively or has special medical problems (eg, exudative dermatitis or open skin lesions) that increase the risk of exposure to that attendee's blood or secretions.

Hemodialysis Patients. Vaccination is recommended for susceptible hemodialysis patients. Identification of patients with renal disease for vaccination early in the course of their disease is encouraged because the immunologic response in patients with uremia who are vaccinated before they require dialysis is better than after dialysis is required.

Patients With Bleeding Disorders Who Receive Clotting Factor Concentrates. Vaccination is recommended as soon as the specific clotting disorder is diagnosed. Prevaccination testing for HBsAg and anti-HBc is recommended for patients who already have received multiple infusions of these products.

Household Contacts and Sexual Partners of HBV Carriers. Household and sexual contacts of HBV carriers identified through prenatal screening, donor screening, or diagnostic or other serologic testing should be vaccinated.

Adoptees, and Their Household Contacts, From Countries Where HBV Infection Is Endemic. Adoptees from countries where HBV infection is endemic should be screened for HBsAg. If the adoptee is HBsAg-positive, previously unimmunized family members and other household contacts should be vaccinated, preferably before the adoption.

International Travelers. Those traveling to areas in which HBV infection is of high or intermediate endemicity (see Epidemiology, p 247) who will have close contact with the local population, or who likely will have contact with blood (eg, in a medical setting) or sexual contact with residents should be vaccinated. Vaccination should begin at least 4 to 6 months before travel, in order that a three-dose regimen can be completed (see Pre-exposure Vaccination, p 253). For those in whom vaccination is initiated at less than 4 months before departure, the alternative four-dose schedule of 0, 1, 2, and 12 months (see Table 3.16) should provide protection if the first three doses can be delivered before travel. If departure is within less than 2 months, an incomplete regimen, nevertheless, will provide partial protection; additional dose(s) to complete the three-dose regimen should be given subsequently (see Lapsed Immunizations, p 22).

These and additional indications for immunization of high-risk persons are given in Table 3.17, p 254.

Care of Exposed Persons (Postexposure Immunoprophylaxis) (see also Table 3.18, p 257).

Prevention of Perinatal HBV Infection. Transmission of perinatal HBV infection can be prevented in approximately 95% of infants born to HBsAg-positive mothers by early active and passive immunoprophylaxis of the infants, ie, vaccination and HBIG administration. Vaccination subsequently should be completed in the first 6 months of life. Hepatitis B vaccination only, initiated at or shortly after birth, also is highly effective in preventing perinatal HBV infections (and may be as effective as vaccine in combination with HBIG).

Serologic Screening of Pregnant Women. Prenatal HBsAg testing of all pregnant women is recommended to identify newborns who require immediate postexposure prophylaxis and because selective testing fails to detect more than 50% of women who are HBsAg-positive. Testing should be accomplished during an early prenatal visit in each pregnancy and should be repeated late in pregnancy for HBsAg-negative women who are at high risk for HBV infection (eg, intravenous drug users and those with intercurrent sexually transmitted diseases) or who have had clinical hepatitis. Household contacts and sexual partners of HBsAg-positive women identified through prenatal screening should be vaccinated if susceptible or judged likely to be susceptible to infection.

Management of Infants Born to HBsAg-Positive Women. Infants born to HBsAg-positive mothers, including preterm infants, should receive the initial dose of hepatitis B vaccine within 12 hours of birth (see Table 3.16 for appropriate dosages) and HBIG (0.5 mL) should be given concurrently at a different site. Subsequent doses of vaccine should be given as recommended in Table 3.19 (p 258). For preterm infants who weigh less than 2 kg at birth, the initial vaccine dose should not be

Table 3.18. Guide to Postexposure Immunoprophylaxis for Hepatitis B Infection*

Type of Exposure	Immunoprophylaxis†	Refer to:
Accidental percutaneous or permucosal	Vaccination + HBIG	p 259 (see Table 3.20)
Household contact chronic carrier	Vaccination	p 256
Household contact acute case with identifiable blood exposure	Vaccination + HBIG	p 258
Perinatal	Vaccination + HBIG	p 256
Sexual, acute infection	Vaccination + HBIG	p 259
Sexual, chronic carrier	Vaccination	p 256

* HBIG indicates hepatitis B immune globulin.
† For susceptible patients (eg, previously unvaccinated).

counted in the required three-dose schedule and the subsequent three doses should be given in accordance with schedule for immunization of preterm infants (see Preterm Infants, p 254). Thus, a total of four doses are recommended in this circumstance.

These infants should be serologically tested for anti-HBs and HBsAg 1 to 3 months after completion of the vaccination series. Testing for HBsAg will identify those infants who become chronically infected and will aid in their long-term medical management. Infants with anti-HBs concentrations of less than 10 mIU/mL and who are HBsAg-negative should receive three additional doses of vaccine in a 0-, 1-, and 6-month schedule followed by testing for anti-HBs 1 month after the third dose. Alternatively, additional doses (one to three) of vaccine can be administered, followed by testing for anti-HBs 1 month after each dose to determine if subsequent doses are needed.

Infants Born to Mothers Not Tested During Pregnancy for HBsAg. Pregnant women whose HBsAg status is unknown at delivery should have their blood drawn for testing as soon as possible. While awaiting results, the infant should receive hepatitis B vaccine within 12 hours of birth in the dose recommended for infants born to HBsAg-positive mothers (see Table 3.16). Because HBV vaccine when given at birth is highly effective in preventing perinatal infection in term infants, the possible added value and the cost of HBIG do not warrant its use when the mother's HBsAg status is not known. If the woman is determined to be HBsAg-positive, the infant should receive HBIG (0.5 mL) as soon as possible, but within 7 days of birth; and subsequently vaccinated as recommended for infants of HBsAg-positive mothers (see Table 3.16). If HBIG is unavailable, the infant should still receive the two subsequent doses of hepatitis B vaccine at 1 to 2 and 6 months of age (see Table 3.19, p 258). If the mother is HBsAg-negative, hepatitis B vaccination in the dose and schedule recommended for infants born to HBsAg-negative women should be completed (see Table 3.16).

Preterm Infants Born to Mothers Not Tested During Pregnancy for HBsAg. For preterm infants who weigh less than 2 kg at birth, the maternal HBsAg status should be determined as soon as possible and the infant should receive hepatitis B vaccine, as recommended for term infants in this category. If the mother's HBsAg

Table 3.19. Recommended Schedule of Hepatitis B Immunoprophylaxis to Prevent Perinatal Transmission*

Infant Born to Mother Known To Be HBsAg Positive[†]

Vaccine Dose[‡] and HBIG	Age
First	Birth (within 12 h)
HBIG[§]	Birth (within 12 h)
Second	1–2 mo
Third	6 mo

Infant Born to Mother Not Screened for HBsAg[||]

Vaccine Dose and HBIG	Age
First[¶]	Birth (within 12 h)
HBIG[§]	If mother is HBsAg-positive, give 0.5 mL as soon as possible, not later than 1 wk after birth[||]
Second	1–2 mo
Third	6–18 mo**

* HBsAg indicates hepatitis B surface antigen; HBIG, hepatitis B immune globulin.
[†] See text (p 256) for recommendations for subsequent serological testing.
[‡] See Table 3.16 for appropriate vaccine dose.
[§] HBIG (0.5 mL) given intramuscularly at a site different from that used for vaccine.
[||] See text (p 257) for vaccination recommendations for preterm infants.
[¶] First dose is same as that for infant of HBsAg-positive mother (see Table 3.16). Subsequent doses and schedules are determined by maternal HBsAg status (see p 256 and Table 3.16).
** Infants of HBsAg-positive mothers should be vaccinated at 6 months of age.

status cannot be determined within the initial 12 hours of birth, HBIG (0.5 mL) should be given. As recommended for term infants, the maternal HBsAg status will determine the subsequent dosages and schedule for completion of hepatitis B vaccination. However, if the mother is found to be HBsAg-positive, the initial vaccine dose should not be counted in the required three doses to complete the immunization series. The subsequent three doses (for a total of four doses) are given in accordance with the recommendations for the immunization of preterm infants of birth weights less than 2 kg born to HBsAg-negative women (see Preterm Infants, p 254).

Breastfeeding. Breastfeeding of the infant by a HBsAg-positive mother poses no additional risk for acquisition of HBV infection by the infant (see Human Milk, p 73).

Household Contacts of Persons With Acute HBV Infection. Infants (ie, less than 12 months of age) who have close contact with primary caregivers with acute infection and who have not been vaccinated against hepatitis B, ie, not completed the 3-dose series, should receive HBIG and hepatitis vaccine should be given in accordance with the routinely recommended 3-dose schedule (see Pre-exposure Vaccination, p 253).

Prophylaxis with HBIG for other unimmunized household contacts of persons with acute HBV infection is not indicated unless they have identifiable blood exposure to the index patient, such as by sharing of toothbrushes or razors. Such exposures should be treated as in sexual exposures. All such persons, however, should be immunized as soon as possible against hepatitis B because of the possibility of future household exposures and in accordance with the national goal of universal immunization.

Sexual Partners of Persons With Acute HBV Infection. Susceptible sex partners should receive a single dose of HBIG (0.06 mL/kg) and should begin the hepatitis B vaccine series. Sexual partners of persons with acute HBV infection are at increased risk for infection, and HBIG is 75% effective in preventing these infections. The period after sexual exposure during which HBIG is effective is unknown, but is unlikely to exceed 14 days.

Acute Exposure to Blood That Contains (or Might Contain) HBsAg. For inadvertent percutaneous (eg, needle stick, laceration, or bite) or permucosal (eg, ocular or mucous membrane) exposure to blood, the decision to give HBIG prophylaxis and to vaccinate the patient includes consideration of whether the HBsAg status of the person who was the source of the exposure is available and the hepatitis B vaccination and response status of the exposed person. Vaccination is recommended for any exposure of a person not previously vaccinated. If possible, a blood sample from the person who was the source of the exposure should be tested for HBsAg and appropriate prophylaxis administered according to the hepatitis B vaccination status and anti-HBs response status (if known) of the exposed person (see Table 3.20, p 260, and Injuries From Discarded Needles in the Community, p 120).

Detailed guidelines on the management of health care workers and other persons exposed to blood that is or might be HBsAg-positive is provided in the recommendations of the Advisory Committee of the Immunization Practices (ACIP) of the Centers for Disease Control and Prevention (see also Table 3.20).*

Child Care. All children, including those in child care, should receive hepatitis B vaccine as part of their routine immunization schedule. Immunization not only will reduce the potential for transmission after bites but also will allay anxiety about transmission from attendees who may be HBV carriers.

Children who are HBV carriers and who have no behavioral or medical risk factors, such as unusually aggressive behavior (eg, biting), generalized dermatitis, or a bleeding problem, should be admitted to child care without restrictions. The risk of HBV transmission in child care appears to be negligible. Routine screening for HBsAg is not warranted. Admission of HBV carrier children with behavioral or medical risk factors should be assessed on an individual basis by the child's physician, the program director, and the responsible public health authorities (for further discussion, see Children in Out-of-Home Child Care, p 80).

---

* Centers for Disease Control and Prevention. Hepatitis B virus infection: a comprehensive immunization strategy to eliminate transmission in the United States — 1997 Update: recommendations of the Advisory Committee on Immunization Practices (ACIP). *MMWR.* In press.

Table 3.20. **Recommendations for Hepatitis B Prophylaxis After Percutaneous Exposure to Blood That Contains (or Might Contain) HBsAg***

Exposed Person	Treatment When Source Is		
	HBsAg-Positive	HBsAg-Negative	Unknown or Not Tested
Unvaccinated	Administer HBIG,[†] 1 dose and initiate hepatitis B vaccine	Initiate hepatitis B vaccine	Initiate hepatitis B vaccine
Previously vaccinated			
Known responder	No treatment	No treatment	No treatment
Known nonresponder	HBIG, 2 doses or HBIG, 1 dose **and** initiate revaccination	No treatment	If known high-risk source, treat as if source were HBsAg positive
Response unknown	Test exposed person for anti-HBs[‡] • If inadequate HBIG,[†] 1 dose **and** initiate revaccination • If adequate, no treatment	No treatment	Test exposed person for anti-HBs[‡] • If inadequate, initiate revaccination • If adequate, no treatment

* Modified from the Centers for Disease Control and Prevention. Hepatitis B virus infection: a comprehensive immunization strategy to eliminate transmission in the United States — 1997 Update: recommendations of the Advisory Committee on Immunization Practices (ACIP). *MMWR*. In press. HBsAg indicates hepatitis B surface antigen; HBIG, hepatitis B immune globulin; anti-HBs, antibody to HBsAg.
† Dose of HBIG, 0.06 mL/kg, intramuscularly.
‡ Adequate anti-HBs is ≥10 mIU/mL.

Hepatitis C

CLINICAL MANIFESTATIONS: The signs and symptoms of hepatitis C infection are often indistinguishable from those of hepatitis A or B infection. Acute disease tends to be mild and insidious in onset and in children most infections are asymptomatic. Jaundice occurs in only 25% of patients, and abnormalities in liver function tests generally are less than those in patients with hepatitis B infection. Persistent infection occurs in at least 85%, even in the absence of biochemical evidence of liver disease. Most children with chronic infection are asymptomatic. Approximately 65% to 70% of patients develop chronic hepatitis and 20% develop cirrhosis; primary hepatocellular carcinoma can occur in these patients.

ETIOLOGY: Hepatitis C virus (HCV) is a small, single stranded RNA virus with a lipid envelope and is a member of the Flavivirus family. Multiple HCV genotypes exist which fail to elicit cross-neutralizing antibodies in animal models.

EPIDEMIOLOGY: The prevalence of HCV infection in the general population of the United States is estimated at 1.8%, and based on limited testing, an average of 150 000 infections occur each year. In children the seroprevalence rate in those without known risk factors is 0.2% for those less than 12 years old and 0.4% for those 12 to 19 years old. Seroprevalence rates among individuals vary according to their associated risk factors.

Infection is spread primarily by parenteral exposure to blood and blood products from HCV-infected persons. The current risk of HCV infection following blood transfusion is estimated at 0.1% or less per recipient in the United States because of the exclusion of high-risk individuals from the pool of blood donors and by the screening of donors with first- and second-generation assays for HCV antibody. Some transfusion-associated HCV infections continue to occur because currently available serological assays do not detect anti-HCV antibody in approximately 5% of infected persons and rare donations of blood are made by persons in the period of infectivity before anti-HCV antibody is detectable. Outbreaks of HCV associated with contaminated intravenous immunoglobulin products have occurred in Sweden and in 1994 in the United States. The latter was associated with a specific product, administered between April 1, 1993, and February 23, 1994, when the contaminated lots were withdrawn. Currently all intravenous and intramuscular immunoglobulin products available commercially in the United States undergo an inactivation procedure for HCV and are documented to be HCV RNA-negative before release.

The highest seroprevalence rates of infection (60% to 90%) occur in persons with large or repeated direct percutaneous exposure to blood or blood products, such as injection drug users and patients with hemophilia who have received multiple blood transfusions. Rates are moderately high among those with smaller but repeated direct or inapparent percutaneous exposures, such as hemodialysis patients (20%); and lower rates are found among those with inapparent parenteral or mucosal exposures, such as persons with high-risk sexual behaviors and sexual and household contacts of infected persons (1% to 10%), as well as among those with sporadic percutaneous exposures, such as health care workers (1%).

Other body fluids contaminated with infected blood also can be sources of infection. Intranasal cocaine users have a high rate of infection, presumably resulting from epistaxis and shared equipment. Sexual transmission is uncommon except in circumstances of promiscuity. Transmission among family contacts without other risk factors is also low, averaging 4%, and in some studies no intrafamilial transmission has been documented in the absence of other risk factors. In persons with no risk factors, seroprevalence rates are less than 0.5%. For most infected children and adolescents, no specific source of infection can be identified.

Seroprevalence among pregnant women in the United States has been estimated at 1% to 2%, but maternal-fetal (vertical) transmission is only 5% (range 0% to 25%). Maternal coinfection with HIV has been associated with increased risk of perinatal transmission of HCV and may depend in part on the HCV genotype and the serum titer of maternal HCV RNA. Serum anti-HCV antibody and HCV RNA have been detected in colostrum, but HCV transmission by breastfeeding to infants in the limited number of patients studied has not been demonstrated. The rate of transmission among breastfed infants has been the same as that among bottle-fed infants.

All individuals with HCV antibody and/or HCV-RNA in their blood are considered to be infectious.

The **incubation period** for HCV infection averages 6 to 7 weeks with a range of 2 weeks to 6 months.

DIAGNOSTIC TESTS: The two major types of tests currently available for the laboratory diagnosis of HCV infections are (1) antibody assays for anti-HCV and (2) those for detecting and quantitating HCV nucleic acid (RNA). No antigen detection tests are available yet. Diagnosis by antibody assays involves an initial screening enzyme immunoassay (EIA); repeated positive results are confirmed by a recombinant immunoblot assay (RIBA), analogous to testing for HIV infection. Both assays detect IgG antibody; no IgM assays are available currently. The current EIA and RIBA assays (which are second-generation tests) are 95% sensitive and 95% specific. False-negative results early in the course of acute infection result from the prolonged interval between onset of illness and seroconversion that may occur. Within 5 to 6 weeks after the onset of hepatitis, however, 80% of patients will be positive for serum anti-HCV antibody.

Highly sensitive polymerase chain reaction (PCR) assays for detection and quantitation of HCV RNA and other nucleic acid-based amplification tests are available from several commercial laboratories for investigational testing but are costly, not standardized and, thus, limited in use. False-positive and false-negative results can occur from improper handling, storage, and contamination of the test samples. Viral RNA may be detected intermittently and, thus, a single negative PCR assay result is not conclusive. The clinical value of these assays is not yet established, but they have been used in the early diagnosis of infection, monitoring patients receiving antiviral therapy, and identifying infection in infants early in life (ie, maternal-fetal transmission) when maternal serum antibody interferes with the ability to detect antibody produced by the infant.

TREATMENT: Interferon-α is the only treatment currently available for chronic HCV infection in adults, but 20% or less of patients have had a sustained response. Interferon therapy is not approved by the Food and Drug Administration for those less than 18 years of age. Limited experience in children with interferon-α therapy suggests efficacy similar to that observed in adults. Children with severe disease or histologically advanced pathology (bridging necrosis or active cirrhosis) should be referred to a specialist in the management of chronic HCV infection.

Persons with chronic HCV infection should be vaccinated against hepatitis A and B infections (unless they have previously been demonstrated to be nonsusceptible).

Management of Chronic HCV Infection. Persons who have chronic HCV infection are at risk for development of serious liver disease, including primary hepatocellular carcinoma (PHC) with advancing age. However, PHC from chronic HCV infection has been only reported, to date, in adults. Children with chronic infection should be screened periodically for chronic hepatitis with serum liver function tests because of their potential long-term risk for chronic liver disease. Definitive recommendations on frequency have not been established. Children with persistently elevated serum transaminases concentrations (exceeding twice the upper limits of normal) should be referred to a gastroenterology specialist for further management.

The need for testing for α–fetoprotein concentration and of abdominal ultrasonography in children has not been determined.

ISOLATION OF THE HOSPITALIZED PATIENT: Standard precautions are recommended.

CONTROL MEASURES:

Care of Exposed Persons.

Immunoprophylaxis. Based on the lack of clinical efficacy in humans and on data from studies using animals, the use of immune globulin for postexposure prophylaxis against hepatitis C infection is not recommended by the Centers for Disease Control and Prevention. Furthermore, immune globulin is manufactured currently from plasma documented to be negative for anti-HCV antibodies.

Breastfeeding. Mothers infected with HCV should be advised that transmission of HCV by breastfeeding is possible but has not been documented. According to current guidelines of the US Public Health Service, maternal HCV infection is not a contraindication to breastfeeding. The decision to do so should be based on an informed discussion between the mother and the health care provider.

Child Care. Exclusion of children with HCV infection from out-of-home child care is not indicated.

Serologic Testing for HCV Infection.

Persons Who Have Risk Factor(s) for HCV Infection. These persons, such as injection drug users, recipients of 1 or more units of blood or blood products prior to 1990, or those receiving hemodialysis, should be tested.

Screening of Pregnant Women. Routine serologic testing of pregnant women for HCV infection is not recommended. Testing should be reserved for those whose history suggests an increased risk for HCV infection.

Infants Born to Women With HCV Infection. Serologic testing for anti-HCV of children born to women previously identified to be HCV-infected is recommended because approximately 5% will acquire the infection. The duration of passive maternal antibody in infants is unknown, but is unlikely to be more than 12 months in most cases. Therefore, testing for anti-HCV should not be performed until after 12 months of age. Testing by PCR generally is not available and is not recommended for routine use in these children.

Adoptees. Routine serologic testing of adoptees, either domestic or international, is not recommended. Testing is indicated, however, if the biological mother has an increased risk of HCV infection.

Recipients of Immune Globulin Intravenous (IGIV). The US Public Health Service recommends that persons who received Gammagard (produced by Baxter Healthcare Corporation) between April 1, 1993, and February 23, 1994, should be offered serologic testing for aminotransferase (ALT) concentrations and for anti-HCV. Because of concerns that anti-HCV may not be detectable in persons who are immunocompromised, PCR testing for HCV RNA is recommended for persons with elevated ALT concentrations who are negative for anti-HCV on repeated testing. Screening of children who have received other IGIV products is not indicated.

Counseling of Patients With HCV Infection. All persons with HCV infection should be considered infectious, informed of the possibility of transmission to others, and should refrain from donating blood, organs, tissues, or semen, or sharing toothbrushes and razors.

Infected persons should be counseled to avoid hepatotoxic medications, particularly if to be given for prolonged periods and whenever feasible, and of the risks of alcohol use. Patients with chronic liver disease, if susceptible, should be vaccinated against hepatitis A and B.

Changes in sexual practices of infected persons with a steady partner are not currently recommended. They, however, should be informed of the possible risks and use of precautions to prevent transmission. Persons with multiple partners should be advised to reduce the number of partners and to use condoms to prevent transmission. No data currently exist to support counseling a woman against pregnancy.

Hepatitis D

CLINICAL MANIFESTATIONS: Hepatitis D virus infection causes hepatitis, but only in individuals with acute or chronic hepatitis B virus infection. Infection in a person with chronic hepatitis B infection results in higher rates of acute fulminant hepatitis and chronic hepatitis that may progress to cirrhosis than those with acute hepatitis B infection.

ETIOLOGY: Hepatitis D virus (HDV) is a 35- to 37-nm particle consisting of an RNA genome and a delta protein antigen (HDAg), both of which are coated with hepatitis B surface antigen (HBsAg). Hepatitis D virus requires HBV as a helper virus and cannot produce infection in the absence of HBV.

EPIDEMIOLOGY: Hepatitis D virus can cause an infection at the same time as the initial hepatitis B infection (coinfection), or it can infect an individual already chronically infected (superinfection). Acquisition of HDV is similar to that of hepatitis B virus (HBV), ie, by parenteral, percutaneous, or mucous membrane inoculation. Hepatitis D virus can be transmitted by blood or blood products, injection drug use, or sexual contact as long as HBV also is present in the patient. Transmission from mother to newborn infant is uncommon. Intrafamilial spread can occur among HBsAg carriers. High-prevalence areas include southern Italy and parts of Eastern Europe, South America, Africa, and the Middle East. In contrast to HBV, HDV infection is uncommon in the Far East. In the United States, HDV infection is found most frequently in parenteral drug abusers, hemophiliacs, and persons immigrating from endemic areas.

The **incubation period** for HDV superinfection, estimated from inoculation of animals, is approximately 2 to 8 weeks. When hepatitis B and D viruses infect simultaneously, the incubation period is similar to that of hepatitis B (45 to 160 days; average 120 days).

DIAGNOSTIC TESTS: A test for anti-HDV antibody is commercially available, usually at referral laboratories. Tests for IgM-specific anti-HDV antibody and HDAg are research procedures at present. If markers for HDV infection exist, coinfection with hepatitis B virus can usually be differentiated from superinfection of an established HBsAg carrier by testing for IgM hepatitis B core antibody; absence of this core antibody suggests that the person is an HBsAg carrier.

TREATMENT: Supportive.

ISOLATION OF THE HOSPITALIZED PATIENT: Standard precautions are recommended.

CONTROL MEASURES: The same control and preventive measures as for HBV infection are indicated. Because HDV cannot be transmitted in the absence of HBV infection, hepatitis B immunization protects against HDV infection. Carriers of HBsAg should take extreme care to avoid exposure to HDV because no currently available immunobiological exists for prevention of HDV superinfection.

Hepatitis E
(Enterically Transmitted Non-A, Non-B Hepatitis)

CLINICAL MANIFESTATIONS: Hepatitis E is an acute illness with jaundice, malaise, anorexia, fever, abdominal pain, and arthralgia.

ETIOLOGY: The hepatitis E virus (HEV) is a single-stranded RNA virus that is structurally similar to a calicivirus.

EPIDEMIOLOGY: Transmission of HEV is by the fecal-oral route. Disease is more common in adults than in children, and it has an unusually high case-fatality rate in pregnant women. Cases have been reported in epidemics or sporadically in parts of Asia, Africa, and Mexico and have usually been related to contaminated water. Endemic HEV transmission has not been recognized in Western Europe or the United States, but cases have occurred in travelers to endemic areas. The period of communicability after acute infection is unknown, but fecal shedding of the virus and viremia occur commonly for at least 2 weeks. Chronic infection does not appear to occur.

The mean **incubation period** is approximately 40 days, with a range of 15 to 60 days.

DIAGNOSTIC TESTS: No serologic test is commercially available. The diagnosis is established usually by exclusion of acute hepatitis A, B, C, D, and other viral causes of acute hepatitis. Serologic assays (eg, enzyme immunoassay, Western blot, and fluorescent antibody blocking assay) that detect antibody to HEV have been developed in research laboratories; viral RNA can be identified in stool and serum by the polymerase chain reaction (PCR). Health care professionals who require information about serologic and PCR testing of persons with evidence of non-A, non-B, non-C hepatitis should contact the Centers for Disease Control and Prevention

(CDC).* IgG antibody test for anti-HEV is available as an investigational test at the Center for Blood Research at the Sacramento Medical Foundation in California.

TREATMENT: Supportive.

ISOLATION OF THE HOSPITALIZED PATIENT†: Contact precautions are recommended.

CONTROL MEASURES: Good sanitation and not ingesting potentially contaminated food and water are the most effective measures. Passive immunoprophylaxis against hepatitis E with immune globulin prepared in the United States has not been proved effective.

Herpes Simplex

CLINICAL MANIFESTATIONS:

Neonatal. In newborn infants, herpes simplex virus (HSV) infection can manifest as (1) generalized, systemic infection involving the liver and other organs, including the central nervous system (CNS), encephalitis; (2) localized CNS disease; or (3) disease localized to the skin, eyes, and mouth (SEM). Ocular manifestations include conjunctivitis, keratitis, and chorioretinitis. Typical vesicular skin lesions are helpful diagnostically, if present. In approximately one third of the patients, SEM involvement is the first indication of the infection. In another one third of the patients, other evidence of systemic or CNS disease can occur before the appearance of SEM lesions. Central nervous system disease also occurs frequently in the absence of SEM manifestations. Another one third of the infants with systemic or localized encephalitis will not have SEM involvement. In the absence of the more characteristic SEM lesions (such as vesicles or keratitis), the differential diagnosis in infants with respiratory distress, sepsis, and convulsions in newborn infants must include HSV infection. Although asymptomatic HSV infection is common in older children, in neonates it probably occurs rarely, if at all.

Neonatal herpetic infections are frequently severe, with a high mortality rate and substantial neurologic and/or ocular impairment in survivors, particularly in the absence of antiviral therapy. Recurrent skin lesions are frequent in surviving infants and are associated with sequelae if they occur more than three times in the first 6 months of life.

Initial symptoms of HSV infection can occur at birth or as late as 4 to 6 weeks after birth. Disseminated disease usually occurs during the first 2 weeks of life; disease localized to the CNS or to the SEM more often occurs during the second or third week.

Children and Infants Beyond the Neonatal Period. Gingivostomatitis is the most commonly recognized manifestation of primary HSV infection. Gingivostomatitis is characterized by fever, irritability, and an ulcerative enanthem involving the gingiva

---

* Hepatitis Branch, National Center for Infectious Diseases, CDC, Atlanta, Ga (see Directory of Telephone Numbers, p 667).
† In addition to standard precautions.

and the mucous membranes of the mouth. Most HSV infections, however, at this age are asymptomatic.

Genital herpes, which is the most common manifestation of HSV infection in adolescents and adults, is characterized by vesicular or ulcerative lesions of the male or female genital organs and/or perineum.

Eczema herpeticum with vesicular lesions concentrated in the areas of eczematous involvement can develop in patients who are infected with HSV.

In immunocompromised patients, severe local lesions and, less commonly, disseminated HSV infection with generalized vesicular skin lesions and visceral involvement can occur.

Herpes simplex virus persists in a latent form after primary infection. Reactivation of latent virus most often is manifested by cold sores (herpes labialis), which appear as single or grouped vesicles in the perioral region, usually on the vermilion border of the lips. Reactivation of genital HSV infection on the penis, scrotum, vulva, cervix, buttocks, and perianal areas, or on the thighs or back can also occur.

Eye infections can be a primary manifestation of HSV infection or a recurrence. They vary in severity from a superficial conjunctivitis to involvement of the deeper layers of the cornea. Herpetic whitlow consists of single or multiple vesicular lesions on the distal parts of fingers. Herpes simplex virus infection has been implicated as a precipitating factor in erythema multiforme.

Herpes simplex virus encephalitis can result from primary or recurrent infection and is associated with fever, alterations in the state of consciousness, personality changes, convulsions, and usually focal neurologic findings. Encephalitis frequently has an acute onset with a fulminant course, leading to coma and death in untreated patients. Cerebrospinal fluid (CSF) pleocytosis with both lymphocytes and erythrocytes is usual. Herpes simplex virus infection can also cause meningitis with nonspecific clinical manifestations that are usually mild and self-limited. Meningitis usually is associated with primary HSV-2 genital infection.

ETIOLOGY: Herpes simplex viruses are large, enveloped DNA viruses. The two types have major genomic and antigenic differences. Type 1 (HSV-1) usually involves the face and skin above the waist; however, an increasing number of genital herpes cases are attributable to HSV-1. Type 2 (HSV-2) usually involves the genitalia and skin below the waist in sexually active adolescents and adults and is the most common cause of disease in neonates. Either type of virus, however, can be found in either site, depending on the source of the infection.

EPIDEMIOLOGY:

Neonatal. The incidence of neonatal HSV infection is low, with estimates ranging from 1 per 3000 to 1 per 20 000 live births. Infants in whom HSV infection develops are significantly more likely to be born prematurely. Herpes simplex virus is transmitted most frequently to an infant during birth through an infected maternal genital tract or by an ascending infection, sometimes through apparently intact membranes. Most neonatal infections, thus, are caused by HSV-2, but 15% to 20% are HSV-1 infections. Late intrauterine infections that manifest soon after birth are not infrequent. Intrauterine infections causing congenital malformations have been implicated in rare cases. Other less common sources of neonatal infection include postnatal transmission (1) from the mother or father, most often from a nongenital infection (eg, mouth, hands, or around the nipples); or (2) in the nursery from another infected infant, probably via the hands of personnel attending the infants. Postnatal transmission from nursery personnel with fever blisters to neonates has been extremely rare.

The risk of HSV infection in an infant born vaginally to a mother with a first episode, or primary genital infection is high and has been estimated to be at least 33% to 50%. The risk to an infant born to a mother with recurrent HSV infection at delivery is much lower, at most 3% to 5%. Distinguishing between primary and recurrent HSV infections in women by history or physical examination may not be possible. Surveys suggest that 0.01% to 0.39% of American women shed HSV at delivery. Either primary or recurrent infection can be present without signs or symptoms or with nonspecific findings (eg, vaginal discharge, genital pain, or shallow ulcers). Most infants in whom HSV infection develops have been born to women without a history or clinical findings suggestive of active infection during pregnancy.

Children and Infants Beyond the Neonatal Period. Herpes simplex virus infections are ubiquitous and are transmitted from persons who are symptomatic or asymptomatic with primary or recurrent infections. Infection with HSV-1 results primarily from direct contact with infected oral secretions or lesions. Infection with HSV-2 usually results from direct contact with infected genital secretions or lesions through sexual activity. Type 1 strains can be recovered from the genital tract; type 2 strains probably can be recovered from the pharynx as a result of oral-genital sexual activity. Type 1 HSV genital infections in children also can result from autoinoculation of virus from the mouth. Sexual abuse nevertheless must always be considered in prepubertal children with genital herpes.

Type 1 HSV usually is contracted during the first few years of life in infected individuals in lower socioeconomic groups. In higher socioeconomic groups, more than half of infected individuals do not contract HSV-1 until after they reach adulthood. Children in child care centers may have high rates of HSV-1 acquisition. The frequency of HSV-2 infection correlates with sexual activity and in association with other sexually transmitted diseases.

Direct inoculation of skin can occur, such as among wrestlers (herpes gladiatorum), or cause herpetic whitlows of the fingers, usually from hand contact with HSV-containing oral or genital secretions.

Herpes simplex virus can be transmitted during primary and recurrent infection, regardless of whether clinical manifestations are present. The period of time that patients with primary gingivostomatitis or primary genital HSV can transmit infection is not well defined. Virus can usually be isolated for at least 1 week, and occasionally for several weeks. Thereafter, HSV may be shed intermittently from the mouth, genital tract, and other mucosal sites in the absence of clinical manifestations and for years after initial infection. In addition, viral DNA can be detected by polymerase chain reaction (PCR) for prolonged periods of time after primary infection, implying a chronic infection rather than an intermittent recurrent one. Most primary infections and recurrences are asymptomatic or are associated with minor intraoral or genital lesions. In recurrent lesions, virus is present in the highest concentrations in the first 24 hours after the appearance of vesicles, rapidly decreases in the next 24 hours, and usually cannot be recovered after 5 days.

Genital HSV-2 and HSV-1 infections are commonly transmitted during sexual intercourse and by oral-genital sexual activity. Many primary infections are asymptomatic. Some individuals may not have recurrences; in others, recurrences can occur as often as every month. Genital HSV-2 infections are more likely to recur than those caused by HSV-1. Viral shedding during recurrences also can occur in the absence of clinical signs.

The **incubation period** for primary infection, other than in neonates, varies with estimates of 2 days to 2 weeks. Neonatal HSV infection may be manifest at birth or as late as 4 to 6 weeks of age.

DIAGNOSTIC TESTS: Herpes simplex virus can be recovered in cell culture relatively easily. Special transport media are available for specimens that cannot be inoculated into susceptible cell culture immediately. Viral detection usually requires 1 to 3 days after inoculation. Newer diagnostic techniques, such as direct fluorescent antibody staining of vesicle scrapings or enzyme immunoassay detection of HSV antigens, offer more rapid diagnosis. These techniques are as specific but less sensitive than culture. A variety of techniques are available for distinguishing HSV-1 from HSV-2 isolates. Polymerase chain reaction (PCR), which currently is available only in research or specialized microbiology laboratories, is a very sensitive method for detecting HSV DNA; its prime limitation is the possibility of a false-positive result. Determination of the presence of HSV by culture or by PCR in a mucosal lesion (except in newborns and young infants) does not necessarily confirm an etiological association, as intermittent excretion of virus from mucous membrane sites can persist for life following primary infection (see Epidemiology, p 267).

For the diagnosis of neonatal HSV infection, specimens for culture are obtained from skin vesicles, mouth or nasopharynx, eyes, urine, blood, stool or rectum, and cerebrospinal fluid (CSF). Positive swab cultures obtained from the conjunctiva, nasopharynx, mouth, stool, or rectum of infants longer than 24 to 48 hours after birth are more likely to indicate viral replication and infant infection than transient colonization from intrapartum exposure. The most sensitive technique for detecting genital HSV infection in symptomatic pregnant women is culture of labial or cervical lesions or, in the absence of lesions, culture of the cervix and vulva. The presence of multinucleated giant cells and eosinophilic intranuclear inclusions in Papanicolaou-stained smears of the cervix indicate probable HSV infection, but this method is less sensitive than viral isolation.

Acute and convalescent sera can be tested for rises in HSV antibody titers to confirm acute primary infection, but serologic diagnosis is less helpful than viral isolation, as sera that confirm acute infection often are obtained late in the course of illness. Serologic responses are of no value in considering the need for antiviral therapy. Rises in antibody titer are not frequently demonstrable during recurrences. Tests available only in research laboratories are reliable in differentiating HSV-1 from HSV-2 antibodies.

In children with suspected HSV encephalitis, a brain biopsy may be useful before (or soon after) therapy is initiated to identify other treatable causes of encephalitis or to confirm a diagnosis of HSV infection. Detection of HSV DNA by PCR in the CSF of patients with HSV encephalitis is the diagnostic method of choice and may obviate the need for a brain biopsy, but it currently is available only in research and other specialized laboratories and in a few commercial laboratories.

TREATMENT: Acyclovir is the treatment of choice for HSV infections, including potentially serious infections, as occur in neonates and immunocompromised patients and, in less serious, noninvasive infections. However, its use in the latter has been limited primarily to adults, and information on children is limited. For recommended antiviral dosages and duration of therapy, see Antiviral Drugs for Non-HIV Infections (p 634).

Neonatal. Acyclovir should be administered to all infants with neonatal HSV infection, irrespective of the presenting clinical findings. The highest success rate is achieved in the treatment of disease localized to the skin, eyes, and mouth and to a lesser extent in the treatment of localized CNS disease, and least successful in the treatment of generalized, systemic infection. Initiation of therapy early in the course of the disease may enhance its efficacy. The dose of acyclovir that has been demonstrated to be effective is 30 mg/kg per day in three divided doses, given intravenously, but most experts recommend higher dosages (45 to 60 mg/kg per day). Data supporting the use of these higher dosages, however, are not currently available. The optimal duration of therapy has not been established; the recommended minimal duration is 14 days. Courses as long as 21 days may be indicated in some cases. A collaborative, multi-institutional trial is in progress to determine whether 21 days of therapy improves outcome. Relapse of disease after cessation of treatment can occur and most often appears to be related to host factors. The need for retreatment of infants with recurrent skin lesions is under study. Prolonged oral administration of acyclovir has been associated with neutropenia.

Infants with ocular involvement due to HSV infection should receive a topical ophthalmic drug (specifically, 1% to 2% trifluridine, 1% iododeoxyuridine, or 3% vidarabine), as well as parenteral antiviral therapy. Ophthalmologic consultation is strongly advised.

Genital Infection.

Primary. In adults, acyclovir, valacyclovir, and famciclovir diminish the duration of symptoms and viral shedding in primary genital herpes. Oral acyclovir initiated within 6 days of onset of the disease has been demonstrated to shorten the median duration of the signs and symptoms and viral shedding from primary lesions by approximately 3 to 5 days. The oral administration of valacyclovir or famciclovir does not appear to provide improved efficacy when compared with acyclovir for the treatment of primary genital herpes, but valacyclovir and famciclovir do have the advantage of less frequent dosing. However, no pediatric formulation of either drug is currently available. Intravenous acyclovir for primary genital herpes only is indicated in patients with a severe or complicated course that requires hospitalization. Topical acyclovir (5%) ointment applied to primary genital herpes minimally reduces viral shedding and symptoms, and is not recommended. Systemic or topical treatment of primary herpetic lesions does not affect the subsequent risk or severity of recurrences.

Recurrent. Antiviral therapy has minimal effect on recurrent genital herpes. Oral acyclovir initiated within 2 days of the onset of symptoms shortens the mean clinical course by 1 day. Valacyclovir and famciclovir are licensed for the treatment of recurrent genital herpes; however, no data exist for the treatment of adolescent or pediatric disease. Topical acyclovir is not beneficial in immunocompetent hosts.

Oral acyclovir administered daily to adults for suppressive therapy has been effective in decreasing the frequency of recurrences of active disease in persons with frequent recurrences (six or more episodes per year) of genital HSV infection. After 1 year of continuous daily therapy, acyclovir should be discontinued and the patient's recurrence rate should be assessed. Usually, however, the disease recurs at the same frequency as before the course of suppressive therapy. Acyclovir seems to be safe in adults receiving the drug for up to 6 years, but the long-term effects are unknown. No data exist for suppressive therapy with valacyclovir or famciclovir.

Acyclovir is not recommended for pregnant women unless disease is life-threatening.

Other Mucocutaneous HSV Infections.

Immunocompromised Hosts. Intravenous acyclovir is effective in the treatment and prevention of dissemination of mucocutaneous HSV infections. Topical acyclovir also may accelerate the healing of recurrent lesions in immunocompromised patients. Both oral and intravenous acyclovir have been beneficial in reducing the rate of recurrences during, but not after, the course of therapy.

In the immunocompromised patient who has received prolonged or recurrent treatment with acyclovir for HSV infection, acyclovir-resistant HSV may be isolated from unresponsive lesions or lesions that occur or expand while the patient is receiving acyclovir. In this circumstance, foscarnet is the drug of choice.

Immunocompetent Hosts. Insufficient information is available to determine whether the effects of acyclovir on primary or recurrent nongenital mucocutaneous herpetic disease are similar to those for genital HSV infections. In adults, minimal therapeutic benefit has been demonstrated from use of oral acyclovir in individuals with recurrent herpes labialis (cold sores). Children with primary gingivostomatitis have been treated with acyclovir, but definitive data on efficacy are lacking.

In a small, controlled study in adults with recurrent herpes labialis (six or more episodes per year), prophylactic acyclovir given in a dose of 400 mg twice a day was effective in reducing the frequency of recurrent episodes.

Encephalitis. Patients with HSV encephalitis should be treated for 14 to 21 days with intravenous acyclovir as early in the illness as possible. Therapy is less effective in adults than in children and in those who have become comatose or semicomatose.

Ocular. Treatment of eye lesions should be undertaken in conjunction with an ophthalmologist. Multiple DNA inhibitor drugs, such as 1% to 2% trifluridine, 1% iododeoxyuridine, and 3% vidarabine, have been successful for topical therapy for superficial keratitis. Topical corticosteroids are contraindicated in suspected HSV conjunctivitis; however, ophthalmologists may choose to use corticosteroids in conjunction with antiviral drugs to treat more locally invasive infections.

ISOLATION OF THE HOSPITALIZED PATIENT*:

Neonates With HSV Infection. Neonates with HSV infection, or with positive cultures in the absence of disease, should be hospitalized in a private room, if possible, and managed with contact precautions for the duration of the illness.

---

* In addition to standard precautions.

Neonates Exposed to HSV During Delivery. Neonates with documented perinatal exposure to HSV may be in the incubation phase of infection and should be observed carefully. One method of infection control is to have the infant continuously in a private room with the mother. Infants born vaginally, or by cesarean delivery if membranes have been ruptured for more than 4 to 6 hours, to a mother with active HSV lesions should be separated physically from other infants and managed with contact precautions if they are hospitalized in the nursery during the incubation period. Some experts recommend separation of infants born by cesarean delivery irrespective of the duration of ruptured membranes before delivery. The risk of HSV infection in possibly exposed infants (eg, those born to a mother with a history of recurrent genital herpes) is low. Although expert opinion varies, standard precautions only are recommended for these infants.

Women in Labor and Postpartum Women With HSV Infection. Women in labor who have active HSV lesions, or whose viral cultures or Papanicolaou smear is positive, should be managed during labor, delivery, and the postpartum period with contact precautions if infection is severe or likely to be primary. In other circumstances, standard precautions only are acceptable. These women should be instructed in the importance of careful hand washing before and after caring for their infant. A clean covering gown may be used to help avoid contact of the infant with the lesions or infectious secretions. A mother with herpes labialis (cold sores) or stomatitis should wear a disposable surgical mask when touching her newborn until the lesions have crusted and dried. She should not kiss or nuzzle her newborn until the lesions have cleared. Herpetic lesions on other skin sites should be covered.

Breastfeeding is acceptable if no lesions are present on the breast and if active lesions elsewhere on the mother are covered (see Human Milk, p 73).

Children With Mucocutaneous HSV Infection. For patients with severe mucocutaneous HSV infection, contact precautions are recommended. Patients with localized recurrent lesions should be managed with standard precautions.

Patients With Central Nervous System HSV Infection. Standard precautions are recommended for patients with infection limited to the CNS.

CONTROL MEASURES:

Prevention of Neonatal Infection. Expert opinion on the appropriate management of pregnant women to minimize the risk of neonatal HSV infection has changed considerably in the past 15 years. Weekly HSV cultures during pregnancy are no longer recommended, and women with a history of genital HSV infection and signs or symptoms of infection during pregnancy, or those whose sexual partners have genital HSV infection, are recognized to be at low (albeit somewhat increased) risk of transmitting HSV to their infants (see Epidemiology, p 267). In addition, intrapartum cultures have not had sufficient predictive value to be useful.

Experts differ about the recommendations for the prevention of neonatal infection. In particular, management of the infant exposed to HSV during delivery will differ according to the status of the mother's infection, mode of delivery, and expert opinion (see Care of Newborns Whose Mothers Have Active Genital Lesions, p 273). Current recommendations for management of pregnant women for the prevention of HSV infection include the following:

- *During pregnancy.* All pregnant women should be questioned during a prenatal visit for a history of HSV infection in themselves or in their sexual partners, and signs and symptoms of current infection should be sought as part of prenatal care.
- *Women in labor.* During labor, all women should be questioned about recent and current HSV symptoms and carefully examined for evidence of genital HSV infection. Cesarean delivery in women who have clinically apparent HSV infection (particularly primary infection) may reduce the risk of neonatal HSV infection unless the membranes have been ruptured for more than 4 to 6 hours. The risk when the membranes have been ruptured for longer periods is uncertain. Many experts recommend that infants should be delivered by cesarean section whenever the birth canal is infected even if the membranes have been ruptured for 6 or more hours. However, a recent cost-benefit analysis has suggested that cesarean delivery is not indicated in the woman with an active recurrent infection. A history of genital HSV for a woman in labor is not an indication for cesarean section. Scalp monitors should be avoided when possible in infants of women suspected of having HSV infection.

A cesarean section should be performed immediately on a woman who presents with ruptured membranes and active genital lesions at term, or at a time when the fetal lung is known to be mature. In a woman who presents with ruptured membranes and active genital lesions at a time when the fetal lung is immature, the appropriate course of action is not clear. The options include (1) expectant management (ie, labor is allowed to follow its natural course), with or without administration of intravenous acyclovir (15 mg/kg in three divided doses) to the mother; (2) delay of delivery until betamethasone can be given to enhance the maturity of the fetal lungs; and, (3) cesarean delivery with administration of topical surfactant to the infant. The value and risks of acyclovir in this situation of expectant management are unknown. Use of acyclovir in this circumstance is not approved by the Food and Drug Administration, and cannot be recommended for routine use. Acyclovir given to the mother may decrease the duration of viral shedding and does result in appreciable drug concentrations in the fetus, which may reduce the risk of HSV disease in the infant.

If acyclovir is administered to pregnant women, physicians are encouraged to report patients to the Acyclovir in Pregnancy Registry.*

Care of Newborns Whose Mothers Have Active Genital Lesions.†

By Vaginal Delivery. Because the risk to infants exposed to HSV lesions during delivery varies in different circumstances from less than 5% to 50% or more, the decision to treat the asymptomatic, exposed infant empirically with intravenous

---

* Burroughs Welcome Co in conjunction with the Centers for Disease Control and Prevention maintains a registry to monitor fetal and maternal outcomes of pregnant women given systemic acyclovir. Physicians are encouraged to register pregnant women treated with acyclovir by calling 800-722-9292, ext 39437.
† For further information and the recommendations of the Infectious Disease Society of America, see Prober CG, Corey L, Brown ZA, et al. The management of pregnancies complicated by genital infections with herpes simplex virus. *Clin Infect Dis.* 1992;15:1031-1038.

acyclovir is controversial. The infection rate of infants born to mothers with active recurrent genital herpes infections is 5% or less. Most experts would not treat empirically these infants with acyclovir. The infant's parents or caregivers, however, should be educated about the signs and symptoms of neonatal HSV infection.

For those infants born of mothers with a first-episode, primary genital infection, the risk of infection is high (at least 33% to 50%), and is increased for exposed infants born prematurely, who required instrumentation, or those in whom lacerations occurred during delivery. Most experts, therefore, recommend empiric acyclovir treatment at birth after HSV cultures have been obtained (see Recommendations, below) for infants who are exposed intrapartum to maternal HSV infection when signs and symptoms suggest primary or first-episode infection and who have one or more of the aforementioned risk factors. Some experts, if the infant is asymptomatic, would obtain HSV cultures 24 to 48 hours after delivery, and initiate acyclovir therapy only if HSV is identified by the cultures. However, if the infant has symptoms suggestive of HSV infection, such as skin or scalp rashes (especially vesicular lesions) and/or unexplained clinical manifestations (such as those of sepsis), cultures should be obtained, irrespective of age, and acyclovir therapy should be initiated immediately.

In assessing the risk of HSV infection for the exposed infant, differentiation of primary, first-episode genital infection from recurrent HSV infection in the mother is helpful, but is often difficult or impossible. In addition, primary infection and first-episode infection are not necessarily the same, as some primary infections are asymptomatic, in which case the first symptomatic episode is a secondary (recurrent) infection. In selected instances, serologic testing can be useful. For example, a woman with herpetic lesions who is seronegative for HSV antibody by any standard serologic assay has primary infection, and her infant has a high risk of infection if born vaginally. Assessment of seropositive women, however, necessitates differentiation of HSV-1 antibodies from HSV-2 antibodies. In the future, reliable type-specific antibody assays may allow the determination of the presence or absence of HSV-2 antibodies to assist in the categorizing of maternal infection.

Recommendations. In the management of exposed, asymptomatic infants, those who were delivered vaginally of mothers with active genital lesions can be categorized according to the type of maternal infection as follows:

- Mother with primary, first-episode infection.
- Mother with known, recurrent lesions.
- Mother whose status (primary vs recurrent) is not known.

Infants in each category should have cultures obtained for HSV at 24 to 48 hours after birth (and sooner if symptoms develop and/or acyclovir therapy is initiated before then), including swabs or specimens of the urine, stool or rectum, mouth, and nasopharynx (see Diagnostic Tests, p 269). For infants whose mothers have primary, first-episode infection, most experts would recommend empiric acyclovir treatment at birth, although no data exist to prove the efficacy of such an approach.

The infant whose mother has known, recurrent genital lesions should be observed carefully for skin or scalp rashes, especially vesicular lesions and unexplained clinical manifestations including respiratory distress, seizures, and signs of sepsis. Education of the parents or caregivers regarding the signs and symptoms of neonatal HSV infection is essential. An infant with any of these manifestations should be evaluated as soon as possible for possible HSV infection as well as for bacterial infection. Skin lesions, conjunctiva, nasopharynx, mouth, cerebrospinal fluid (CSF), stool or rectum, and urine should be cultured for HSV. Acyclovir therapy should be initiated if culture(s) from the infant become positive, if the CSF findings are abnormal, or if HSV infection otherwise is suspected strongly while awaiting culture results (assuming bacterial culture results are negative or pending, and no other causes of the infant's clinical manifestations are found).

Infants born to mothers in whom the differentiation between primary and recurrent infection cannot be made should be managed as recommended for those born to mothers with recurrent infection.

By Cesarean Delivery. Infants born by cesarean delivery to a mother with herpetic lesions (primary, secondary, or unknown in status) should be observed carefully, and cultures performed, as recommended for the potentially exposed infant born by vaginal delivery. Similarly, antiviral therapy should be initiated if cultures from the infant are positive, or if HSV is suspected strongly while awaiting culture results (assuming other causes of the infant's manifestations are not identified). Data confirming the benefit or need for antiviral therapy in these circumstances of the exposed infant born by vaginal or cesarean delivery are not yet available.

Care of Infants Born to Mothers With a History of Genital HSV but No Active Lesions at Delivery. These infants should be evaluated carefully for manifestations of neonatal HSV infection. No data support the value of obtaining the intrapartum cultures from these women. Most experts would not culture asymptomatic infants born to those women free of active lesions. A positive culture obtained from the mother or infant at the time of birth indicates only exposure and does not necessarily indicate infection.

Other Recommendations.

- The length of in-hospital observation for infants at increased risk for neonatal HSV is empiric and based on factors specific to the infant and local resources, such as the family's ability to observe the infant at home, availability of follow-up care, and clinical assessment.
- Delay of elective or ritual circumcision for approximately 1 month after birth for infants at highest risk of disease is prudent.
- Neonatal HSV infection can occur as late as 6 weeks after delivery; physicians must be vigilant and not ignore a new rash or symptoms that may be caused by HSV.

Infected Hospital Personnel. Transmission of HSV in newborn nurseries from infected personnel to newborn infants has been documented rarely. The risk of transmission to infants by personnel who have labial HSV infection (cold sores) or who are asymptomatic oral shedders of the virus is low. Compromising patient care by excluding personnel with cold sores who are essential for the operation of the nursery must be weighed against the potential risk of infecting newborn infants. Personnel with cold sores who have contact with infants (1) should cover and not touch their lesions, (2) should carefully observe hand washing policies, and (3) must not kiss or nuzzle newborn infants or children with dermatitis. Transmission of HSV infection from personnel with genital lesions is not likely as long as hand washing policies are carefully observed. Personnel with active herpetic whitlow should not have responsibility for direct care of neonates, immunocompromised patients, or patients in an intensive care unit.

Household Contacts of Infected Persons With Newborns. Intrafamilial transmission of HSV to newborns on rare occasions has occurred. Hence, household members with herpetic skin lesions (eg, herpes labialis or herpetic whitlow) should be counseled about the risk and avoid contact of their lesions with newborns by taking the same measures as recommended for infected hospital personnel.

Care of Persons With Dermatitis. Patients with dermatitis are at risk of developing eczema herpeticum. If these patients are hospitalized, special care should be taken to avoid exposure to HSV. They should not be kissed by persons with cold sores or handled by people with herpetic whitlow.

Care of Children With Mucocutaneous Infections Who Are in Child Care or School. Oral HSV infections are common in children who are in child care or school. Most of these infections are asymptomatic. In addition, recurrent shedding of virus in saliva in the absence of clinical disease is common. Only those children with HSV gingivostomatitis (ie, primary infection) who do not have control of oral secretions should be excluded from child care. Exclusion of children with cold sores (ie, recurrent infection) from child care or school is not indicated (see Children in Out-of-Home Child Care, p 80).

Children with uncovered lesions on exposed surfaces and who were infected with HSV as newborn infants or as a result of sexual abuse pose a small potential risk to contacts. If children are certified by a physician to have recurrent HSV infection, covering the active lesions with clothing, a bandage, or an appropriate dressing when they attend child care or school is sufficient.

HSV Infections in Wrestlers and Rugby Players. Herpes simplex virus type 1 infection has been transmitted during athletic competition involving close physical contact and frequent skin abrasions, such as wrestling (herpes gladiatorum) and rugby (herpes rugbiaforum or scrum pox). Competitors often do not recognize or may deny possible infection. Transmission of these infections can be limited or prevented by the following: (1) examination of wrestlers and rugby players dressed in underwear or competition outfits for vesicular or ulcerative lesions on exposed areas of their bodies and around their mouths or eyes before practice or competition by a person familiar with the appearance of different mucocutaneous infections (including HSV, herpes zoster, and impetigo); (2) exclusion of athletes with these conditions from competition or practice until healing occurs or a physicians' note declaring their condition noninfectious is obtained; and (3) wiping of wrestling mats with a freshly prepared solution of $\frac{1}{64}$ household bleach ($\frac{1}{4}$ cup diluted to 1 gallon of water) at least daily, and preferably between matches. However, HSV spread during wrestling and other sports involving close, personal contact still can occur through contact with saliva of asymptomatic persons.

Histoplasmosis

CLINICAL MANIFESTATIONS: Histoplasmosis encompasses a spectrum of clinical diseases. Acute pulmonary histoplasmosis is an influenza-like illness with pulmonary infiltrates and hilar adenopathy. Chronic pulmonary histoplasmosis which, clinically, resembles tuberculosis in adults, is uncommon in children. Primary cutaneous infections can occur after trauma.

Acute disseminated histoplasmosis is most frequent in immunosuppressed hosts, including patients with HIV infection, and in children younger than 2 years. Symptoms include fever, cough, hepatosplenomegaly, adenopathy, pneumonitis, skin lesions and diarrhea. Pancytopenia, resembling acute lymphatic leukemia, can occur. Central nervous system involvement is common. Chronic disseminated infection is rare in children.

ETIOLOGY: *Histoplasma capsulatum* is a dimorphic fungus. In soil, it exists in the mycelial phase, but it converts to a yeast phase at the body temperature (37°C) of mammals.

EPIDEMIOLOGY: *Histoplasma capsulatum* is encountered in many parts of the world and is endemic in the eastern and central United States, particularly the Mississippi and Ohio River valleys. Infection is acquired through inhalation of airborne spores (conidia) from mycelia. The quantity of inhaled inoculum and the immune status of the host affect the degree of symptomatology; more than 95% of infections are asymptomatic. The source of the organism is soil or dust in barnyards and other locations that harbor bat and bird droppings. Histoplasmosis is not transmitted from person to person.

The **incubation period** is variable but is usually 1 to 3 weeks from the time of exposure.

DIAGNOSTIC TESTS: Culture is the definitive method of diagnosis. *Histoplasma capsulatum* grows on standard mycologic media and most nonselective bacterial media at room temperature, requiring usually 2 to 6 weeks. Bone marrow, blood, sputum, and material from lesions may be cultured. The lysis-centrifugation method is preferred for blood cultures. A chemiluminescent DNA probe is available for identification of cultures of *H capsulatum*. The procedure can be applied to non-sporulating cultures, thereby reducing the risk of exposure of laboratory personnel to infectious spores of the fungi.

Direct demonstration of intracellular yeast in smears of bone marrow or biopsy material from infected tissues is helpful in diagnosing disseminated or chronic histoplasmosis. Hematoxylin and eosin, Wright, and Giemsa stains are usually adequate, but the Gomori methenamine silver stain is more likely to detect sparse organisms.

Detection of *H capsulatum* polysaccharide antigen in urine or serum by radioimmunoassay is a specific sensitive and rapid method for the diagnosis of disseminated histoplasmosis in immunocompromised patients, including those infected with HIV.

Both mycelial-phase (histoplasmin) and yeast-phase antigens are used in serologic testing for complement-fixing antibodies to *H capsulatum*. Low titers are often present in healthy persons living in endemic areas. A fourfold rise in yeast-phase titers or a single high titer of 1:32 or greater is presumptive evidence of active infection. Cross-reacting antibodies can result from *Blastomyces dermatiditis* and *Coccidioides immitis* infections. Serum titers of mycelial but not the yeast-phase antibodies can increase slightly after skin testing with mycelium-derived histoplasmin. In the immunodiffusion antibody test, H bands, although rarely encountered, are highly suggestive of active infection. The immunodiffusion test is more specific than the complement fixation test, whereas the complement fixation test is more sensitive.

A positive reaction to the histoplasmin skin test indicates current or previous infection with *Histoplasma* species. It is not recommended for diagnostic purposes.

TREATMENT: Uncomplicated, primary pulmonary histoplasmosis usually requires no specific therapy. Indications for antifungal therapy include a progressive, disseminated disease and acute infection in immunocompromised patients, such as those with HIV infection.

Amphotericin B is effective and recommended for disseminated disease (see Systemic Treatment With Amphotericin B, p 630). In other circumstances in which antifungal therapy is warranted, ketoconazole, fluconazole, and itraconazole also have been effective. The safety and efficacy of itraconazole in children has not been established, but in otherwise healthy adults, it has been demonstrated to be at least as effective as ketoconazole and is better tolerated with lower or negligible toxicity. Itraconazole also has proven effective in the treatment of mild disseminated histoplasmosis in HIV-infected patients.

Duration of treatment with amphotericin B is 6 weeks or longer and is determined by clinical and laboratory evidence that active infection has subsided. Patients with HIV infection require lifelong suppressive therapy. Amphotericin B, fluconazole, and itraconazole have been used successfully. In adults, itraconazole is the drug of choice for suppressive therapy.

ISOLATION OF THE HOSPITALIZED PATIENT: Standard precautions are recommended.

CONTROL MEASURES: Investigation for the common source of infection in outbreaks is indicated. Exposure to soil and dust from areas with significant accumulations of bird and bat droppings should be avoided or, if unavoidable, controlled through use of masks, gloves, and disposable clothing.

HIV Infection*

CLINICAL MANIFESTATIONS: Human immunodeficiency virus (HIV) infection in children causes a broad spectrum of disease and a varied clinical course. Acquired immunodeficiency syndrome (AIDS) represents the most severe end of the clinical spectrum. The current surveillance definitions of the Centers for Disease Control and Prevention (CDC) for AIDS in adults and adolescents and the pediatric classification system of CDC for children younger than 13 years who are born to HIV-infected mothers or who are known to be infected with HIV are given in Tables 3.21 and 3.22, respectively.[†‡] Although this pediatric classification system was established for surveillance of HIV infection, its clinical categories (see Table 3.23) are used to define progression of disease. This system also emphasizes the importance of the CD4+ T-lymphocyte count as an immunological surrogate and prognosis marker.

The manifestations of HIV infection include generalized lymphadenopathy, hepatomegaly, splenomegaly, failure to thrive, oral candidiasis, recurrent diarrhea, parotitis, cardiomyopathy, hepatitis, nephropathy, central nervous system (CNS) disease (including developmental delay, which can be progressive), lymphoid interstitial pneumonia, recurrent invasive bacterial infections, opportunistic infections, and specified malignancies.

Pneumocystis carinii pneumonia (PCP) is the most common, serious opportunistic infection in children with HIV infection and is associated with high mortality (see *Pneumocystis carinii* Infections, p 419). *Pneumocystis carinii* pneumonia occurs most frequently in infants between 3 and 6 months of age who acquired infection before or at birth, but it can occur in younger infants, beginning as early as 4 to 6 weeks. Other common opportunistic infections in children include *Candida* esophagitis, disseminated cytomegalovirus infection, and chronic or disseminated herpes simplex and varicella-zoster virus infections and, less commonly, *Mycobacterium tuberculosis, Mycobacterium avium* complex (MAC) infection, chronic enteritis caused by *Cryptosporidium* or other agents, and disseminated or central nervous system (CNS) cryptococcal or *Toxoplasma gondii* infection.

Malignancies in pediatric HIV infection have been relatively uncommon to date, but leiomyosarcomas and certain lymphomas, including those of the CNS and non-Hodgkin's B-cell lymphomas of the Burkitt's type, occur much more frequently in children with HIV infection than in nonimmunocompromised children. Kaposi's sarcoma is very rare in children.

The development of opportunistic infections, particularly PCP, progressive neurologic disease, and severe wasting is associated with a poor prognosis. The prognosis for survival is also poor in children infected perinatally in whom virus may be

---

* For a complete listing of current Academy guidelines, see *Pediatric Human Immunodeficiency Virus (HIV) Infection — A Compendium of AAP Guidelines or Pediatric HIV Infection*. Elk Grove Village, Ill: American Academy of Pediatrics; In press.

† Centers for Disease Control and Prevention. 1993 revised classification system for HIV infection and expanded case surveillance definition for AIDS among adolescents and adults. *MMWR.* 1992;41(No. RR-17):1-19.

‡ Centers for Disease Control and Prevention. 1994 revised classification system for human immunodeficiency virus infection in children less than 13 years of age. Official authorized addenda: human immunodeficiency virus infection codes and official guidelines for coding and reporting ICD-9-CM. *MMWR.* 1994;43(No. RR-12):1-19.

detected early (ie, 7 days of life) and in those who become symptomatic in the first year of life. With earlier and more effective treatment, survival is likely to improve.

Laboratory Findings. The most notable finding, particularly as the disease progresses, is an increasing loss of cell-mediated immunity. The peripheral blood lymphocyte count initially can be normal, but eventually lymphopenia develops because of a decrease in the total number of circulating T-lymphocytes. The cells most affected are the T-helper CD4+ lymphocytes. The T-suppressor CD8+ lymphocytes usually increase in number initially and are not depleted until late in the course of the infection. These changes in cell populations result in a decrease of the normal CD4+ to CD8+ cell ratio. This nonspecific finding, although characteristic of HIV infection, also occurs with other acute viral infections, such as those caused by cytomegalovirus or Epstein-Barr virus. The normal values for peripheral CD4+ T-lymphocyte counts and percentages are age-related and the lower limits of normal are given in Table 3.22. Response of T-lymphocytes to plant lectin mitogens (phytohemagglutinin, concanavalin A, and particularly pokeweed) are decreased or absent, and patients may be anergic to skin test antigens such as mumps, *Candida, Trichophyton,* tetanus, and tuberculin (purified protein derivative [PPD]).

Although B-lymphocyte numbers remain normal or are somewhat increased, humoral immune dysfunction accompanies cellular dysfunction. Serum immunoglobulin concentrations, particularly IgG and IgA, frequently are elevated. Some patients will develop panhypogammaglobulinemia. Specific antibody responses to antigens to which the patient has not previously been exposed can be abnormal. Measuring the serum antibody response to measles vaccine administered to children 12 months of age or older, or to tetanus after three doses of DTaP or DTP can be useful for assessing humoral responsiveness. Circulating concentrations of virus (termed viral load) in children younger than 12 months are very high (mean of approximately 300 000 RNA copies/mL). By 24 months of age, viral concentrations decrease (to a mean of approximately 40 000 RNA copies/mL). Recent data suggest that plasma viral concentration determinations in conjunction with CD4+ cell count determinations are more accurate predictors than each marker alone of prognosis and of survival. Guidelines for the use of viral load determinations in the treatment of children, however, have not yet been formulated.

ETIOLOGY: Infection is caused by RNA cytopathic human retroviruses, human immunodeficiency virus type 1 (HIV-1) and, less commonly, HIV-2, a related virus that is extremely uncommon in the United States but more common in West Africa. Human immunodeficiency virus is particularly tropic for T-helper CD4+ lymphocytes and other cells such as monocytes and macrophages and for CNS cells that have CD4+ receptors (eg, glial cells). The role of cofactors, such as simultaneous infection with other infectious agents, such cytomegalovirus or malnutrition, in the natural history of HIV infection is not known.

EPIDEMIOLOGY: Humans are the only known reservoir of HIV, although related viruses have been identified in monkeys. Since retroviruses integrate into the target cell genome as proviruses and the viral genome is copied during cell replication, the virus persists in infected persons for life. Human immunodeficiency virus has been isolated from blood (including lymphocytes, macrophages, and plasma) and from

Table 3.21. **1993 Revised Case Definition of AIDS-Defining Conditions for Adults and Adolescents 13 Years of Age and Older***

- Candidiasis of bronchi, trachea, or lungs
- Candidiasis, esophageal
- Cervical cancer, invasive
- Coccidioidomycosis, disseminated or extrapulmonary
- Cryptococcosis, extrapulmonary
- Cryptosporidiosis, chronic intestinal (>1 month's duration)
- Cytomegalovirus disease (other than liver, spleen, or nodes)
- Cytomegalovirus retinitis (with loss of vision)
- Encephalopathy, HIV-related
- Herpes simplex: chronic ulcer(s) (>1 month's duration); or bronchitis, pneumonitis, or esophagitis
- Histoplasmosis, disseminated or extrapulmonary
- Isosporiasis, chronic intestinal (>1 month's duration)
- Kaposi's sarcoma
- Lymphoma, Burkitt's (or equivalent term)
- Lymphoma, immunoblastic (or equivalent term)
- Lymphoma, primary or brain
- *Mycobacterium avium* complex or *M kansasii,* disseminated or extrapulmonary
- *Mycobacterium tuberculosis,* any site, pulmonary or extrapulmonary
- *Mycobacterium,* other species or unidentified species, disseminated or extrapulmonary
- *Pneumocystis carinii* pneumonia
- Pneumonia, recurrent
- Progressive multifocal leukoencephalopathy
- *Salmonella* septicemia, recurrent
- Toxoplasmosis of brain
- Wasting syndrome due to HIV
- CD4+ T-lymphocyte count less than 200 cells/μL or CD4+ percentage less than 15%

* Modified from Centers for Disease Control and Prevention. 1993 revised classification system for HIV infection and expanded case surveillance definition for AIDS among adolescents and adults. *MMWR.* 1992;41(No. RR-17):1-19.

other body fluids such as cerebrospinal fluid, pleural fluids, human milk, semen, cervical secretions, saliva, urine, and tears. Only blood, semen, cervical secretions, and human milk, however, have been implicated epidemiologically in the transmission of infection.

The established modes of HIV transmission in the United States are via (1) sexual contact (both homosexual and heterosexual); (2) percutaneous (from needles or other sharp instruments) or mucous membrane exposure to contaminated blood or other

Table 3.22. **Pediatric HIV Classification for Children Less Than 13 Years of Age***

Immunologic Definitions	Immunological Categories Age-specific. CD4+ T-Lymphocyte Count and % of Total Lymphocytes						Clinical Classifications†			
	< 12 mo		1–5 y		6–12 y		N: No Signs/ Symptoms	A: Mild Signs/ Symptoms	B: Moderate Signs/Symptoms‡	C: Severe Signs/Symptoms‡
	µL	%	µL	%	µL	%				
1: No evidence of suppression	≥1500	≥25	≥1000	≥25	≥500	≥25	N1	A1	B1	C1
2: Evidence of moderate suppression	750–1499	15–24	500–999	15–24	200–499	15–24	N2	A2	B2	C2
3: Severe suppression	<750	<15	<500	<15	<200	<15	N3	A3	B3	C3

* Modified from Centers for Disease Control and Prevention. 1994 revised classification system for human immunodeficiency virus infection in children less than 13 years of age. Official authorized addenda: human immunodeficiency virus infection codes and official guidelines for coding and reporting ICD-9-CM. *MMWR*. 1994;43(No. RR-12):1-19.

† Children whose HIV infection status is not confirmed are classified by using this grid with a letter E (for perinatally exposed) placed before the appropriate classification code (eg, EN2).

‡ Lymphoid interstitial pneumonitis in Category B or Category C is reportable to state and local health departments as AIDS (see Table 3.23 for further definition of clinical categories).

Table 3.23. Clinical Categories for Children Less Than 13 Years of Age With HIV Infection*

Category N: Not Symptomatic

Children who have no signs or symptoms considered to be the result of HIV infection or have only one of the conditions listed in Category A.

Category A: Mildly Symptomatic

Children with two or more of the conditions listed below but none of the conditions listed in Categories B and C.

- Lymphadenopathy (≥0.5 cm at more than two sites; bilateral = one site)
- Hepatomegaly
- Splenomegaly
- Dermatitis
- Parotitis
- Recurrent or persistent upper respiratory tract infection, sinusitis, or otitis media

Category B: Moderately Symptomatic

Children who have symptomatic conditions other than those listed for Category A or C which are attributed to HIV infection. Examples of conditions in clinical Category B include but are not limited to the following:

- Anemia (<8 g/dL), neutropenia (<1000/mm³), and/or thrombocytopenia (<100 000/mm³) persisting ≥30 d
- Bacterial meningitis, pneumonia, or sepsis (single episode)
- Candidiasis, oropharyngeal (thrush), persisting (>2 mo) in children >6 mo of age
- Cardiomyopathy
- Cytomegalovirus infection, with onset before 1 mo of age
- Diarrhea, recurrent or chronic
- Hepatitis
- Herpes simplex virus (HSV) stomatitis, recurrent (>2 episodes within 1 year)
- HSV bronchitis, pneumonitis, or esophagitis with onset before 1 mo of age
- Herpes zoster (shingles) involving at least 2 distinct episodes or more than 1 dermatome
- Leiomyosarcoma
- Lymphoid interstitial pneumonia (LIP) or pulmonary lymphoid hyperplasia complex
- Nephropathy
- Nocardiosis
- Persistent fever (lasting >1 mo)
- Toxoplasmosis, onset before 1 mo of age
- Varicella, disseminated (complicated chickenpox)

Category C: Severely Symptomatic

- Serious bacterial infections, multiple or recurrent (ie, any combination of at least two culture-confirmed infections within a 2-y period), of the following types: septicemia, pneumonia, meningitis, bone or joint infection, or abscess of an internal organ or body cavity (excluding otitis media, superficial skin or mucosal abscesses, and indwelling catheter-related infections)

Table 3.23. Clinical Categories for Children Less Than 13 Years of Age With HIV Infection, continued

- Candidiasis, esophageal or pulmonary (bronchi, trachea, lungs)
- Coccidioidomycosis, disseminated (at site other than or in addition to lungs or cervical or hilar lymph nodes)
- Cryptococcosis, extrapulmonary
- Cryptosporidiosis or isospsoriasis with diarrhea persisting >1 mo
- Cytomegalovirus disease with onset of symptoms at age >1 mo (at a site other than liver, spleen, or lymph nodes)
- Encephalopathy (at least one of the following progressive findings present for at least 2 mo in the absence of a concurrent illness other than HIV infection which could explain the findings): (1) failure to attain or loss of developmental milestones or loss of intellectual ability, verified by standard developmental scale or neuro-psychological tests; (2) impaired brain growth or acquired microcephaly demon-strated by head circumference measurements or brain atrophy demonstrated by computed tomography or magnetic resonance imaging (serial imaging is required for children <2 y of age); (3) acquired symmetric motor deficit manifested by 2 or more of the following: paresis, pathologic reflexes, ataxia, or gait disturbance
- Herpes simplex viral infection causing a mucocutaneous ulcer that persists for >1 mo; or bronchitis, pneumonitis, or esophagitis for any duration affecting a child >1 mo of age
- Histoplasmosis, disseminated (at a site other than or in addition to lungs or cervical or hilar lymph nodes)
- Kaposi's sarcoma
- Lymphoma, primary, in brain
- Lymphoma, small, noncleaved cell (Burkitt's), or immunoblastic, or large-cell lymphoma of B-cell or unknown immunologic phenotype
- *Mycobacterium tuberculosis*, disseminated or extrapulmonary
- *Mycobacterium*, other species or unidentified species, disseminated (at a site other than or in addition to lungs, skin or cervical or hilar lymph nodes)
- *Pneumocystis carinii* pneumonia
- Progressive multifocal leukoencephalopathy
- *Salmonella* (nontyphoid) septicemia, recurrent
- Toxoplasmosis of the brain with onset at >1 mo of age
- Wasting syndrome in the absence of a concurrent illness other than HIV infection that could explain the following findings: (1) persistent weight loss >10% of base-line OR (2) downward crossing of at least 2 of the following percentile lines on the weight-for-age chart (eg, 95th, 75th, 50th, 25th, 5th) in a child ≥1 y of age OR (3) <5th percentile on weight-for-height chart on 2 consecutive measurements, ≥30 d apart PLUS (1) chronic diarrhea (ie, at least 2 loose stools per day for ≥ 30 d) OR (2) documented fever (for ≥30 d, intermittent or constant)

* Centers for Disease Control and Prevention. 1994 revised classification system for human immuno-deficiency virus infection in children less than 13 years of age. Official authorized addenda: human immunodeficiency virus infection codes and official guidelines for coding and reporting ICD-9-CM. *MMWR*. 1994;43(No. RR-12):1-19.

body fluids with high titers of HIV; (3) mother-to-infant (ie, vertical) transmission before or around the time of birth; and (4) breastfeeding. Transfusion of blood, blood components, or clotting factor concentrates is now rarely a mode of HIV transmission in this country because of exclusion of infected donors, viral inactivation treatment of clotting factor concentrates, and the availability of recombinant clotting factors. In the absence of documented parenteral, mucous membrane, or skin contact with blood, transmission of HIV rarely has been demonstrated to occur in families or households, in schools or child care settings, or with routine care in hospitals or clinics.

Accidental exposure of health care personnel to HIV, such as from needle stick injuries or HIV-infected blood, rarely has resulted in HIV infection. The risk of infection varies according to the severity and type of exposure. The risk of infection after a percutaneous exposure to HIV-infected blood is 0.3%. The risk after mucous membrane and from skin exposure to HIV-infected blood is 0.1% and less than 0.1%, respectively. Many of the known cases may have been prevented by careful adherence to infection control measures (see Control Measures, p 296).

Cases of AIDS in children have accounted for 2% of all reported cases in the United States. The total number of reported cases of AIDS in children and adolescents, however, continues to increase, and acquisition of HIV during adolescence significantly contributes to the large number of cases in young adults. Routes of transmission of HIV in adolescents are similar to those for adults.

More than 90% of infected children in the United States acquired their infection from their mother. The remainder, including patients with hemophilia or other coagulation disorders, received contaminated blood, its components, or clotting factor concentrates. A few cases of HIV infection in children have resulted from sexual abuse by an HIV-seropositive individual. Less than 5% of cases have been reported to have no identifiable risk factor, and after careful investigation, most are reclassified into one of the established risk factor groups. Vertically acquired infection now accounts for almost all new infections in pre-adolescent children.

The risk of infection for an infant born to an HIV-seropositive mother who did not receive antiretroviral therapy during pregnancy is estimated to be between 13% and 39%. The exact timing of transmission from an infected mother to her infant is uncertain, but evidence suggests that transmission may occur in utero, around the time of delivery, or postpartum through breastfeeding. The available evidence suggests that the majority of infections occur close to the time of or during delivery. Some studies suggest higher rates of perinatal transmission in women who seroconvert during pregnancy and those with advanced disease, low peripheral CD4+ T-lymphocyte counts, prolonged rupture of membranes, and/or high viral concentrations as evidenced by HIV p24 antigenemia or quantitative viral culture or RNA concentration (load). In vaginal deliveries, a first-born twin is at greater risk of HIV infection than a second-born twin. Prevention of transmission by cesarean section has not been proven. Vertical transmission, however, can be reduced significantly by the use of zidovudine therapy of pregnant women and their newborn infants (see Control Measures, p 296).

Human immunodeficiency virus genomes have been detected in both the cellular and cell-free fractions of human breast milk, and breastfeeding has been implicated in the transmission of HIV infection. High maternal plasma viral concentration (load) also may be a factor in the frequency of transmission by breastfeeding.

Incubation Period: HIV-infected infants usually are asymptomatic during the first few months of life. Although the median age of onset of symptoms is estimated to be 3 years for infants infected perinatally, increasing numbers of children are remaining asymptomatic for more than 5 years. Two categories of infection based on incubation period and progression of symptoms have been recognized. Approximately 10% to 15% of children die before 4 years of age, most of whom succumb before 18 months of age, whereas the majority of children survive beyond 5 years of age. Other than infants born of infected mothers, persons infected with HIV usually develop serum antibody to HIV by 6 to 12 weeks after infection.

DIAGNOSTIC TESTS: Diagnosis of HIV infection usually is made by serum antibody tests except in children younger than 18 months in whom passively acquired maternal antibody may be present.

Enzyme immunoassays (EIA) are used most widely to screen for serum HIV antibody. These tests are highly sensitive and specific, but false-positive results occur in a small percentage of cases. Repeat EIA testing of initially reactive specimens is required to reduce the likelihood of laboratory error; repeatedly reactive tests are highly reliable. Western blot or immunofluorescent antibody tests should be used for confirmation. A positive HIV antibody test in a child 18 months of age or older usually is indicative of infection.

Serum antibodies to HIV are present in almost all infected persons, although some patients with AIDS become seronegative late in disease. Occasional children with HIV infection may lack HIV antibody because they have hypogammaglobulinemia, or may be unable to produce antibody if they have advanced disease. Very rarely an HIV-infected child is antibody negative by EIA testing but positive on Western blot or positive by other virologic tests, such as culture or polymerase chain reaction (PCR).

Diagnosis in Infants Born to HIV-Seropositive Women (see Table 3.24). These infants pose a special diagnostic challenge since they are almost always seropositive at birth, whether or not they are infected, as the result of transplacental acquisition of maternal antibody which can be detectable in the infant for as long as 18 months after birth. IgG antibody tests for HIV, thus, are not useful for diagnosis in children younger than 18 months. The preferred tests are HIV culture and detection of HIV genomic sequences by using the PCR, which are the most sensitive and specific tests to detect HIV infection in children born to HIV-infected mothers.*

Using these assays (culture or PCR), only approximately 30% to 50% of infected newborns will be diagnosed at birth, but nearly 100% of infected infants can be diagnosed by 4 to 6 months of age. For an infant born to an HIV-seropositive mother, an initial diagnostic assay of PCR or viral culture should be performed by approximately 1 month of age or as soon as possible thereafter. If the assay is negative, testing between 4 and 6 months of age should be repeated. A positive HIV culture, PCR, and/or p24 antigen detection assay constitutes presumptive evidence of HIV infection; a second diagnostic test subsequently should be performed, using either

---

* For additional information, see Centers for Disease Control and Prevention. 1994 revised classification system for human immunodeficiency virus infection in children less than 13 years of age. Official authorized addenda: human immunodeficiency virus infection codes and official guidelines for coding and reporting ICD-9-CM. *MMWR.* 1994;43(No. RR-12):1-19.

Table 3.24. **Diagnosis of HIV Infection in Children Less Than 13 Years of Age***

Diagnosis: HIV Infected

A child <18 mo of age who is known to be HIV seropositive or born to an HIV-infected mother and

- has positive results on 2 separate determinations[†] (excluding cord blood) from 1 or more of the following HIV detection tests:
  —HIV culture
  —HIV polymerase chain reaction
  —HIV antigen (p24)

or

- meets criteria for acquired immunodeficiency syndrome (AIDS) diagnosis based on the 1987 AIDS surveillance case definition.[‡]

A child ≥ 18 mo of age born to an HIV-infected mother or any child infected by blood, blood products, or other known modes of transmission (eg, sexual contact) who:

- is HIV-antibody positive by repeatedly reactive enzyme immunoassay (EIA) and confirmatory test (eg, Western blot or immunofluorescence assay [IFA])

or

- meets any of the criteria above

Diagnosis: Perinatally Exposed (Prefix E[§])

A child who does not meet the above criteria who:

- is HIV seropositive by EIA and confirmatory test (eg, Western blot or IFA) and is <18 mo of age at the time of test

or

- has unknown antibody status, but was born to a mother known to be infected with HIV

Diagnosis: Seroreverter

A child who is born to an HIV-infected mother and who:

- has been documented as HIV-antibody negative (ie, 2 or more negative EIA tests performed 6–18 mo of age or 1 negative EIA test after 18 mo of age)

and

- has had no other laboratory evidence of infection (has not had 2 positive viral detection tests, if performed)

and

- has not had an AIDS-defining condition

---

* Modified from Centers for Disease Control and Prevention. 1994 revised classification system for human immunodeficiency virus infection in children less than 13 years of age. Official authorized addenda: human immunodeficiency virus infection codes and official guidelines for coding and reporting ICD-9-CM. *MMWR.* 1994;43(No. RR-12):1-19.

† Both determinations performed at or beyond 1 month of age and at least one determination at or beyond 4 months of age.

‡ Centers for Disease Control and Prevention. Revision of the CDC surveillance case definition for acquired immunodeficiency syndrome. *MMWR.* 1987;36(suppl1):1S-15S.

§ See Table 3.22.

the same assay or one of the other two assays, to confirm the diagnosis. The modified (ie, after acid dissociation) p24 antigen assay is less sensitive than viral culture or PCR, and should be used only if the other tests are not available. If an infant younger than 18 months who has a positive serologic test for HIV develops an AIDS-defining illness (Category C — see Table 3.23), the diagnosis of HIV infection is established even if virologic tests are negative.

The child who has two negative virologic tests, both of which are performed at 1 month of age or older and one of which is performed at 4 months of age or older, is considered to have had HIV infection reasonably excluded in the absence of any clinical illness. Follow-up serologic tests should be performed to confirm exclusion of HIV infection and seroreversion. Such tests include either two negative EIA tests performed between 6 and 18 months of age or one negative EIA test at more than 18 months of age.* Some experts recommend that the final EIA test be performed at 24 months of age.

Since interpretation of the available diagnostic tests may be complex, the pediatrician should consult with an HIV specialist to assist in the interpretation of diagnostic assays.

Perinatal HIV Serologic Testing. The Academy recommendations include the following*:

- On the basis of recent advances in therapy to reduce the rate of perinatal HIV transmission and the continued occurrence of life-threatening illness in young infants with unrecognized HIV infection, the Academy recommends documented, routine HIV education, and routine testing with consent for all pregnant women in the United States (see Informed Consent for HIV Serologic Testing). Documented consent for maternal and/or newborn HIV testing may be obtained in a variety of ways, including by right of refusal (documented patient education, with testing to take place unless rejected in writing by the patient). The Academy supports utilization of consent procedures that facilitate rapid incorporation of HIV education and testing into the routine medical care setting.
- Routine education about HIV infection and testing needs to be a part of a comprehensive program of health care for women, particularly for women of child-bearing age.
- All testing programs for the detection of HIV infection should evaluate periodically the proportion of women who refuse HIV testing following HIV education. Those programs in which a proportionately low number of women receive HIV testing should examine the reasons for poor acceptance, with appropriate program modifications made as needed.
- For women who are seen by a health care professional for the first time in labor and who have either not received prenatal care or have previously tested negative, but have not been tested for HIV infection during the current pregnancy, education about HIV infection and maternal HIV testing are recommended during the perinatal period.

---

* For further information, see American Academy of Pediatrics, Provisional Committee on Pediatric AIDS. Perinatal human immunodeficiency virus testing. *Pediatrics*. 1995;95:303-307.

- For newborns whose mother's HIV serostatus was not determined during the recent pregnancy or the postpartum period, the infant's health care provider should educate the mother concerning the potential benefits of HIV testing for her infant and the possible risks and benefits to herself of knowing the child's serostatus, and recommend HIV testing for the newborn.
- In the absence of parental availability for consent to test the newborn for HIV antibody, procedures need to be established to facilitate the rapid evaluation and testing of the infant.
- The health care provider for the infant needs to be informed of maternal HIV serostatus so that appropriate care and testing of the infant can be accomplished. Similarly, if the infant is found to be seropositive when maternal serostatus is unknown, the health care provider for the child should ensure that information about the serostatus and its significance be provided to the mother and, with her consent, to her health care provider. The mother should be referred to an appropriate HIV-related service for adults.
- Comprehensive, HIV-related medical services should be accessible to all infected mothers, their infants, and other family members.
- The Academy supports legislation and public policy directed toward eliminating any form of discrimination based on HIV serostatus.

Informed Consent for HIV Serologic Testing. Testing for HIV infection is unlike most routine blood testing in that substantial psychosocial risks can be incurred. Before testing an infant or child, the parents or other primary caregivers, and the patient, if old enough to comprehend, should be counseled about the possible risks and benefits of testing and the consequences of HIV infection. Oral consent should be obtained from the parent or legal guardian and recorded in the patient's chart. Special written consent procedures for HIV testing should be discouraged as they can inhibit the performance of testing without adding significant benefit. State and local laws and hospital regulations, nevertheless, should be considered in deciding whether written consent is required. The necessity for counseling and consent should not deter efforts to undertake appropriate diagnostic testing for HIV infection. Refusal of parents or patients to give consent does not relieve physicians of the professional and legal responsibilities to their patients. If the physician believes that testing is essential to the child's health, authorization for testing will need to be obtained by other means. The results of serologic tests should be discussed in person with the family, primary caregiver, and, if appropriate according to age, the patient; if positive, appropriate counseling and subsequent follow-up care must be provided. Maintaining confidentiality in all cases is essential to preserving patient and parent trust and consent.

Treatment (see Table 3.25 for a list of antiretroviral drugs and their recommended dosage). Primary care physicians are encouraged to participate actively in the care of HIV-infected patients in consultation with specialists who have expertise in the care of HIV-infected children and adolescents. Expert opinions and knowledge about diagnostic and therapeutic strategies are changing rapidly. In areas of the United States in which enrollment into clinical trials is possible, enrollment of the HIV-infected child into available clinical trials should be encouraged. Information

Table 3.25. **Dosage and Administration of Antiretroviral Drugs for Children***

Drug Name [Trade Name]	Recommended Dosage[†]	
Zidovudine (ZDV, AZT, azidothymidine) [Retrovir]	0–6 wk:	2 mg/kg/dose every 6 h
	4 wk–13 y:	90-180 mg/M^2/dose every 6 h
	≥ 13 y:	100 mg/dose 5 times a day or 200 mg/dose every 8 h
Didanosine (ddI, dideoxyinosine) [Videx]	< 13 y:	90–135 mg/M^2/dose every 12 h
	≥ 13 y:	<60 kg: tablets, 125 mg every 12 h buffered powder, 167 mg every 12 h
		≥60 kg: tablets, 200 mg every 12 h buffered powder, 250 mg every 12 h
Zalcitabine (ddC, dideoxycytidine) [Hivid]	< 13 y:	0.01 mg/kg/dose every 8 h
	≥ 13 y:	0.75 mg every 8 h
Stavudine (d4T) [Zerit]	< 13 y:	1 mg/kg/dose every 12 h
	≥ 13 y:	30–40 mg every 12 h
Lamivudine (3TC) [Epivir]	3 mo–12 y:	4 mg/kg/dose every 12 h twice a day
	≥ 12 y:	150 mg/dose every 12 h twice a day
Saquinavir (SQV) [Invirase]	< 13 y:	dosage not established
	≥ 13 y:	600 mg/dose every 8 h
Indinavir (IDV) [Crixivan]	< 13 y:	dosage not established
	≥ 13 y:	800 mg/dose every 8 h
Ritonavir (RTV) [Norvir]	< 13 y:	350 mg/M^2/dose every 12 h[‡]
	≥ 13 y:	600 mg/dose every 12 h

* Modified from Havens PL, Waters DA, Cuene BA, McIntosh K, Yogev R. Caring for infants, children, adolescents and families with HIV infection. *Wisconsin State Guide*, 1995.
† All dosages listed are by mouth.
‡ Based on preliminary pharmacokinetic data.

about trials for adolescents and children can be obtained by calling the Pediatric Clinical Trials Group.*

Antiretroviral therapy is the standard of care for HIV-infected children. Initiation of antiretroviral therapy depends upon virologic, immunologic, and clinical criteria. The pediatric classification system (see Tables 3.22 and 3.23) can be used as a reference for this criteria. Antiretroviral therapy should be initiated in HIV-infected children with moderate or severe immunosuppression and in those with moderate or severe signs and symptoms of the disease, as defined in Tables 3.22 and 3.23, respectively. Because preliminary data in asymptomatic adults suggest a clinical benefit of therapy with a reduction of viral concentration (load) and a lessened decline in the CD4+ cell count, consideration should be given to initiation of therapy in HIV-infected children who are asymptomatic or mildly symptomatic (ie, categories N or A in Table 3.22) with no evidence of immune suppression (see Table 3.22). The utilization of viral concentration (load) determinations in therapeutic decisions for children is not yet routine, as a specific viral criterion that would indicate a need for initiation or change in therapy has not been defined.

* See Directory of Telephone Numbers, p 667.

Oral zidovudine given alone has been the antiretroviral therapy of choice, but recent data suggest that zidovudine alone is less effective than didanosine alone or the combination of zidovudine plus didanosine. Although many experts recommend combination therapy, didanosine monotherapy for patients with mild clinical symptoms and/or mild immunosuppression is reasonable. This option is particularly appropriate for patients who cannot tolerate or refuse to take zidovudine. Monotherapy also allows the addition of other nucleoside analogs (eg, zalcitabine, lamivudine, and stavudine) when clinical, immunological, or virological deterioration occurs. Only limited data, however, are available regarding the efficacy of such regimens.

Clinical and laboratory monitoring are important to identify both drug toxicity (see Table 3.26) and therapeutic failure indicating disease progression. In the absence of definitive information, the combination of zidovudine and didanosine also may be used to treat children with more advanced disease (ie, in Table 3.22, Category C and immunologic categories 2 and 3). Other nucleoside analog combinations (eg, zidovudine and lamivudine, didanosine and stavudine, or lamivudine and stavudine) may be used, but published data regarding their efficacy in patients with pediatric AIDS are not available. Preliminary data in adults receiving triple drug regimens (ie, zidovudine, lamivudine and a protease inhibitor [eg, ritonavir and indinavir]) have demonstrated a sustained and marked decline in circulating viral concentration (load). As further data accrue on the safety, dosing, and effectiveness of protease inhibitor drugs in children, these agents may prove to enhance the effectiveness in children of antiretroviral drug regimens.

Changing antiretroviral therapy should be considered if (1) the current therapy failed (ie, disease progression occurs); (2) the patient develops a toxic reaction or intolerance to the drug; or (3) if new data prove that the given therapy is suboptimal for the patient's condition. When considering a change in therapy, the reason for the change (ie, failure, intolerance, or suboptimal therapy), the patient's clinical condition (ie, clinical, immunological, and virological status), and concomitant medications (which may interact with certain antiretroviral drugs) should be considered. Consultation with a pediatric subspecialist who has extensive experience in the care of HIV-infected children is strongly recommended.

Other new antiretroviral drugs, immunomodulators, and vaccines for therapeutic use are under evaluation. Further information on therapeutic trials in HIV-infected children can be obtained from the Pediatric Clinical Trials Group.*

The value of immune globulin intravenous (IGIV) in children with HIV infection has been evaluated in several trials. The Working Group on Antiretroviral Therapy has recommended routine IGIV therapy in combination with an antiviral agent for children with humoral immunodeficiency including (1) hypogammaglobulinemia (IgG less than 250 mg/dL); (2) recurrent, serious bacterial infections (defined as two or more serious bacterial infections such as bacteremia, meningitis, or pneumonia in a 1-year period); (3) children who fail to form antibodies to common antigens; and/ or (4) children living in areas where measles is highly prevalent who have not developed an antibody response after two doses (1 month or more apart) of MMR.† The

---

* See Directory of Telephone Numbers, p 667.

† Working Group on Antiretroviral Therapy: National Pediatric HIV Resource Center. Antiretroviral therapy and medical management of the human immunodeficiency virus-infected child. *Pediatr Infect Dis J.* 1993;12:513-522.

Table 3.26. Summary of Incidence of Adverse Events From Antiretroviral Drugs in Children*

Drug Name	Hematologic	Hepatic	Pancreatic	Neurologic	Comments
Zidovudine	>20%	5%–10%	Rare	0%–10%	Anemia, granulocytopenia, increased alanine aminotransferase concentrations are most common. Macrocytosis occurs in nearly 100% of recipients. Nausea, vomiting, xerostomia, headache, malaise, myositis, and lactic acidosis also occur.
Didanosine	1%–5%	13%	5%–17%	10%–34%	Pancreatitis and peripheral neuropathy are most common. Retinitis, diarrhea, and nausea also occur.
Zalcitabine	0%–10%	5%	<1%	15%–30%	Peripheral neuropathy is most common. Mouth sores, dysphagia, abdominal pain, rash, and headache also occur. Pancreatitis risk is 3% if prior pancreatitis.
Stavudine	Minimal	10%	<1%	15%–20%	Peripheral neuropathy is most common. Nausea, vomiting, abdominal pain, diarrhea, and pancreatitis can occur. Sleep disorders, increased energy, and mania also have been observed.
Lamivudine†	22%	4%	15%	13%	These incidences are for patients with normal baseline laboratory test results, receiving lamivudine alone. With prior abnormalities, incidences are as follows: decreased leukocyte count, 40%; anemia, 24%; decreased platelets, 25%; and increased serum amylase, 23%. Gastrointestinal symptoms, headache, and fatigue occur.
Saquinavir‡	Minimal	Minimal	Minimal	5%–8%	Increased creatine phosphokinase concentrations, 7%–10%, occur when given in combination with zidovudine or zalcitabine. Nausea, vomiting, and diarrhea occur in 1%–3% of cases. Fatigue, rash, and hemolytic anemia have been observed.
Indinavir‡	Minimal	3%–5%	2%–4%	5%–8%	Nephrolithiasis occurs in 4%; hyperbilirubinemia in 10%; abdominal pain in 10%; and nausea in 10%. Some drug interactions have been reported. Drinking liberal quantities of water to avoid nephrolithiasis is recommended.
Ritonavir‡	Minimal	3%–5%	Minimal	5%–7%	Increased creatine phosphokinase concentrations in 7%; nausea in 40%–50%; vomiting in 20%; diarrhea in 15%; and anorexia in 7% occur. Multiple drug interactions have been observed.

* Modified from Havens PL, Waters DA, Cuene BA, McIntosh K, Yogev R. Caring for infants, children, adolescents and families with HIV infection. *Wisconsin State Guide*, 1995.

† Incidence is based on studies of very few pediatric patients, many with late-stage infection which may predispose to complications of therapy.

‡ Incidence is based on studies of adult patients. Virtually no data are available in pediatric patients.

dose of IGIV is 400 mg/kg per dose given every 4 weeks. Immune globulin intravenous may also be useful in the treatment of HIV-associated thrombocytopenia in a dose of 500 to 1000 mg/kg per day for 3 to 5 days. In addition, children with bronchiectasis despite treatment with the standard medical regimen of cyclic antibiotics and aggressive respiratory therapy may benefit from adjunctive IGIV therapy at 600 mg/kg per dose, given monthly.

Early diagnosis and aggressive treatment of opportunistic infections may prolong survival. Since *Pneumocystis carinii* pneumonia (PCP) can be an early complication of perinatally acquired HIV infection and mortality is high, chemoprophylaxis should be given to HIV-exposed children at risk for PCP (see *Pneumocystis carinii* Infections, p 421). For infants younger than 1 year with possible or proven HIV infection, PCP prophylaxis should be administered beginning at 4 to 6 weeks of age and continued for the first year of life unless HIV infection is reasonably excluded by two negative HIV diagnostic tests (ie, HIV culture or PCR). The need for PCP prophylaxis in HIV-infected children 1 year of age and older is determined by CD4+ T-lymphocyte counts (see *Pneumocystis carinii* Infections, p 419).

Chemoprophylaxis also may be warranted for *Mycobacterium avium* complex (MAC) infections (see Diseases Caused By Nontuberculous Mycobacteria, p 563), and possibly other opportunistic infections such as cytomegalovirus and disease and toxoplasmic encephalitis.*

Immunization Recommendations (see also Immunodeficient and Immunosuppressed Children, p 50, and Table 3.27, p 294).

Children With Symptomatic HIV Infection. In general, live-virus (eg, oral poliovirus, varicella) vaccines and live-bacterial (eg, bacillus Calmette-Guerin) vaccines should not be given to patients with AIDS or other clinical manifestations of HIV infection indicative of immunosuppression. Measles-mumps-rubella (MMR) vaccine in patients who are not severely immunocompromised is an exception. Children receiving IGIV prophylaxis may not respond to MMR vaccine (see Measles, p 352). Other routinely recommended vaccines, ie, DTaP (or DTP), hepatitis B, *Haemophilus influenzae* type b conjugate, and inactivated poliovirus (IPV), should be given according to the usual immunization schedule (see Fig 1.1, p 18, and Table 1.3, p 20). Pneumococcal vaccine at 2 years of age and yearly influenza vaccination beginning at age 6 months also are recommended.

As the result of the occurrence of severe measles in symptomatic HIV-infected children and the lack of reported serious or unusual reactions to immunization with MMR, measles immunization (given as MMR) of HIV-infected children is recommended unless they are severely immunocompromised. Vaccine should be given at 12 months of age in order to enhance the likelihood of an immune response, ie, before deterioration of the immune system, if possible. The second dose may be administered as soon as 1 month (4 weeks) later in an attempt to induce seroconversion as early as possible. If the risk of exposure to measles is increased, such as during an outbreak, vaccination at an earlier age, such as at 6 to 9 months, is indicated (see Measles, p 355).

---

* See Centers for Disease Control and Prevention. USPHS/IDSA guidelines for the prevention of opportunistic infections in persons infected with human immunodeficiency virus: a summary. *MMWR.* 1995;44(No. RR-8):1-34.

Table 3.27. Recommendations for Routine Immunization of HIV-Infected Children in the United States*

Vaccines[†]	Known Asymptomatic HIV Infection	Symptomatic HIV Infection
Hepatitis B	Yes	Yes
DTaP (or DTP)	Yes	Yes
IPV[‡]	Yes	Yes
MMR	Yes	Yes[§]
Hib	Yes	Yes
Pneumococcal[‖]	Yes	Yes
Influenza[¶]	Yes	Yes
Varicella[#]	No	No

* See Fig 1.1 (p 18) and disease-specific chapters for age at which specific vaccines are indicated.
† DTP indicates diphtheria and tetanus toxoids and pertussis vaccine; DTaP, diphtheria and tetanus toxoids acellular pertussis vaccine; IPV, inactivated poliovirus vaccine; MMR, live-virus measles, mumps, and rubella; Hib, *Haemophilus influenzae* type b conjugate.
‡ Only inactivated polio vaccine (IPV) should be used for HIV-infected children, HIV-exposed infants whose status is indeterminate and household contacts of HIV-infected persons.
§ **Severely immunocompromised HIV-infected children should not receive MMR vaccine (see text).**
‖ Pneumococcal vaccine should be administered at 2 years of age to all HIV-infected children. Children who are older than 2 years of age should receive pneumococcal vaccine at the time of diagnosis. Revaccination after 3 to 5 years is recommended in either circumstance.
¶ Influenza vaccine should be provided each fall and repeated annually for HIV-exposed infants 6 months of age and older, HIV-infected children, and adolescents, and for household contacts of HIV-infected persons.
# Varicella vaccine is not currently indicated for HIV-exposed or HIV-infected persons, but studies are in progress to determine safety and possible indication.

Based on the case report of HIV-infected adolescents with severe immunocompromise who developed severe pneumonitis associated with measles vaccine virus, MMR vaccine is contraindicated in severely immunocompromised (as defined in Table 3.22) persons with HIV infection.

In general, children with symptomatic HIV infection have poor immunologic responses to vaccines. Hence, such children, when exposed to a vaccine-preventable disease such as measles or tetanus, should be considered susceptible regardless of the history of vaccination, and should receive, if indicated, passive immunoprophylaxis (see Passive Immunization of Children With HIV Infection, p 295). Immune globulin (IG) also should be given to any unimmunized household member who is exposed to measles infection.

Children With Asymptomatic HIV Infection. Children with asymptomatic HIV infection should receive DTaP or DTP, IPV, *Haemophilus influenzae* type b conjugate, hepatitis B, IPV, and MMR vaccines, according to the usual immunization schedules (see Fig 1.1, p 18 and Table 1.3, p 20). Although oral poliovirus vaccine (OPV) has been given to these patients without adverse effect, IPV is recommended because both the child and family members may be immunosuppressed as the result of HIV infection and, therefore, may be at risk for vaccine-associated paralytic poliomyelitis.

Varicella vaccine is currently contraindicated in persons with known HIV infection, regardless of the presence or absence of symptoms (see Varicella-Zoster Infections, p 583). The only exception is participants in studies to assess the safety and efficacy of varicella vaccine in HIV-infected persons.

Pneumococcal vaccination is indicated for HIV-infected children 2 years and older as they are at increased risk of invasive pneumococcal infection. Revaccination after 3 to 5 years is recommended. Yearly influenza vaccination is indicated for HIV-infected children 6 months of age or older.

In the United States and in areas of low prevalence of tuberculosis, BCG is not recommended. However, in developing countries where the prevalence of tuberculosis is high, the World Health Organization recommends that BCG should be given to all infants at birth if they are asymptomatic, regardless of maternal HIV infection.

Seronegative Children Residing in the Household of a Patient With Symptomatic HIV Infection. In a household with an adult or child immunocompromised as the result of HIV infection, seronegative as well as seropositive children should receive IPV vaccine because the live polioviruses in OPV can be excreted and transmitted to immunosuppressed contacts. MMR may be given because these vaccine viruses are not transmitted. To reduce the risk of transmission of influenza to patients with symptomatic HIV infection, yearly influenza vaccination is indicated for their household contacts (see Influenza, p 307).

Although person-to-person transmission of the varicella vaccine virus has been reported rarely, varicella vaccination of siblings and susceptible adult caregivers of patients with HIV infection is strongly encouraged to prevent acquisition of the wild-type varicella-zoster infection, which can cause severe disease in immunocompromised hosts.

Passive Immunization of Children With HIV Infection.
- **Measles** (see Measles, p 344). Symptomatic HIV-infected children who are exposed to measles should receive immune globulin (IG) prophylaxis (0.5 mL/kg, maximum 15 mL), regardless of vaccination status. Exposed, asymptomatic HIV-infected patients who are susceptible should also receive IG; the recommended dose is 0.25 mL/kg. Children who have received IGIV within 3 weeks of exposure do not require additional passive immunization.
- **Tetanus.** In the management of wounds classified as tetanus prone (see Tetanus, p 518, and Table 3.58, p 520), children with HIV infection should receive tetanus immune globulin (TIG) regardless of vaccination status.
- **Varicella.** Children infected with HIV who are exposed to varicella or zoster and who are susceptible should receive Varicella-Zoster Immune Globulin (VZIG) (see Varicella-Zoster Infections, p 573). Children who have received IGIV or VZIG within 3 weeks of exposure do not require additional passive immunization.

ISOLATION OF THE HOSPITALIZED PATIENT: Standard precautions should be followed scrupulously by all hospital personnel. The risk to health care personnel of acquiring HIV infection from a patient is minimal, even after accidental exposure from a needle stick injury (see Epidemiology). Every effort, nevertheless, should be made to avoid exposures to blood and other body fluids that could contain HIV.

CONTROL MEASURES:

Reduction of Perinatal HIV Transmission. * Zidovudine therapy of selected HIV-infected pregnant women and their newborns reduces by approximately two-thirds the risk of perinatal transmission. The treatment regimen demonstrated to be effective in the AIDS Clinical Trials Group Protocol 076 is oral administration of zidovudine to pregnant women beginning at 14 to 34 weeks' gestation and continuing throughout pregnancy, intravenous administration of zidovudine during labor until delivery (ie, intrapartum), and oral administration of zidovudine to the newborn for the first 6 weeks of life (see Table 3.28). Women for whom this protocol has been established to be effective are those who are not otherwise receiving antiretroviral therapy, do not have clinical indications for therapy, and have peripheral CD4+ T-lymphocyte counts of 200 cells/μL or greater at the time zidovudine is begun (ie, between 14 and 34 weeks of gestation).

Prophylaxis is recommended for women who meet these aforementioned criteria. In addition, zidovudine prophylaxis should be offered to HIV-infected pregnant women whose gestation is beyond 34 weeks and to newborns whose mothers did not receive zidovudine, because it may still be effective in reducing the transmission rate. The pregnant woman and her health care provider should consider the possible benefits and risks of such therapy in the absence of efficacy data for the specific clinical circumstance.

Breastfeeding (see also Human Milk, p 73). Transmission of HIV by breastfeeding, especially from mothers who acquire infection during the postpartum period, has been demonstrated. In the United States, where safe and alternative sources of feeding are readily available and affordable, HIV-infected women should be counseled not to breastfeed their infants or donate to milk banks. The World Health Organization has recommended that mothers residing in areas where infectious disease and malnutrition are an important cause of mortality early in life should be advised to breastfeed their infants regardless of the mother's HIV serologic status. The Academy guidelines for women in the United States are as follows[†]:

- Women and their health care providers need to be aware of the potential risk of transmission of HIV infection to infants during pregnancy and in the peripartum period, as well as through human milk.
- Documented, routine HIV education and routine testing with consent of all women seeking prenatal care are strongly recommended in order that each woman knows her HIV status and the methods available both to prevent the

---

* For further information, see Centers for Disease Control and Prevention. Recommendations for the use of zidovudine to reduce perinatal transmission of human immunodeficiency virus. *MMWR.* 1994; 43(No. RR-11):1-20; Connor EM, Mofenson LM. Zidovudine for the reduction of perinatal human immunodeficiency virus transmission: Pediatric AIDS Clinical Trials Group Protocol 076—results and recommendations. *Pediatr Infect Dis J.* 1995;14:536-541; and American Academy of Pediatrics, Provisional Committee on Pediatric AIDS. Perinatal human immunodeficiency virus testing. *Pediatrics.* 1995;95:303-307.

† American Academy of Pediatrics, Committee on Pediatric AIDS. Human milk, breast-feeding, and transmission of human immunodeficiency virus in the United States. *Pediatrics* 1995;96:977-979.

Table 3.28. **Zidovudine Regimen for the Reduction of Perinatal Transmission of HIV***

Period of Time	Route	Dosage
During pregnancy, initiate at 14 and 34 wk of gestation	Oral	100 mg 5 times a day[†]
During labor and delivery	Intravenous	2 mg/kg during the first hour, then 1 mg/kg/h until delivery
For the newborn, beginning 8–12 h after birth until 6 wk of age	Oral	2 mg/kg 4 times a day

* AIDS Clinical Trials Group Protocol (Centers for Disease Control and Prevention). Recommendations for the use of zidovudine to reduce perinatal transmission of human immunodeficiency virus. *MMWR.* 1994;43(No. RR-11):1-20.
† Some experts recommend 200 mg three times a day.

acquisition and transmission of HIV and to determine whether breastfeeding is appropriate.

- At the time of delivery, provision of education about HIV and testing with consent of all women whose HIV status during this pregnancy is unknown are strongly recommended. Knowledge of the woman's HIV status assists in counseling on breastfeeding and helps each woman understand the benefits to herself and her infant of knowing her serostatus and the behaviors that would decrease the likelihood of acquisition and transmission of HIV.
- Women who are known to be HIV-infected must be counseled not to breast-feed or provide their milk for the nutrition of their own or other infants.
- In general, women who are known to be HIV-seronegative should be encouraged to breastfeed. However, women who are HIV-seronegative but at particularly high risk of seroconversion (eg, injection drug users and sexual partners of known HIV-positive persons or active drug users) should be educated about HIV with an individualized recommendation concerning the appropriateness of breastfeeding. In addition, during the perinatal period, information should be provided on the potential risk of transmitting HIV through human milk and about methods to reduce the risk of acquiring HIV infection.
- Each woman whose HIV status is unknown should be informed of the potential for HIV-infected women to transmit HIV during the peripartum period and through human milk and the potential benefits to her and her infant of knowing her HIV status and how HIV is acquired and transmitted. The health care provider needs to make an individualized recommendation to assist the woman in deciding whether to breastfeed.
- Neonatal intensive care units should develop policies that are consistent with these recommendations for the use of expressed human milk for neonates. Current standards of the Occupational Safety and Health Administration (OSHA) do not require gloves for the routine handling of expressed human milk. Gloves, however, should be worn by health care workers in situations

where exposure to breast milk might be frequent or prolonged, such as in milk banking.

- Human milk banks should follow the guidelines developed by the United States Public Health Service, which includes screening all donors for HIV infection and assessing risk factors that predispose to infection, as well as pasteurization of all milk specimens.

Adolescent Education. Adolescents are at special risk for HIV infection; they should be educated about this disease and have access to HIV testing and knowledge of their serostatus. Particular efforts should be targeted for those adolescents with known risk factors for the acquisition of HIV infection. Informed consent for either testing or the release of information regarding serostatus is necessary. Decisions regarding the disclosure of HIV status to a sexual partner without the consent of the patient should be based on several factors, including whether the partner has a reasonable cause to suspect the risk and to take precautions without specific warning, the likelihood that the partner is at risk, relevant law that may prohibit or require such disclosure, and the possible effects of such disclosure on future relationships.

Specific Academy recommendations for pediatricians caring for adolescents are as follows*:

- Information regarding HIV infection and AIDS should be regarded as an important component of the anticipatory guidance provided by pediatricians to their adolescent patients. This guidance should include information about transmission, implications of infection, and strategies for prevention including abstinence from behaviors that place adolescents at risk and safer sex practices for those who decide to be sexually active.
- Adolescents should be considered potentially at risk for HIV infection and should be offered educational and counseling services. Diagnostic testing should be available and offered. Parental involvement in adolescent health care is a desirable goal. The consent of the adolescent alone, however, should be sufficient to provide evaluation and treatment for suspected or confirmed HIV infection.
- The maintenance of confidentiality regarding HIV status is of great importance. Respecting this confidentiality, the pediatrician should use all reasonable means to persuade an infected adolescent to inform his or her sexual partner(s) on a voluntary basis. Involuntary disclosure is a complex question that should be decided on the basis of local law, the relationship between the physician and the patient, the relationship of the physician to the partner, and the degree of perceived risk to the unsuspecting sexual partner.
- All sexually active adolescents should be counseled about the correct and consistent use of condoms to reduce the risk of infection (see Sexually Transmitted Diseases, p 108).

School Attendance and Education of Children With HIV Infection. In the absence of blood exposure, HIV infection is not acquired through the types of contact that usually occur in a school setting, including contact with saliva or tears. Hence, children with HIV infection should not be excluded from school for the protection of

---

* For further information, see American Academy of Pediatrics, Task Force on Pediatric AIDS. Adolescents and human immunodeficiency virus infection: the role of the pediatrician in prevention and intervention. *Pediatrics.* 1993;92:626-630.

other children or personnel. Specific recommendations concerning school attendance of children and adolescents with HIV infection are the following:

- Most school-age children and adolescents infected with HIV should be allowed to attend school without restrictions, provided the child's physician gives approval.
- The need for a more restricted school environment for some infected children should be evaluated on a case-by-case basis with consideration of conditions that may pose an increased risk to others, such as aggressive biting behavior or the presence of exudative, weeping skin lesions that cannot be covered.
- Only the child's parents, other guardians, and physician have an absolute need to know that the child is HIV-infected. The number of personnel aware of the child's condition should be kept to the minimum needed to ensure proper care of the child. The family has the right to inform the school. Persons involved in the care and education of an infected student must respect the student's right to privacy.
- All schools should adopt routine procedures for handling blood or blood-contaminated fluids, including the disposal of sanitary napkins, regardless of whether students with HIV infection are known to be in attendance. School health care workers, teachers, administrators, and other employees should be educated about procedures (see Housekeeping Procedures for Blood and Body Fluids, p 300).
- Children infected with HIV develop progressive immunodeficiency, which increases their risk of experiencing severe complications from infections such as varicella, tuberculosis, measles, cytomegalovirus, and herpes simplex virus. The child's physician should regularly assess the risk of an unrestricted environment on the health of the HIV-infected student, including evaluation of possible contagious diseases in the school (eg, measles, varicella, tuberculosis).
- Routine screening of schoolchildren for HIV infection is not recommended.

As the life expectancy of HIV-infected children and adolescents increases, the school population of children and adolescents with this disease also will increase. An understanding of the effect of chronic illness and the recognition of neurodevelopmental problems in these children are essential to provide appropriate educational programs. The Academy recommendations regarding the education of children with HIV infection are as follows*:

- All children with HIV infection should receive an appropriate education that is adapted to their evolving special needs. The spectrum of needs differs with the stage of the disease.
- HIV infection should be treated like other chronic illnesses that require special education and other related services.
- Continuity of education must be assured whether at school or at home.
- Because of the stigmata associated with this disease, maintaining confidentiality is essential. Disclosures of information should be only with the informed consent of the parents or legal guardians and age-appropriate assent of the student.

---

* For further information, see American Academy of Pediatrics, Task Force on Pediatric AIDS. Education of children with human immunodeficiency virus infection. *Pediatrics.* 1991;88:645-648.

Child Care and Foster Care*. Current Academy recommendations are as follows[†]:

- No reason exists to restrict foster care or adoptive placement of children who have HIV infection to protect the health of other family members. The risk of transmission of HIV infection in family environments is negligible.
- No need exists to restrict the placement of HIV-infected children in child care settings to protect personnel or other children because the risk of transmission of HIV in these settings is negligible.
- Child care personnel need not be informed of the HIV status of a child to protect the health of caregivers or other children in the child care environment. In some jurisdictions, the child's diagnosis cannot be divulged without the written consent of the parent or legal guardian. Parents may choose to inform the child care provider of the child's diagnosis in order to support a request that the caregiver observe the child closely for signs of illness that may require medical attention and assist the parents with the child's special emotional and social needs.
- The recommended standard precautions should be followed in all child care settings when blood or bloody fluids are handled to minimize the possibility of transmission of any blood-borne disease (see Housekeeping Procedures for Blood and Body Fluids, below).
- All preschool child care programs routinely should inform all families whenever a highly contagious illness, such as varicella or measles, occurs in any child in that setting. This process will help families protect their immunodeficient children.
- To facilitate foster care or adoptive placement, courts should adopt methods for rapid processing of court orders to allow HIV testing of infants and young children whenever such testing would promote placement. Placement would be promoted most clearly when such court-ordered testing is pursued in areas of high seroprevalence or when the child comes from a high-risk setting.

Adults With HIV Infection Working in Child Care or Schools. Asymptomatic HIV-infected adults may care for children in school or child care settings provided that they do not have exudative skin lesions or other conditions that would allow contact with their body fluids. No data indicate that HIV-infected adults have transmitted HIV in the course of normal child care or school responsibilities.

Adults with symptomatic HIV infection are immunocompromised and at increased risk from infectious diseases of young children. They should consult their physicians regarding the safety of their continuing work.

Housekeeping Procedures for Blood and Body Fluids. In general, routine housekeeping procedures using a commercially available cleaner (detergents, disinfectant-detergents, or chemical germicides) compatible with most surfaces are satisfactory for cleaning spills of vomitus, urine, and feces. Nasal secretions can be removed with tissues and discarded in routine waste containers. For spills involving blood or other body fluids: organic material should be removed, then the surface disinfected with freshly diluted bleach (ie, 1:10 to 1:100). A 1:64 dilution is ¼ cup bleach diluted in

---

[*] For additional discussion of recommendations for child care, see Children in Out-of-Home Child Care, p 80.

[†] Adapted from American Academy of Pediatrics, Task Force on Pediatric AIDS. Guidelines for human immunodeficiency virus (HIV)-infected children and their foster families. *Pediatrics.* 1992;89:681-683.

1 gallon (16 cups) of water. Reusable rubber gloves should be used for cleaning large spills to avoid contamination of the hands of the person cleaning the spill, but gloves are not essential for cleaning small amounts of blood that can be contained easily by the material used for cleaning. Persons involved in cleaning contaminated surfaces should avoid exposure of open skin lesions or mucous membranes to blood or bloody fluids. Whenever possible, disposable towels or tissues should be used and properly discarded, and mops should be rinsed in the disinfectant. After clean-up and after removal of gloves, hands should be washed thoroughly with soap and water.

Management and Counseling of Families. * Infection acquired by children before or during birth is a disease of the family. Serologic screening of siblings and parents is recommended. In each case, the physician needs to provide education and ongoing counseling regarding HIV and its transmission, and to outline precautions to be taken within the household and the community to prevent spread of this virus.

Infected women need to be made aware of the risk of having an infected child if they become pregnant, and they should be referred for family planning counseling. Infected persons should not donate blood, plasma, sperm, organs, corneas, bone, other tissues, or breast milk.

The infected child should be taught good hygiene and behavior. How much he or she is told about the illness will depend on age and maturity. Older children and adolescents should be made aware that the disease can be transmitted sexually and should be provided with appropriate counseling. Most families are not willing to share the diagnosis with others because it can create social isolation. Feelings of guilt are common. Family members, including children, can become clinically depressed and require psychiatric counseling.

Sexual Abuse. After sexual abuse by a person with or at risk for HIV infection, the child should be tested serologically at the time of abuse and at 6 weeks, 3 months, and 6 months after sexual contact (see Sexual Abuse, p 112). If feasible, serologic evaluation of the abuser for HIV infection should be obtained. Counseling of the child and family needs to be provided.

Blood, Blood Components, and Clotting Factors. † Screening blood and plasma for HIV antibody has reduced dramatically the risk of infection through transfusion. Nevertheless, careful scrutiny of the requirements of each patient for blood, its components, or clotting factors is important.

Transmission of HIV through contaminated clotting-factor concentrates has been virtually eliminated in the United States. All plasma-derived factor VIII and factor IX concentrates currently available in the United States are manufactured from plasma screened for HIV antibody. Additionally, the concentrates are treated with heat or solvent/detergent for inactivation of HIV (as well as other agents including hepatitis B and hepatitis C viruses). Some concentrates also undergo monoclonal antibody purification. Cryoprecipitate from single-donor plasma is screened for anti-HIV antibody by testing the individual donor's plasma, but does not undergo any

---

* For further information, see Centers for Disease Control and Prevention. *HIV Counseling, Testing, and Referral Standards and Guidelines.* Atlanta, Ga: Dept of Health and Human Services, Public Health Service; 1994.

† For further information, see Centers for Disease Control and Prevention. US Public Health Service guidelines for testing and counseling blood and plasma donors for human immunodeficiency virus type 1 antigen. *MMWR.* 1996;45(No. RR-2):1-9.

process to inactivate HIV or other viruses. Patients with hemophilia should be managed in consultation with specialists familiar with current aspects of treatment, such as desmopressin for the treatment of persons with mild or moderate factor VIII deficiency. Recombinant factor replacement is now available.

HIV-Exposed Health Care Workers. A health care worker who has had a percutaneous or mucous membrane exposure to blood or bloody secretions from an HIV-seropositive patient should receive counseling and medical evaluation as soon as possible after the exposure. A baseline HIV antibody test should be performed and the HIV status of the blood source should be investigated. If the health care worker is seronegative, he or she should be retested 6 weeks, 3 months, and 6 months after exposure to determine whether transmission has occurred. Most exposed persons who have been infected will seroconvert during the first 3 months after exposure.

Current recommendations for postexposure prophylaxis (PEP) were issued by the US Public Health Service in 1996 and are provisional because they are based on limited data regarding the efficacy and toxicity of PEP and the risk for HIV infection after different types of exposure.* Since most exposed health care workers do not develop HIV infection, the potential toxicity of the prophylactic treatment should be considered carefully in relation to its potential benefits and workers counseled accordingly. These recommendations are as follows (also see Table 3.29):

- Chemoprophylaxis (ie, PEP) should be recommended to exposed workers after occupational exposures associated with the highest risk for HIV transmission (see Table 3.29). For exposures with a lower, but nonnegligible risk, PEP should be offered, balancing the lower risk against the use of drugs having uncertain efficacy and toxicity. For exposures with negligible risk, PEP is not justified. Exposed workers should be informed that (1) knowledge about the efficacy and toxicity of PEP is limited; (2) for agents other than zidovudine, data are limited regarding toxicity in persons without HIV infection or who are pregnant; and (3) any or all drugs for PEP may be declined by the exposed worker.

- At present, zidovudine should be considered for all PEP regimens because it is the only agent for which data support the efficacy of PEP in the clinical setting. Lamivudine usually should be added to zidovudine for increased antiretroviral activity and activity against many zidovudine-resistant strains. A protease inhibitor (preferably indinavir) should be added for exposures with the highest risk for HIV transmission (see Table 3.29). Adding a protease inhibitor also may be considered for lower risk exposures if zidovudine-resistant strains are likely, although whether the potential additional toxicity of a third drug is justified for lower risk exposures is uncertain. For HIV strains resistant to both zidovudine and lamivudine or resistant to a protease inhibitor, or if these drugs are contraindicated or poorly tolerated, the optimal PEP regimen is uncertain; and expert consultation is advised.†

---

* For further information, see Centers for Disease Control and Prevention. Update: Provisional Public Health Service recommendations for chemoprophylaxis after occupational exposure to HIV. *MMWR.* 1996;45:468-472.

† An HIV strain is more likely to be resistant to a specific antiretroviral agent if it is derived from a patient who has been exposed to the agent for a prolonged period of time (eg, 6 to 12 months or longer). In general, resistance develops more readily in persons with more advanced HIV infection (eg, CD4+ T-lymphocyte count of <200 cells/mm^3), reflecting the increasing rate of viral replication during later stages of the illness.

Table 3.29. Provisional Public Health Service Recommendations for Chemoprophylaxis After Occupational Exposure to HIV, by Type of Exposure and Source Material—1996*

Type of Exposure	Source Material[†]	Antiretroviral Prophylaxis[‡]	Antiretroviral Regimen[§]
Percutaneous	Blood[‖]		
	Highest risk	Recommend	Zidovudine plus lamivudine plus indinavir
	Increased risk	Recommend	Zidovudine plus lamivudine with or without indinavir[¶]
	No increased risk	Offer	Zidovudine plus lamivudine
	Fluid containing visible blood, other potentially infectious fluid,[#] or tissue	Offer	Zidovudine plus lamivudine
	Other body fluid (eg, urine)	Not offer	
Mucous membrane	Blood	Offer	Zidovudine plus lamivudine with or without indinavir[¶]
	Fluid containing visible blood, other potentially infectious fluid,[#] or tissue	Offer	Zidovudine with or without lamivudine
	Other body fluid (eg, urine)	Not offer	
Skin, increased risk**	Blood	Offer	Zidovudine plus lamivudine with or without indinavir[¶]
	Fluid containing visible blood, other potentially infectious fluid,[#] or tissue	Offer	Zidovudine with or without lamivudine
	Other body fluid (eg, urine)	Not offer	

* Centers for Disease Control and Prevention. Update: Provisional Public Health Service recommendations for chemoprophylaxis after exposure to HIV. *MMWR.* 1996;45:468-472.

† Any exposure to concentrated HIV (eg, in a research laboratory or production facility) is treated as percutaneous exposure to blood with highest risk.

‡ *Recommend*—Postexposure prophylaxis (PEP) should be recommended to the exposed worker with counseling. *Offer*—PEP should be offered to the exposed worker with counseling. *Not offer*—PEP should not be offered because it is not an occupational exposure to HIV.

§ Regimens for adults: zidovudine, 200 mg three times a day; lamivudine, 150 mg twice a day; indinavir, 800 mg three times a day (if indinavir is not available, ritonavir, 600 mg twice a day, or saquinavir, 600 mg three times a day, may be used). Prophylaxis is given for 4 weeks. For full prescribing information, see package inserts.

‖ *Highest risk*—Exposure that involves BOTH a larger volume of blood (eg, deep injury with large diameter hollow needle previously in source patient's vein or artery, especially involving an injection of source-patient's blood) AND blood containing a high titer of HIV (eg, source with acute retroviral illness or end-stage AIDS; viral load measurement may be considered, but its use in relation to PEP has not been evaluated). *Increased risk*—EITHER exposure to a larger volume of blood OR blood with a high titer of HIV. *No increased risk*—NEITHER exposure to larger volume of blood NOR blood with a high titer of HIV (eg, solid suture needle injury from source patient with asymptomatic HIV infection).

¶ Possible toxicity from this additional drug may not be warranted (see text).

Includes semen; vaginal secretions; cerebrospinal, synovial, pleural, peritoneal, pericardial, and amniotic fluids.

** For skin, risk is increased for exposures involving a high titer of HIV, prolonged contact, an extensive area, or an area in which skin integrity is visibly compromised. For skin exposures without increased risk, the risk for drug toxicity outweighs the benefit of PEP.

- Postexposure prophylaxis (PEP) should be initiated promptly, preferably within 1 to 2 hours after exposure. Although studies using animals suggest that PEP probably is not effective when started later than 24 to 36 hours after exposure, the interval after which no benefit exists from PEP for humans is undefined. Initiating therapy after a longer interval (eg, 1 to 2 weeks) may be considered for the highest risk exposures; even if infection is not prevented, early treatment of acute HIV infection may be beneficial. The optimal duration of PEP is unknown; because 4 weeks of zidovudine appeared protective, PEP probably should be administered 4 weeks, if tolerated.
- If the source patient or the patient's HIV status is unknown, initiating PEP should be decided on a case-by-case basis, based on the exposure risk and likelihood of HIV infection in known or possible source patients. If additional information becomes available, decisions about PEP can be modified.
- If PEP is used, drug-toxicity monitoring should include a complete blood count and renal and hepatic chemical function tests at baseline and 2 weeks after starting PEP. If subjective or objective toxicity is noted, dose reduction or drug substitution should be considered with expert consultation, and further diagnostic studies may be indicated.

HIV-Exposed Children. Although data on the efficacy of chemoprophylaxis in children exposed to HIV (except for perinatal exposure) are not available, these recommendations on postexposure prophylaxis for HIV-exposed health care workers are reasonable for the management of pediatric injuries (eg, from discarded needles). The exception is that if a decision is made to use a protease inhibitor, ritonavir (350 mg/M^2/dose given every 12 hours) is preferred for younger children because it is currently the only protease inhibitor available in a suspension formulation.

Reporting of Cases. Patients meeting the criteria for AIDS (see Tables 3.21 and 3.22) must be reported to the appropriate public health department. In many states, HIV infection also must be reported.

Hookworm Infections
(*Ancylostoma duodenale* and *Necator americanus*)

CLINICAL MANIFESTATIONS: After contact with contaminated soil, initial skin penetration of larvae, usually involving the feet, causes stinging or burning followed by pruritus and a papulovesicular rash persisting for 1 to 2 weeks. Pneumonitis associated with migrating larvae in this phase is uncommon and usually mild, except in severe infections. Disease after oral ingestion of infectious *Ancylostoma duodenale* larvae can present with pharyngeal itching, hoarseness, nausea, and vomiting shortly after ingestion. Colicky abdominal pain with diarrhea and marked eosinophilia can develop 29 to 38 days after exposure. Chronic infection is a common cause of hypochromic, microcytic anemia in persons living in tropical, developing countries, and severe infection can cause hypoproteinemia and edema secondary to blood loss. Cardiac decompensation occasionally develops in children with hemoglobin concentrations of less than 6 g/dL.

ETIOLOGY: Infection is caused by *Ancylostoma duodenale* and *Necator americanus*, two worms with similar life cycles.

EPIDEMIOLOGY: Humans are the major reservoir. Well-nourished, lightly infected individuals are often asymptomatic. Hookworms are prominent in rural, tropical, and subtropical areas where soil contamination with human feces is common. Larvae and eggs survive in loose, sandy, moist, shady, well-aerated, warm soil (optimal temperature 23° to 33°C). Although both worms are equally prevalent in many areas, *A duodenale* is the predominant species in Europe, the Mediterranean region, northern Asia, and the west coast of South America, and *N americanus* is predominant in the Western hemisphere, sub-Saharan Africa, southeast Asia, and a number of Pacific islands. Percutaneous infection occurs after exposure to infectious larvae. Peroral and possibly transmammary infection can occur with *A duodenale*. Infectious larvae are found in contaminated soil within 5 to 7 days, and can persist for weeks to months. Untreated infected patients who do not become reinfected can harbor worms for 5 to 15 years, but a reduction in worm burden of at least 70% generally occurs within 1 to 2 years.

The **incubation period**, the time from exposure to eggs in the stool (prepatent period), is 4 to 6 weeks.

DIAGNOSTIC TESTS: The microscopic demonstration of hookworm eggs in the feces is diagnostic. Adult worms or larvae are seen rarely. During the acute infection, eggs will not be present in the stool. A direct stool smear with potassium iodide saturated with iodine is adequate for the diagnosis of significant hookworm infection; light infections require concentration techniques. Quantification techniques are necessary to determine the clinical significance of infection (see Table 3.30).

TREATMENT: Mebendazole or pyrantel pamoate is the drug of choice. Albendazole is also effective. In children younger than 2 years, in whom experience with these drugs is limited, the risks and benefits of therapy should be considered before drug administration. In pregnancy, mebendazole is not recommended and pyrantel pamoate has not been adequately studied. Therefore, adequate protein and iron nutrition should be maintained throughout pregnancy and treatment is delayed until after delivery. A repeat stool examination, using a concentration technique, should be performed 2 weeks posttreatment, and, if positive, retreatment is indicated. Nutritional supplementation, including iron, is important when anemia is present. Severely affected children may require blood transfusion.

Table 3.30. Intensity of Infection (Beaver Technique)

Egg Count per mg of Stool	Clinical Significance
≥50 eggs	Massive infection
≥20 eggs	Anemia in well-nourished patients
≥5 eggs	Anemia in malnourished patients
<5 eggs	Minimal clinical significance

ISOLATION OF THE HOSPITALIZED PATIENT: Standard precautions are recommended.

CONTROL MEASURES: Sanitary disposal of feces to prevent contamination of the soil, particularly in endemic areas, is necessary but rarely accomplished. Treatment of all known infected patients and screening of high-risk groups (ie, children and agricultural workers) in endemic areas can help reduce environmental contamination. Wearing shoes is also helpful.

Human Herpesvirus 6 (Including Roseola)

CLINICAL MANIFESTATIONS: Major clinical manifestations of primary infection in children younger than 3 years of age are variable. They include roseola (exanthem subitum, sixth disease) in approximately 20% of cases, undifferentiated febrile illness without rash or localizing signs, and other acute febrile illnesses, often accompanied by cervical and postoccipital lymphadenopathy, gastrointestinal or respiratory signs, and inflamed tympanic membranes. Fever is characteristically high, lasting 3 to 7 days. In roseola, fever is followed by an erythematous maculopapular rash lasting hours to days. Seizures occur during the febrile period in approximately 10% to 15% of primary infections. A bulging anterior fontanelle and encephalopathy occur occasionally.

The virus persists and may reactivate subsequently. The clinical circumstances and manifestations of reactivation in healthy persons are currently unclear. Illness associated with reactivation has been described primarily in immunosuppressed hosts in whom manifestations, such as fever, hepatitis, bone marrow suppression, and pneumonia, occasionally have been reported.

ETIOLOGY: Human herpesvirus 6 (HHV-6) is a newly identified member of the family *Herpesviridae*, which contains a large, double-stranded DNA genome. Strains may be divided into two major groups, variants A and B. Nearly all primary infections in children appear to be caused by variant B strains.

EPIDEMIOLOGY: Humans are the only known natural hosts. Transmission to the infant most likely occurs via the asymptomatic shedding of persistent virus in the secretions of a family member, caregiver, or other close contact. During the febrile phase of primary infection, HHV-6 can be isolated from peripheral blood lymphocytes in which it may persist subsequently, as well as from other sites, including saliva and cerebrospinal fluid. In healthy individuals, isolation of the virus at any time after primary infection is rare, despite detectable viral persistence. The attack rate is highest in children between the ages of 6 and 24 months. Infection within the first few months of age also occurs, but is relatively uncommon before 3 months or after 3 years of age. Serum virus-specific maternal antibody is present uniformly in infants at birth and affords some protection. As maternal antibody declines during the first year of life, the rate of infection increases rapidly and almost all children are seropositive by 2 years of age. Infections occur throughout the year without a distinct seasonal pattern. Secondary cases rarely are identified, although occasional outbreaks of roseola have been reported.

The mean **incubation period**, based on experimental infection, is estimated to be approximately 9 to 10 days.

DIAGNOSTIC TESTS: The diagnosis of primary HHV-6 infection currently necessitates the use of research techniques to isolate the virus from peripheral blood as well as for demonstration of seroconversion. A fourfold rise in serum antibody alone does not necessarily indicate new infection, as a rise in the titer also may occur with reactivation and in association with other infections. Commercial assays for antibody and antigen detection are in development, but so far do not reliably differentiate between primary infection and viral persistence or reactivation.

TREATMENT: Supportive.

ISOLATION OF THE HOSPITALIZED PATIENT: Standard precautions are recommended.

CONTROL MEASURES: None.

Influenza

CLINICAL MANIFESTATIONS: Influenza is characterized by the sudden onset of fever, frequently with chills or rigors, headache, malaise, diffuse myalgia, and a dry cough. Subsequently, the respiratory signs of sore throat, nasal congestion, and cough become more prominent. Conjunctival infection, abdominal pain, nausea, and vomiting can be present. In some children, influenza can appear as a simple upper respiratory tract infection or as a febrile illness with few respiratory signs. In young infants, influenza can produce a sepsislike picture and occasionally cause croup or pneumonia. Acute myositis characterized by calf tenderness and refusal to walk may develop after several days of influenza, especially type B infection. Reye syndrome has been associated primarily with influenza B, but also with influenza A infection. Influenza can alter the metabolism of certain medications, especially theophylline, possibly resulting in the development of toxicity from high serum concentrations.

ETIOLOGY: Influenza viruses are orthomyxoviruses of three antigenic types (A, B, and C). Epidemic disease is caused by types A and B. Influenza A strains are subclassified by two antigens, hemagglutinin (H) and neuraminidase (N). Three immunologically distinct hemagglutinin subtypes (H1, H2, and H3) and two neuraminidases (N1 and N2) have been recognized as causing human infection. Specific antibodies to these various antigens are important determinants of immunity. Major changes in the predominant strain in either of these antigens, such as H1 to H2, are called antigenic shifts; minor variations within the same subtypes are called antigenic drifts. Antigenic shift has occurred only with influenza A, usually at intervals of 10 or more years. Antigenic drift, which occurs almost annually in both influenza A and B viruses, can result in susceptibility to infection with a type of influenza with which persons were previously infected or immunized.

EPIDEMIOLOGY: Influenza is spread from person to person by direct contact, large droplet infection, or articles recently contaminated by nasopharyngeal secretions. In some explosive outbreaks, airborne spread by small-particle aerosols has appeared to be an important mode of transmission. During an outbreak of influenza, the highest attack rates occur in school-age children. Secondary spread to adults and other children within the family is common. The attack rates depend in part on the immunity developed by previous experience (either by natural disease or immunization) with the circulating strain or a related strain. Antigenic shift or major drift in the circulating strain is most likely to produce widespread epidemics. In temperate climates, epidemics usually occur during the winter months, and within a community, peak within 2 weeks of onset and last 4 to 8 weeks or longer. In recent years, activity of two or three types of influenza virus in a community has been common and associated with a prolongation of the influenza season to 3 months or more. Influenza is highly contagious, especially among institutionalized populations. Patients are most infectious in the 24 hours before the onset of symptoms and during the period of peak symptoms. Viral shedding in the nasal secretions usually ceases within 7 days of the onset of illness, but it can last longer in young children and immunodeficient patients.

The impact of influenza on children is appreciable during interepidemic years as well as epidemic years in both healthy children and those with underlying high-risk conditions. Attack rates in healthy children recently have been estimated at 10% to 40% each year, and approximately 1% of these infections can result in hospitalization. The risk of lower respiratory tract disease complicating influenza infection, in children primarily pneumonia and bronchiolitis, has ranged from 0.2% to 25%. A wide spectrum of complications, such as Reye syndrome, myositis, and central nervous system (CNS) manifestations can occur. The risk of Reye syndrome, which occurs primarily in school-age children, has decreased in recent years. Respiratory viruses other than influenza (eg, respiratory syncytial virus and the parainfluenza viruses) more commonly produce life-threatening illness in young children than in adults, and, as a result, morbidity and mortality rates in children for influenza and the effect of control measures are more difficult to determine.

Excess rates of hospitalization have been documented for neonates with influenza or children who have sickle cell disease, bronchopulmonary dysplasia, asthma, cystic fibrosis, malignancies, diabetes, or chronic renal disease. Pulmonary complications such as bronchitis and pneumonia seem to be more common in these children. Influenza in neonates has been associated with considerable morbidity, including a sepsislike syndrome, apnea, and lower respiratory tract disease.

The **incubation period** is usually 1 to 3 days.

DIAGNOSTIC TESTS: Viral cultures, when performed, should be obtained during the first 72 hours of illness because the quantity of virus shed subsequently decreases rapidly. Nasopharyngeal secretions obtained by swab or aspirate should be placed in appropriate transport media for culture. After inoculation into eggs or cell culture, virus can usually be isolated within 2 to 6 days. The sensitivity of rapid diagnostic tests for identification of influenza antigen in nasopharyngeal specimens has been variable. Serologic diagnosis can be made retrospectively by a significant change in antibody titer between acute and convalescent sera, as determined by complement fixation, hemagglutination inhibition, neutralization, or enzyme immunoassay tests.

TREATMENT: Both amantadine and its closely related analogue rimantadine are approved by the Food and Drug Administration (FDA) for prophylaxis against influenza A infection in children and adults. Currently only amantadine is approved for treatment in children. Studies evaluating the efficacy of amantadine and rimantadine in children are limited, but they indicate that treatment with either drug diminished the severity of the signs and symptoms of influenza A infection when administered within 48 hours of the onset of illness. Amantadine and rimantadine are not effective against influenza B infections and are not FDA-approved for use in infants (ie, children younger than 1 year).

Influenza A therapy with amantadine or rimantadine should be considered for (1) patients in whom the amelioration of clinical symptoms may be particularly beneficial, such as those with underlying conditions that predispose them for to severe or complicated influenza infection; (2) otherwise healthy children with severe illness; and (3) those with special environmental, family, or social situations, such as examinations in school and athletic competitions. Influenza A virus may become resistant to amantadine and rimantadine after several days of treatment, but development of resistance during treatment has not affected the clinical benefits of therapy. Resistant virus has not been demonstrated to spread more easily or cause more serious disease than susceptible virus and does not persist in the population in the absence of antiviral drug therapy. Nevertheless, the epidemiologic implications of influenza A antiviral drug resistance are not yet clear, and any influenza A isolate obtained from a patient receiving amantadine or rimantadine should be reported to the Centers for Disease Control and Prevention (CDC) through the state health department, and the isolate should be submitted for antiviral testing.

If antiviral therapy is indicated, treatment should be started as soon as possible after the onset of symptoms and, in immunocompetent patients, continued for 2 to 5 days or for 24 to 48 hours after the person becomes asymptomatic. Immunocompromised patients may require a longer course of therapy. Little information is available on the use of amantadine or rimantadine in children younger than 1 year. The recommended dosages for amantadine and rimantadine in children are given in Table 3.31. Dosage should be reduced in patients with severe renal insufficiency. Either drug may cause CNS symptoms, which resolve with discontinuation of the drug. The incidence of CNS-related adverse events appears to be higher in amantadine recipients than in those receiving rimantadine. An increased incidence of convulsions has been reported in children with epilepsy who receive amantadine. Seizures or seizure-like activity also has been observed in a small number of patients while taking rimantadine who have a history of convulsions; however, the incidence has not been evaluated adequately.

Both influenza A and B viruses are sensitive in vitro to ribavirin. In placebo-controlled clinical trials of healthy, young adults with natural influenza A and B infections, therapy with a short course of aerosolized ribavirin has been associated with a modest shortening of clinical symptoms. Currently, however, ribavirin is not approved for the treatment of influenza infections.

Control of fever with acetaminophen or other appropriate antipyretic may be important in young children because the fever of influenza can precipitate febrile convulsions. **Children and teenagers with influenza should not receive salicylates because of the resulting increased risk of developing Reye syndrome.**

Table 3.31. Dosage Recommendations for Amantadine and Rimantadine*†‡

	Age		
	1–9	≥10	
		Weight <40 kg	Weight ≥ 40 kg
Treatment	5 mg/kg/d, maximum 150 mg/d, in 1 or 2 divided doses	5 mg/kg/d in 1 or 2 divided doses	200 mg/d in 1 or 2 divided doses
Prophylaxis	Dosages may be the same as those for treatment. An alternative and equally acceptable dosage is 100 mg/d for children weighing >20 kg and adults. For either regimen, the total daily dosage may be given in 1 or 2 divided doses.		

* Amantadine and rimantadine are not FDA-approved for use in children younger than 1 year.
† Rimantadine is FDA-approved for prophylaxis but not for treatment of children.
‡ Patients, including elderly persons, with any degree of renal insufficiency should be monitored for adverse effects, and the dosage reduced or the drug discontinued as necessary (see product label for further information).

ISOLATION OF THE HOSPITALIZED PATIENT*: For children hospitalized with influenza or an influenza-like illness, droplet precautions are recommended for the duration of the illness. Respiratory secretions should be considered infectious, and strict hand washing procedures should be used.

CONTROL MEASURES:

Influenza Vaccine. The current influenza vaccines produced in embryonated eggs are immunogenic, safe, and associated with minimal side effects. These multivalent vaccines contain different viral subtypes; their composition is periodically changed in anticipation of the expected prevalent influenza strains. The preparations currently in use include inactivated whole-virus vaccine prepared from the intact, purified virus particles; the subvirion vaccine prepared by the additional step of disrupting the lipid-containing membrane of the virus; and purified surface-antigen vaccine. Only the subvirion or purified surface-antigen vaccines, ie, those termed "split-virus" vaccines, should be administered to children younger than 13 years. The whole-virus vaccines are associated with higher rates of adverse effects in young children.

Immunogenicity in Children. In children with little previous experience with influenza, two doses of vaccine administered 1 month apart are necessary to produce a satisfactory antibody response (see Table 3.32, p 311). Children previously primed with a related strain of influenza by infection or vaccination exhibit almost uniformly a brisk antibody response to one dose of the vaccine.

Vaccine Efficacy. The impact of influenza immunization on acute respiratory illness is less likely to be evident in pediatric than adult populations because of the frequency of upper respiratory tract infections and influenza-like illness caused by other viral agents in young children. The efficacy of the currently available inactivated viral vaccines also has been difficult to assess because of yearly variation in the strains of the circulating viruses and their resulting variation in similarity to the antigens contained in the available vaccines. The protection in healthy subjects from

* In addition to standard precautions.

Table 3.32. **Schedule for Influenza Immunization***

Age	Recommended Vaccine[†]	Dose, mL[‡]	No. of Doses
6–35 mo	Split virus only	0.25	1–2[§]
3–8 y	Split virus only	0.5	1–2[§]
9–12 y	Split virus only	0.5	1
>12 y	Whole or split virus	0.5	1

* Vaccine is administered intramuscularly.
† Split-virus vaccine may be termed "split," "subvirion," or "purified surface-antigen" vaccine.
‡ Dosages are those recommended in recent years. Physicians should refer to the product circular each year to ensure that the appropriate dosage is given.
§ Two doses administered at least 1 month apart are recommended for children who are receiving influenza vaccine for the first time.

either the whole-virus or split-virus vaccines against homologous viral-type challenge is usually 70% to 80%, with a range of 50% to 95%. The duration of protection from vaccination is brief, usually presumed to be less than 1 year. Efficacy has not been evaluated in infants vaccinated in the first 6 months of life.

Special Considerations.

• In immunosuppressed children receiving chemotherapy, influenza immunization with a new vaccine antigen results in a sufficient immune response in only a minority of children. The optimal time to immunize children with malignancies who must undergo chemotherapy is 3 to 4 weeks after chemotherapy has been discontinued and the peripheral granulocyte and lymphocyte counts are greater than 1000/mm³. Children who are no longer receiving chemotherapy generally have high rates of seroconversion.

• Children with hemodynamically unstable cardiac disease constitute a large group of children potentially at high risk for complications of influenza. The immune response and safety of influenza vaccine in these children are comparable to those in healthy children.

• Corticosteroids administered for brief periods or every other day appear to have only a minimal effect on the serum antibody response to influenza vaccine. Brief or intermittent courses of high-dose corticosteroids, particularly in children with asthma who require frequent corticosteroid therapy, does not necessitate deferring administration of influenza vaccine. Prolonged administration of high doses of corticosteroids (ie, a dose equivalent to either 2 mg/kg or greater, or a total of 20 mg/d of prednisone), however, may impair antibody responses to other vaccines, particularly in unvaccinated or previously uninfected persons. Hence, influenza vaccination could be deferred temporarily during the time of receipt of high-dose corticosteroids, provided deferral does not compromise the likelihood of immunization before the start of the influenza season (see Vaccine Administration, p 8).

• Infants younger than 6 months with high-risk conditions, especially those with cardiopulmonary compromise, may have the same or greater risk as older children. Insufficient information, however, is available about the reactivity, immunogenicity, and efficacy of the influenza vaccines in infants during the first 6 months of life. The effect of influenza antigens in an inactivated vaccine on the infant's future immune response to influenza also is not established. Because rimantadine and amantadine are not licensed for use in young infants, immunization and chemoprophylaxis of adults who are in close contact with high-risk infants is an important means of their protection (see Recommendations for Influenza Immunization and for Chemoprophylaxis, p 314).

- Preliminary studies indicate that influenza vaccine may reduce the incidence of acute otitis media in children in child care centers. Before use of vaccine for this purpose can be recommended, further studies are necessary.

Recommendations for Influenza Immunization.

Targeted High-Risk Children and Adolescents. Yearly immunization, administered in the fall (see Vaccine Administration, p 313), is recommended for children 6 months of age and older with one or more specific risk factors. Data on the severity of influenza in several of these groups of children are limited. Infancy alone may be a risk factor for more severe infection, as children younger than 1 year have higher rates of hospitalization due to influenza than older children. On the basis of available data and knowledge of the pathophysiology of these disorders, children at risk who warrant immunization are those who have needed regular medical follow-up and/or hospitalization during the preceding year because of one or more of the following risk factors:

- Asthma and other chronic pulmonary diseases.
- Hemodynamically significant cardiac disease.
- Immunosuppressive disorders and therapy (see Special Considerations, p 311).
- HIV infection (see HIV Infection, p 279).
- Sickle cell anemia and other hemoglobinopathies.
- Diseases requiring long-term aspirin therapy, such as rheumatoid arthritis or Kawasaki disease which may increase the risk for development of Reye syndrome following influenza.

Other High-Risk Children and Adolescents. Children and adolescents who should be considered potentially at increased risk for complicated influenza illness and who may benefit from influenza immunization are those with one or more of the following conditions:

- Diabetes mellitus.
- Chronic renal disease.
- Chronic metabolic disease.
- Any underlying condition that marginally may compromise children, including young age, as previously noted, because even uncomplicated influenza can produce adverse effects on the course of an underlying disease.
- Pregnancy. Pregnant women with medical conditions that increase the risk of complications from influenza should receive influenza vaccine before the onset of the influenza season. Although increased mortality among pregnant women has not been observed except during the pandemics of 1918–1919 and 1957–1958, case reports and recent studies indicate that women in the second and third trimesters of pregnancy or early puerperium, even in the absence of other risk factors, are at increased risk of complications and hospitalization from influenza. As a result, the Advisory Committee on

Immunization Practices (ACIP) of the Centers for Disease Control and Prevention (CDC) recommends that influenza vaccination of all women who will be beyond 14 weeks of pregnancy or early puerperium during the influenza season.

Close Contacts of High-Risk Patients. Immunization and chemoprophylaxis of adults who are in close contact with high-risk children may be an important means of protection for these children, especially for infants younger than 6 months or other children for whom vaccination may not be appropriate or is contraindicated. In addition, immunization of pregnant women may be beneficial to their unborn infants because transplacentally acquired antibody appears to protect them from infection with influenza A virus. The following is recommended:

- Immunization of health care personnel in contact with pediatric patients should be encouraged.
- Household contacts, including siblings and primary caregivers of high-risk children, should be immunized.
- Children who are members of households with high-risk adults, including those with symptomatic HIV infection, should be immunized.

Foreign Travel. Persons traveling to foreign areas in which influenza outbreaks that are or may be occurring should be considered for vaccination because of the increased likelihood of exposure to influenza. The decision to vaccinate will depend on the person's destination, duration of travel, and risk of acquiring influenza (such as the season of the year and other factors) and the possible consequences.

Other Children. Vaccination should be considered for groups of individuals whose close contact facilitates rapid transmission and spread of infection that may result in disruption of routine activities, such as students in colleges, schools, and other institutions of learning, particularly those who reside in dormitories or who are members of athletic teams, and persons living in residential institutions.

Influenza vaccine may be administered to any healthy child or adolescent. The morbidity from influenza in healthy children can be appreciable, but currently routine immunization of all healthy children is not feasible.

Vaccine Administration. Influenza vaccine should be administered in the fall before the start of the influenza season at the time specified in the yearly recommendations of the CDC. The optimal time in recent years has been from the beginning of October through mid-November. However, persons may be vaccinated in September when the vaccine for the forthcoming influenza season becomes available. The recommended vaccine, dose, and schedule for different age groups are given in Table 3.32 (p 311).

Annual vaccination is recommended because of declining immunity in the year after vaccination, and in most years at least one of the antigens is changed to increase the antigenic similarity between the vaccine and circulating strains.

Influenza vaccine may be administered simultaneously (but at a separate site and with a different syringe) with other routine vaccinations in children, including pertussis vaccine (DTaP or DTP). Both influenza and whole-cell pertussis vaccines can cause fever; therefore acellular pertussis vaccine (DTaP) should be given when both need to be administered at the same time.

Reactions, Adverse Effects, and Contraindications. In children younger than 13 years of age, febrile reactions are infrequent, especially after split-virus vaccine administration. Fever occurs primarily 6 to 24 hours after vaccination in children younger than 24 months of age. For children older than 12 years and for adults, the side effects and immunogenicity of the whole- and split-virus vaccines are similar when used at the recommended doses (see Table 3.32, p 311). Local reactions are infrequent in children younger than 13 years. In children 13 years or older, local reactions occur in approximately 10% after immunization with either whole- or split-virus vaccine.

Unlike the 1976–1977 swine influenza vaccine, subsequent vaccines prepared from other influenza strains have not been associated clearly with an increased frequency of Guillain-Barré syndrome (GBS). Estimating the precise risk for a rare condition such as GBS, however, is difficult. During at least 1 year, a small increase may have occurred in the number of GBS cases in vaccinated persons 18 to 64 years of age, but not in those aged 65 years or older or those younger than 18 years; and no overall increase in frequency of GBS among vaccine recipients was observed. Even if GBS were a casually related adverse effect, the very low estimated risk of GBS is less than that of severe influenza that could be prevented by immunization. In addition, GBS has **not** been associated with influenza immunization of children.

Immunization of children who have asthma with the currently available influenza vaccines is not associated with a detectable increase in adverse reactions, such as bronchial hyperreactivity and leukocyte histamine release.

Children demonstrating severe anaphylactic reaction to chickens or egg protein can experience, on rare occasion, a similar type of reaction to killed influenza vaccines. Although influenza vaccine has been administered safely to such children after skin testing and even desensitization, they generally should not receive influenza vaccine because of their risk of reactions, the likely need for yearly vaccination, and the availability of chemoprophylaxis against influenza A infection.

Immunization of pregnant women is considered safe at any stage of pregnancy.

Chemoprophylaxis: An Alternative Method of Protecting Children Against Influenza.

Most studies demonstrating the efficacy of amantadine or rimantadine as a chemoprophylactic agent against influenza A infection have been performed in adults and have demonstrated an approximate 70% to 90% effectiveness in preventing illness from influenza A strains. Asymptomatic infection, nevertheless, may occur. Several studies in children have indicated a similar beneficial effect in diminishing the spread of influenza among institutionalized children and family members and in pediatric hospitals. Both drugs are FDA-approved for prophylaxis in children and adults. The usual recommended doses of rimantadine and amantadine for prophylaxis are the same as those for treatment. Studies have demonstrated, however, that a dose of 100 mg/d for prophylaxis in adults and in children weighing more than 20 kg is as effective as the recommended dose of 200 mg/d for treatment and may be associated with fewer side effects. This dosage of 100 mg/d, given in one or two divided doses, thus, is also acceptable. The prophylactic dosages for children are given in Table 3.31 (p 310).

Indications. Persons for whom chemoprophylaxis is or may be indicated are as follows:

- Children* and adolescents at high risk who were vaccinated after circulation of influenza A in the community has begun. Chemoprophylaxis can be beneficial during the interval before a vaccine response (2 weeks after the recommended vaccine schedule of one or two doses has been completed).
- Unimmunized persons providing care to high-risk individuals.
- Immunodeficient persons whose antibody response to vaccine is likely to be poor.
- Persons at high risk for whom vaccine is contraindicated, specifically those with anaphylactic hypersensitivity to egg protein who do not receive desensitization (see Reactions, Adverse Effects, and Contraindications, p 313).
- Chemoprophylaxis with amantadine or rimantadine also may be administered at the discretion of the physician and parent to any healthy child older than 1 year of age for whom the prevention of influenza is considered particularly desirable. These children also should be immunized.

Chemoprophylaxis should not be considered as a substitute for vaccination. Chemoprophylaxis in vaccinated persons does not interfere with the immune response to the vaccine and may provide additional protection.

Isosporiasis
(Isospora belli)

CLINICAL MANIFESTATIONS: Protracted watery diarrhea is the most common presenting symptom. Manifestations are similar to those caused by *Cryptosporidium* and include abdominal pain, anorexia, and weight loss. Infection can be life-threatening in immunocompromised patients, particularly those with HIV infection. Fever, malaise, vomiting, and headache have all been reported.

ETIOLOGY: *Isospora belli* is a coccidian protozoan.

EPIDEMIOLOGY: Humans are the only known host for *I belli*. The frequency of this parasite, especially in asymptomatic persons, is unknown. Infection is more common in tropical and subtropical climates than in temperate climates and in areas of poor sanitary conditions. Human infection probably occurs by the oral-fecal route. *Isospora belli* has been reported as an etiologic agent of travelers' diarrhea in visitors to endemic areas. Oocysts are resistant to most disinfectants and may remain viable for months in a cool, moist environment.

The **incubation period** is estimated to be 8 to 14 days, based on a small number of persons who had laboratory exposure to the organism.

DIAGNOSTIC TESTS: Demonstration of oocysts in feces or in duodenal aspirates or finding developmental stages of the parasite in biopsy specimens of the small intestine is diagnostic. Oocysts in stool can be distinguished by their size, which is 10 times larger than *Cryptosporidium*, and by their oval shape. Oocysts can be

---

* Use of amantadine and rimantadine in infants (ie, children younger than 1 year) has not been adequately evaluated and neither drug is FDA-approved for use in infants.

detected by a modified Kinyoun carbolfuchsin stain and by auramine-rhodamine stains. Concentration techniques may be needed prior to staining because organisms are often present in small numbers.

TREATMENT: Trimethoprim-sulfamethoxazole or pyrimethamine-sulfadoxine are effective. In HIV-infected patients who are allergic to sulfonamides, treatment of adults with pyrimethamine (50 to 75 mg/d), followed by daily prophylactic administration of pyrimethamine (25 mg/d) has been effective. Antimicrobial prophylaxis may be indicated in HIV-infected persons to prevent recurrent disease.

ISOLATION OF THE HOSPITALIZED PATIENT*: Enteric precautions are recommended, but the risk of nosocomial infection is unknown.

CONTROL MEASURES: None.

Kawasaki Disease

CLINICAL MANIFESTATIONS: Kawasaki disease is a febrile, exanthematous, multisystem illness in which the acute phase is self-limited. It occurs predominantly in children younger than 5 years of age. Within 3 days of the abrupt onset of fever, the other characteristic features of the illness usually appear, including (1) discrete bulbar conjunctival injection without exudate; (2) erythematous mouth and pharynx, strawberry tongue, and red, cracked lips; (3) a polymorphous generalized erythematous rash that can be morbilliform, maculopapular, scarlatiniform, or may resemble erythema multiforme; (4) changes in the peripheral extremities consisting of induration of the hands and feet with erythematous palms and soles; and (5) a usually solitary, frequently unilateral cervical lymph node enlarged to more than 1.5 cm in diameter. These early manifestations progress with drying, cracking, and fissuring of the lips, usually apparent by the sixth day of illness. Periungual desquamation and peeling of the palms and, to a lesser extent, soles, occur during the second to third week. For the diagnosis to be made, patients should have fever and at least four of these five features. Patients with fever and fewer than four of these manifestations, usually infants, can be diagnosed as having atypical Kawasaki disease when coronary artery disease is detected. Extreme irritability, severe abdominal pain, diarrhea, and vomiting are common associated features. Other findings include urethritis with sterile pyuria (70% of cases), hepatic dysfunction (40%), arthritis or arthralgias (35%), aseptic meningitis (25%), pericardial effusion or arrhythmias (20%), gallbladder hydrops (less than 10%), and carditis with congestive heart failure (less than 5%).

Without aspirin or intravenous immunoglobulin therapy, the mean duration of fever is 12 days. After the fever resolves, patients can remain anorectic or irritable for 2 to 3 weeks. During this subacute phase, the characteristic peripheral desquamation can occur, usually between days 10 and 20 of the illness. Recurrence (ie, second episodes) occur rarely.

---

* In addition to standard precautions.

Routine two-dimensional echocardiography or angiography demonstrates coronary aneurysm(s) in approximately 20% of untreated patients. Patients at increased risk for development of coronary aneurysms include males, infants (ie, younger than 12 months), those whose fever persists for more than 10 days, those with low serum albumin and/or hemoglobin concentrations, and those who manifest signs or symptoms of cardiac involvement (such as arrhythmias or pericardial effusion). Coronary aneurysms have been detected as early as 3 days after the onset of symptoms, but in most cases appear 1 to 2 weeks later. The peak prevalence of coronary aneurysms and coronary dilation is approximately 2 to 4 weeks after onset of disease; their appearance after more than 6 weeks is uncommon. Other arterial aneurysms (eg, iliac, femoral, renal, and axillary vessels) can occur. In addition to coronary artery disease, carditis can involve the pericardium, myocardium, or endocardium, and mitral and aortic regurgitation can develop. Carditis can occur at any time during the first 3 weeks of illness and generally resolves by 6 to 8 weeks.

In some children with mild coronary dilation, the coronary artery size returns to baseline by 8 weeks after the onset of disease. Although coronary aneurysms frequently regress to normal lumen size within 1 to 2 years, this process may be accompanied by coronary stenosis and aneurysm regression does not always result in a normal blood vessel.

The current mortality rate in the United States is less than 0.1%. Death results from myocardial infarction with coronary occlusion due to thrombosis or progressive stenosis. Seventy-five percent of fatalities occur within 6 weeks of the onset of symptoms, but myocardial infarction and sudden death can occur months to years after the acute episode. Long-term prognosis is unknown. Second episodes occur rarely in previously affected children. The vasculitis of Kawasaki disease may be a risk factor for subsequent atherosclerotic disease.

ETIOLOGY: The etiology is unknown. However, the epidemiology and clinical presentation suggest an infectious cause.

EPIDEMIOLOGY: Peak age of occurrence in the United States is between 18 and 24 months. Fifty percent of patients are younger than 2 years and 80% are younger than 5 years; children older than 8 years rarely have the disease. The male-to-female ratio is 1.6:1. The incidence is highest in Asians; 3000 to 3500 cases are estimated to occur annually in the United States. Kawasaki disease was first described in Japan, where a pattern of endemic occurrence with superimposed epidemic outbreaks has emerged. A similar pattern of steady or increasing endemic disease with sharply defined community-wide epidemics has been recognized in diverse locations in North America and Hawaii. Epidemics generally occur during the winter and spring at 2- to 3-year intervals. No evidence indicates person-to-person or common-source spread, although the incidence is higher in siblings of children with the disease.

The **incubation period** is unknown.

DIAGNOSTIC TESTS: No specific tests are available. The diagnosis is established by fulfillment of the clinical criteria (see Clinical Manifestations, p 316) and exclusion of other possible illnesses, including measles, streptococcal infections (ie, scarlet fever), viral and rickettsial exanthems, drug reactions (eg, Stevens-Johnson syndrome), staphylococcal scalded skin syndrome, toxic shock syndrome, juvenile rheumatoid arthritis, leptospirosis, and mercury poisoning.* An elevated sedimentation rate and serum C-reactive protein concentration during the first 2 weeks of illness and an elevated platelet count (greater than 450 000/mm³) after the 10th day of illness are common laboratory features. These values usually return to normal within 6 to 8 weeks.

TREATMENT: Management consists of supportive care, detection of coronary artery disease, and anti-inflammatory therapy. **Specific therapy should be initiated when the diagnosis is established or strongly suspected.** Specific recommendations are as follows:

Immune Globulin Intravenous (IGIV). High-dose IGIV therapy initiated within 10 days of the onset of fever in conjunction with aspirin decreases the prevalence of coronary artery dilation and aneurysms detected 2 and 7 weeks later in comparison to treatment with aspirin alone. Significant and rapid resolution of fever and other indicators of acute inflammation also have been demonstrated. Therapy with IGIV should be initiated as soon as possible; efficacy if initiated later than 10 days after onset of illness or after aneurysms have been detected has not been evaluated. Therapy with IGIV, however, should be considered for those patients diagnosed after day 10 who have manifestations of continuing inflammation (eg, fever and increased sedimentation rate) or of evolving coronary artery disease.

Dosage. The optimal therapeutic dose of IGIV is not known. A dosage schedule of 2 g/kg as a single dose, given during 10 to 12 hours, is recommended. Few complications occur from this regimen.

Retreatment. Approximately 10% of children with Kawasaki disease treated with IGIV may not respond to the initial dose and may experience persistent (for more than 48 to 72 hours) or recrudescent fever. Other clinical indications of inflammation, such as conjunctivitis and rash, also may persist or recur. If the diagnosis remains likely, retreatment with a second infusion of 2 g/kg, given during 10 to 12 hours, should be considered.

Aspirin. Aspirin usually is given initially in high dosage for its anti-inflammatory effect, and, subsequently, in low dosage to reduce the likelihood of spontaneous coronary thrombosis through its antiplatelet aggregation action. A dose of 80 to 100 mg/kg per day in four divided doses reduces the duration of fever if started during the first week of the illness. Monitoring of serum salicylate concentrations during high-dose therapy may be helpful in apparent nonresponders because gastrointestinal absorption is highly variable. The dosage of aspirin in the acute phase of the illness does not appear to affect the subsequent incidence of coronary artery aneurysms. After fever is controlled, the aspirin doses should be decreased. A suggested dose is 3 to 5 mg/kg per day in one dose. In patients with no coronary artery abnormalities detected on echocardiography, this regimen should be maintained for 6 to 8 weeks or until both the platelet count and erythrocyte sedimentation rate return to normal. Low-dose aspirin therapy should be continued indefinitely for those in whom coronary artery abnormalities are present. Because of the potential risk of Reye syndrome in patients with influenza or varicella receiving salicydates, parents of children receiv-

---

* For further information on the diagnosis of this disease, see the recommendations of the American Heart Association in Dajani AS, Taubert KA, Gerber MA, et al. Diagnosis and therapy of Kawasaki disease in children. *Circulation.* 1993;87:1776-1780.

ing aspirin should be instructed to contact their child's physician promptly if the child develops symptoms of or is exposed to either disease.

Cardiac Care. * An echocardiogram should be obtained early in the acute phase of the illness, approximately 3 weeks and 8 weeks after onset. **The care of patients with carditis should involve a cardiologist experienced in the management of patients with Kawasaki disease and in echocardiographic studies of coronary arteries in children.** Long-term management of patients with Kawasaki disease should be based on the degree of coronary artery involvement. Children must be examined repeatedly during the first 2 months to detect arrhythmias, congestive heart failure, valvular insufficiency, and myocarditis. In addition to prolonged low-dose aspirin therapy to suppress platelet aggregation in patients with persistent coronary artery abnormalities, some experts recommend 4 mg/kg per day of dipyridamole, given in three divided doses. Development of giant coronary artery aneurysms may require the addition of anticoagulant therapy to prevent thrombosis.

Subsequent Immunization. Measles vaccination in children who have received high-dose IGIV for treatment of Kawasaki disease should be deferred for 11 months after IGIV administration (see Measles, p 344). If the child's risk of exposure to measles is high, however, he or she should be vaccinated, then revaccinated at or after 11 months following the administration of IGIV unless serologic testing indicates successful immunization by the earlier dose. Varicella vaccine should not be given for at least 5 months after receipt of IGIV or other blood products (see Varicella-Zoster Infections, p 582). The schedule for subsequent administration of other childhood immunizations should not be interrupted. Yearly influenza vaccination is indicated in patients 6 months to 18 years of age who require long-term aspirin therapy because of the possible increased risk of development of Reye syndrome (see Influenza, p 307).

ISOLATION OF THE HOSPITALIZED PATIENT: Standard precautions are indicated.

CONTROL MEASURES: None.

Legionella pneumophila Infections

CLINICAL MANIFESTATIONS: Pneumonia (Legionnaires' disease) varies in severity from a mild to a severe, progressive infection, often with associated gastrointestinal tract, central nervous system, and/or renal manifestations. Respiratory failure and death can occur. In contrast, Pontiac fever is an abrupt-onset, self-limited, influenza-like illness without pneumonia.

ETIOLOGY: *Legionella* species are fastidious, aerobic bacilli that stain Gram-negative after recovery on artificial media. At least 18 different species have been implicated in human disease, but the majority of *Legionella* infections in the United States are caused by *L pneumophila* serogroup 1.

---

* For specific recommendations of the American Heart Association, see Dajani AS, Taubert KA, Takahashi M, et al. Guidelines for long-term management of patients with Kawasaki disease. *Circulation.* 1994;89:916-922.

EPIDEMIOLOGY: Legionnaires' disease is acquired through inhalation of aerosolized water contaminated with *Legionella*. Person-to-person transmission has not been demonstrated. More than 80% of cases are sporadic; the sources of infection for these cases may be related to exposure to *Legionella*-contaminated water in the patient's home, workplace, or location of medical therapy and to aerosol-producing devices in public places. Outbreaks have been ascribed to common-source exposure to contaminated cooling towers, evaporative condensers, potable water systems, whirlpool spas, humidifiers, and respiratory therapy equipment. Outbreaks have occurred in hospitals, hotels, and other large buildings. The disease occurs most commonly in elderly and immunocompromised persons. Infection in children is uncommon and usually is asymptomatic or mild and unrecognized. Severe disease has occurred in children with malignancy, severe combined immunodeficiency, chronic granulomatous disease, organ transplant, underlying pulmonary disease, those treated with corticosteroids, and in neonates.

The **incubation period** for Legionnaires' disease (pneumonia) is 2 to 10 days; for Pontiac fever it is 1 to 2 days.

DIAGNOSTIC TESTS: Recovery of *Legionella* from respiratory tract secretions by culture using special media provides definitive evidence of infection. The bacterium can be demonstrated in these specimens by direct immunofluorescence and by DNA probes, but these tests are less sensitive and specific than culture. Detection of *L pneumophila* serogroup 1 antigens in urine by commercially available radioimmunoassay or enzyme immunoassay (EIA) allows rapid diagnosis of infection due to this subtype. For serologic diagnosis, a fourfold or greater rise in titer of antibody to *L pneumophila* serogroup 1 to 1:128 or greater, measured by an indirect immunofluorescence antibody assay (IFA), also indicates acute infection. Newer serologic assays, such as EIA or tests using *Legionella* antigens other than serogroup 1, are available commercially, but have not been adequately standardized for routine use. The positive predictive value of a single titer of 1:256 or more is low and should not be used for diagnostic purposes except in some outbreak settings. Antibodies to *Mycoplasma pneumoniae* and several Gram-negative organisms including *Campylobacter jejuni, Pseudomonas aeruginosa,* and *Bacteroides fragilis* may cause false-positive IFA test results. Antibody titers usually rise within 1 to 6 weeks after onset of symptoms, but can be delayed for as long as 12 weeks.

TREATMENT: Erythromycin (30 to 60 mg/kg per day; maximum, 2 to 4 g/d in four divided doses) is the drug of choice. Intravenous high-dose therapy generally is given initially. Once the patient is improving, oral therapy can be substituted. The addition of rifampin (15 mg/kg per day; maximum, 600 mg/d) is recommended for patients with confirmed disease who are severely ill, and/or immunocompromised, or do not respond promptly to intravenous erythromycin. Newer antimicrobial agents such as azithromycin, clarithromycin, ciprofloxacin, and ofloxacin also may be effective. Duration of therapy is usually 3 weeks.

ISOLATION OF THE HOSPITALIZED PATIENT: Standard precautions are recommended.

CONTROL MEASURES: Methods for decontaminating water supplies in common-source outbreaks have included hyperchlorination (or other chemical decontaminants) and/or superheating (to 70°C [158°F]) in conjunction with appropriate mechanical cleaning followed by continuous chlorination or maintenance of hot water temperature greater than 50°C (122°F). Insufficient information is available to evaluate the utility of other chemical and physical methods of decontamination.

Leishmaniasis

CLINICAL MANIFESTATIONS: The three major clinical syndromes are as follows:
- *Cutaneous leishmaniasis.* After inoculation by the bite of an infected sand fly, parasites proliferate locally in mononuclear phagocytes, leading to an erythematous macule or nodule that typically forms a shallow ulcer with raised borders. Lesions are commonly located on exposed areas of the face and extremities and may be accompanied by satellite lesions and regional adenopathy. The clinical manifestations of Old World and New World cutaneous leishmaniasis are similar. Spontaneous resolution of lesions may take from weeks to years and usually results in a flat, atrophic scar.
- *Mucosal leishmaniasis (espundia).* From the initial cutaneous infection by *Leishmania braziliensis* or related New World species, parasites may disseminate to midline facial structures, including the oral and nasopharyngeal mucosa. In some patients, granulomatous ulceration follows, leading to facial disfigurement, secondary infection, and mucosal perforation months to years after the cutaneous lesion heals.
- *Visceral leishmaniasis (kala-azar).* After cutaneous inoculation of parasites, organisms spread throughout the mononuclear macrophage system and are concentrated in the spleen, liver, and bone marrow. The resulting clinical illness is marked by fever, anorexia, weight loss, splenomegaly, hepatomegaly, lymphadenopathy (in some geographic areas), anemia, leukopenia, thrombocytopenia with hemorrhage, and hypergammaglobulinemia. Secondary pyogenic, enteric, and mycobacterial infections are common. Active, untreated visceral disease is often fatal. Reactivation of latent visceral leishmaniasis has been reported in patients with concurrent HIV infection or other immunocompromising conditions.

ETIOLOGY: In the human host, *Leishmania* species are obligate intracellular parasites of mononuclear phagocytes. A single *Leishmania* species can produce different clinical syndromes, and each syndrome can be caused by different species. Cutaneous leishmaniasis typically is caused by *L tropica, L major, L aethiopica* (Old World species), and by *L mexicana, L amazonensis, L braziliensis, L panamensis, L guyanensis, L peruviana, L chagasi,* and other New World species. Mucosal leishmaniasis is caused by *L braziliensis* and occasionally other related species. Visceral leishmaniasis is caused by *L donovani, L infantum, L chagasi* as well as *L tropica* and *L amazonensis.*

EPIDEMIOLOGY: Leishmaniasis is a zoonosis with a variety of mammalian reservoir hosts, including canines and rodents. The vectors are phlebotomine sand flies. The distribution of Old World cutaneous leishmaniasis includes the Middle East, some Asian and African countries, India, countries of the former Soviet Union, and, sporadically, southern Europe. New World cutaneous leishmaniasis is found in areas extending from Mexico to northern Argentina, and a few cases have been reported as far north as Texas. Mucosal leishmaniasis occurs primarily in the Amazon basin and the central plains of Brazil, but also has been reported in other countries in South and Central America. The distribution of visceral leishmaniasis in the Old World includes southern Europe, the Mediterranean basin, the Middle East, East Africa, China, and India. Endemic foci are found in South and Central America, particularly in Brazil.

The **incubation period** of the different forms of leishmaniasis ranges from several days to months. In cutaneous leishmaniasis, primary skin lesions typically appear several weeks after parasite inoculation. In visceral infection, the incubation period can vary from 6 weeks to 6 months. However, incubation periods from 10 days to 10 years have been reported and reactivation of previously asymptomatic latent infection can occur in immunosuppressed patients.

DIAGNOSTIC TESTS: Definitive diagnosis usually is established by microscopic identification of intracellular leishmanial organisms on Wright or Giemsa stains of smears or histologic sections of infected tissues. In cutaneous disease, tissue can be obtained by a 3-mm punch biopsy, lesion scrapings, or needle aspiration of the raised nonnecrotic edge of the lesion. In visceral leishmaniasis, the organisms can be isolated from the spleen and less commonly from the bone marrow and liver, and in East Africa, the lymph nodes. Blood cultures have been positive in some Indian patients, and in HIV-infected patients organisms sometimes may be observed in blood smears or buffy-coat preparations. Isolation of parasites by culture of appropriate tissue specimens in specialized media should be attempted, when possible. Culture media and further information can be provided by the Centers for Disease Control and Prevention (CDC).

The diagnosis of visceral leishmaniasis and some cases of cutaneous infection also can be aided by serologic testing available at the CDC. However, a negative serologic test should never be interpreted as excluding the possibility of a leishmanial infection. In addition, occasional false-positive results may occur in sera of patients with other infectious diseases, especially American trypanosomiasis (Chagas' disease).

TREATMENT: Because cutaneous lesions may heal without specific therapy, treatment is not always necessary. Treatment is indicated when the ulcers are disabling or disfiguring, when healing is delayed, or when the patient may be infected with *L braziliensis* or other *Leishmania* species associated with mucosal disease. Drug therapy is always indicated when mucosal or visceral infection is present.

In the United States, the standard drug of choice for leishmaniasis is sodium stibogluconate, a parenteral pentavalent antimonial that usually is given daily for a minimum of 20 days. It is available from the CDC Drug Service (see Directory of Telephone Numbers, p 667). It is generally well tolerated in young, otherwise healthy patients, but cardiac, pancreatic, and hepatic toxicity can occur. Meglumine antimonate (which is not available in the United States) is an alternative drug. For patients with disease refractory to antimonial therapy, amphotericin B, pentamidine, or interferon-gamma in combination with an antimonial should be considered. In selected cases of American cutaneous leishmaniasis, ketoconazole, itraconazole, and allopurinol, as well as local heat, have been used successfully.

ISOLATION OF THE HOSPITALIZED PATIENT: Standard precautions are recommended.

CONTROL MEASURES: Because elimination of infected animal reservoirs and/or sand fly populations is unlikely in most regions that are endemic for leishmaniasis, travelers should be advised to minimize their exposure to sand fly bites by using screened accommodations, fine-mesh bed netting, protective clothing, and insect repellent, and by minimizing outdoor exposures from dusk to dawn. Patients infected with *Leishmania* species should not donate blood or be organ donors.

Leprosy

CLINICAL MANIFESTATIONS: Leprosy is a chronic disease involving mainly skin, peripheral nerves, and the mucosa of the upper respiratory tract. The clinical syndromes of leprosy represent a spectrum that reflects the cellular immune response to *Mycobacterium leprae*. Characteristic features are the following:

- *Tuberculoid.* One or few well-demarcated, hypopigmented or erythematous, hypoesthetic or anesthetic skin lesions, frequently with raised, active, spreading edges and central clearing. Cell-mediated immune responses are intact.
- *Lepromatous.* Initial numerous, ill-defined, hypopigmented, or erythematous macules that progress to papules, nodules, or plaques; and late-occurring hypesthesia. Dermal infiltration of the face, hands, and feet in a bilateral and symmetric distribution can occur without preceding maculopapular lesions. *Mycobacterium leprae*-specific, cell-mediated immunity is greatly diminished, but serum antibody responses to *M leprae*-derived antigens may occur, or titers of nonspecific antibodies (such as rheumatoid factor or nontreponemal tests for syphilis) may be elevated.
- *Borderline (dimorphous).* Single or multiple well-defined skin lesions, similar to tuberculoid, but with a raised central area; and delayed development of dysesthesia. Borderline disease often is subdivided into borderline lepromatous, borderline, and borderline tuberculoid.
- *Indeterminate.* An early form of leprosy that may develop into any of the other forms; typified by hypopigmented macules with indistinct edges and no associated dysesthesia.

Serious consequences of leprosy occur from nerve involvement with resulting anesthesia, which can lead to repeated, unrecognized trauma, ulcerations, fractures, and bone resorption.

ETIOLOGY: Leprosy is caused by *Mycobacterium leprae.*

EPIDEMIOLOGY: The major mode of transmission is contact with humans who have untreated or drug-resistant multibacillary disease (lepromatous or borderline types). A long duration of exposure, such as to a household contact, is common. However, 70% to 80% of cases in endemic areas do not have a history of household exposure or other contact with a known or suspected case of leprosy, suggesting the possibility of other sources of infection. The major source of infectious material is probably nasal secretions from patients with untreated multibacillary disease, from whom organisms are excreted in large numbers. Little shedding of *M leprae* from patients' intact skin occurs. In the United States, 90% of reported cases are imported, occurring in immigrants and refugees from areas endemic for leprosy, particularly Mexico and Southeast Asia. Indigenous cases continue to occur in Texas, California, Louisiana, and Hawaii. The infectivity of lepromatous patients probably ceases soon after treatment is instituted, frequently within a few days or weeks of initiating rifampin therapy or about 3 months after initiating therapy with dapsone or clofazimine.

The **incubation period** ranges from 1 to many years; but usually is 3 to 5 years. The incubation period of tuberculoid cases tends to be shorter than that for lepromatous cases.

DIAGNOSTIC TESTS: Histopathologic examination by an experienced pathologist is the best method for establishing the diagnosis and is the basis for the classification of leprosy. Acid-fast bacilli (AFB) may be found in slit-smears or biopsies from skin lesions, but rarely from patients with the tuberculoid and indeterminate forms of disease. Organisms have not been successfully cultured in vitro. Drug resistance is tested by the mouse footpad inoculation test. However, since this test is only performed in specialized laboratories and results are not available for at least 6 months, changes in medication are usually based on clinical findings. The demonstration of morphologically normal bacilli, ie, organisms with solid staining of the capsule on AFB stains, despite usually effective therapy, should suggest possible drug resistance (or poor compliance with therapy), indicating the possible need for a change in therapy.

High titers of predominantly IgM serum antibodies against phenolic glycolipid-1 of *M leprae* have been detected in untreated patients with lepromatous or borderline disease. Because elevated antibody titers frequently occur in persons without disease, this test is not diagnostic for leprosy. Titers of these antibodies slowly decrease after years of therapy. This test is experimental and available only in a few reference laboratories.

TREATMENT: Therapy for patients with leprosy should be undertaken in consultation with an expert in leprosy. The Gillis W. Long Hansen's Disease Center (GWLHDC), Carville, La (800-642-2477), provides consultation on clinical and pathologic issues and can provide information about local Hansen's disease clinics and/or clinicians who have experience with the disease.

Dapsone is one of the primary drugs used in the treatment of leprosy. It is usually administered in a dose of 100 mg/d for adults and 1 mg/kg/d for children. Persons in high-risk groups for glucose-6-phosphate dehydrogenase deficiency should be tested for this disorder before administration. Because primary dapsone resistance of *M leprae* has been reported, dapsone should not be used as monotherapy. To reduce the risk of drug resistance and possibly to shorten the duration of therapy, multidrug therapy is necessary in all patients. Rifampin (600 mg/d for adults or 10 mg/kg per day for children) should be given with dapsone for 6 months for paucibacillary (indeterminate, tuberculoid, and borderline tuberculoid) disease, with close follow-up to detect relapses. Clofazimine (50 mg/d for adults or 1 mg/kg per day for children) should be added for multibacillary (borderline, borderline lepromatous, and lepromatous) disease and continued for at least 2 years and until skin smears are negative. Other drugs including ofloxacin, minocycline, and clarithromycin have been demonstrated to have activity against *M leprae* and could be considered for therapy in patients with intolerance to routine drugs or with drug-resistant infections. All clinically compatible patients with demonstrable AFB organisms on skin biopsy or smear should be treated for presumptive multi-bacillary leprosy. Corticosteroids are used to treat erythema nodosum leprosum (ENL), which commonly occurs in patients with multibacillary disease after drug therapy is initiated. Occasionally, ENL occurs in untreated patients as well. Short-term, high-dose corticosteroids, followed by maintenance thalidomide, are often useful for managing severe or recurrent ENL reactions. Thalidomide is available from the GWLHDC as an experimental drug for selected patients and should never be given to a woman of childbearing age unless she is following a reliable means of contraception. Other agents, including clofazimine, can also be used to treat ENL.

Another type of reaction seen primarily in patients with borderline disease is the reversal reaction, which is characterized by delayed type hypersensitivity reactions at the site of current or former leprosy lesions and/or acute neuropathies. Reversal reactions, especially those with neuropathies, should be treated aggressively with corticosteroids to avoid permanent neurologic sequelae.

Most patients can be treated as outpatients. Rehabilitative measures, including surgery and physical therapy, may be necessary in some patients.

ISOLATION OF THE HOSPITALIZED PATIENT: Standard precautions are indicated.

CONTROL MEASURES: Hand washing is recommended for all persons in contact with a lepromatous patient. Disinfection of nasal secretions, handkerchiefs, and other fomites should be considered until treatment is established. Household contacts, particularly those with multibacillary disease, should be examined initially and then annually for at least 5 years. Household contacts of patients with borderline or lepromatous leprosy who are younger than 25 years should be treated prophylactically with dapsone for 3 years at the same doses as for treatment. Local public health department regulations for leprosy vary and should be consulted.

Newly diagnosed cases of leprosy should be reported to the regional public health department.

Leptospirosis

CLINICAL MANIFESTATIONS: The onset of leptospirosis is usually abrupt, with nonspecific, influenza-like, constitutional symptoms of fever, chills, headache, severe myalgia, and malaise. Gastrointestinal tract symptoms also can occur. The clinical course frequently is biphasic and protean, and can result in hepatic (abnormal liver function tests, hepatomegaly, jaundice, and liver failure), renal (abnormal urinalysis, azotemia, and renal failure), and central nervous system (aseptic meningitis and altered sensorium) involvement. Myositis is common. Weil's syndrome refers to severe leptospirosis with jaundice. Conjunctival suffusion, the most characteristic physical finding, occurs in less than half the patients. The duration of illness varies from less than 1 week to 3 weeks.

ETIOLOGY: The etiologic agent is the spirochete, *Leptospira interrogans.* Approximately 250 serotypes (serovars) comprising 19 serogroups have been recognized. Leptospirosis in the United States has been caused by more than 10 serotypes, the most common of which are *L iterohaemorrhagiae* and *L canicola.*

EPIDEMIOLOGY: The sources for human infection include many species of wild and domestic mammals, particularly dogs, rats, and livestock, that excrete *Leptospira* organisms in the urine. Most cases in the United States probably result from recreational exposure. Disease occurs most commonly in the summer among teenagers and adults, especially in the tropics. Persons predisposed by occupation include abattoir and sewer workers, veterinarians, farmers, and field workers. Transmission is zoonotic, either by direct or indirect contact of mucosal surfaces or abraded or traumatized skin with urine or carcasses of infected animals. Indirect contact occurs from swimming, wading, or splashing in pools, streams, or puddles contaminated by urine from infected animals and, occasionally, causes common-source outbreaks. Asymptomatic and symptomatic human infections occur. Communicability in infected animals exists during the 1-month to more than 3-month phase of prolonged leptospiruria. Humans with leptospirosis usually excrete the organism in urine for 4 to 6 weeks and occasionally for as long as 18 weeks. Person-to-person transmission is rare.

The **incubation period** is usually 7 to 13 days, with a range of 2 to 26 days.

DIAGNOSTIC TESTS: Blood and cerebrospinal fluid in the first 7 to 10 days of illness, and urine after the first week and during convalescence, should be cultured on special media. Because such media are not available routinely, laboratory personnel should be consulted in cases of suspected leptospirosis. The organism also can be recovered by inoculation of body fluids into guinea pigs. Serum antibody measured by enzyme immunoassay or agglutination reactions develop in the second week of illness, but titer rises can be delayed or absent in some patients. Microscopic agglutination is the confirmatory serologic test and is performed in reference laboratories. Direct darkfield examination of blood and other body fluids has pitfalls that obviate its usefulness, and is not recommended.

TREATMENT: Penicillin is the drug of choice for severely ill patients. High-dose penicillin (1.5 million units given every 6 hours to adults) administered intravenously for 7 days appears to be effective even in patients in whom therapy is not started until after the fourth day of the illness. Oral doxycycline therapy in persons with mild illness also appears to shorten the course of illness and reduces the frequency of convalescent leptospiruria. Tetracycline drugs should not be given to children younger than 8 years unless the benefits of therapy justify the risk of dental staining (see Antimicrobials and Related Therapy, p 606).

ISOLATION OF THE HOSPITALIZED PATIENT: Standard precautions are recommended. These precautions also include urine, which potentially is infectious in persons with leptospirosis.

CONTROL MEASURES:
- Vaccination of dogs and livestock prevents disease but not infection (ie, leptospiruria) in animals but the effect of vaccination of dogs and livestock on prevention of human disease is unproven, since vaccinated animals may transmit the organism to humans.
- Protective clothing, boots, and gloves should be worn to reduce occupational exposure.
- Rodent control is indicated.
- Doxycycline, 200 mg, given orally once a week to adults, is effective prophylaxis and should be considered for high-risk occupational groups with short-term exposure. However, indications for doxycycline use in children have not been established. Tetracycline drugs generally should not be given to children younger than 8 years (see Antimicrobials and Related Therapy, p 606).

Listeria monocytogenes Infections
(Listeriosis)

CLINICAL MANIFESTATIONS: *Listeria* infections are relatively uncommon; those affecting children are categorized as maternal, neonatal, or childhood with or without associated predisposing conditions. Neonatal illness has early onset and late-onset syndromes similar to those of group B streptococcal infections. Pneumonia, septicemia, and associated maternal symptoms of *Listeria* infection are common in early onset disease; granulomatosis infantisepticum, characterized by disseminated granulomas, occurs less frequently. Late-onset infection occurs after the first week of life, and usually results in meningitis. Maternal infection can be associated with an influenza-like illness, fever, malaise, headache, gastrointestinal tract symptoms, and back pain. Approximately 65% of women experience a symptomatic prodromal illness before diagnosis of listeriosis in their fetus or newborn infant. Amnionitis during labor or asymptomatic infection can occur. Infection occurs most commonly in the perinatal period and in patients with decreased cell-mediated immunity resulting from cancer chemotherapy, corticosteroid therapy, congenital immunodeficiency, hepatic or renal disease, or HIV infection. In childhood infections, most patients have meningitis and nearly half do not have an underlying, predisposing condition. *Listeria* rarely causes a diffuse encephalitis.

ETIOLOGY: *Listeria monocytogenes* is a small, aerobic, non-spore-forming, motile Gram-positive bacillus that produces a narrow zone of hemolysis on blood agar.

EPIDEMIOLOGY: *Listeria monocytogenes* is distributed widely in the environment, especially in the food chain. Food-borne transmission causes epidemics and sporadic infections. Incriminated foods include unpasteurized milk, soft cheeses and other dairy products, undercooked poultry, prepared meats such as paté, and unwashed raw vegetables. Asymptomatic fecal and vaginal carriage in pregnant women can result in sporadic neonatal disease from transplacental or ascending routes of infection or from exposure during delivery. Maternal infection has been associated with abortion, preterm delivery, and other obstetric complications. Late-onset neonatal infection can result from acquisition of the organism during passage through the birth canal or from environmental sources, and then hematogenous invasion of the organism from intestine. Nosocomial nursery outbreaks also have occurred.

The median **incubation period** for food-borne transmission is 21 days.

DIAGNOSTIC TESTS: The organism can be recovered on blood agar media from cultures of blood, cerebrospinal fluid (CSF), meconium, gastric washings, placenta, amniotic fluid, and other infected tissues. Special techniques (eg, enrichment and selective media) may be needed to recover *Listeria* from sites with mixed flora (eg, vagina and rectum). Gram staining of gastric aspirate or CSF from an infected newborn infant may demonstrate the organism. As the result of morphologic similarity to diphtheroids and streptococci, a culture isolate of *Listeria* mistakenly can be considered a contaminant or saprophyte. The value of serologic tests is not established.

TREATMENT:
- Initial therapy with intravenous ampicillin and an aminoglycoside, usually gentamicin, is recommended for severe infections. This combination is more effective than ampicillin alone in animal models of *Listeria* infection. After clinical response occurs, or for less severe infections in normal hosts, ampicillin or penicillin alone may be given. The optimal therapeutic regimen, however, has not been established. For the penicillin-allergic patient, the alternative regimen is trimethoprim-sulfamethoxazole. Cephalosporins, including the newer derivatives, are not active against *Listeria.*
- In invasive infections without associated meningitis, 10 to 14 days of treatment usually is satisfactory. For *Listeria* meningitis, most experts recommend 14 to 21 days of treatment.
- The usefulness of culturing the vagina and stool of the mother of an infected infant and treatment of the mother, if either culture is positive, has not been established. Similarly, no data suggest that reculturing during a subsequent pregnancy has any value.

ISOLATION OF THE HOSPITALIZED PATIENT: Standard precautions are required.

CONTROL MEASURES:
- Antimicrobial therapy of infection diagnosed during pregnancy may prevent fetal or perinatal infection and its consequences.

- The existence of listeriosis in herds of sheep or cattle should preclude use of untreated manure on crops destined for human consumption.
- Pregnant women and immunosuppressed patients should avoid unpasteurized dairy products, soft cheeses, undercooked meats, and ready-to-eat foods (eg, hot dogs) left for an extended period of time at room temperature unless they are re-heated until steaming hot. Raw vegetables should be thoroughly washed before eating.
- Cases of listeriosis should be reported to the regional health department to facilitate early recognition and control of common-source outbreaks.

Lyme Disease
(Borrelia burgdorferi)

CLINICAL MANIFESTATIONS: The clinical manifestations are divided into the three following stages: early localized, early disseminated, and late disease. Early localized disease is manifest by a distinctive rash, termed erythema migrans, at the site of a recent tick bite. Erythema migrans begins as a red macule or papule, and usually expands during days to weeks to form a large annular erythematous lesion that is 5 cm or more in diameter (median, 15 cm), sometimes with partial central clearing. Localized erythema migrans can vary greatly in size and shape and may have vesicular or necrotic areas in its center. Fever, malaise, headache, mild neck stiffness, and arthralgia often accompany the rash. In untreated persons, these associated symptoms may be intermittent and variable during a period of several weeks.

The most common manifestation of early disseminated disease is multiple erythema migrans. This rash usually occurs 3 to 5 weeks after the tick bite, and consists of secondary annular erythematous lesions similar to, but usually smaller than, the primary lesion. These lesions reflect a spirochetemia with dermal dissemination. Other common manifestations of early disseminated illness (which may occur with or without rash) are palsies of the cranial nerves (especially seventh nerve palsy, ie, Bell's palsy), meningitis and conjunctivitis. Systemic symptoms, such as arthralgia, myalgia, headache and fatigue also are common in the early disseminated stage. Carditis, which usually is manifested by various degrees of heart block, occurs rarely.

Late disease is characterized most commonly by recurrent arthritis that usually is pauciarticular and affects the large joints, in particular the knees. Chronic arthritis is uncommon in children who are treated with antimicrobial agents in the early stage of the disease. Arthritis may occur without a history of manifestations of earlier stages of illness (including erythema migrans). Central nervous system manifestations also occur in late disease, and include encephalopathology and neuropathy, including one or more peripheral nerves.

No casual relationship between maternal Lyme disease and abnormalities of pregnancy or congenital disease caused by *Borrelia burgdorferi* have been documented, although transplacental transmission of *B burgdorferi* has been reported. No evidence exists that Lyme disease can be transmitted via human milk.

ETIOLOGY: The cause is the spirochete *Borrelia burgdorferi*.

EPIDEMIOLOGY: Lyme disease occurs primarily in three distinct geographic regions of the United States. Most cases are reported in the Northeast from Massachusetts to Maryland. The disease also occurs, but with lower frequency, in the upper Midwest, especially in Wisconsin and Minnesota, and, less commonly, in the West Coast, especially northern California. The occurrence of cases in the United States correlates with the distribution and frequency of infected tick vectors (*Ixodes scapularis* [previously known as *Ixodes dammini*] in the East and Midwest; *Ixodes pacificus* in the West). However, cases of Lyme disease have been reported by 48 states, many of which are outside the usual range of habitation for these ticks, and the identity of infected vectors in these areas has not been established. Reported cases in states without known enzootic risks may be imported, or, in many cases, may be misdiagnoses resulting from false-positive serologic test results. Endemic Lyme disease also has been reported in Canada, Europe, states of the former Soviet Union, China, and Japan. Most cases occur between April and October. Persons of all ages may be affected.

The **incubation period** from tick bite to appearance of erythema migrans ranges from 3 to 31 days and is typically from 7 to 14 days. Late manifestations occur several months to more than 1 year later.

DIAGNOSTIC TESTS: Diagnosis is made clinically in the early stages of Lyme disease if erythema migrans is present. While cultures of a biopsy specimen of the perimeter of this lesion frequently yields the organism, *Borrelia* cultures (which require special media) are not commercially available. In patients without a rash who manifest symptoms and signs of a later stage of Lyme disease, diagnosis also should be based on clinical findings, using serologic tests as an adjunct.

The diagnosis of Lyme disease can be difficult in part because of poor standardization and the inappropriate use of serological diagnostic tests that were developed for surveillance of serum to establish a clinical diagnosis. The IgM-specific antibody titer usually peaks between weeks 3 and 6 after the onset of disease; specific IgG antibody titers usually rise slowly and generally are highest weeks to months later. Localized erythema migrans typically occurs 1 to 2 weeks after the tick bite; therefore antibodies against *B burgdorferi* will not be detectable in most patients with early localized Lyme disease. Some patients who are treated early with antimicrobial agents never develop antibodies against *B burgdorferi*. However, most patients with early disseminated disease and virtually all patients with late disease will have antibodies against *B burgdorferi*. As with other infections, once such antibodies develop, they may persist for many years despite cure of the disease. Consequently, tests for antibodies should not be used to assess treatment of Lyme disease. Because of the poor sensitivity and specificity of the serologic testing for *B burgdorferi* that is currently available in many commercial laboratories, testing for serum antibodies against *B burgdorferi* when possible, should be performed in a reference laboratory. Physicians should contact their state health departments for additional information if they are not familiar with the reference laboratories in their area.

The enzyme immunosorbent assay (EIA) is the most commonly used test for detection of antibodies against *B burgdorferi*. This test and the immunofluoresence assay (IFA) may give false-positive serological results because of cross-reactive serum antibodies in patients with other spirochetal infections (eg, syphilis, leptospirosis, and relapsing fever), certain viral infections (eg, varicella), and certain autoimmune diseases (eg, syphilis and systemic lupus erythematosus). While *B burgdorfen* antibody cross-reacts with other spirochetes, including *Treponema pallidum*, patients with Lyme disease do not have positive nontreponemal syphilis tests such as the VDRL or RPR. In addition, antibodies directed against in the normal oral flora may cross-react with antigens of *B burgdorferi* and produce a false-positive test result.

Currently, the immunoblot test is most useful for corroborating positive or equivocal EIA or IFA serological results and, as a result, a two-test approach is recommended for confirming the diagnosis of active disease and previous infection. Sera that are positive or equivocal by a sensitive EIA or IFA should be tested by a standardized Western immunoblot for the presence of antibodies against proteins specific for *B burgdorferi*; those that are negative by a sensitive EIA or IFA do not require immunoblot testing. When sera from a patient in the first 4 weeks of disease onset (early disease) is tested by Western immunoblot, both IgM and IgG procedures should be performed. IgM testing is not recommended for determining active disease in persons with illness of greater than 1 month's duration. If a patient with suspected early disease has a negative serology, evidence of infection is best obtained by testing of paired acute- and convalescent-phase sera. Persons with early disseminated or late-stage Lyme disease almost always have a robust IgG response to *B burgdorferi* antigens.

Suspected central nervous system involvement with Lyme disease can be confirmed by demonstration of intrathecal production of antibodies against *B burgdorferi*. However, interpretation of antibody tests of cerebrospinal fluid is complex, and physicians should seek the advice of a specialist experienced in the management of patients with Lyme disease to assist them in interpreting results of these tests.

The widespread practice of ordering serologic tests in patients with nonspecific symptoms (such as fatigue or arthralgia) who have a low probability of having Lyme disease is a major problem. Nearly all positive serologic test results in these patients are false-positive. Patients with acute Lyme disease almost always have objective signs of infection (eg, erythema migrans, facial nerve palsy, and/or arthritis). Nonspecific symptoms commonly accompany these specific signs, often in persons with neurologic manifestations of chronic Lyme disease, but are almost never the only evidence of Lyme disease.

New, more sensitive and more specific diagnostic tests, such as the polymerase chain reaction, which may be able to identify the presence of even small quantities of spirochetal DNA, are in development. However, physicians should be cautious when interpreting results of these investigational tests until their clinical utility has been proven.

TREATMENT: See Table 3.33, p 332.

Early Localized Disease. Doxycycline is the drug of choice for children 8 years of age and older. Precautions to avoid exposure to the sun (eg, the use of sunscreen) should be taken because a rash develops in 20% of persons who take doxycycline in sun-exposed areas. For children younger than 8 years of age, amoxicillin is recommended. For patients allergic to penicillin, alternative drugs are cefuroxime axetil and erythromycin, although erythromycin may be less effective. Most experts treat persons with early Lyme disease for 14 to 21 days, but information is limited about the optimal duration of treatment.

Table 3.33. Recommended Treatment of Lyme Disease in Children

Disease Category	Drug(s) and Dose*
Early localized disease*	
≥8 y	Doxycycline, oral regimen, 100 mg twice a day for 14-21 d
All ages	Amoxicillin, oral regimen, 25–50 mg/kg/d, divided into 3 doses (maximum, 2 g/d) for 14–21 d
Early disseminated and late disease	
Multiple erythema migrans	Same oral regimen as for early disease but for 21 d
Isolated facial palsy	Same oral regimen as for early disease but for 21–28 d[†‡]
Arthritis	Same oral regimen as for early disease but for 28 d
Persistent or recurrent arthritis[§]	Ceftriaxone, 75–100 mg/kg, IV or IM, once a day (maximum, 2 g/d) for 14-21 d; or penicillin, 300 000 U/kg/d, IV, given in divided doses every 4 h (maximum, 20 million U/d) for 14–21 d
Carditis	Ceftriaxone, 75-100 mg/kg, IV or IM, once a day (maximum, 2 g/d); or penicillin, 300 000 U/kg/d, IV, given in divided doses every 4 h (maximum, 20 million U/d) for 14–21 d
Meningitis or encephalitis	Ceftriaxone, 75-100 mg/kg, IV or IM, once a day (maximum, 2 g/d); or penicillin, 300 000 U/kg/d, IV, given in divided doses every 4 h (maximum, 20 million U/d) for 14–21 d

* For patients who are allergic to penicillin, cefuroxime axetil and erythromycin are alternative drugs. IV indicates intravenously; IM, intramuscularly.

† Corticosteroids should not be given.

‡ Treatment has no effect on the resolution of the nerve palsy; its purpose is to prevent late disease.

§ Arthritis is not considered persistent or recurrent unless objective evidence of synovitis exists at least 2 months after treatment is initiated. Some experts administer a second course of an oral agent before using an intravenously administered antimicrobial agent.

Treatment of erythema migrans almost always prevents development of later stages of Lyme disease. Clinical response to therapy is often slow, and signs and symptoms may persist for several weeks even in successfully treated patients. Erythema migrans resolves within several days following treatment.

Early Disseminated and Late Disease. Multiple erythema migrans and arthritis should be treated with orally administered antimicrobial agents. Most experts also recommend orally administered antimicrobial agents for seventh-nerve palsy, although some experts recommend a lumbar puncture if central nervous system involvement is suspected, and if cerebrospinal fluid pleocytosis is found, recommend parenterally administered antimicrobial therapy as for meningitis. Recurrent or persistent arthritis and meningitis should be treated with parenterally administered antimicrobial drugs. Carditis also is usually treated with parenteral therapy, although some experts treat mild carditis with oral doxycycline or amoxicillin. The optimal duration of therapy for these different manifestations is not well established, but no evidence indicates that children with any manifestation of Lyme disease benefit from either prolonged or repeated courses of parenterally administered antimicrobial agents. Accordingly, the maximum duration of a single course of therapy is 4 weeks.

The Jarisch-Herxheimer reaction, with increased fever, chills, and malaise, can occur transiently when therapy is initiated. Nonsteroidal anti-inflammatory agents may be beneficial and the antimicrobial agent should be continued.

Pregnancy. Tetracyclines are contraindicated. Otherwise, therapy is the same as for nonpregnant persons.

ISOLATION OF THE HOSPITALIZED PATIENT: Standard precautions are recommended.

CONTROL MEASURES:

Ticks. Avoidance of tick-infested areas is the best preventive measure. In a tick-infested area, clothing should cover as much of the arms and legs as possible. Permethrin can be sprayed on clothing to prevent tick attachment. Tick repellents containing DEET* can be applied to the exposed skin. These repellents should be used sparingly, however, because of rare reports of serious neurologic complications in children resulting from the frequent and excessive application of deet-containing repellents, and they should be applied only to exposed skin and not to the child's face, hands, or irritated or abraded skin. After the child returns indoors, treated skin should be washed with soap and water. Daily self-inspection, inspection of family members, and prompt removal of ticks are recommended (see also Control Measures for Prevention of Tick-Borne Infections, p 126).

Chemoprophylaxis. The risk of infection with *B burgdorferi* after a recognized deer tick bite, even in highly endemic areas, is sufficiently low that prophylactic antimicrobial treatment after a tick bite is not indicated routinely. In addition, animal studies indicate that transmission of *B burgdorferi* from infected ticks requires a prolonged duration (24 to 48 hours) of tick attachment. However, factors such as a long duration of feeding by a tick (eg, as indicated by removal of an engorged tick) or pregnancy may alter the decision not to administer prophylactic antimicrobial therapy. Analysis of ticks to determine whether they are infected also is not indicated because the predictive values of such tests in terms of association with human disease are unknown.

Blood Donation. Patients with active disease should not donate blood because spirochetemia occurs in early Lyme disease. Patients who have been treated for Lyme disease can be considered for blood donation.

Vaccines. Investigational vaccines to prevent Lyme disease have been developed and clinical trials are in progress.

---

* Diethyltoluamide

Lymphocytic Choriomeningitis

CLINICAL MANIFESTATIONS: Infection may result in a mild to severe nonspecific illness, including fever, malaise, myalgia, retro-orbital headache, photophobia, anorexia, and nausea. Fever usually lasts 1 to 3 weeks. A biphasic febrile course is frequent. Neurologic manifestations varying from aseptic meningitis to severe encephalitis can occur. Arthralgia or arthritis, respiratory symptoms, orchitis, and leukopenia occasionally develop. Infection during pregnancy has been associated with abortion and with hydrocephalus and chorioretinitis in the fetus.

ETIOLOGY: Lymphocytic choriomeningitis (LCM) virus is an arenavirus.

EPIDEMIOLOGY: Lymphocytic choriomeningitis is a chronic infection of the common house mouse. These mice are often asymptomatically infected in nature. In addition, laboratory mice and colonized golden hamsters can be infected with significant viral shedding. Pet hamsters also have been a source of infection. Humans are infected incidentally by inhalation or ingestion of dust or food contaminated with the virus from the urine, feces, blood, or nasopharyngeal secretions of infected rodents. The disease is most prevalent in young adults. Human-to-human spread of the virus has not been reported.

The **incubation period** is usually 6 to 13 days and occasionally as long as 3 weeks.

DIAGNOSTIC TESTS: The cerebrospinal fluid (CSF) may contain hundreds to thousands of white blood cells, predominantly lymphocytes, and hypoglycorrhachia can occur. The LCM virus can be isolated from blood, CSF, urine, and/or, rarely, nasopharyngeal secretions. Acute and convalescent sera can be tested for increases in antibody titers; demonstration of virus-specific IgM antibodies in serum and cerebrospinal fluid is useful. Infection of mice trapped in or around houses may be identified by demonstrating serum antibody or viral antigen in liver impression smears.

TREATMENT: Supportive.

ISOLATION OF THE HOSPITALIZED PATIENT: Standard precautions are recommended.

CONTROL MEASURES: Infection can be controlled by preventing rodent infestation in animal and food storage areas of wholesalers and others dealing in the sale of mice, hamsters, or other rodents. Because the virus is excreted by rodent hosts for long periods, attempts should be made to monitor colonies for infection. Pet rodents or wild mice in the patient's home should be considered likely sources of infection. Pregnant women in particular should avoid exposure to rodents and their aerosolized excreta.

Malaria

CLINICAL MANIFESTATIONS: The classic symptoms are high fever with chills, rigor, sweats, and headache, which may be paroxysmal. As the infection becomes synchronized, the fever and paroxysms generally occur in a cyclic pattern. Depending on the infecting species, fever may appear every other or every third day. Other manifestations can include nausea, vomiting, diarrhea, cough, arthralgia, and abdominal and back pain. Pallor and jaundice caused by hemolysis also may be present. Hepatosplenomegaly may be present and is more prominent in chronic infections.

Infection by *Plasmodium falciparum* is potentially fatal and most commonly manifests as a febrile illness without specific or localizing signs. With more severe disease, however, *P falciparum* infection may be manifest by one of the following clinical syndromes:

- *Cerebral malaria*, which may have variable neurologic manifestations including seizures, signs of increased intracranial pressure, confusion, and progression to stupor, coma, and death
- *Severe anemia*, due to high parasitemia and consequent hemolysis
- *Hypoglycemia*, sometimes associated with quinine treatment, requiring urgent correction
- *Respiratory failure and metabolic acidosis*, without pulmonary edema
- *Pulmonary edema*, which is difficult to manage and may be fatal (rare in children)
- *Renal failure*, caused by acute tubular necrosis (rare in children younger than 8 years)
- *Vascular collapse and shock*, associated with hypothermia and adrenal insufficiency

Children with asplenia are at high risk of death from malaria and children who have chronic hepatitis B infection are at increased risk of severe disease.

Syndromes primarily associated with *P vivax* and *P ovale* are as follows:

- *Hypersplenism*, with danger of late splenic rupture
- *Anemia* due to acute parasitemia
- *Relapse*, for as long as 3 to 5 years after the primary infection, due to latent hepatic stages.

Syndromes associated with *P malariae* infection are as follows:

- *Nephrotic syndrome*, from the deposition of immune complexes in the kidney
- *Chronic asymptomatic parasitemia*, for as long as several years after the last exposure

Congenital malaria secondary to perinatal transmission may occur rarely. Most congenital cases have been caused by *P vivax* and *P falciparum; P malariae* and *P ovale* account for less than 20% of such cases. Manifestations can resemble those of neonatal sepsis, including fever and non-specific symptoms of poor appetite, irritability, and lethargy.

ETIOLOGY: The *Plasmodium* species infecting humans are *P vivax, P malariae, P ovale,* and *P falciparum.*

EPIDEMIOLOGY: Malaria is endemic throughout the tropical areas of the world and is acquired from the bite of female *Anopheles* mosquitoes. One-half of the world's population lives in areas where transmission occurs. Areas of highest prevalence include sub-Saharan Africa, parts of Central and South America, and parts of Oceania and Southeast Asia. Transmission is possible in more temperate climates, including areas in the United States where *Anopheles* mosquitoes are present. Mosquitoes in airplanes flying from tropical climates have been the source of occasional cases in persons working or residing near international airports. However, nearly all of the approximately 1000 annual reported cases in the United States are imported and infection was acquired abroad. Transmission also can be congenital, through transfusions or the use of contaminated needles.

  Plasmodium vivax and *P falciparum* are the most common species worldwide. *P vivax* malaria is prevalent on the Indian subcontinent and in Central America, and *P falciparum* is prevalent in Africa, Haiti, and New Guinea. Both *P vivax* and *P falciparum* are common in Southeast Asia, Oceania, and South America. *Plasmodium malariae*, although less common, has a wide distribution. *P ovale* occurs most often in West Africa, but has been reported from other areas. Relapses may occur in *P vivax* and *P ovale* malaria because of a persistent hepatic stage of the infection. Recrudescence of *P falciparum* and *P malariae* infection occurs when a persistent low-concentration parasitemia causes a recurrence of the disease. In hyperendemic areas of Africa and Asia, reinfection in persons with partial immunity often results in a high prevalence of asymptomatic parasitemia. The spread of strains throughout the world of chloroquine-resistant *P falciparum* is of increasing importance. Resistance to other antimalarial drugs is now occurring in many areas where the drugs are widely used. Chloroquine-resistant *P vivax* recently has been reported in Oceania.

DIAGNOSTIC TESTS: Definitive diagnosis relies on identification of the parasite on stained blood films. Both thick and thin blood films should be examined. The thick film allows for concentration of the blood to find the parasite that may be present in small numbers whereas the thin film is most useful in species identification and determination of parasitemia (the percentage of erythrocytes harboring parasites). If the initial blood smears are negative for *Plasmodium* species but malaria remains a possibility, the smear should be repeated every 12 to 24 hours during a 72-hour period. A rapid screening test for malarial parasites, the quantitative buffy coat analysis (QBC), is available, but blood smears should continue to be performed because the data are insufficient to justify using only QBC. In hyperendemic areas, the presence of malaria on a blood smear is not conclusive evidence of malaria as a cause of the presenting illness as other infections are often superimposed upon low-concentration parasitemia in children with partial immunity. Confirmation and identification of the species of malaria parasites on the blood smear is important in guiding therapy. Serology generally is not helpful, except in epidemiologic surveys. New diagnostic tests in development, including those using polymerase chain reaction, DNA probes, and malarial ribosomal RNA, may provide rapid and accurate diagnosis in the future.

TREATMENT: Chemotherapy is based on the infecting species, possible drug resistance, and the severity of disease (see Table 3.34, p 337). Severe malaria is

Table 3.34. **Treatment of Malaria**

Drug	Adult Dosage	Pediatric Dosage
All *Plasmodium* species except chloroquine-resistant *Plasmodium falciparum*		
Oral drug of choice		
Chloroquine phosphate	600 mg base (1 g), then 300 mg base, (500 mg) 6 h later, and 300 mg base (500 mg) at 24 and 48 h	10 mg base/kg (maximum, 600 mg base), then 5 mg base/kg 6 h later (maximum, 300 mg base), and 5 mg base/kg/d at 24 and 48 h (maximum, 300 mg base)
Parenteral drug of choice		
Quinidine gluconate*	10 mg/kg loading dose, IV (maximum, 600 mg) during 1–2 h, then 0.02 mg/kg/min contin-uous infusion until oral therapy can be started	Same as adult
OR		
Quinine dihydrochloride*†	600 mg in 300 mL of normal saline IV during 2–4 h; repeat every 8 h (maximum, 1800 mg/d) until oral therapy can be started	30 mg/kg/d; give ⅓ of daily dose over 2-4 h; repeat every 8 h until oral therapy can be started (maximum, 1800 mg/d)
***P falciparum* acquired in areas of known chloroquine resistance**		
Oral regimen of choice‡		
Quinine sulfate§	650 mg 3 times a day for 3–7 d	30 mg/kg/d in 3 doses for 3–7 d
PLUS		
Tetracycline‖	250 mg 4 times a day for 7 d	5 mg/kg 4 times a day for 7 d (maximum, 250 mg 4 times a day)
Alternative regimen		
Oral: Quinine sulfate	650 mg/3 times a day for 3–7 d	30 mg/kg in 3 doses for 3 d
Parenteral: Quinidine gluconate*	Same as above	Same as above
or		
Quinine dihydrochloride*†	Same as above	Same as above
PLUS		

Table 3.34. **Treatment of Malaria, continued**

Drug	Adult Dosage	Pediatric Dosage
Pyrimethamine- sulfadoxine (Fansidar)¶	Single dose of 3 tablets on last day of quinine therapy	<1 y of age, single dose of ¼ tablet; 1-3 y of age, single dose of ½ tablet; 4–8 y of age, single dose of 1 tablet; 9–14 y of age, single dose of 2 tablets; >14 y of age, single dose of 3 tablets
or		
Mefloquine hydrochloride#**	Single dose of 15 to 25 mg/kg (maximum, 1250 mg)	15–25 mg/kg in a single dose** (maximum, 1250 mg)

Prevention of relapses: *Plasmodium vivax* and *Plasmodium ovale* only

Primaquine phosphate‡‡	15 mg base (26.3 mg)/d for 14 d or 45 mg base (79 mg)/wk for 8 wk	0.3 mg base/kg/d for 14 d (maximum, 26.3 mg/d)

* Electrocardiogram monitoring is recommended to detect arrhythmias, widening QRS complex, or prolonged QT interval. Patients should also be monitored for hypotension. IV indicates intravenously.
† Not available in the United States.
‡ The combination of quinine sulfate and tetracycline is the most efficacious regimen for all chloroquine-resistant *P falciparum* infections.
§ For treatment of *P falciparum* infections acquired in Southeast Asia and possibly in other areas such as South America, quinine sulfate should be continued for 7 days.
‖ Physicians must weigh the benefits of tetracycline therapy against the possibility of dental staining in children younger than 8 years (see Antimicrobials and Related Therapy, p 606).
¶ Use of Fansidar, which contains 25 mg pyrimethamine and 500 mg sulfadoxine per tablet, is contraindicated in patients with a history of sulfonamide or pyrimethamine intolerance, in infants younger than 2 months and in pregnant women at term. Pregnant women should be administered chloroquine, or if chloroquine-resistant malaria is suspected, quinine or mefloquine. Resistance to pyrimethamine-sulfadoxine has been reported from Southeast Asia and the Amazon Basin, and therefore, this drug should not be used for treatment of malaria acquired in these areas.
# Mefloquine is not licensed by the Food and Drug Administration for children who weigh less than 15 kg, but recent Center for Disease Control and Prevention recommendations allow use of the drug to be considered in children without weight restrictions when travel to chloroquine-resistant *P falciparum* areas cannot be avoided. Mefloquine is *contraindicated* for use by travelers with a known hypersensitivity to mefloquine, or for travelers with a history of epilepsy or severe psychiatric disorders. A review of available data suggests that mefloquine may be administered to persons concurrently receiving ß-blockers if they have no underlying arrhythmia. However, mefloquine is not recommended for persons with cardiac conduction abnormalities until additional data are available. Caution may be advised for persons involved in tasks requiring fine coordination and spatial discrimination, such as airline pilots. Quinidine or quinine may exacerbate the known side effects of mefloquine; patients not responding to mefloquine therapy or failing mefloquine prophylaxis should be monitored closely if they are treated with quinidine or quinine.
** For most patients, 15 mg/kg in a single dose is effective therapy, except for those who acquired infection in the areas of the Amazon basin, or the Thailand-Cambodian and Thailand-Myanmar borders (see ‡footnote).
‡‡ Primaquine phosphate can cause hemolytic anemia in patients with glucose-6-phosphate dehydrogenase (G6PD) deficiency. A G6PD screen should be done before initiating treatment. Pregnant women should not be administered primaquine.

defined as a parasitemia greater than 5%, signs of central nervous system or other end-organ involvement, shock, acidosis, and/or hypoglycemia. Patients with severe malaria require intensive care and parenteral treatment until they are able to tolerate oral therapy. Exchange transfusion may be warranted when parasitemia exceeds 10%. Other adjunctive therapies, such as iron chelation, are under investigation but are not yet recommended. In patients with *P falciparum* malaria, sequential blood smears are indicated to monitor the treatment.

ISOLATION OF THE HOSPITALIZED PATIENT: Standard precautions are recommended.

CONTROL MEASURES: Control of the *Anopheles* mosquito population, chemotherapy of infected persons, and chemoprophylaxis of travelers in endemic areas are effective. Measures to prevent contact with mosquitoes, especially from dusk to dawn (because of the nocturnal biting habits of the *Anopheles* mosquito) through use of bed nets impregnated with insecticide, mosquito repellents, and protective clothing also are beneficial. The most current information on risks, drug resistance, and resulting recommendations for travelers can be obtained by contacting the 24-hour service of the Centers for Disease Control and Prevention (CDC, see Directory of Telephone Numbers, p 667).

Chemoprophylaxis for Travelers to Endemic Areas.* The appropriate chemoprophylactic regimen is determined by the traveler's risk of acquiring malaria in the area(s) to be visited and by the risk of exposure to chloroquine-resistant *P falciparum*. Indications for prophylaxis for children are identical to those for adults. Chemoprophylaxis should begin 1 week before arrival in the endemic area, allowing time for development of adequate blood concentration of the drug and evaluation of any adverse reactions.

Chloroquine-resistant *P falciparum* has not yet been reported in Haiti, the Dominican Republic, Central America west of the Panama Canal, and the Middle East, including Egypt. Travelers to areas where chloroquine-resistant malaria species have not been reported should take chloroquine, once weekly, for the duration of exposure and for 4 weeks after departure from the endemic area.

Travelers to areas where chloroquine-resistant *P falciparum* exists should take mefloquine, once weekly, starting 1 week before travel, continuing weekly during travel, and for 4 weeks after travel has concluded (see Table 3.35, p 341). Mefloquine is not approved by the Food and Drug Administration (FDA) for children who weigh less than 15 kg (33 lb), but recent recommendations of the Center for Disease Control and Prevention (CDC) allow it to be considered for use in children without weight or age restrictions when travel to areas of chloroquine-resistant *P falciparum* cannot be avoided. Mefloquine is contraindicated for use by travelers with a known hypersensitivity to mefloquine and should only be used with caution in travelers with a history of epilepsy or severe psychiatric disorders. Although a warning about such is given in the product labeling, a review of available data suggest that mefloquine may be used in persons concurrently receiving beta blockers if they have no

---

* For further information on prevention of malaria in travelers, see the annual publication of the US Public Health Service, *Health Information for International Travel,* Superintendent of Documents, US Government Printing Office, Washington, DC.

underlying arrhythmia. However, mefloquine is not recommended for persons with cardiac conduction abnormalities until additional data are available. Caution may be advised for travelers involved in tasks requiring fine coordination and spatial discrimination, such as airline pilots. Patients in whom the response to mefloquine therapy is inadequate or in whom mefloquine prophylaxis fails should be monitored closely if they are treated with quinidine or quinine because quinidine or quinine may exacerbate the known side effects of mefloquine. Because of the frequency of side effects, mefloquine should not be used for presumptive self-treatment.

For short-term travelers unable to take mefloquine, doxycycline alone is the preferred alternative regimen (see Table 3.35, p 341). Travelers taking doxycycline should be advised of the need for strict compliance with daily dosing (in a single dose), as well as the possible side effects, including diarrhea, photosensitivity, and increased risk of monilial vaginitis. Use of doxycycline should be avoided in pregnant women and usually in children younger than 8 years because of the risk of dental staining (see Antimicrobials and Related Therapy, p 606).

Children who cannot take mefloquine or doxycycline can be given chloroquine (with proquanil for travel to sub-Saharan Africa) for prophylaxis. Children should avoid travel to areas with chloroquine-resistant *P falciparum*, unless they can take a highly effective drug, such as mefloquine or doxycycline.

Prophylaxis During Pregnancy. Malaria infection in pregnant women may be more severe than in nonpregnant women. Malaria may increase the risk of adverse outcomes in pregnancy, including prematurity, abortion, and stillbirth. For these reasons and because no chemoprophylactic regimen is completely effective, women who are pregnant or likely to become pregnant should avoid travel to areas where they could contract malaria. Women traveling to areas where drug-resistant *P falciparum* has not been reported may take chloroquine prophylaxis. Harmful effects on the fetus have not been demonstrated when chloroquine is given in the recommended doses for malaria prophylaxis. Pregnancy, therefore, is not a contraindication for malaria prophylaxis with chloroquine.

Mefloquine, according to the FDA-approved product labeling, is not recommended for use during pregnancy. However, a review of data from clinical trials and reports of inadvertent use of mefloquine during pregnancy suggests that its use is not associated with adverse fetal or pregnancy outcomes such as birth defects, stillbirths, and spontaneous abortions. Consequently, mefloquine may be considered for prophylactic use in women who are pregnant or likely to become so when exposure to chloroquine-resistant *P falciparum* is unavoidable. Because information on the use of mefloquine in the first trimester is limited, women who receive mefloquine during the first trimester of pregnancy or their health care providers are asked to report the exposure to the CDC Malaria Section (770-488-7760) for inclusion in a registry to assess pregnancy outcomes.

In other travelers for whom mefloquine is contraindicated and doxycycline is inappropriate (eg, for reasons of age), chloroquine alone or chloroquine plus proguanil have been used as alternatives but are less effective (see Table 3.35). In addition, such travelers should carry pyrimethamine-sulfadoxine for use as presumptive self-treatment if a febrile illness develops while taking chloroquine and professional medical care is not readily available. Resistance to pyrimethamine-

Table 3.35. **Prevention of Malaria***

Drug[†]	Adult Dosage	Pediatric Dosage
Chloroquine-Sensitive Areas		
Chloroquine phosphate	300 mg base (500 mg salt), orally, once per wk beginning 1 wk before exposure, and continuing for 4 wk after last exposure	5 mg/kg base (8.3 mg/kg salt) once per wk (maximum, 300 mg base)
Chloroquine-Resistant Areas		
Mefloquine[‡]	250 mg salt (equal to 228 mg base) orally, once per wk, beginning 1 wk before travel and continuing for 4 wk after last exposure	15–19 kg, ¼ tablet per wk; 20–30 kg, ½ tablet per wk; 31–45 kg, ¾ tablet per wk; >45 kg, 1 tablet per wk
Alternatives		
Doxycycline[§]	100 mg/d, starting 1–2 d before exposure and continuing for 4 wk after last exposure	>8 y of age, 2 mg/kg/d orally (maximum, 100 mg/d)
OR		
Chloroquine phosphate **with or without**	Same as above	
Proguanil[‖]	200 mg/d during exposure and for 4 wk after last exposure	<2 y of age, 50 mg/d; 2–6 y of age, 100 mg/d; 7–10 y of age, 150 mg/d; >10 y of age, 200 mg/d
plus		
Pyrimethamine-sulfadoxine (Fansidar) for presumptive treatment[¶]	Carry a single dose (3 tablets) for self-treatment of febrile illness when medical care is not immediately available	Used as for adults in the following doses: <1 y of age, ¼ tablet; 1–3 y of age, ½ tablet; 4–8 y of age, 1 tablet; 9–14 y of age, 2 tablets; >14 y of age, 3 tablets

* Currently, no drug regimen guarantees protection against malaria. Travelers to countries with risk of malaria should be advised to avoid mosquito bites by using personal protective measures (see text).

† All drugs should be continued for 4 weeks after last exposure.

‡ Mefloquine is not licensed by the Food and Drug Administration for children weighing less than 15 kg, but recent recommendations from the Centers for Disease Control and Prevention allow use of the drug to be considered in children without weight restrictions when travel to chloroquine-resistant *P falciparum* areas cannot be avoided. Mefloquine is *contraindicated* for use by travelers with a known hypersensitivity to mefloquine and travelers with a history of epilepsy or severe psychiatric disorders. A review of available data suggests that mefloquine may be administered to persons concurrently receiving ß-blockers if they have no underlying arrhythmia. However, mefloquine is not recommended for persons with cardiac conduction abnormalities until additional data are available. Caution may be advised for persons involved in tasks requiring fine coordination and spatial discrimi-

Table 3.35. **Prevention of Malaria*, continued**

Drug†	Adult Dosage	Pediatric Dosage

nation, such as airline pilots. Quinidine or quinine may exacerbate the known side effects of mefloquine; patients not responding to mefloquine therapy or failing mefloquine prophylaxis should be closely monitored if they are treated with quinidine or quinine.

§ Physicians who prescribe doxycycline as malaria chemoprophylaxis should advise patients to limit their exposure to direct sunlight to minimize the possibility of photosensitivity reaction. Use of doxycycline is contraindicated in pregnant women and usually in children younger than 8 years. Physicians must weigh the benefits of doxycycline therapy against the possibility of dental staining in children younger than 8 years (see Antimicrobial and Related Therapy, p 606).

‖ Proguanil (chloroguanide hydrochloride) is not available in the United States but is widely available overseas. It is recommended primarily for use in Africa south of the Sahara. Failures in prophylaxis with chloroquine and chloroguanide have been reported commonly, however, as they are only 40% to 60% effective.

¶ Use of Fansidar, which contains 25 mg pyrimethamine and 500 mg sulfadoxine per tablet, is contraindicated in patients with a history of sulfonamide or pyrimethamine intolerance, in infants younger than 2 months, and in pregnant women at term. Resistance to pyrimethamine-sulfadoxine has been reported from Southeast Asia and the Amazon Basin and therefore should not be used for treatment of malaria acquired in these areas.

sulfadoxine (Fansidar) has been reported from Southeast Asia and the Amazon Basin and, therefore, should not be used for treatment of malaria acquired in these areas. Travelers should be advised that self-treatment should not be considered a replacement for seeking prompt medical help. Pyrimethamine-sulfadoxine (Fansidar) should not be taken for routine prophylaxis or by patients with known intolerance to either drug, infants younger than 2 months, or by pregnant women at term, unless circumstances suggest the potential benefit outweighs the possible risk of hyperbilirubinemia in the infant.

Prevention of Relapses. To prevent relapses of *P vivax* or *P ovale* infection after departure from areas where these species are endemic, use of primaquine phosphate should be considered. Primaquine can cause hemolysis in patients with glucose-6-phosphate dehydrogenase deficiency; thus, all patients should be screened for this condition before primaquine therapy is initiated.

Protective Measures. All travelers to areas where malaria is endemic should be advised to use personal protective measures including (1) using insecticide-impregnated mosquito nets while sleeping, (2) remaining in well-screened areas, (3) wearing protective clothing, and (4) using mosquito repellents containing DEET.* To be effective, most of these repellents require reapplication every 1 to 2 hours. Since adverse reactions have been reported with deet on children and include toxic encephalopathy and seizures and skin rashes; it should be used according to the product label, sparingly on exposed skin, and, where possible, on clothing to limit skin exposure. Travelers, particularly children, should be advised against using products containing high concentrations of deet directly on skin because the risks of serious adverse effects is exceedingly low when used according to FDA-approved product label instructions.

---

* Diethyltoluamide.

Malassezia furfur Invasive Infections

CLINICAL MANIFESTATIONS: Neonates with fungemia have fever, pneumonitis, apnea, bradycardia, leukocytosis, and thrombocytopenia. Other serious illnesses, resulting in fungemia, chronic sinusitis, peritonitis, and/or life-threatening pulmonary infections, and infarction, occur primarily in patients with central venous catheters, but can occur in patients with central nervous system catheters, those undergoing continuous peritoneal dialysis, and patients who are immunosuppressed. Locally invasive infection is rare, but includes dacryocystitis, folliculitis, and mastitis.

ETIOLOGY: *Malassezia furfur* is a dimorphic lipid-dependent yeast. It also causes superficial skin infection (see Tinea Versicolor, p 529).

EPIDEMIOLOGY: Hematogenously disseminated infection occurs primarily in neonates receiving parenteral nutrition that includes fat emulsions. Increased neonatal colonization is correlated with a lower gestational age and prolonged hospitalization. In one study, 64% of neonates in an intensive care unit had skin colonization with *M furfur*, whereas only 3% of healthy infants did. Nosocomial colonization provides the likely source of invading strains that colonize the catheter, leading to hematogenous dissemination of the organism.

The **incubation period** is unknown.

DIAGNOSTIC TESTS: The diagnosis can be made from scale scrapings or smears of skin lesions. In potassium hydroxide preparations or methylene blue–stained smears, short septate hyphae of variable length plus clusters of 4- to 8-μm oval or budding yeasts are diagnostic. Routine media may not support growth of this organism because medium- and long-chain fatty acids are required. Sabouraud's dextrose agar medium overlaid with sterile olive oil provides an effective culture system.

TREATMENT: Removal of catheters and temporary cessation of lipid infusions are usually adequate therapy. Although the organism is frequently susceptible to antifungal agents, treatment with these drugs without catheter removal is usually not successful. The need for antifungal therapy in addition to catheter removal in patients with cultures positive for *M furfur* from sites other than blood has not been determined.

ISOLATION OF THE HOSPITALIZED PATIENT: Standard precautions are recommended.

CONTROL MEASURES: Strict adherence to routine infection control measures, such as hand washing, is essential. In addition, aseptic technique when managing intravascular, central nervous system, and intraperitoneal catheters and devices, particularly when administering hyperalimentation fluids, is indicated in neonatal nursery outbreaks.

Measles

CLINICAL MANIFESTATIONS: Measles is an acute disease characterized by fever, cough, coryza, conjunctivitis, an erythematous maculopapular rash, and a pathognomonic enanthem (Koplik spots). Complications such as otitis media, bronchopneumonia, laryngotracheobronchitis (croup), and diarrhea occur more commonly in young children. Acute encephalitis, which frequently results in permanent brain damage, occurs in approximately 1 of every 1000 cases. Death, predominantly due to respiratory and neurologic complications, occurs in 1 to 2 of every 1000 cases reported in the United States. Case-fatality rates are increased in immunocompromised children, including those with leukemia and HIV infection; the characteristic rash sometimes does not develop in these patients.

Subacute sclerosing panencephalitis (SSPE), a rare degenerative central nervous system disease characterized by behavioral and intellectual deterioration and convulsions, is a result of a persistent measles virus infection that develops years after the original infection. Widespread measles vaccination has led to its virtual disappearance in the United States.

ETIOLOGY: Measles virus is an RNA virus with one serotype, classified as *Morbillivirus* in the *Paramyxovirus* family.

EPIDEMIOLOGY: Measles is transmitted by direct contact with infectious droplets or, less commonly, by airborne spread. In temperate areas, the peak incidence of infection usually occurs during the winter and spring. In the prevaccine era, measles was an epidemic disease with biennial cycles in urban areas. Most cases occurred in preschool- and young school-age children, and few persons were still susceptible by age 20 years. The childhood immunization program in the United States has resulted in a greater than 99% reduction in the reported incidence of measles. Since 1963 when measles vaccine was first licensed, the incidence of measles has decreased dramatically in all age groups. The decline has been greatest in children 5 to 14 years of age.

From 1989 to 1991, the incidence of measles in the United States increased, especially in preschool-age children (younger than 5 years) in large, urban settings. The greatest relative increase occurred among children too young (less than 15 months of age) to be immunized according to routine recommendations at that time. The majority of cases in children 15 months to 4 years of age were in vaccine-eligible, unvaccinated children. The major factor contributing to this recrudescence of measles was low immunization rates in preschool-age children, especially in urban areas. Outbreaks involving children and young adults 5 to 24 years old became less prominent in the early 1990s than they were in the 1980s, during which time outbreaks occurred in junior and senior high schools and on college campuses, primarily among vaccinated adolescents who had received a single dose of vaccine. Since 1992, the incidence of measles in the United States has been very low (less than 1000 reported cases per year in 1993 through 1995), and indigenous measles transmission was likely interrupted in 1993. Cases of measles also occur from importation of the virus from other countries.

Vaccine failure occurs in as many as 5% of individuals vaccinated at 12 months of age or older. Although possible waning immunity after vaccination may be a factor in some cases, most cases of measles in previously vaccinated children appear to occur in those in whom response to the vaccine was inadequate, ie, primary vaccine failures.

Patients are contagious from 1 to 2 days before the onset of symptoms (3 to 5 days before the rash) to 4 days after the appearance of the rash. Immunocompromised patients who may have prolonged excretion of the virus in respiratory secretions can be contagious for the duration of the illness. Patients with SSPE are not contagious.

The **incubation period** is generally 8 to 12 days from exposure to onset of symptoms; the average interval from exposure to appearance of the rash is 14 days. In family studies, the average interval between appearance of rash in the source case and subsequent cases is 14 days, with a range of 7 to 18 days. In SSPE, the mean incubation period of 84 cases reported between 1976 and 1983 was 10.8 years.

DIAGNOSTIC TESTS: Measles virus infection can be diagnosed by viral isolation in cell culture from nasopharyngeal secretions, conjunctiva, blood, and/or urine during the febrile phase of the illness. However, virus isolation is technically difficult and often not available. Nevertheless, attempts to isolate the virus are useful in the public health efforts to control and eliminate measles transmission. Detected viruses can be identified by nucleic acid and sequencing, thereby helping to trace the spread of measles strains within the United States and document importation from other countries. Many measles cases can be diagnosed by comparing the serum antibody concentration from a person shortly after appearance of the rash (ie, acute phase) with that in the patient's convalescent sera, obtained as early as 1, but preferably 2 to 4, weeks later. Some patients will already have experienced a substantial rise in antibody titer if the initial serum is obtained 4 or more days after the onset of rash. Some laboratories, however, use a single specimen to detect the presence of measles-specific IgM antibody. Correct interpretation of serologic data requires knowledge of the time at which specimens were obtained relative to the onset of the rash and the characteristics of the antibody assay. Measle-specific IgM antibody may not be detectable in the first 72 hours after the onset of the rash and is usually undetectable 30 to 60 days after the onset of the rash. Some IgM-specific antibody tests may not be positive even in confirmed cases, and some assays have had a relatively high rate of false-positive results.

In SSPE, high titers of measles antibody are found in serum and cerebrospinal fluid.

TREATMENT: No specific antiviral therapy is available. Measles virus is susceptible in vitro to ribavirin, which has been given by the intravenous and/or aerosol route to treat severely affected and immunocompromised children with measles. However, no controlled trials have been conducted, and ribavirin is not approved by the Food and Drug Administration for the treatment of measles.

Vitamin A. The World Health Organization (WHO) and the United Nations International Children's Emergency Fund (UNICEF) recommend administration of vitamin A to all children diagnosed with measles in communities where vitamin A deficiency is a recognized problem and where mortality related to measles is 1% or greater. Several recent investigations indicate that vitamin A treatment of children with measles in developing countries has been associated with reduction in morbidity and mortality.

Although vitamin A deficiency is not recognized as a major problem in the United States, low serum concentrations of vitamin A have been found in children with more severe measles. Hence, although the available data are incomplete and insufficient to determine the appropriate use of vitamin A for all children with measles, vitamin A supplementation should be considered in the following circumstances:

- Patients 6 months to 2 years of age hospitalized with measles and its complications (eg, croup, pneumonia, and diarrhea). Limited data are available regarding the safety and need for vitamin A supplementation for infants younger than 6 months of age.
- Patients older than 6 months with measles who have any of the following risk factors and who are not already receiving vitamin A:
  — Immunodeficiency (eg, HIV infection, congenital immunodeficiencies, and immunosuppressive therapy).
  — Ophthalmologic evidence of vitamin A deficiency, including night blindness, Bitot's spots (grayish white deposits on the bulbar conjunctiva adjacent to the cornea), or xerophthalmia.
  — Impaired intestinal absorption (eg, biliary obstruction, short bowel syndrome, or cystic fibrosis).
  — Moderate to severe malnutrition, including that associated with eating disorders.
  — Recent immigration from areas where high mortality rates due to measles have been observed.

The available vitamin A oral formulation in the United States is a solution, 50 000 IU/mL. The recommended dosage is similar to that recommended by the WHO and UNICEF, and is as follows:

- Single dose of 200 000 IU, orally, for children 1 year and older (100 000 IU for children 6 months to 1 year of age). The higher dose may be associated with vomiting and headache for a few hours.
- The dose should be repeated the next day and at 4 weeks for children with ophthalmologic evidence of vitamin A deficiency.

ISOLATION OF THE HOSPITALIZED PATIENT*: Airborne precautions are indicated for 4 days after the onset of the rash in otherwise healthy children and for the duration of the illness in immunocompromised patients.

CONTROL MEASURES:

Care of Exposed Persons.

Use of Vaccine. Exposure to measles is not a contraindication to vaccination. Available data suggest that live-virus measles vaccine, if given within 72 hours of measles exposure, will provide protection in some cases. If the exposure does not result in infection, the vaccine should induce protection against subsequent

---

* In addition to standard precautions.

measles infection. Vaccine is the intervention of choice for control of measles outbreaks in schools and child care centers. For susceptible household contacts who are at least 6 months of age and are not immunocompromised or pregnant, vaccine is acceptable only if it can be given within 72 hours of exposure, which is usually not possible (since diagnostic findings generally do not occur in the index case until the third or fourth day of the illness). Hence immune globulin is recommended in this circumstance.

Use of Immune Globulin (IG). Immune globulin can be given to prevent or modify measles in a susceptible person within 6 days of exposure. The usual recommended dose is 0.25 mL/kg of body weight given intramuscularly; immunocompromised children should receive 0.5 mL/kg (the maximum dose in either instance is 15 mL). Immune globulin is indicated for susceptible household contacts of patients with measles, particularly contacts younger than 1 year, pregnant women, and immunocompromised persons for whom the risk of complications is highest. Infants younger than 5 months usually have partial or complete protection from passively acquired measles antibodies. However, infants who are less than 6 months of age whose mother develop measles also should receive IG because they are not protected by passive immunity.

Immune globulin is not indicated for household contacts who have received one dose of vaccine at 12 months of age or older unless they are immunocompromised.

Intravenous immune globulin (IGIV) preparations generally contain measles antibodies at approximately the same concentration per gram of protein as IG, although the concentration may vary by lot and manufacturer. For patients who regularly receive IGIV, the usual dose of 100 to 400 mg/kg should be more than sufficient for measles prophylaxis after exposures occurring within 3 weeks of receiving IGIV.

For children who receive IG for modification or prevention of measles after exposure, measles vaccine (if not contraindicated) should be given 5 months (if the dose was 0.25 mL/kg) or 6 months (if the dose was 0.5 mL/kg) after IG administration, provided that the child is at least 12 months old. Longer intervals are required after larger doses of IGIV (see Precautions and Contraindications, p 352).

HIV Infection. Children and adolescents with symptomatic HIV infection who are exposed to measles should receive IG prophylaxis (0.5 mL/kg), regardless of vaccination status (see HIV Infection, p 279). An exception is the patient receiving IGIV at regular intervals whose last dose was received within 3 weeks of exposure. Immune globulin is also indicated for measles-susceptible household contacts with asymptomatic HIV infection, particularly those younger than 1 year.

Hospital Personnel. To decrease nosocomial infection, vaccination programs should be established to ensure that health care personnel who will be in contact with patients with measles are immune to the disease (see Health Care Personnel, p 65).

Measles Vaccine. The only measles vaccine currently licensed in the United States is a live further-attenuated strain prepared in chick embryo cell culture. Measles vaccines provided through the Expanded Programme on Immunization in developing countries meet the WHO standards and are usually comparable to the vaccine available in the United States. Measles vaccine is available in monovalent (measles only) formulation and in combination formulations, ie, measles-rubella (MR) and measles-mumps-rubella (MMR) vaccines.

MMR vaccine is the recommended product of choice in most circumstances, especially when administered at 12 months of age or older and including the routinely recommended second dose of measles vaccine, in order to also provide optimal protection against mumps and rubella. Vaccine (as a combination or monovalent product) in a dose of 0.5 mL is given subcutaneously. Measles and measles-containing vaccines can be given simultaneously with other vaccines (see Simultaneous Administration of Multiple Vaccines, p 21).

Serum measles antibodies develop in approximately 95% of children vaccinated at 12 months of age and 98% of those vaccinated at 15 months of age. Protection conferred by a single dose is durable in most persons. However, a very small percentage of vaccinated individuals may lose protection after several years. More than 99% of persons who receive two doses separated by at least 1 month (4 weeks) and on or after their first birthday develop serologic evidence of measles immunity. Measles vaccination of seronegative persons causes a mild or inapparent, noncommunicable infection. Vaccination is not deleterious for individuals who are already immune.

Improperly stored vaccine may fail to protect against measles. Since 1979, an improved stabilizer has been added to the vaccine that makes it more resistant to heat inactivation. However, during storage before reconstitution, measles vaccine should be kept at 2° to 8°C or colder. Freezing is not harmful to the lyophilized vaccine. Measles vaccine also must be protected from ultraviolet light (especially after reconstitution), which can inactivate the virus. Vaccine should be shipped at 10°C or colder and may be shipped on dry ice. The vaccine diluent (sterile water) vials may break if frozen. Therefore, the diluent should not be frozen. Reconstituted vaccine should be stored in a refrigerator and discarded if not used within 8 hours.

Vaccine Recommendations (see Table 3.36, p 349, for summary).

General. Effective measles control necessitates identification and immunization of all susceptible persons, especially preschool-age children. Because of the continuing occurrence of cases in older children and young adults, emphasis must be placed on identifying and appropriately immunizing potentially susceptible adolescents and young adults in high school, college, and health care settings. Special emphasis should be placed on the administration of the first dose of vaccine by 15 months of age. Delays in administering the first dose contributed to large outbreaks from 1989 to 1991.

By 12 years of age, persons should have received two doses of live-virus measles vaccine, the first of which should be given on or after the first birthday. Prior recommendations for routine reimmunization allowed for flexibility in the age of administration of the second dose—specifically, administration at either 11 to 12 years of age (as recommended by the Academy), at entry to junior high school or middle school, or at 4 to 6 years of age at school entry (as recommended by the Centers for Disease Control and Prevention). As of 1997, however, the second dose is now also recommended at school entry by the Academy. By 2001, the national goal is that all school-age children will have received two doses of measles-containing vaccine.

Persons should be considered susceptible unless they have documentation of appropriate vaccination, physician-diagnosed measles, laboratory evidence of immu-

Table 3.36. **Recommendations for Measles Vaccination***

Category	Recommendations
Unvaccinated, no history of measles (12–15 mo)	A 2-dose schedule (with MMR) is recommended if born after 1956. The first dose is recommended at 12–15 mo; the second is recommended at 4–6 y
Children 12 mo in areas of recurrent measles transmission	Vaccinate; a second dose is indicated at 4–6 y (at school entry)
Children 6–11 mo in epidemic situations[†]	Vaccinate (with monovalent measles vaccine or, if not available, MMR); revaccination (with MMR) at 12–15 mo is necessary and a third dose is indicated at 4–6 y
Children 11–12 y who have received 1 dose of measles vaccine at ≥12 mo	Revaccinate (1 dose)
Students in college and other post-high school institutions who have received 1 dose of measles vaccine at ≥12 mo	Revaccinate (1 dose)
History of vaccination before the first birthday	Consider susceptible and vaccinate (2 doses)
Unknown vaccine, 1963–1967	Consider susceptible and vaccinate (2 doses)
Further attenuated or unknown vaccine given with IG	Consider susceptible and vaccinate (2 doses)
Egg allergy	Vaccinate; no reactions likely (see text for details)
Neomycin allergy, nonanaphylactic	Vaccinate; no reactions likely
Tuberculosis	Vaccinate; vaccine does not exacerbate infection
Measles exposure	Vaccinate or give IG, depending on circumstances (see text, p 347)
HIV-infected	Vaccinate (2 doses) unless severely compromised (see text, p 347)
Immunoglobulin or blood product received	Vaccinate at the appropriate interval (see Table 3.37, p 353)

* See text for details. MMR indicates measles-mumps-rubella vaccine; IG, immune globulin.
† See Outbreak Control (p 355).

nity to measles, or were born before 1957. For children, adolescents, and adults born after 1956, two doses of measles vaccine are required for evidence of immunity.

A parental report of immunization is not considered adequate documentation. Physicians should provide an immunization record for patients only if they have administered the vaccine or have seen a record documenting vaccination.

Age of Routine Vaccination. The first dose should be given at age 12 to 15 months. The second dose is routinely recommended by the Academy at school entry (ie, 4 to 6 years of age). Those children who were not revaccinated at school entry should receive the second dose by 11 to 12 years of age. The second dose also may be given at any age before 4 to 6 years of age (eg, during an outbreak or before international travel), provided the interval between the first and second doses is at least 1 month (4 weeks). If the child receives a dose of measles vaccine before 12 months of age, two additional doses are required beginning at 12 to 15 months.

Colleges and Other Institutions for Education Beyond High School. Colleges and other institutions should require that all entering students have documentation of physician-diagnosed measles, serologic evidence of immunity, birth before 1957, or receipt of two doses of measles-containing vaccines. Students without documentation of any measles vaccination or immunity should receive a dose on entry, followed by a repeat dose 1 or more months (4 weeks) later.

Vaccination of Preschool-age Children in Areas of Recurrent Measles Transmission. Initial vaccination at 12 months of age is recommended for preschool-age children in high-risk areas, especially large urban areas.

During an outbreak, monovalent measles vaccine may be given to infants as young as 6 months (see Outbreak Control, p 355). If monovalent vaccine is not available, MMR may be given. However, seroconversion rates following measles, mumps, and rubella vaccination are significantly lower in children vaccinated before the first birthday than are seroconversion rates in those vaccinated after the first birthday. Children, therefore, vaccinated before their first birthday should be vaccinated with MMR vaccine at 12 to 15 months and again at school entry (4 to 6 years).

International Travel. Persons traveling to foreign countries should be immune to measles. For young children traveling to areas where measles is endemic or epidemic, the age for initial measles vaccination may need to be lowered. Children 12 to 15 months old should be given their first dose of MMR vaccine before departure. Infants 6 to 11 months old should receive a dose of monovalent measles (or MMR) vaccine before departure; they should be revaccinated with MMR vaccine (at least 1 month [4 weeks] after the initial measles vaccination); at 12 to 15 months and again at 4 to 6 years of age in accordance with the requirements for routine measles vaccination. Children 12 months of age and older who have received one dose and are traveling to areas where measles is endemic or epidemic should receive their second dose before departure, provided the interval between dosages is 1 month (4 weeks) or more.

Medical Facilities. Evidence of having had measles, measles immunity, or receipt of two measles vaccinations is recommended before beginning employment for nurses and nursing and medical students, residents, and other staff born after 1956 (see Health Care Personnel, p 65). For recommendations during an outbreak, see Outbreak Control (p 355).

Adverse Events. A fever of 39.4°C (103°F) or higher develops in approximately 5% to 15% of susceptible vaccinees, usually beginning 7 to 12 days after MMR vaccination; the fever generally lasts 1 to 2 days (and for as many as 5 days). Most persons with fever are otherwise asymptomatic. Transient rashes have been reported in approximately 5% of vaccinees. Transient thrombocytopenia has occurred after administration of measles-containing vaccines, specifically MMR (see Thrombocytopenia, p 351). The reported frequency of central nervous system conditions, including encephalitis and encephalopathy, is less than one per million doses administered in the United States. Because the incidence of encephalitis or encephalopathy after measles vaccination in the United States is lower than the observed incidence of encephalitis of unknown etiology, some or most of the reported severe neurologic disorders may be only temporally, rather than causally, related to measles vaccination. After revaccination, reactions are expected to be clinically similar but much less frequent in occurrence because most of these vaccine recipients already are immune.

Very high-titer vaccines have been associated in several developing countries with increased mortality in females several months to years after vaccination. These high-titer vaccines were never licensed in the United States and are no longer in use in foreign countries.

Allergic Reactions. Hypersensitivity reactions occur rarely, usually are minor, and consist of wheal and flare reactions or urticaria at the injection site. Reactions have been attributed to trace amounts of neomycin or gelatin, or some other component in the vaccine formulation. Anaphylaxis is extremely rare. Measles vaccine is produced in chick embryo cell culture and does not contain significant amounts of egg cross-reacting proteins. Recent studies indicate that children with egg allergy are at low risk for anaphylactic reactions to measles-containing (including MMR) vaccines and that skin testing of children allergic to eggs is not predictive of reactions to MMR vaccine.

Seizures. As with any condition that induces fever during the second year of life, children predisposed to febrile seizures can experience seizures after measles immunization. Most of these seizures are simple febrile seizures and do not increase the risk of subsequent epilepsy or other neurologic disorders. Studies have suggested an increased risk of seizures after administration of measles-containing vaccines to children who have a history of seizures or whose first-degree family members have a history of seizures. Although the exact risk cannot be determined, it appears to be low. Children with personal histories of seizures or those whose first-degree relatives have histories of seizures should be immunized because the benefits greatly outweigh the risks. This recommendation is based on the risks from measles disease, the large number of children with personal or family history of seizures (5% to 7%), the low incidence of seizures after measles vaccination, and the lack of association of these seizures with permanent brain damage.

Thrombocytopenia. Reports of adverse reactions in the United States and other countries indicate that MMR vaccine rarely can cause clinically apparent thrombocytopenia within 2 months. Reported cases generally have been transient and benign in outcome. In prospective studies, the reported number has ranged from 1 case per 25 000 vaccinated children to 1 case in 40 000 with a temporal clustering of cases 2 to 3 weeks after vaccination. By passive surveillance, the reported incidence was approximately 1 per 100 000 doses distributed in Canada and 1 per 2 million doses distributed in the United States. The risks of thrombocytopenia from measles or rubella infection is much greater. Based on case reports, the risk of vaccine-associated thrombocytopenia may be higher for those who previously experienced thrombocytopenia, especially when it occurred in temporal association with earlier MMR vaccination.

Subacute Sclerosing Panencephalitis (SSPE). Measles vaccine, by protecting against measles, significantly reduces the possibility of developing SSPE. The marked decline in the number of SSPE cases after the introduction of measles vaccine is additional strong evidence of a protective effect of measles vaccination. Subacute sclerosing panencephalitis has been rarely reported in children with no history of natural measles but with a history of receiving measles vaccine, and SSPE has developed in other children without a history of having had measles or measles vaccine. Some of these children have had unrecognized measles and some children with a history of receiving measles vaccine have been exposed to measles or have had measles-like illnesses before vaccination. However, the risk of SSPE is not enhanced from live-virus measles vaccine given to individuals who previously received live-virus measles vaccine or had natural measles infection.

Precautions and Contraindications (see also Table 3.37 p 353).

Febrile Illnesses. Children with minor illnesses, with or without fever, such as upper respiratory tract infections, may be vaccinated (see Vaccine Safety and Contraindications, p 26). Fever per se is not a contraindication to immunization. However, if other manifestations suggest a more serious illness, the child should not be vaccinated until recovery. Most studies have demonstrated that children with afebrile upper respiratory infections had serologic responses similar to those in well children after measles vaccination.

Allergies. Hypersensitivity reactions rarely follow the administration of measles vaccine (see Adverse Events, p 350). Most children with a history of anaphylactic reactions to eggs have no untoward reactions to measles or MMR vaccine. Persons are not at increased risk if they have egg allergies that are not anaphylactic, and they should be vaccinated in the usual manner. In addition, skin testing of egg-allergic children with vaccine has not been predictive of which children will have an immediate hypersensitivity reaction (see Hypersensitivity Reactions to Vaccine Constituents, p 32). Children who have had a hypersensitivity reaction following the first dose of measles vaccine should be skin tested before receiving the second dose, or they can be tested for serum antibodies to measles to determine the need for a second dose. Children who have had an anaphylactic reaction to prior vaccination should be vaccinated only in settings in which a life-threatening, immediate hypersensitivity reaction can be adequately managed. Persons with allergies to chickens or feathers are not at increased risk of reaction to the vaccine.

Persons who have experienced anaphylactic reactions to topically or systemically administered neomycin should not receive measles vaccine. Most often, however, neomycin allergy manifests as a contact dermatitis, which is a delayed-type (cell-mediated) immune response rather than anaphylaxis. In such persons, an adverse reaction to neomycin in the vaccine would be an erythematous, pruritic nodule or papule 48 to 96 hours after vaccination. A history of contact dermatitis to neomycin is not a contraindication to receiving measles vaccine.

Thrombocytopenia. The risk for developing clinically apparent thrombocytopenia following vaccination with MMR may be increased in children with a history of previous thrombocytopenia or thrombocytopenia purpura. The decision to vaccinate, therefore, should be based on the benefits of protection against measles, mumps, and rubella in comparison to the risks of a recurrence of thrombocytopenia after vaccination and those from measles or rubella. In most cases, the benefits of vaccination outweigh the risks, especially in view of the greater risk of thrombocytopenia with natural infection. However, if an episode of thrombocytopenia occurred in close temporal proximity to vaccination, not giving a subsequent dose may be prudent. Serological testing for immunity to measles and rubella also can be considered in deciding whether to administer the second dose. While thrombocytopenia can be

Table 3.37. **Suggested Intervals Between Immunoglobulin Administration and Measles Vaccination (MMR or Monovalent Measles Vaccine)***

Indication for Immunoglobulin	Route	Dose		Interval, mo[†]
		U or mL	mg IgG/kg	
Tetanus (as TIG)	IM	250 U	~10	3
Hepatitis A prophylaxis (as IG)				
Contact prophylaxis	IM	0.02 mL/kg	3.3	3
International travel	IM	0.06 mL/kg	10	3
Hepatitis B prophylaxis (as HBIG)	IM	0.06 mL/kg	10	3
Rabies prophylaxis (as RIG)	IM	20 IU/kg	22	4
Measles prophylaxis (as IG)				
Standard	IM	0.25 mL/kg	40	5
Immunocompromised host	IM	0.50 mL/kg	80	6
Varicella prophylaxis (as VZIG)	IM	125 U/10 kg (maximum, 625 U)	20–39	5
Blood transfusion				
Washed RBCs	IV	10 mL/kg	Negligible	0
RBCs, adenine-saline added	IV	10 mL/kg	10	3
Packed RBCs	IV	10 mL/kg	20–60	5
Whole blood	IV	10 mL/kg	80–100	6
Plasma or platelet products	IV	10 mL/kg	160	7
Replacement (or therapy) of immune deficiencies (as IGIV)	IV	...	300–400	8
ITP (as IGIV)	IV	...	400	8
RSV-IGIV	IV	...	750	9
ITP	IV	...	1000	10
ITP or Kawasaki disease	IV	...	1600–2000	11

* IG indicates immune globulin; TIG, tetanus IG; IM, intramuscular; HBIG, hepatitis B IG; RIG, rabies IG; VZIG, varicella-zoster IG; IV, intravenous; IGIV, intravenous IG; ITP, immune (formerly termed "idiopathic") thrombocytopenic purpura; and RSV-IGIV, respiratory syncytial virus IGIV.

† These intervals should provide sufficient time for decreases in passive antibodies in all children to allow for an adequate response to measles vaccine. Physicians should not assume that children are fully protected against measles during these intervals. Additional doses of IG or measles vaccine may be indicated after exposure to measles (see text).

life threatening, no reports of thrombocytopenia associated with receipt of MMR vaccine have resulted in death.

Recent Administration of Immune Globulin. Immune globulin preparations interfere with the serologic response to measles vaccine for variable periods depending on the dose administered. For example, vaccination should be deferred for 3 months after a person has received IG for postexposure prophylaxis against hepatitis A, but substantially longer intervals are indicated after larger doses of IG, IGIV, or other

IgG-containing products, such as in the case of patients with immune (formerly termed "idiopathic") thrombocytopenia or Kawasaki disease. Suggested intervals between immune globulin or blood product administration and measles vaccination are given in Table 3.37 (p 353). If vaccine is given at less than the indicated intervals, as may be warranted if the risk of exposure to measles is imminent, the child should be revaccinated at or after the appropriate interval for immunization unless serologic testing indicates that measles-specific antibodies were produced (ie, the child was successfully immunized by the earlier dose of vaccine).

If IG is to be administered in preparation for international travel, administration of vaccine should precede receipt of IG by at least 2 weeks to preclude interference with replication of the vaccine virus.

Tuberculosis. Tuberculin skin testing is not a prerequisite for measles vaccination. Although tuberculosis may be exacerbated by natural measles infection, live-virus measles vaccine is not known to have a deleterious effect, and the value of protection against natural measles far outweighs the theoretical hazard of possible exacerbation of unsuspected tuberculosis. If tuberculin skin testing is otherwise indicated, it can be done on the day of vaccination. Otherwise, it should be postponed for 4 to 6 weeks because measles vaccination may temporarily suppress tuberculin skin test reactivity.

Altered Immunity. Significantly immunocompromised patients should not be given live-virus measles vaccine (see Immunodeficient and Immunosuppressed Children, p 50). Replication of the measles vaccine virus can be potentiated in patients with immunodeficiency diseases and by the suppressed immune responses associated with leukemia, lymphoma, or generalized malignancy, or resulting from therapy with alkylating drugs, antimetabolites, radiation, or large systemic doses of corticosteroids. Patients with such conditions should not be vaccinated with live-virus measles vaccine (see Immunodeficient and Immunosuppressed Children, p 51). Their risk of exposure to measles can be reduced by vaccinating their close susceptible contacts. Vaccinated persons do not transmit vaccine virus. Management of immunodeficient patients exposed to measles can be facilitated by prior knowledge of their immune status. Susceptible patients with immunodeficiencies should receive IG after measles exposure (see Care of Exposed Persons, p 346).

After cessation of immunosuppressive therapy, live-virus measles vaccine in most circumstances is withheld for an interval of at least 3 months (with the exception of corticosteroid recipients, see below). This interval is based on the assumption that immunologic responsiveness will have been restored in 3 months and the underlying disease for which immunosuppressive therapy was given is in remission or under control. However, because the interval can vary with the intensity and type of immunosuppressive therapy, radiation therapy, underlying disease, and other factors, a definitive recommendation for an interval after cessation of immunosuppressive therapy when measles vaccine can be safely and effectively administered is often not possible.

Corticosteroids. For patients who have received high doses of corticosteroids for 14 days or more, and who are not otherwise immunocompromised, the recommended interval is at least 1 month (see Immunodeficient and Immunosuppressed Children, see p 51).

HIV Infection. Measles vaccination (given as MMR vaccine) is recommended at the usual ages for persons with asymptomatic HIV infection and for those with symptomatic infection who are not severely immunocompromised. These recommendations are based on reports of severe and often fatal measles and the lack of complications from live-virus vaccination in HIV-infected patients (see HIV Infection, p 279). However, a case of vaccine-related measles pneumonitis in a severely immunocompromised patient has been recently reported. Hence, in severely immunocompromised patients with HIV infection, as defined by low CD4+ T-lymphocyte counts or percentage of total lymphocytes, should not receive measles vaccine (see HIV Infection, p 293).

Regardless of vaccination status, symptomatic HIV-infected patients who are exposed to measles should receive IG prophylaxis because vaccination may not provide protection (see Care of Exposed Persons, p 346). An exception is the patient receiving IGIV at regular intervals whose last dose was received within 3 weeks of exposure.

Personal or Family History of Seizures. Children with this history should be vaccinated after discussion of the risks and benefits of immunization with the parent or guardian (see Adverse Events, p 350). The parents or guardians of children who have a personal or immediate family history of seizures should be advised that such children have a slightly increased risk of seizures after measles vaccination. Because fever induced by measles vaccine usually occurs between 7 and 12 days after immunization, prevention of vaccine-related febrile seizures is difficult. Parents should be alert to the occurrence of fever after vaccination and should treat their children appropriately. Children who are receiving anticonvulsants should continue to take such therapy after measles vaccination. However, prophylactic use of anticonvulsants may not be feasible, as therapeutic concentrations of many of the currently prescribed anticonvulsants (eg, phenobarbital) are not achieved for some time after the initiation of therapy.

Pregnancy. Live-virus measles vaccine, when given as a component of MR or MMR, should not be given to women known to be pregnant or who are considering becoming pregnant within 3 months of vaccination. Women who are given monovalent measles vaccine should not become pregnant for at least 30 days. This precaution is based on the theoretical risk of fetal infection, which applies to the administration of any live-virus vaccine to women who might be pregnant or who might become pregnant shortly after vaccination. No evidence, however, substantiates this theoretical risk. In the immunization of adolescents and young adults against measles, asking women if they are pregnant, excluding those who are, and explaining the theoretical risks to the others are recommended precautions.

Outbreak Control (see Table 3.38, p 356, for summary). All reports of suspected measles cases should be investigated promptly. A measles outbreak exists in a community whenever one case of measles is confirmed. Subsequent prevention of the spread of measles depends on the prompt vaccination of exposed and potentially exposed persons who cannot readily provide documentation of measles immunity, including the date of vaccination (see p 346). Such persons who have been exempted from measles vaccination for medical, religious, or other reasons, if not vaccinated within 72 hours of exposure, should be excluded from the setting until at least 2 weeks after the onset of rash in the last case of measles.

Table 3.38. **Recommendations for Control of Measles Outbreaks**

Setting	Control Measures
Outbreaks in preschool-age children	Age for vaccination should be lowered to 6 mo in outbreak area if cases are occurring in children <1 y.*
Outbreaks in institutions: child care centers, K-12th grades, colleges, and other institutions	All students, their siblings, and school personnel born after 1956 who do not have documentation of immunity to measles[†] should have received 2 doses of measles vaccine.
Outbreaks in medical facilities	Revaccination of all medical workers born after 1956 who have direct patient contact and who do not have proof of immunity to measles.[†] Vaccination may also be considered for workers born before 1957.
	Susceptible personnel who have been exposed should be relieved from direct patient contact from the 5th to the 21st day after exposure (regardless of whether they received measles vaccine or IG) or, if they become ill, for 4 d after rash develops.

* Children initially vaccinated before the first birthday should be revaccinated at 12 to 15 months of age. A third dose should be administered at 4 to 6 years of age.
† Proof consists of documentation of physician-diagnosed measles disease, serologic evidence of immunity to measles, or documentation of receipt of 2 doses of measles vaccine on or after the first birthday.

Schools and Child Care Centers. A program of revaccination with MMR vaccine is recommended during outbreaks in child care centers; elementary, middle, junior, and senior high schools; and colleges and other institutions of higher education. Consideration should be given to revaccination in unaffected schools that may be at risk of measles transmission. Revaccination should include all students and their siblings and personnel born after 1956 who cannot provide documentation that they received two doses of measles-containing vaccine on or after their first birthday or other evidence of measles immunity. Persons revaccinated, as well as unvaccinated persons receiving their first dose as part of the outbreak control program, may be immediately readmitted to school. Mass revaccination of entire communities is not necessary.

Imposing quarantine measures for outbreak control is difficult and disruptive to schools and other organizations. Under special circumstances, restriction of an event might be warranted; however, such action is not recommended as a routine measure for outbreak control.

Children Younger Than 1 Year. The risk of complications from measles is high among infants younger than 1 year. Therefore, considering the benefits and risks, vaccination with monovalent measles vaccine (or MMR if monovalent vaccine is not available) is recommended for infants as young as 6 months when exposure to natural measles is considered likely. Children vaccinated before the first birthday should be revaccinated with MMR when they are 12 to 15 months and again at school entry (see Vaccine Recommendations, p 348).

Medical Settings. If an outbreak occurs in an area served by a hospital or within a hospital, all employees with direct patient contact who were born after 1956 who cannot provide documentation that they have received two doses of measles vaccine on or after their first birthday or other evidence of immunity to measles should receive a dose of measles vaccine. Because some health care personnel who have acquired measles in medical facilities were born before 1957, vaccination of older employees who may have occupational exposure to measles should also be considered. Susceptible personnel who have been exposed should be relieved from direct patient contact from the fifth to the 21st day after exposure regardless of whether they received vaccine or IG after the exposure. Personnel who become ill should be relieved from patient contact for 4 days after rash develops.

Meningococcal Infections*

CLINICAL MANIFESTATIONS: Invasive infection usually results in meningococcemia and/or meningitis. Onset is abrupt in meningococcemia with fever, chills, malaise, prostration, and a rash that initially may be urticarial, maculopapular, or petechial. In fulminant cases, purpura, disseminated intravascular coagulation, shock, coma, and death (Waterhouse-Friderichsen syndrome) can ensue within several hours despite appropriate therapy. The signs of meningococcal meningitis are indistinguishable from those of acute meningitis caused by *Haemophilus influenzae* type b, *Streptococcus pneumoniae,* and other bacterial pathogens. Invasive meningococcal infections can be complicated by arthritis, myocarditis, pericarditis, endophthalmitis, or pneumonia. Less common diseases include pneumonia, occult febrile bacteremia, conjunctivitis, and chronic meningococcemia.

ETIOLOGY: *Neisseria meningitidis* is a Gram-negative diplococcus with multiple serogroups known to cause invasive disease (A, B, C, X, Y, Z, W-135, and L). Serogroups B and C are currently the most prevalent in the United States, each accounting for approximately 45% of reported cases. Group A has been associated frequently with epidemics elsewhere in the world.

EPIDEMIOLOGY: Asymptomatic colonization of the upper respiratory tract is frequent and provides the focus from which the organism is spread. Transmission is from person to person through droplets of respiratory tract secretions. Since the introduction of *H influenza* type b vaccination of infants, *N meningitidis* has become one of the two leading causes of bacterial meningitis in young children and remains an important cause of septicemia. Disease occurs most often in children younger than 5 years; the peak attack rate occurs in the 3- to 5-month age group. Close contacts of patients with meningococcal disease are at an increased risk for developing infection. Outbreaks have occurred in semiclosed communities, including child care centers, schools, colleges, and military recruit camps. Onset of an outbreak is often heralded by a shift in the age distribution of cases to an older age group. Patients

---

* For further information, see American Academy of Pediatrics, Committee on Infectious Diseases. Meningococcal disease prevention and control strategies for practice-based physicians *Pediatrics.* 1996;97:404-412.

with deficiency of a terminal complement component (C5-9), properdin deficiencies, and those with anatomic or functional asplenia are at particular risk for invasive and recurrent meningococcal disease. Patients are considered capable of transmitting infection for approximately 24 hours after initiation of effective treatment.

The **incubation period** is from 1 to 10 days, most commonly less than 4 days.

DIAGNOSTIC TESTS: Cultures of blood and cerebrospinal fluid (CSF) are indicated in all patients with suspected invasive meningococcal disease. Cultures of petechial scraping, synovial fluid, sputum, and other body fluids are positive in some patients. A Gram stain of a petechial scraping, CSF, and buffy coat of blood can be helpful on occasion. Since *N meningitidis* can be part of the normal nasopharyngeal flora, isolation of this organism from the throat is not helpful in determining the cause of invasive disease. Bacterial antigen detection tests, such as by latex agglutination, are of limited value in rapid diagnosis. Detection of meningococcal polysaccharide antigens by a latex agglutination test in urine is not helpful in case identification because false-positive as well as false-negative results can occur. The sensitivity and specificity are less than 50%. In contrast, a positive antigen detection test of CSF or serum has better sensitivity and specificity, and supports the diagnosis of a probable case if the clinical illness is consistent with meningococcal disease, particularly during an outbreak or a cluster of cases. These tests also may be useful in patients in whom antibiotics were administered before specimens for culture were obtained. Rapid antigen tests for group B *N meningitidis* may be unreliable because group B meningococcal antisera also reacts with *Escherichia coli* K1 antigen. A polymerase chain reaction test has been used in research laboratories to detect and type *N meningitidis* from clinical specimens. Multilocus enzyme electrophoresis can be used to detect divergence among strains as an epidemiologic marker during a suspected outbreak.

Case definitions for invasive disease are given in Table 3.39, p 359.

TREATMENT:
- Penicillin G should be administered intravenously in a high dose every 4 to 6 hours for patients with invasive disease. Cefotaxime and ceftriaxone are acceptable alternatives. In a patient with anaphylactoid-type penicillin allergy, chloramphenicol is indicated. Five to 7 days of antibiotic therapy usually is adequate for most cases of invasive meningococcal disease. In the few areas (Spain and parts of Africa) where in vitro penicillin resistance has been reported, cefotaxime, ceftriaxone, or chloramphenicol is recommended.
- Dexamethasone therapy should be considered in infants and children 2 months or older with bacterial meningitis after consideration of the possible benefits and risks (see Dexamethasone Therapy for Bacterial Meningitis in Infants and Children, p 620).

ISOLATION OF THE HOSPITALIZED PATIENT*: Droplet precautions are recommended until 24 hours after initiation of effective therapy.

---

* In addition to standard precautions.

Table 3.39. Case Definitions for Invasive Meningococcal Disease

Confirmed

• Isolation of *N meningitidis* from a usually sterile site, eg:
  Blood
  Cerebrospinal fluid
  Synovial fluid
  Pleural fluid
  Pericardial fluid
  Petechial or purpuric lesion

Presumptive

• Gram-negative diplococci in any sterile fluid, such as cerebrospinal fluid, synovial fluid, or aspirate from a petechial or purpuric lesion

Probable

• A positive antigen test for *N meningitidis* in blood or cerebrospinal fluid in the absence of a positive sterile site culture in the setting of a clinical illness consistent with meningococcal disease

CONTROL MEASURES:

Care of Exposed Persons.

Careful observation. Exposed household, school, or child care contacts must be carefully observed. Exposed individuals who develop a febrile illness should receive prompt medical evaluation. If indicated, antimicrobial therapy appropriate for invasive meningococcal infections should be administered, pending results of blood and CSF cultures.

Chemoprophylaxis. The risk of contracting invasive meningococcal disease among contacts of cases is the determining factor in the decision to give chemoprophylaxis (see Table 3.40, p 360). Close contacts of all persons with invasive disease, whether sporadic or in a cluster or an outbreak, are at increased risk and should receive prophylaxis as soon as possible, preferably within 24 hours of the diagnosis of the primary case. Throat and nasopharyngeal cultures are not of value in deciding who should receive prophylaxis.

Household, child care center, and nursery school contacts. Household, child care, and nursery school contacts are at increased risk, with attack rates more than 300 times higher than those in the general population.

Other contacts. Prophylaxis is warranted for persons who have had contact with the patient's oral secretions through kissing or sharing of food or beverages during the 7 days before onset of disease in the index case. In addition, persons who frequently eat or sleep in the same dwelling within this period of time should receive chemoprophylaxis. Prophylaxis is not recommended routinely for medical personnel except those who have had intimate exposure, such as occurs with unprotected mouth-to-mouth resuscitation, intubation, or suctioning, before antibiotic therapy was begun.

Antibiotic regimens (see Table 3.41, p 361). The drug of choice in most instances is rifampin. The recommended regimen for rifampin prophylaxis is 10 mg/kg (maxi-

Table 3.40. **Disease Risk for Contacts of Index Cases of Invasive Meningococcal Disease***

High risk: chemoprophylaxis recommended

- Household contact: especially young children
- Child care or nursery school contact in previous 7 d
- Direct exposure to index patient's secretions through kissing or sharing toothbrushes or eating utensils
- Mouth-to-mouth resuscitation, unprotected contact during endotracheal intubation in 7 d before onset of the illness
- Frequently sleeps or eats in same dwelling as index patient

Low risk: chemoprophylaxis not recommended

- Casual contact: no history of direct exposure to index patient's oral secretions, eg, school or work mate
- Indirect contact: only contact is with a high-risk contact, no direct contact with the index patient
- Medical personnel without direct exposure to patient's oral secretions

In outbreak or cluster

- Chemoprophylaxis for persons other than those at high risk should be given only after consultation with the local public health authorities

* Nasopharyngeal aspirate to throat swab cultures are **not** useful in determining risk.

mum, 600 mg) every 12 hours, for a total of four doses in 2 days. Some experts recommend reducing the dose to 5 mg/kg for infants younger than 1 month. A liquid preparation can be formulated or the powder can be mixed with other vehicles such as applesauce. For adults, each dose is 600 mg. The 4-day rifampin regimen, given for prophylaxis of *Haemophilus influenzae* type b disease, of 20 mg/kg (maximum, 600 mg) once a day for 4 days, also is effective for meningococcal prophylaxis.

Ceftriaxone given in a single intramuscular dose (125 mg for children younger than 12 years; 250 mg for children older than 12 years and for adults) has been demonstrated to be more effective than oral rifampin in eradicating pharyngeal carriage of group A meningococci. Although ceftriaxone is not recommended routinely for prophylaxis because its efficacy has been confirmed only for group A strains, its effect is likely to be similar for other strains. It has the advantages of easier dosage administration and safety in pregnancy in comparison to rifampin.

Ciprofloxacin given to adults in a single, oral dose of 500 mg also is effective in eradicating meningococcal carriage. At present, ciprofloxacin is not recommended for persons younger than 18 years or for pregnant women (see Antimicrobials and Related Therapy, p 605).

Sulfisoxazole may be used when an isolate is known to be susceptible to sulfonamides. The dose is 500 mg/d for infants younger than 1 year, 500 mg every 12 hours for children 1 to 12 years, and 1 g every 12 hours for children older than 12 years and for adults. The duration of therapy is 2 days.

The **index case** also should receive chemoprophylactic antibiotics before hospital discharge unless the infection was treated with ceftriaxone or cefotaxime.

Table 3.41. Recommended Chemoprophylaxis Regimens for High-Risk Contacts and Index Cases of Invasive Meningococcal Disease*

Infants, Children, and Adults	Dose	Duration	% Efficacy	Cautions
Rifampin†				
≤1 mo	5 mg/kg orally every 12 h	2 d	72–90	May interfere with efficacy of oral contraceptives, some seizure prevention, and anticoagulant medications; may stain soft contact lenses
>1 mo	10 mg/kg (maximum, 600 mg) orally every 12 h	2 d		
	20 mg/kg (maximum, 600 mg) orally every 24 h	4 d		
Ceftriaxone				
≤12 y	125 mg intramuscularly	Single dose	97	To decrease pain at injection site, dilute with 1% lidocaine
> 12 y	250 mg intramuscularly	Single dose		
Ciprofloxacin†				
≥ 18 y	500 mg orally	Single dose	90-95	Not recommended for use in children

* Oral sulfisoxazole may be used if the organism is known to be susceptible. The dosage is as follows: <1 year of age, 500 mg a day for 2 days; and 1 to 12 years of age, 500 mg every 12 hours for 2 days; >12 years of age, 1 g every 12 hours for 2 days.
† Not for use in pregnant women.

Immunoprophylaxis. Because secondary cases can occur several weeks or more after onset of disease in the index case, meningococcal vaccine is a possible adjunct to chemoprophylaxis when the outbreak is caused by a serogroup contained in the vaccine.

Meningococcal Vaccine. A serogroup-specific quadrivalent meningococcal vaccine against groups A, C, Y, and W-135 *N meningitidis* is approved in the United States for use in children 2 years of age and older. The vaccine consists of 50 µg each of the respective purified bacterial capsular polysaccharides. It is administered subcutaneously as a single 0.5-mL dose and can be given concurrently with other vaccines but at a different site. No vaccine is available for the prevention of group B disease due to the poor immunogenicity of unconjugated group B meningococcal polysaccharide.

The group A meningococcal vaccine is immunogenic in children 3 months and older, although a response comparable to that seen in adults is not achieved until

4 or 5 years of age. For children younger than 18 months, two doses 3 months apart have been given in epidemic control. When the quadrivalent vaccine is given to infants in a group A outbreak, response to the other meningococcal group polysaccharides usually is poor. The serogroup C polysaccharide does not induce an immunogenic antibody response before age 24 months. The groups Y and W135 vaccine polysaccharides have been demonstrated to be immunogenic and safe in children 2 years of age and older.

Indications. Routine immunization of children with meningococcal vaccine is not recommended. However, immunization is recommended for children 2 years and older in high-risk groups, including those with functional or anatomic asplenia (see Asplenic Children, p 56), and those with terminal complement component or properdin deficiencies. Vaccination can be used as an adjunct to chemoprophylaxis (see Care of Exposed Persons, p 359). The vaccine is indicated to control outbreaks of disease caused by one of the serogroups (ie, A, C, Y and W-135) represented in the vaccine. Vaccination may be beneficial for travelers to countries recognized to have hyperendemic or epidemic meningococcal disease caused by a vaccine-preventable serogroup. The vaccine currently is given to all military recruits in the United States.

Revaccination. Little information is available to determine the need for or timing of reimmunization when the risk of disease continues or recurs. The duration of protection from the initial vaccination is not established. Serum meningococcal antibody in vaccinated adults appears to persist for as long as 10 years but in children, especially those initially immunized when younger than 4 years, antibody concentrations decline markedly during the first 3 years after vaccination. Hence, if new or continued risk of exposure occurs, reimmunization of children against group C infection should be considered after 1 year if the child was first immunized at younger than 4 years and after 5 years for children first immunized at 4 years of age or older. Reimmunization of adults before 5 years after initial immunization does not appear to be necessary even if a new risk of exposure occurs.

Adverse reactions and precautions. Infrequent and mild adverse reactions occur, the most common of which is localized erythema for 1 to 2 days. The safety of the vaccine in pregnant women has not been established, and pregnant women should be immunized only if they have a substantial risk of infection.

Reporting. All confirmed, presumptive, and probable cases of invasive meningococcal disease must be reported to the regional public health department. Timely reporting can facilitate early recognition of clusters of cases and outbreaks so that appropriate prevention programs can be implemented quickly.

Counseling and Public Education. When a case of invasive meningococcal disease is detected, the physician needs to provide accurate and timely information about meningococcal disease and the risk of transmission to families and contacts of the index case, including health care workers. Public health questions, such as whether a mass vaccination program is needed are best referred to the local public health department, which also can be helpful in alerting other physicians in the community and in handling questions from the media. In appropriate situations, early provision of information in collaboration with the local health department to schools or other groups at increased risk and to the media may help minimize public anxiety and unrealistic or inappropriate demands for intervention.

Microsporidia Infections
(Microsporidiosis)

CLINICAL MANIFESTATIONS: Patients with intestinal infection have watery, nonbloody diarrhea. Fever is uncommon. Intestinal infection is most common in immunocompromised persons, especially those who are HIV-infected, resulting often in chronic diarrhea. The clinical course is complicated by malnutrition and progressive weight loss. Chronic infection in immunocompetent persons is rare. Other clinical syndromes that can occur in HIV-infected and immunocompetent patients include keratoconjunctivitis, nephritis, hepatitis, cholangitis, and peritonitis, but they occur infrequently.

ETIOLOGY: *Microsporidia* are intracellular protozoa. The following genera infect humans: *Encephalitozoon, Septata, Enterocytozoon, Pleistophora,* and *Nosema,* as well as unclassified microsporidia. *Enterocytozoon bieneusi* and *S intestinalis* are important causes of chronic diarrhea in HIV-infected patients.

EPIDEMIOLOGY: Information about the epidemiology and mode of transmission is limited. In animals, transmission occurs by ingestion of *Microsporidia* spores in food or contact with spores shed into the environment through stools or urine. In humans, fecal-oral contact may have a role in transmission.

The **incubation period** is not known.

DIAGNOSTIC TESTS: Infection with *Microsporidia* can be documented by identification of organisms in biopsy specimens from the small intestine. *Microsporidia* spores also can be detected in formalin-fixed stool specimens or duodenal aspirates stained with a chromotrope-based stain, which is a modification of the trichrome stain, and viewed by light microscopy. Gram, acid-fast, periodic acid–Schiff, and Giemsa stains also can be used to detect organisms in tissue sections. The organisms often are not noticed because they are small, stain poorly, and evoke minimal inflammatory response. Use of one of the stool concentration techniques does not appear to improve the ability to detect *E bieneusi* spores. Identification for classification purposes and diagnostic confirmation of species requires electron microscopy.

TREATMENT: No effective therapy is known. In a limited number of patients, albendazole or metronidazole have been reported to decrease diarrhea, but without eradication of the organism. Albendazole appears to be more effective in cases due to *S intestinalis*. Recurrence of diarrhea is common after therapy is stopped.

ISOLATION OF THE HOSPITALIZED PATIENT*: Contact precautions are recommended for diapered and/or incontinent children for the duration of illness.

CONTROL MEASURES: None.

---

* In addition to standard precautions.

Molluscum Contagiosum

CLINICAL MANIFESTATIONS: Molluscum contagiosum is a benign, usually asymptomatic viral disease of the skin. It is characterized by relatively few (usually 2 to 20) discrete, papular, waxy lesions, some with central umbilication, in a generalized distribution. An eczematous reaction may encircle the lesions in about 10% of patients. It has no systemic manifestations. Patients with eczema and immunosuppressed individuals, including those with HIV infection, tend to have more intense and widespread eruptions.

ETIOLOGY: The cause is a poxvirus.

EPIDEMIOLOGY: Humans are the only known source of the virus. It is spread by direct contact, including sexual contact, or by fomites such as towels. The infectivity is generally low, but occasional outbreaks have been reported. The period of communicability is unknown.

The **incubation period** seems to vary between 2 and 7 weeks but may be as long as 6 months.

DIAGNOSTIC TESTS: The diagnosis can usually be made from the characteristic appearance of the lesions. Wright or Giemsa staining of material expressed from the central core of the lesions reveals characteristic intracytoplasmic inclusions. Electron microscopic examination will identify the typical poxvirus particles.

TREATMENT: Mechanical removal of the central core of each lesion usually results in resolution; EMLA* cream, a topical anesthetic, may be applied 30 minutes before the procedure. Alternatively, topical application of cantharidin (0.7% in collodion), peeling agents such as salicylic and lactic acid preparations, or liquid nitrogen may be successful. Although lesions can regress spontaneously, removal is advisable, when possible, to prevent autoinoculation and spread to other individuals. Scarring does not occur.

ISOLATION OF THE HOSPITALIZED PATIENT: Standard precautions are recommended.

CONTROL MEASURES: No control measures are known for isolated cases. For outbreaks, such as are commonly found in the tropics, restricting direct body contact and sharing of potentially contaminated fomites (eg, towels and washcloths) between affected and unaffected persons can reduce the spread.

---

* Eutetic mixture of local anesthetics.

Moraxella catarrhalis Infections

CLINICAL MANIFESTATIONS: Common infections include acute otitis media and paranasal sinusitis in children. Bronchopulmonary infection, often occurring in patients with chronic lung disease, can occur. Rare manifestations are bacteremia in healthy or immunocompromised children (sometimes associated with focal infections such as osteomyelitis, septic arthritis or abscesses, or a rash indistinguishable from that observed in meningococcemia) and conjunctivitis in neonates.

ETIOLOGY: *Moraxella catarrhalis* (formerly called *Branhamella catarrhalis*) is a Gram-negative diplococcus. Nearly 100% of strains produce ß-lactamase that mediates resistance to penicillins.

EPIDEMIOLOGY: *Moraxella catarrhalis* is part of the normal flora of the upper respiratory tract of humans. The mode of transmission is presumed to be direct contact with contaminated respiratory tract secretions and/or droplet spread. Infection is most frequent in infants but occurs at all ages. Transmission in families, schools, and child care centers has not been studied. The duration of carriage by infected and colonized children and the period of communicability are unknown.

The **incubation period** is unknown.

DIAGNOSTIC TESTS: The organism can be isolated readily on common culture media (blood or chocolate agar) after incubation in air or with increased CO_2 (candle jar). Culture of middle ear or sinus aspirates is indicated in patients with unusually severe infection, some who fail to respond to treatment, and neonates or other highly susceptible children. Concomitant recovery of *M catarrhalis* with other pathogens (*Streptococcus pneumoniae* or *Haemophilus influenzae*) can occur and indicates a mixed infection.

TREATMENT: Although most strains of *Moraxella* produce ß-lactamase and are resistant to amoxicillin in vitro, this agent remains effective as empiric therapy for otitis media and other respiratory tract infections. When *Moraxella* is isolated from appropriately obtained specimens (middle ear fluid, sinus aspirates, or lower respiratory secretions), or when initial therapy has been unsuccessful, appropriate antibiotic choices include amoxicillin-clavulanate, cefixime, cefaclor, cefuroxime, erythromycin, clarithromycin, azithromycin, dirithromycin, and trimethoprim-sulfamethoxazole. If parenteral drugs are needed to treat *M catarrhalis* infection, in vitro data indicate that the following drugs will be effective: cefuroxime, cefotaxime, ceftriaxone, ceftazidime, chloramphenicol, and trimethoprim-sulfamethoxazole.

ISOLATION OF THE HOSPITALIZED PATIENT: Standard precautions are recommended.

CONTROL MEASURES: None.

Mumps

CLINICAL MANIFESTATIONS: Mumps is a systemic disease characterized by swelling of the salivary glands. Approximately one third of infections, however, do not cause clinically apparent salivary gland swelling. Meningeal signs are common. Encephalitis occurs rarely, and permanent sequelae or death is uncommon. Orchitis is a common complication after puberty, but sterility rarely occurs. Other rare complications include arthritis, renal involvement, thyroiditis, mastitis, pancreatitis, and hearing impairment.

ETIOLOGY: Mumps is caused by a paramyxovirus.

EPIDEMIOLOGY: Humans are the only known natural hosts. The virus is spread by direct contact via the respiratory route. Infection occurs throughout childhood. During adulthood, infection is likely to produce more severe disease, including orchitis. Death due to mumps is rare; more than half the fatalities occur in persons older than 19 years. Mumps infection during the first trimester of pregnancy can increase the rate of spontaneous abortion. Although mumps virus can cross the placenta, no evidence exists that mumps infection in pregnancy causes congenital malformations. The infection is more common during late winter and spring. The incidence has declined markedly since the introduction of the mumps vaccine. While a minor resurgence of mumps occurred in 1986-1987 in the United States, the incidence since has declined substantially to about 1500 cases per year in recent years. Incidence rates are currently highest in children 5 to 9 years of age followed by those 1 to 4 and 10 to 14 years of age. However, many cases of parotitis can be caused by agents other than mumps, especially in vaccinated children. Outbreaks can occur in highly vaccinated populations, indicating that mumps transmission can be sustained among the few persons not protected by vaccination. The period of communicability usually is from 1 to 2 days after onset (but occasionally as long as 7 days) before the onset of parotid swelling to as long as 9 days.

The **incubation period** is usually from 16 to 18 days, but cases may occur from 12 to 25 days after exposure.

DIAGNOSTIC TESTS: Children with parotitis should have diagnostic testing to confirm mumps virus as the cause, since mumps is now a rare infection and parotitis may be caused by other agents. Mumps virus can be isolated in cell culture inoculated with throat washings, urine, or spinal fluid. The complement fixation (CF), neutralization, or hemagglutination inhibition (HAI) test or an enzyme immunoassay (EIA) can be used to serologically confirm infection or vaccination. Although paired sera are desirable, a single serum specimen containing complement-fixing antibody against the soluble component of mumps virus suggests recent infection. Immunity is assessed by an EIA or neutralization test, although the latter test is not always readily available; CF or HAI tests are unreliable for this purpose. Skin tests also are unreliable and should not be used to test immune status.

TREATMENT: Supportive.

ISOLATION OF THE HOSPITALIZED PATIENT*: Droplet precautions are recommended until 9 days after the onset of parotid swelling.

CONTROL MEASURES:

School and Child Care. Children should be excluded for 9 days from the onset of parotid gland swelling. For control measures during an outbreak, see Outbreak Control, p 369.

Care of Exposed Persons. Mumps vaccine has not been demonstrated to be effective in preventing infection after exposure. However, mumps vaccine can be given after exposure, as immunization will provide protection against subsequent exposures. No increased risk of reactions or contraindications exist after vaccination of a person during the incubation period of mumps or from vaccination of a person who is already immune. Because approximately 90% of adults who have no knowledge of past infection are immune by serologic testing, mumps vaccine is not routinely advised for those born before 1957 unless they are proven to be susceptible (ie, seronegative). Mumps immune globulin is of no value and is no longer manufactured or licensed in the United States.

Mumps Vaccine. Live-virus vaccine is prepared in chick embryo cell cultures. Vaccine is administered by subcutaneous injection of 0.5 mL, either alone as a monovalent vaccine or preferably as the combined vaccine containing measles, mumps, and rubella vaccines (MMR). Antibody develops in more than 95% of all susceptible persons after a single dose. Serologic and epidemiologic evidence extending for more than 25 years indicates that vaccine-induced immunity is long lasting.

Vaccine Recommendations.
- Mumps vaccine should be given as MMR routinely to children at 12 to 15 months of age. A second dose of MMR is recommended at 4 to 6 years of age in accordance with recommendations for routine measles vaccination; those who have not received this dose at school entry should be vaccinated by or before 12 years of age (see Measles, p 344). Revaccination for mumps can be important because mumps can occur in highly vaccinated populations, including individuals with a history of mumps vaccination. Administration of MMR is not harmful if given to an individual already immune to one or more of the viruses (from infection or vaccination).
- Mumps vaccination is of particular importance for children approaching puberty, adolescents, and adults who have not had mumps or mumps vaccine. At office visits of prepubertal children and adolescents, the status of immunity to mumps should be assessed. Persons should be considered susceptible unless they have documentation of at least one dose of vaccine on or after the first birthday, documentation of physician-diagnosed mumps, serologic evidence of immunity, or were born before 1957.

---

* In addition to standard precautions.

- Susceptible children, adolescents, and adults born after 1956 should be offered mumps vaccination (usually as MMR) before beginning travel. Although vaccination against mumps is not a requirement for entry into any country, mumps is still endemic throughout most of the world. Because of concern about inadequate seroconversion related to persisting maternal antibodies and because the risk of serious disease from mumps infection is relatively low, persons younger than 12 months need not be given mumps vaccine before travel.
- Mumps vaccine is not routinely advised for those born before 1957 unless they are considered susceptible, as defined by seronegativity. However, vaccination is not contraindicated in these persons if their serologic status is unknown.
- Mumps vaccine can be given simultaneously with other vaccines (see Simultaneous Administration of Multiple Vaccines, p 21).

Adverse Reactions. Adverse reactions attributed to mumps live-virus vaccine are extremely rare. Temporally related reactions, including febrile seizures, nerve deafness, parotitis, meningitis, encephalitis, rash, pruritus, and purpura, may not be causally related. In the United States, the frequency of central nervous system complications after mumps vaccination has been lower than the observed incidence in the normal (ie, unvaccinated) population. Orchitis and parotitis have been reported rarely. Allergic reactions are also rare (see Precautions and Contraindications, below). Other reactions that occur following vaccination with MMR are attributable to the measles and rubella components of the vaccine (see Measles, p 350, and Rubella, p 459).

Reimmunization with mumps vaccine (monovalent or MMR) is not associated with an increased incidence of reactions. Reactions might be expected only among those not protected by the first dose.

Precautions and Contraindications.

Febrile Illness. Children with minor illnesses with or without fever, such as upper respiratory tract infections, may be vaccinated (see Vaccine Safety and Contraindications, p 26). Fever per se is not a contraindication to immunization. However, if other manifestations suggest a more serious illness, the child should not be vaccinated until recovery.

Allergies. The widespread use of the mumps vaccine since 1967 has resulted in only rare, isolated reports of allergic reactions. Allergic reactions to components of the vaccine occasionally may occur. Severe allergic reactions, such as anaphylaxis, are rarely reported. Most children with egg hypersensitivity can be safely immunized with MMR. Skin testing with MMR vaccine does not reliably predict which children will have a hypersensitivity reaction following the administration of MMR vaccine (see Measles, p 344).

Recent Administration of Immune Globulin. Live mumps vaccine should be given at least 2 weeks before or at least 3 months after administration of IG or blood transfusion because of the theoretical possibility that antibody will neutralize vaccine virus and inhibit a successful immunization. Because mumps vaccine is usually given as MMR, and high doses of IG (such as those given for the treatment of Kawasaki disease) can inhibit the response to measles vaccine for longer intervals, mumps vaccination with MMR also should be deferred for longer periods in such circumstances (see Measles, p 344).

Altered Immunity. Patients with immunodeficiency diseases and those receiving immunosuppressive therapy (eg, patients with leukemia, lymphoma, or generalized malignancy), including large systemic doses of corticosteroids, alkylating agents, antimetabolites, or radiation, or who are otherwise immunocompromised should not receive live-virus mumps vaccine (see Immunodeficient and Immunosuppressed Children, p 50). The exceptions are patients with symptomatic HIV infection who are not severely immunocompromised; these patients should be vaccinated against mumps with MMR (see HIV Infection, p 279). The risk of mumps exposure for patients with altered immunity can be reduced by vaccinating their close, susceptible contacts. Vaccinated persons do not transmit mumps vaccine virus.

After cessation of immunosuppressive therapy, live-virus mumps vaccine in most circumstances is withheld for an interval of at least 3 months (with the exception of corticosteroid recipients, see below). This interval is based on the assumption that immunologic responsiveness will have been restored in 3 months and the underlying disease for which immunosuppressive therapy was given is in remission or under control. However, because the interval can vary with the intensity and type of immunosuppressive therapy, radiation therapy, underlying disease, and other factors, a definitive recommendation for an interval after cessation of immunosuppressive therapy when mumps vaccine can be safely and effectively administered is often not possible.

Corticosteroids. For patients who have received high doses of corticosteroids for 14 days or more, and who are not otherwise immunocompromised, the recommended interval is at least 1 month (see Immunodeficient and Immunosuppressed Children, p 51).

Pregnancy. Susceptible postpubertal females should not be vaccinated if they are known to be pregnant, and before vaccination they should be counseled about the potential hazard of fetal infection with vaccine virus. Live-virus mumps vaccine can infect the placenta, but the virus has not been isolated from fetal tissues of susceptible females who received vaccine and underwent elective abortions. In view of the theoretical risk, however, conception should be avoided for 3 months after mumps vaccination with MMR vaccine (see Measles, p 352). Women given monovalent mumps vaccine should not become pregnant for at least 30 days.

Outbreak Control. In determining means to control outbreaks, exclusion of susceptible students from affected schools and schools judged by local public health authorities to be at risk for transmission should be considered. Such exclusion should be an effective means of terminating school outbreaks and rapidly increasing rates of immunization. Excluded students can be readmitted immediately after vaccination. Pupils who have been exempted from mumps vaccination because of medical, religious, or other reasons should be excluded until at least 26 days after the onset of parotitis in the last person with mumps in the affected school. Experience with outbreak control for other vaccine-preventable diseases indicates that this strategy has been highly effective.

Mycoplasma pneumoniae Infections

CLINICAL MANIFESTATIONS: Initial symptoms in patients who develop pneumonia, the most prominent infection, are malaise, fever, and, in some cases, headache. Cough, usually associated with widespread rales on physical examination, develops within a few days and lasts for 3 to 4 weeks. Nonproductive at first, the cough later may become productive, particularly in older children and adolescents. Approximately 10% of children with pneumonia exhibit a rash, most often maculopapular. Roentgenographic abnormalities vary, but bilateral, diffuse infiltrates are common.

The most common clinical syndromes are acute bronchitis and upper respiratory tract infections, including pharyngitis, and, occasionally, otitis media or myringitis, which may be bullous. Coryza (ie, the common cold), sinusitis, and croup are infrequent.

Unusual manifestations are aseptic meningitis, encephalitis, cerebellar ataxia, peripheral neuropathy, myocarditis, pericarditis, polymorphous mucocutaneous eruptions (including Stevens-Johnson syndrome), hemolytic anemia, and arthritis. Patients with sickle cell disease, immunodeficiencies, and chronic cardiorespiratory disease can develop severe pneumonia with pleural effusion.

ETIOLOGY: The mycoplasmas, including *Mycoplasma pneumoniae*, are the smallest free-living microorganisms. These organisms lack a cell wall and are pleomorphic.

EPIDEMIOLOGY: Infected humans are the only known source of infection. *Mycoplasma pneumoniae* is highly transmissible; acquisition is most likely from symptomatic patients and is presumed to be by droplet spread. Persons of any age can be infected, but specific disease syndromes are age-related. *M pneumoniae* is an uncommon cause of infection in children younger than 5 years but is the leading cause of pneumonia in school-age children and young adults. Military and college populations have a high incidence of the disease. Infections occur throughout the world, in any season, and in all geographic settings. Community-wide epidemics may occur every 4 to 8 years. Familial spread frequently continues for many months, resulting in cumulative household attack rates that approach 100%. Clinical illness within a group, particularly a family, can range from tracheobronchitis to pneumonia. Asymptomatic carriage after infection can occur for prolonged intervals, commonly for weeks, but has not been associated with transmission of illness. Immunity after infection is not long-lasting.

The **incubation period** is 1 to 4 weeks.

DIAGNOSTIC TESTS: Recovery of *M pneumoniae* in cultures requires special media (which is not widely available), is successful in only 40% to 90% of cases, and takes 7 to 21 days. Isolation of *M pneumoniae* in a patient with compatible clinical manifestations suggests causation. Because this organism can be excreted from the respiratory tract for several weeks after an acute infection despite appropriate therapy, isolation of the organism, however, may not indicate acute infection. A polymerase chain reaction test for *M pneumoniae* also has been developed but is not yet widely available.

Serological diagnosis can be made by demonstrating a fourfold or greater increase in titer between acute and convalescent sera. The complement fixation (CF) and immunofluorescent (IF) methods are most widely used. Several enzyme immuno-assay (EIA) antibody tests also are available. Several rapid diagnostic tests for detection of *M pneumoniae* antibodies are available, including a slide agglutination reaction and a 5-minute EIA. The IF test is capable of detecting *Mycoplasma*-specific IgM and IgG antibodies. Although the presence of IgM antibodies confirms recent *M pneumoniae* infection, they persist in serum for several months and do not necessarily indicate current infection. Since *M pneumoniae* CF and EIA antibodies cross-react with some other antigens, particularly with those of other mycoplasmas, results of these tests should be interpreted cautiously in evaluating febrile illnesses of unknown origin. However, no cross-reactivity with other respiratory pathogens causing diseases clinically similar to those caused by *M pneumoniae* exists. False-negative results also occur with both assays.

Serum cold hemagglutinin titers of 1:32 or more are present in more than 50% of patients with pneumonia by the beginning of the second week of illness. Fourfold increases in hemagglutinin titer between acute and convalescent sera occur more often in patients with severe *M pneumoniae* than in those with less severe disease. This test has low specificity for *Mycoplasma* infection, however, and other agents, including adenoviruses, Epstein-Barr virus, and measles, can cause illnesses in infants or children associated with a rise in titer of cold hemagglutinins. A negative test for cold agglutinins does not exclude the diagnosis of mycoplasmal infection.

Since infections are common and resulting antibodies persist for months or years, measurement of antibody in a single serum sample is of little diagnostic value. However, a CF titer of 1:32 or greater during an acute respiratory illness is suggestive of *M pneumoniae* infection.

TREATMENT: Acute bronchitis and upper respiratory tract illness caused by *M pneumoniae* are generally mild and resolve without antibiotic therapy. Erythromycin is the preferred antimicrobial agent for treatment of pneumonia and otitis media in children younger than 8 years. Other new macrolides, such as clarithromycin and azithromycin, are also likely to be effective. Tetracycline is equally effective and may be used in children 8 years of age and older. Most studies with these antimicrobial agents have been conducted in adults, and definitive evidence of their efficacy in children with *M pneumoniae* infection is lacking.

ISOLATION OF THE HOSPITALIZED PATIENT*: Droplet precautions are recommended for the duration of illness.

CONTROL MEASURES: Diagnosis of an infected patient should lead to an increased index of suspicion for *Mycoplasma* infection in household members and close contacts. Case finding should be instituted if infection has occurred in many persons in a group. Therapy for each contact should be given if a compatible clinical illness occurs.

Antibiotic prophylaxis for exposed contacts is not routinely recommended. The benefit of chemoprophylaxis has not been adequately assessed, but limited

---

* In addition to standard precautions.

data suggested that prophylaxis may reduce the rate of transmission within families. Hence, households where patients with underlying conditions that predispose to severe *Mycoplasma* infection, such as sickle cell disease, are intimately exposed to infection, prophylaxis with erythromycin or tetracycline may be of value during the acute phase of illness in a household member.

Nocardiosis

CLINICAL MANIFESTATIONS: A common presentation in nonimmunocompromised children is cutaneous or lymphocutaneous disease after contamination of an abrasion. Usually in these cases the lesions remain localized. Invasive disease occurs most commonly in immunocompromised patients, particularly those with chronic granulomatous disease or HIV infection. Infection characteristically begins in the lung, with hematogenous spread to the liver, brain, kidneys, and other organs. Pulmonary disease resembles that of tuberculosis and systemic fungal infection.

ETIOLOGY: *Nocardia* species are funguslike bacteria. Disease is caused most commonly by *Nocardia asteroides*, less frequently by *Nocardia braziliensis*, and occasionally by other *Nocardia* species.

EPIDEMIOLOGY: *Nocardia* species are free living in nature, soil, and compost, and are found worldwide. Infectious particles are airborne, and the lung is the probable portal of entry. Direct skin inoculation occurs, often as the result of minor trauma and/or soil contamination. Person-to-person transmission does not occur.

The **incubation period** is unknown.

DIAGNOSTIC TESTS: Stained smears of sputum, cerebrospinal fluid, or pus can demonstrate beaded, branched, weakly Gram-positive rods that are variably acid fast. The Brown and Brenn and the methenamine silver stains are recommended for demonstrating microorganisms in tissue. Growth of typical colonies occurs on Sabouraud's dextrose agar without added antibiotics. Blood specimens should be cultured on brain-heart infusion media. These organisms are slow growing; therefore, cultures should be maintained for 7 to 10 days.

TREATMENT: Trimethoprim-sulfamethoxazole or a sulfonamide (eg, sulfadiazine, sulfisoxazole, or triple sulfonamide combinations) is the drug of choice. Blood concentrations of the sulfonamide should be maintained at 15 to 20 mg/dL. Immunocompetent patients with lymphocutaneous disease usually respond after 6 to 12 weeks of therapy. Immunocompromised patients and those with invasive disease should be treated for 6 to 12 months and for at least 3 months after apparent cure because of the tendency for relapse or the appearance of metastatic abscesses that can recur months or years after therapy. Patients with AIDS may need even longer therapy. Patients with meningitis or brain abscess should be monitored with serial imaging studies of the brain. If response to trimethoprim-sulfamethoxazole or sulfadiazine drugs does not occur, gentamicin, amikacin, minocycline, cycloserine, ampicillin, imipenem, amoxicillin/clavulanate, or an extended-spectrum cephalosporin may be of benefit. Tetracycline antibiotics generally are not recommended for children younger than 8 years of age (see Antimicrobials and Related Therapy, p 606). Incision and drainage of abscesses are beneficial.

ISOLATION OF THE HOSPITALIZED PATIENT: Standard precautions are recommended.

CONTROL MEASURES: None.

Onchocerciasis
(River Blindness, Filariasis)

CLINICAL MANIFESTATIONS: The disease involves the skin, subcutaneous tissues, lymphatics, and eyes. Subcutaneous nodules of varying sizes, containing adult worms, develop 6 to 12 months after the initial infection. In patients in Africa, the nodules tend to be found on the lower torso, pelvis, and lower extremities, whereas in patients in Central America, the nodules are more often located on the upper body (the head and torso). After the worms mature, microfilariae are produced and migrate in the tissues, and may cause a chronic, generalized, pruritic dermatitis. After a period of years, the skin can become lichenified and hypopigmented or hyperpigmented. The presence of microfilariae, living or dead, in the ocular structures, leads to photophobia and inflammation of the cornea, iris, ciliary body, retina, choroid, and optic nerve. Blindness can result if the disease is untreated.

ETIOLOGY: *Onchocerca volvulus* is a filarial nematode.

EPIDEMIOLOGY: The larvae are transmitted by the bites of an infected Simulium black fly that breeds in fast-flowing streams and rivers (hence the colloquial name of the disease, "river blindness"). The disease occurs primarily in equatorial Africa, but small foci are found in southern Mexico, Guatemala, northern South America, and Yemen. Prevalence is greatest among those who live near vector-breeding areas. The adult worms continue to produce microfilariae capable of infecting flies for as long as a decade. The infection is not transmissible by person-to-person contact or blood transfusion.

The **incubation period** from larval inoculation to microfilariae in the skin is approximately 6 to 12 months.

DIAGNOSTIC TESTS: Direct examination of a shave biopsy of the epidermis (taken from scapular or posterior hip area) usually will reveal microfilariae. Specimens should be incubated in saline solution overnight and examined unstained under a microscope. A slit-lamp examination of the anterior chamber of the eye may reveal motile microfilariae or corneal lesions typical of onchocerciasis. Microfilariae are rarely found in blood. Eosinophilia is common. Specific serologic tests and polymerase chain reaction techniques for detection of microfilariae in skin are available only at selected research laboratories.

TREATMENT: Ivermectin, a microfilaricidal agent, is the drug of choice for treatment of onchocerciasis and is available from the manufacturer.* Treatment reduces dermatitis and the risk of developing ocular disease, but it does not kill the adult worms and, thus, is not curative. A single oral dose (150 mg/kg) should be given annually for 5 to 10 years. Adverse reactions are caused by the death of the microfilariae and include rash, edema, fever, exacerbation of asthma, and hypotension (which is rarely severe). Contraindications to treatment include pregnancy, central nervous system disorders, and body weight less than 15 kg.

ISOLATION OF THE HOSPITALIZED PATIENT: Standard precautions are recommended.

CONTROL MEASURES: Repellents and protective clothing (long sleeves and pants) can reduce exposure to black fly bites. Treatment of vector breeding sites with larvicides has been effective for controlling black fly populations, particularly in West Africa. A major initiative to distribute ivermectin to all infected communities to interrupt transmission of the parasite has been undertaken.

Papillomaviruses

CLINICAL MANIFESTATIONS: Human papillomaviruses (HPV) produce epithelial tumors (warts) of the skin and mucous membranes. Cutaneous nongenital warts include common skin warts, plantar warts, flat warts, thread-like (filiform) warts, and epidermodysplasia verruciformis. Those affecting the mucous membranes include anogenital, oral, nasal, and conjunctival warts, and respiratory papillomatosis.

Common skin warts are dome-shaped with conical projections that give the surface a rough appearance. They are usually asymptomatic and multiple, occurring on the hands and around or under the nails. When small dermal vessels thrombose, black dots appear in the warts. Plantar warts on the foot can be painful and are characterized by marked hyperkeratosis, sometimes with black dots.

Flat warts ("juvenile warts") are commonly found on the face and extremities of children and adolescents. They are usually small, multiple, and flat topped; they seldom exhibit papillomatosis and rarely cause pain. Filiform warts occur on the face and neck. Cutaneous warts are benign.

The manifestations of anogenital HPV infection range from asymptomatic infection to condylomata acuminata, skin-colored growths with a cauliflower-like surface that vary from a few millimeters to several centimeters in diameter. In males, such warts may be found on the shaft of the penis, penile meatus, scrotum, and perianal areas. In females, warts are seen on the labia and perianal areas; asymptomatic nonverrucous infections occur in the vagina and on the cervix. Most anogenital warts are asymptomatic but occasionally cause itching, burning, local pain, or bleeding. Some HPV types are associated with genital dysplasia and carcinoma, including carcinoma of the cervix.

---

* Merck and Co, West Point, Pa.

Laryngeal papillomas are rare. They are found mostly in children around 3 years of age, and are manifested by a voice change or abnormal cry. When occurring in infancy, they have been associated with respiratory obstruction.

Epidermodysplasia verruciformis is a rare, lifelong, severe papillomavirus infection, believed to be a consequence of an inherited deficiency of cell-mediated immunity. The lesions can resemble flat warts but are often similar to tinea versicolor, covering the torso and upper extremities. Most appear in the first decade of life, but malignant transformation, which occurs in approximately one third of affected persons, is usually delayed until adulthood.

ETIOLOGY: Human papillomaviruses are members of the *Papovaviridae* family and are DNA viruses. More than 70 types have been identified, but a small number of HPV types account for most warts. Those causing nongenital warts are distinct from those causing anogenital infections. Of the latter, only a small number have been associated with malignancies.

EPIDEMIOLOGY: Papillomaviruses are widely distributed among mammals but are species-specific. Cutaneous warts occur frequently among school-age children; prevalence rates are as high as 50%. Human papillomavirus infections are thought to be transmitted from person to person by close contact. Nongenital warts are acquired through minor trauma to the skin. An increase in the incidence of plantar warts has been associated with swimming in public pools. The intense and often widespread appearance of warts in patients with compromised cellular immunity (particularly patients who have undergone transplantation and those with HIV infection) suggests that alterations in immunity may predispose to the reactivation of latent intraepithelial infection.

Anogenital warts are primarily transmitted by sexual contact but can be acquired at the time of delivery. When they are found in a prepubertal child beyond infancy, sexual abuse must be considered. Evidence of genital HPV infection has been detected in as many as 38% of sexually active adolescent females. Anogenital HPV infection is the most common viral sexually transmitted disease in the United States.

Laryngeal papillomas are believed to be transmitted through aspiration of infectious secretions during passage through the infected birth canal.

The **incubation period** is unknown but is estimated to range from 3 months to several years. Papillomavirus acquired by a neonate at the time of delivery may not cause clinical manifestations for several years.

DIAGNOSTIC TESTS: Most cutaneous and anogenital warts are diagnosed by clinical inspection. Detection of cervical HPV infection can be enhanced by use of culdoscopy with application of 3% to 5% acetic acid (vinegar), which causes the lesion to turn white. This characteristic, however, is not specific for HPV infection and false-positive test results are common. When the diagnosis is questionable, histologic examination of a biopsy or cytology specimen (for Papanicolaou smear) can be diagnostic.

No culture for HPV is available. Tests for the detection of HPV nucleic acids in cervical cells are available in some centers.

TREATMENT: Most nongenital warts eventually regress spontaneously, but may persist for months or years. The optimal treatment for warts that do not resolve spontaneously has not been identified. Most methods of treatment rely on chemical or physical destruction of the infected epithelium, such as the application of salicylic acid products or cryotherapy with liquid nitrogen. Daily treatment with tretinoin has been found useful for treatment of widespread flat warts in children. Care must be taken to avoid a deleterious cosmetic result of therapy.

The optimal treatment for anogenital (exophytic) warts has not been identified. Approximately 25% regress spontaneously within 3 months. The application of podophyllum resin or patient-applied podofilox (the major cytotoxic ingredient of podophyllum resin) is often the initial therapy of choice. Neither agent has been tested for safety and efficacy in children, and their use is contraindicated in pregnancy. Other treatment modalities are cryotherapy, trichloracetic acid, electrocautery, laser surgery, and surgical excision. Although most forms of therapy are successful in the initial removal of warts, treatment does not eradicate HPV infection from the surrounding normal tissue. Recurrences are, therefore, common and probably due to reactivation rather than reinfection.

Both genital warts and asymptomatic HPV infection of the cervix in adolescents can be associated with epithelial dysplasia. Hence, the care of patients with these conditions requires a physician who is knowledgeable in their diagnosis, treatment, and prognosis.

Laryngeal papillomas are difficult to treat. Local recurrence is common, and repeated surgical procedures for removal are usually necessary. Extension or dissemination of laryngeal papillomas into the trachea, bronchi, or lung parenchyma results in increased morbidity and mortality. Interferon has been used as an investigational treatment and may be of benefit for patients with frequent recurrences.

Oral warts can be removed through cryotherapy, electrocautery, or surgical excision.

ISOLATION OF THE HOSPITALIZED PATIENT: Standard precautions are recommended.

CONTROL MEASURES: Suspected child abuse should be reported to the appropriate local agency. Sexual transmission of anogenital warts can be decreased by using condoms or refraining from intercourse until therapy is completed and lesions have healed. Although HPV infection is postulated to persist for life, the degree and duration of contagiousness in patients with a history of genital infection is unknown.

Examination of sex partners is unnecessary. The majority are probably already infected with HPV and no practical test for asymptomatic infection is available.

Although laryngeal papillomatosis is believed to be acquired in most cases during passage through the birth canal, this condition has occurred among infants delivered by cesarean section. Because the preventive value of cesarean delivery is unknown, it should not be performed to prevent transmission of HPV to the newborn.

Paracoccidioidomycosis
(South American Blastomycosis)

CLINICAL MANIFESTATIONS: Disease occurs primarily in adults; it is rare in children. Primary infection is thought to occur in the lung. Involvement of lymph nodes and visceral dissemination (ie, adrenals, spleen, liver, and kidney) are common features of the illness in children. Chronic granulomatous lesions of the mucous membranes, especially of the mouth, the skin adjacent to the mouth, and the rectum, are typical, although infrequent, findings. Infection may remain latent for many years before causing illness.

ETIOLOGY: *Paracoccidioides brasiliensis* is a dimorphic fungus with a yeast and a mycelial (mold) phase.

EPIDEMIOLOGY: The infection occurs primarily in South America, where it is endemic and the predominant systemic fungal disease. Cases also have been reported in Central America and Mexico. The natural reservoir is not known, although soil is suspected. The mode of transmission is also unknown; person-to-person transmission does not occur.

The **incubation period** is highly variable, ranging from 1 month to many years.

DIAGNOSTIC TESTS: Round, multiple-budding cells may be seen in 10% potassium hydroxide preparations of sputum or material from lesions, or by histopathological examination. The organism can be cultured easily on most enriched media, including blood agar at 37°C and Sabouraud's dextrose agar (preferably with added cycloheximide) at room temperature. Complement fixation, enzyme-linked immunosorbent assay, and immunodiffusion serologic antibody tests are useful diagnostic tests. Skin test hypersensitivity is not reliable in diagnosis because nonreactivity is common at diagnosis and false-positive test results can occur with histoplasmosis; however, hypersensitivity developing during therapy portends a good prognosis.

TREATMENT: Paracoccidioidomycosis can be treated with sulfonamides, amphotericin B, and azole drugs, such as ketoconazole and itraconazole. For acute and severe paracoccidioidomycosis, amphotericin B is usually recommended in combination with a sulfonamide or an azoles (see Systemic Treatment With Amphotericin B, p 630). The treatment of choice in children in other circumstances has been ketoconazole. In adults, itraconazole appears to be equally effective as ketoconazole and to cause fewer side effects. However, the safety and efficacy of itraconazole in children have not been established. Prolonged therapy for at least 6 months is necessary.

ISOLATION OF THE HOSPITALIZED PATIENT: Standard precautions are recommended.

CONTROL MEASURES: None.

Paragonimiasis

CLINICAL MANIFESTATIONS: The disease has an insidious onset and a chronic course. The initial symptom is usually cough, which eventually becomes productive of blood-tinged sputum. Pleural pain and dyspnea follow. Bacterial pneumonitis and lung abscesses can complicate the course. Pleural effusion and pneumothorax have also been reported. Because of pulmonary fibrosis and bronchiectasis, clubbing of the fingers and toes can develop. Abdominal disease, occurring when the worms invade the intestinal wall, is associated with dull pain, nausea, vomiting, and diarrhea. Involvement of the lymph nodes can lead to suppuration and abscesses. Symptoms tend to subside after approximately 5 years, but can persist for as many as 20 years. Invasion of the brain occurs rarely; acutely, it may resemble meningoencephalitis and cause seizures.

ETIOLOGY: The adult *Paragonimus westermani* is a fluke, 10- to 12-mm long and 5- to 7-mm wide. Other species of paragonimiasis are responsible for human infection in the Western hemisphere.

EPIDEMIOLOGY: Transmission occurs when raw or uncooked freshwater crabs or crayfish containing larvae (metacercariae) are ingested. They excyst in the small intestine and penetrate the abdominal cavity, where they undergo further development. After several days, most of the larvae travel to the lungs through the diaphragm, but some remain in the abdomen and others reach aberrant sites. They burrow into the tissues, become encapsulated, and begin laying eggs after approximately 4 to 6 weeks. When sputum that contains eggs is swallowed, the eggs are passed in the stool. Eggs in fresh water hatch within 3 weeks and yield miracidia, which penetrate snails. Cercariae emerge several weeks later and encyst on and within the muscles and viscera of freshwater crustaceans and mature into infective metacercariae.

Areas of the highest prevalence are limited to the Far East, especially Japan, Korea, Taiwan, and the Philippines. The disease is also endemic in West Africa. The Western hemisphere has endemic foci in Colombia, Venezuela, Ecuador, Peru, Costa Rica, and Mexico. Foxes, civets, tigers, leopards, panthers, mongooses, wolves, pigs, dogs, and cats serve as animal reservoirs. No person-to-person transmission occurs.

The **incubation period** is not known.

DIAGNOSTIC TESTS: Microscopic examination of stools, sputum, pleural effusion, cerebrospinal fluid, and other tissue aspirates can reveal the eggs. A Western blot serologic antibody test that is available at the Centers for Disease Control and Prevention (CDC) is sensitive and specific, but the results do not distinguish active from past infection. Charcot-Leyden crystals and eosinophils in sputum are useful diagnostic elements.

TREATMENT: Praziquantel in a 2-day course is the drug of choice. An alternative drug, bithionol, is effective but is associated with side effects that include gastrointestinal disturbances and allergic rashes. It is available from the Drug Service of the CDC (see Directory of Telephone Numbers, p 667).

ISOLATION OF THE HOSPITALIZED PATIENT: Standard precautions are recommended.

CONTROL MEASURES: Boiling of crabs for several minutes until the meat has congealed and turned opaque kills the metacercariae. Complete control is impossible because of the animal reservoirs.

Parainfluenza Viral Infections

CLINICAL MANIFESTATIONS: Parainfluenza viruses are the major cause of laryngotracheobronchitis (croup), but they also frequently result in upper respiratory tract infection, pneumonia, or bronchiolitis. Infections can be particularly severe and persistent in immunodeficient children.

ETIOLOGY: Parainfluenza viruses are large, enveloped RNA viruses classified as paramyxoviruses. Four antigenically distinct types—1, 2, 3, and 4 (with two subtypes, 4A and 4B)—have been identified.

EPIDEMIOLOGY: Parainfluenza viruses are believed to be transmitted from person to person by direct contact and exposure to contaminated nasopharyngeal secretions through respiratory droplets and/or fomites. Parainfluenza viral infections are ubiquitous and are epidemic as well as sporadic. Type 1 viruses tend to produce outbreaks of respiratory illness, usually croup, in the fall of every other year. A major increase in the number of cases of croup in the autumn is indicative of a parainfluenza type 1 outbreak. Type 2 virus can also cause outbreaks of respiratory illness in the fall, often in conjunction with type 1 outbreaks, but type 2 outbreaks tend to be less severe, irregular, and less frequent. Parainfluenza type 3 virus usually causes respiratory illness during the spring and summer in temperate climates. Infections with types 4A and 4B are less commonly recognized, sporadic, and generally clinically mild.

Illness from primary infection with types 1 and 2 occurs predominantly in 2- to 6-year-old children. Infection with type 3 virus usually is acquired initially during the first 2 years of life and is a major cause of lower respiratory tract disease in infants. Reinfections can occur at any age, but they are usually milder, causing primarily upper respiratory tract illness. Immunodeficient individuals can develop severe lower respiratory tract disease, with prolonged shedding of the virus.

Healthy children with primary infection from type 1 shed the virus for an average of 4 to 7 days, but this shedding can last as long as 2 weeks. The average period of shedding for type 3 infections is 8 to 9 days, but can last as long as 3 weeks.

The **incubation period** is from 2 to 6 days.

DIAGNOSTIC TESTS: Virus may be isolated from nasopharyngeal secretions in cultures, usually within 4 to 7 days. More rapid identification of viral antigen in the nasopharyngeal secretions can be accomplished by immunofluorescent and enzyme immunoassay methods, but the sensitivity of the tests can be variable. Serologic diagnosis, made retrospectively by a significant rise in antibody titer between sera obtained during acute infection and convalescence, generally is less helpful and can be confusing, because heterotypic antibody rises from infections caused by other serotypes of parainfluenza and mumps viruses are common. Furthermore, infection may not always be accompanied by a significant homotypic antibody response.

TREATMENT: Racemic epinephrine aerosol is given frequently to severely affected, hospitalized patients with laryngotracheobronchitis to reduce airway obstruction. Parenteral dexamethasone in high doses (greater than 0.3 mg/kg), oral dexamethasone (0.15 to 0.6 mg/kg), and nebulized corticosteroids have been demonstrated to lessen the severity and duration of symptoms in patients with moderate to severe laryngotracheobronchitis compared to similar treatment of placebo-treated patients. However, nebulized dexamethasone in outpatient care does not appear to be effective in reducing the risk of hospitalization or in altering the clinical outcome at 24 hours. Management is otherwise supportive.

ISOLATION OF THE HOSPITALIZED PATIENT*: Contact precautions are recommended for hospitalized infants and young children for the duration of illness. Strict adherence to infection control procedures, including prevention of contamination by respiratory secretions and careful hand washing, should control nosocomial spread.

CONTROL MEASURES: Efforts should be aimed at reducing nosocomial infection. Hand washing should be emphasized.

Parasitic Diseases

Parasitic diseases traditionally have been considered exotic and, therefore, frequently are not included in differential diagnoses in the United States and Europe. Nevertheless, these organisms are among the most common causes of morbidity and mortality in various and diverse geographic locations worldwide. Tourists returning to their own countries, immigrants from endemic areas (eg, refugees from Indochina, Central America, and the Caribbean), and immunosuppressed patients are at risk for having acquired parasitic infections in nonendemic areas. Physicians and clinical laboratories need to be aware of where these infections may be acquired, clinical presentations, and methods of diagnosis so that tourists can be appropriately warned before travel and evaluated upon return to the United States.

Table 3.42 (p 381) gives details on some less commonly encountered parasitic diseases.

Consultation and assistance in the diagnosis and management of parasitic diseases are available from government agencies (eg, Centers for Disease Control and Prevention [CDC] and state health departments) and from university departments of geographic medicine, tropical medicine, infectious disease, international health, and public health.

---

* In addition to standard precautions.

Table 3.42. Additional Parasitic Diseases*

Disease and/or Agent	Where Infection May Be Acquired	Definitive Host	Intermediate Host	Modes of Human Infection	Directly Communicable (Person to Person)	Diagnostic Laboratory Tests in Humans	Causative Form of Parasite	Manifestation in Humans
Angiostrongylus cantonensis	Pacific islands, Eastern Asia, Puerto Rico, Cuba, Africa	Rats	Snails and slugs	Eating uncooked, infected mollusks	No	Eosinophils in CSF; identification of larvae in CSF or at autopsy	Larval worms	Meningo-encephalitis
Angiostrongylus costaricensis	Central and South America	Rodents	Snails and slugs	Eating uncooked, infected mollusks	No	Gel diffusion	Larval worms	Abdominal pain
Anisakiasis	Cosmopolitan, mainly Japan	Marine mammals	Certain saltwater fish, squid or octopus	Eating uncooked, infected fish	No	Identification of recovered larvae in granulomas or vomitus	Larval worms	Acute gastrointestinal disease
Clonorchis sinensis	Far East	Humans, cats, dogs, other animals	Certain fresh-water snails	Eating uncooked, infected freshwater fish	No	Eggs in stool or duodenal fluid	Larvae and mature flukes	Abdominal pain; hepato-biliary disease

Table 3.42. **Additional Parasitic Diseases*, continued**

Disease and/or Agent	Where Infection May Be Acquired	Definitive Host	Intermediate Host	Modes of Human Infection	Directly Communicable (Person to Person)	Diagnostic Laboratory Tests in Humans	Causative Form of Parasite	Manifestation in Humans
Dracontiasis (*Dracunculus medinensis*)	Foci in India, Yemen, Africa, Middle East	Humans	Crustacea copepods	Drinking infected water	No	Adult worm in skin, subcutaneous tissues	Adult female worm	Inflammatory response; systemic and local in skin and subcutaneous tissue
Fascioliasis (*Fasciola hepatica*)	Foci throughout tropics and temperate areas	Humans and many animals	Certain freshwater snails and vegetation	Eating uncooked, infected plants such as watercress	No	Eggs in feces, duodenal fluid or bile	Larvae and mature worms	Disease of liver and biliary tree; acute gastrointestinal disease
Fasciolopsiasis (*Fasciolopsis buski*)	Far East	Humans, pigs, dogs	Certain freshwater snails, plants	Eating uncooked, infected plants	No	Eggs or worm in feces or duodenal fluid	Larvae and mature worms	Diarrhea, constipation vomiting, anorexia, edema of face and legs, ascites
Intestinal capillariasis (*Capillaria philippinensis*)	Philippines, Thailand	Humans	Fish	Ingestion of uncooked, infected fish	Uncertain	Eggs and parasite in feces	Larvae and mature worms	Protein-losing enteropathy, ascites, emaciation

* For recommended drug treatment, see Drugs for Parasitic Infections (p 637). CSF indicates cerebrospinal fluid.

The CDC distributes a number of drugs that are used for treatment of parasitic diseases that are not available commercially in the United States. These drugs are indicated by footnotes in the tables on Drugs for Parasitic Infections (p 637), and in the chapters on specific parasitic infections. To request these drugs, a physician must contact the CDC Drug Service (see Directory of Telephone Numbers, p 667), and provide the following information: (1) the physician's name, address, and telephone number; (2) the type of infection to be treated and the method by which the infection was diagnosed; and (3) the patient's name, age, weight, sex, and, if the patient is a woman, whether she is pregnant. Prior consultation with a medical officer from the CDC may be required.

Important human parasitic infections are discussed in individual chapters in Section 3; the diseases are arranged alphabetically and the discussions include recommendations for drug treatment. **Tables 5.8, 5.9, and 5.10 reproduced from** *The Medical Letter* **(see Drugs for Parasitic Infections, p 637), give specific antiparasitic drugs, dosage recommendations, and other relevant information. Although the recommendations for administration of these drugs given in the disease-specific chapters are similar, they may not be identical in all instances because of differences of opinion among experts. Both sources should be consulted.**

Parvovirus B19
(Erythema Infectiosum, Fifth Disease)

CLINICAL MANIFESTATIONS: Infection is most often recognized as erythema infectiosum (EI), which is characterized by mild systemic symptoms, fever in 15% to 30% of patients, and, frequently, a distinctive rash. Prior to onset of these manifestations, a brief, mild, nonspecific illness consisting of fever, malaise, myalgias, and headache, followed approximately 7 to 10 days later by the characteristic exanthema may occur in some patients. The facial rash is intensely red with a "slapped cheek" appearance and circumoral pallor. A symmetric maculopapular, lacelike rash also occurs on the arms, moving caudally to involve the trunk, buttocks, and thighs. The rash can recur and fluctuate in intensity with environmental changes, such as temperature and exposure to sunlight, for weeks and sometimes months. Arthralgia and arthritis occur infrequently in children but commonly in adults, especially women.

Infection with the etiologic agent of EI, human parvovirus B19, can also cause asymptomatic infection, a mild respiratory illness with no rash, a rash atypical for EI that may be rubelliform or petechial, arthritis in adults (in the absence of manifestations of EI), chronic anemia in immunodeficient patients, and aplastic crisis lasting 7 to 10 days in patients with chronic hemolytic anemias (eg, sickle cell disease) and other conditions requiring increased erythrocyte production. Patients with aplastic crisis may have a prodromal illness with fever, malaise, and myalgia, but rash is usually absent. The red blood cell aplasia is related to lytic infection in erythrocyte precursors.

Parvovirus B19 infection that occurs during pregnancy can cause fetal hydrops and death. The risk of fetal death is less than 10% after proven maternal infection in the first half of pregnancy and is less in the second half. Congenital anomalies have been reported infrequently in newborn infants with fetal B19 infection, but no evidence suggests that the rate of congenital anomalies temporally associated with B19 fetal infection is greater than the background rate for congenital anomalies.

ETIOLOGY: Human parvovirus B19, a small DNA-containing virus, is the cause.

EPIDEMIOLOGY: Humans are the only known hosts. The mode of spread probably involves respiratory secretions and blood. Early in the illness, respiratory secretions have been demonstrated to contain viral DNA, and blood has been found to contain viral particles and DNA. Parvovirus B19 infections are ubiquitous, and cases of EI can occur sporadically or as part of community outbreaks. The outbreaks frequently occur in elementary or junior high schools in spring months. Secondary spread among susceptible household members, adults and children, is common and occurs in about 50% of contacts. Transmission in schools is less, but infection can be an occupational risk for school and child care personnel, affecting 19% of susceptible persons in one outbreak. However, 50% or more of adults have serologic evidence of past infection and are probably not susceptible to reinfection. In young children, only 5% to 10% are immune. The timing of the presence of B19 DNA in serum and respiratory secretions indicates that persons with EI are most infectious before onset of illness and are unlikely to be infectious after onset of the rash and other associated symptoms. In contrast, patients with aplastic crises are contagious from before the onset of symptoms and through the week after onset or even longer. Transmission from patients with aplastic crisis to hospital personnel can occur.

The **incubation period** from acquisition of infection to onset of initial symptoms is usually between 4 and 14 days, but can be as long as 21 days. Rash and joint symptoms occur 2 to 3 weeks after acquisition of infection.

DIAGNOSTIC TESTS: The most feasible method for detecting infection in the healthy host is assaying for serum B19-specific IgM antibody, the presence of which confirms infection within the past several months. Serum IgG antibody indicates previous infection and immunity. These assays are available in commercial laboratories and some state health and research laboratories. Their sensitivity and specificity, especially for IgM antibody, may vary, however. The best method for detecting chronic infection in the immunocompromised patient is to demonstrate virus by nucleic acid hybridization assay or the polymerase chain reaction assay, but these tests are investigational. The virus sometimes can be detected in serum by electron microscopy and viral B19 antigens can be detected by radioimmunoassay or enzyme immunoassay, but these methods generally are insensitive. Parvovirus B19 has not been grown in standard cell culture but has been cultivated in experimental cell culture.

TREATMENT: For most patients, only supportive care is indicated. Patients with aplastic crises may require transfusion. In treating chronic infection in the immunodeficient patient, intravenous immunoglobulin therapy appears to be effective and should be considered. Some cases of B19 infected hydrops fetalis have been treated successfully with intrauterine blood transfusions.

ISOLATION OF THE HOSPITALIZED PATIENT*: Droplet precautions are recommended for those caring for hospitalized children with aplastic crises or immunosuppressed patients with chronic infection and anemia for the duration of hospitalization. For patients with transient aplastic or erythrocyte crisis, these precautions should be maintained for 7 days.

Pregnant health care workers should be informed of the potential risks to the fetus from B19 infections and about preventive measures that may reduce these risks, including not participating in the care of immunosuppressed patients with chronic parvoviral infection or patients with aplastic crises who are highly contagious.

CONTROL MEASURES:
- Women who are exposed to children either at home or at work (eg, teachers or child care workers) are at increased risk of infection with parvovirus B19. However, because of widespread inapparent infection in both adults and children, all women are at some degree of risk of exposure, particularly those with school-age children. In view of the high prevalence of B19, the low incidence of ill effects on the fetus, and the fact that avoidance of child care or teaching can only reduce but not eliminate the risk of exposure, routine exclusion of pregnant women from the workplace where EI is occurring is not recommended. When IgG testing for parvovirus B19 antibody becomes more widely available, women at increased risk may be able to have their susceptibility determined.
- Pregnant women who find that they have been in contact with children who were in the incubation period of EI or who were in aplastic crisis should have the relatively low potential risk explained to them, and the option of serologic testing should be offered, if possible. Fetal ultrasound may be useful when assessing damage to the fetus.
- Children with EI may attend child care or school, as they are not contagious.
- Transmission of infection is likely to be lessened by routine hygienic practices for control of respiratory infections, which include hand washing and the disposal of facial tissues containing respiratory secretions.
- Pediatricians, as school medical advisors, should act as consultants in providing greater access to testing facilities, assistance in interpreting test results, and reassurance to pregnant women.

Pasteurella multocida Infections

CLINICAL MANIFESTATIONS: The most common manifestation in children is cellulitis at the site of a scratch or bite of a cat, dog, or other animal. This finding usually occurs within 24 to 48 hours following the bite or scratch and includes swelling, erythema, tenderness, and serous or sanguinopurulent discharge. Regional lymphadenopathy, chills, and fever can occur. Local complications such as septic arthritis, osteomyelitis, and tenosynovitis are common. Less common complications

---

* In addition to standard precautions.

include meningitis, respiratory tract infections (eg, chronic bronchitis, chronic sinusitis, chronic otitis media, pulmonary abscesses, empyema, and pneumonia), appendicitis, hepatic abscess, spontaneous peritonitis, urinary tract infection, and ocular infections, including conjunctivitis, corneal ulcer, and endophthalmitis.

ETIOLOGY: *Pasteurella multocida* organisms are bipolar staining, Gram-negative coccobacilli.

EPIDEMIOLOGY: The organism is found in the oral flora of 70% to 90% of cats, 25% to 50% of dogs, and the mouths of many other animals. Transmission occurs from the bite or scratch of an infected animal, usually a cat. Respiratory spread from animals to humans also occurs. Human-to-human spread via drainage from a lesion or respiratory discharge has not been documented.

The **incubation period** is usually less than 24 hours.

DIAGNOSTIC TESTS: *Pasteurella multocida* can be isolated from skin lesion drainage or other sites of infection (eg, joint fluid, cerebrospinal fluid, sputum, pleural fluid, or suppurative lymph nodes). The organism resembles several other organisms morphologically (such as *Haemophilus influenzae*, *Neisseria* species, and some enteric organisms), but laboratory differentiation is not difficult.

TREATMENT: The drug of choice is penicillin or ampicillin. In patients allergic to penicillin, either chloramphenicol or tetracycline is effective. Tetracycline drugs should not be given to children younger than 8 years unless the benefits of therapy are considered greater than the risks of dental staining (see Antimicrobial Therapy and Related Infections, p 606). For polymicrobial infection, which frequently occurs with *Staphylococcus aureus*, oral amoxicillin-clavulanate or intravenous ampicillin-sulbactam (for severe infection) can be given. Parenterally administered, broad-spectrum cephalosporins, such as cefotaxime or cefoxitin, are active against *P multocida* in vitro, but the therapeutic experience with these drugs in *P multocida* infections is limited. Broad-spectrum oral cephalosporins, such as cefixime, cefpodoxime, and ceftibuten, may prove effective. The duration of therapy is usually 7 to 10 days for local infections and 10 to 14 days for invasive infections. Wound drainage or debridement may be necessary.

ISOLATION OF THE HOSPITALIZED PATIENT: Standard precautions are recommended for cutaneous infection in which the drainage can be covered and contained adequately; in other circumstances, including culture-proven pneumonia, contact precautions also are indicated.*

---

* In addition to standard precautions.

CONTROL MEASURES: Limiting contact with wild and domestic animals can prevent *Pasteurella* infections. Animal bites and scratches should be promptly irrigated, cleansed, and debrided; whenever possible, surgical closure of the wounds should be avoided. Antimicrobial prophylaxis with penicillin, ampicillin, or amoxicillin-clavulanate may be given, but data supporting the efficacy of prophylaxis are limited.

Pediculosis

CLINICAL MANIFESTATIONS:

Pediculosis Capitis. Itching is the most common symptom of head lice infestation, although some children with light infestations (1 to 5 lice) do not complain. Adult lice or eggs (nits) are found in the hair usually behind the ears and near the nape of the neck. Excoriations and crusting caused by secondary bacterial infection are common and often associated with regional lymphadenopathy. In temperate climates, head lice deposit their eggs on the hair shaft 3 to 4 mm from the scalp. As hair grows at a rate of about 1 cm per month, the duration of infestation can be estimated by the distance of the nit from the scalp.

Pediculosis Pubis. Pruritus of the anogenital area is a common symptom in pubic lice infestations ("crabs"). Many hairy areas of the body can be infested, including the eyelashes, eyebrows, beard, axilla, perianal area, and, rarely, the scalp. A characteristic sign of heavy pubic lice infestation is the presence of bluish or slate-colored macules on the chest, abdomen, or thighs, known as maculae ceruleac.

Pediculosis Corporis. Intense itching, particularly at night, is common with body lice infestations. Body lice and their eggs live on the seams of clothing. Infrequently, a louse can be seen feeding on the skin. Secondary bacterial infection of the skin caused by scratching is common.

ETIOLOGY: The three following species or subspecies of lice infest humans: *Pediculus humanus capitis*, the head louse; *Pediculus humanus corporis* (or *humanus*), the body louse; and *Phthirus pubis*, the pubic or crab louse. Both nymphs and adult lice feed on human blood.

EPIDEMIOLOGY:

Pediculosis Capitis. Head lice infestation in child care and school-age children is common in the United States. All socioeconomic groups are affected. Infestations are less common in blacks than in individuals of other races. Head lice infestation is not influenced by hair length or frequent shampooing or brushing. Head lice are not a health hazard or a sign of uncleanliness, and are not responsible for the spread of any disease. Transmission occurs by direct contact with hair of infested individuals or, possibly, indirectly by contact with their personal belongings such as combs, brushes, and hats. Head lice can survive only 1 to 2 days away from the scalp and their eggs cannot hatch at the lower, ambient temperatures than that close to the scalp.

Pediculosis Pubis. Pubic lice infestations are common in adolescents and young adults and are usually transmitted through sexual contact. The pubic louse can also be transferred by contaminated items such as towels. Pubic lice can be found on the eyelashes of younger children and, while other modes of transmission are possible, may be evidence of sexual abuse. Infested individuals should be investigated for other sexually transmitted diseases, including syphilis, *Neisseria gonorrhoeae*, *Chlamydia trachomatis*, hepatitis B, and HIV infection.

Pediculosis Corporis. Body lice are generally found on persons with poor hygiene. Fomites play a role in their transmission. Body lice cannot survive away from a blood source for longer than 10 days. In contrast to head lice, body lice are well-recognized vectors of disease (eg, epidemic typhus, trench fever, and relapsing fever).

The **incubation period** from laying of the eggs to hatching of the first nymph is 6 to 10 days. Mature adults (lice) capable of reproducing do not appear until 2 to 3 weeks later.

DIAGNOSTIC TESTS: Identification of eggs, nymphs, and lice with the naked eye is possible; the diagnosis can be confirmed by using a hand lens or microscope. Mature lice are seldom seen because they move rapidly and conceal themselves effectively.

TREATMENT:

Pediculosis Capitis. The following agents are effective in treating pediculosis of the scalp, but permethrin has advantages over the other pediculocides:
- ***Permethrin (1%).*** Permethrin is available without a prescription in a 1% cream rinse that is applied to the scalp and hair for 10 minutes. It has low potential for toxicity and a high cure rate, although resistance has been recently reported in other countries. Because permethrin has high ovicidal activity and remains active for 2 weeks or more, a single treatment usually is adequate. Some experts advise a second treatment 7 to 10 days after the first.
- ***Natural pyrethrin-based products.*** These 10-minute shampoos are available without prescription. Ovicidal activity is low and repeat application 7 to 10 days later is necessary to kill newly hatched lice. Resistance to these synergized natural pyrethrins has not been documented. These products are contraindicated in persons allergic to ragweed.
- ***Lindane (1%).*** This 4-minute shampoo, which requires a prescription in the United States, is indicated primarily for patients who have either failed to respond to, or are intolerant of, other approved therapies. Ovicidal activity is low and repeat application 7 to 10 days later is often recommended. Lindane resistance has been reported from a number of countries. It is contraindicated for premature infants, persons with known seizure disorders, and those with hypersensitivity to the product, and should be used with caution in patients with inflamed or traumatized skin and in pregnant or nursing women. Although it has the highest potential toxicity of all pediculocides, serious adverse effects have been rarely reported when used according to product instructions. Toxicity with lindane usually has been associated with misuse, such as ingestion, excessive doses, or prolonged or repeated administration.
- ***Malathion (0.5% and 1%).*** This pesticide is highly effective in the treatment of head lice and is safe when used as directed. However, it is no longer avail-

able in the United States. In other countries, a 1% shampoo, recommended for use in two 10-minute applications approximately 7 days apart is available.

Because pediculocides kill lice shortly after application, the detection of living lice on scalp inspection 24 hours or more after treatment suggests a very heavy infestation, reinfestation, or resistance to therapy. Treatment with a different pediculocide and re-treatment 7 to 10 days later are recommended in this circumstance.

Itching or mild burning of the scalp caused by inflammation of the skin in response to topical therapeutic agents can persist for many days after lice are killed and is not a cause for re-treatment. Topical corticosteroids and oral antihistamines may be beneficial.

Removal of nits after treatment with a pediculocide is not necessary to prevent spread. If removal of nits is attempted for aesthetic reasons, loosening the glue by which the nits are attached may be facilitated by combing with a fine-toothed nit comb following pretreatment with a commercial formic acid rinse designated for this purpose, or soaking the hair with white vinegar (3% to 5% acetic acid) and then applying a damp towel soaked in the same solution for 30 to 60 minutes.

Pediculosis Pubis. Any of the pediculocides for pediculosis capitis are effective in the treatment of pubic lice. Retreatment is recommended 7 to 10 days later. For infestation of eyelashes by pubic lice, 1% mercuric oxide ointment applied 4 times a day for 14 days or petrolatum ointment applied 3 to 4 times daily for 8 to 10 days is effective. Nits should be removed mechanically from the eyelashes.

Pediculosis Corporis. Treatment consists of improving hygiene and cleaning clothes. Infested clothing can be washed and dried at hot temperatures to kill the lice. Pediculocides are not necessary.

ISOLATION OF THE HOSPITALIZED PATIENT*: Contact precautions are recommended until the patient has been treated with an appropriate pediculocide.

CONTROL MEASURES:

Pediculosis Capitis. Household, other close contacts, and classmates should be examined and treated if infested. Differentiation of nits from benign hair casts (a layer of follicular cells that easily slide off the hair shaft), plugs of desquamated epithelial cells, and external debris can be difficult. Bedmates should be treated prophylactically. Children should be allowed to return to school or child care after their first treatment. After proper application of an effective pesticide and the resulting rapid killing of lice, reinfestation of children from an untreated, infested contact is more common than treatment failure.

"No nit" policies requiring that children be free of nits before return to child care or school have not been demonstrated to be effective in controlling head lice transmission. Lice incubating in egg cases ("nits") are so close to the scalp that they are difficult to remove with "nit combs." Egg cases further from the scalp are easier to remove but empty, and, thus, are of no consequence. Combing out of nits after treatment with an appropriate pediculocide, nevertheless, is required by some school officials. Such a policy can lessen the diagnostic confusion that may lead to inappropriate retreatment.

---

* In addition to standard precautions.

Although fomites do not play a major role in transmission of head lice, some parents may wish to disinfest headgear, pillow cases, and towels by washing them in hot water and machine drying (using a hot cycle). Combs and brushes can be washed with a pediculocide shampoo or soaked in hot water. Temperatures exceeding 53.5°C (128.3°F) for 5 minutes are lethal to lice and eggs. Dry cleaning clothing or simply storing contaminated items in well-sealed plastic bags for 10 days is also effective. Disinfesting furniture, such as chairs and sofas, is not necessary. Environmental insecticide sprays, which may increase chemical exposure of household members, have not been demonstrated to be helpful in the control of head lice. Vacuuming is a safe alternative to spraying.

Pediculosis Pubis. All sexual contacts should be treated.

Pediculosis Corporis. The most important factor in the control of body lice infestation is the ability to change and wash clothing. Close contacts should be examined and treated appropriately.

Pelvic Inflammatory Disease

CLINICAL MANIFESTATIONS: Pelvic inflammatory disease (PID) denotes a spectrum of inflammatory disorders of the female upper genital tract including endometritis, parametritis, salpingitis, oophoritis, tubo-ovarian abscess, and pelvic peritonitis. Pelvic inflammatory disease typically presents with continuous bilateral lower abdominal or pelvic pain that may be accompanied by fever, nausea, and vomiting. In many patients, however, infection is asymptomatic (silent PID) or symptoms are vague and mild with abnormal vaginal bleeding, dyspareunia, or unexplained vaginal discharge (atypical PID).

Common findings include lower abdominal or adnexal tenderness (which may be unilateral), tenderness on motion of the cervix, fever, and palpation of an inflammatory mass on bimanual pelvic examination or its demonstration by ultrasonography. The onset of symptoms often follows within a week of onset of menses. Many patients are afebrile, have only mild symptoms, no abnormal vaginal discharge, and normal leukocyte counts. No single historical, physical, or laboratory finding is both sensitive and specific for the diagnosis of acute PID. Combinations of findings that improve sensitivity (ie, detection of more women who have PID) or specificity (ie, exclusion of more women who do not have PID) do so only at the expense of the other. Diagnostic criteria currently recommended by the Centers for Disease Control and Prevention are given in Table 3.43, p 392.

Complications of acute PID include perihepatitis (Fitz-Hugh—Curtis syndrome) in 15% to 30% of patients and tubo-ovarian abscess in 20% of patients. Important long-term sequelae are tubal infertility (in 10% to 30% of patients after a single episode, depending on the severity; in 50% to 75% of patients after three or more episodes), ectopic pregnancy, and chronic pelvic pain.

ETIOLOGY: Sexually transmitted organisms, especially *Neisseria gonorrhoeae* and *Chlamydia trachomatis*, are implicated in most PID cases, but the cause is often polymicrobial. Other organisms isolated from the upper genital tract of patients with PID include multiple anaerobic species (*Bacteroides* and *Peptostreptococcus* species), facultative bacteria (*Gardnerella vaginalis, Streptococcus* species, and coliform bacteria), and genital tract mycoplasmas (eg, *Mycoplasma hominis* and *Ureaplasma urealyticum*). The organisms causing upper tract infection are not reliably predicted by cervical culture or known infection in a sexual partner.

EPIDEMIOLOGY: The incidence of PID is highest among sexually active adolescents. Other risk factors include multiple sexual partners, use of an intrauterine device, douching, and a previous episode of PID. Pelvic inflammatory disease is a frequent complication of common sexually transmitted diseases (STDs), particularly endocervical *N gonorrhoeae* and/or *C trachomatis* infection. Asymptomatic upper genital tract infection is common in apparently uncomplicated chlamydial infection. In prepubertal females, ascending infection resulting in PID is very uncommon.

The **incubation period** varies with the cause (see Gonococcal Infections, p 212, and *Chlamydia trachomatis*, p 170).

DIAGNOSTIC TESTS: The diagnosis is usually based on clinical findings (see Table 3.43) and is supported by evidence of *N gonorrhoeae* or *C trachomatis* in the cervical secretions, increased number of leukocytes in the cervical smear, leukocytosis, and/or an elevated C-reactive protein or erythrocyte sedimentation rate. Endocervical and rectal cultures for *N gonorrhoeae* and an endocervical test for *C trachomatis* should be obtained before treatment. Laparoscopy can be used to definitively diagnose salpingitis, and to obtain a more complete bacteriologic diagnosis, but this procedure will not detect endometritis and is not usually indicated or practical. Because of the increased morbidity associated with PID in pregnancy and other pregnancy-related conditions that can present as abdominal pain (eg, ectopic pregnancy) a pregnancy test is indicated in the management of patients with suspected PID, even if the patient claims her menses are timely and she is using reliable contraception.

TREATMENT: Treatment is empirical and is directed against the common etiologic agents because microbiologic testing cannot determine which organisms are important in an individual patient. Antibiotic treatment should be instituted promptly, based on clinical diagnosis without awaiting culture results, to minimize the risk of progression of the infection and the risk of transmission of the organisms to other sexual partners. No substantial evidence indicates that any one of the current antibiotic regimens decreases the incidence of infertility or ectopic pregnancy more than any other.

Many experts recommend hospitalization for all PID patients, particularly adolescents, in whom the risk of sequelae is high and whose ability to complete a therapeutic regimen may be unpredictable. Hospitalization is indicated if (1) the diagnosis is uncertain and ectopic pregnancy or appendicitis cannot be excluded, (2) compliance with therapy and follow-up within 72 hours cannot be assured, (3) the patient has a pelvic or tubo-ovarian abscess, (4) has overt peritonitis, (5) is pregnant, (6) has HIV infection, (7) has an intrauterine device in place, (8) is unable to follow or tolerate an outpatient regimen, and/or (9) has failed to respond to 48 hours of outpatient management.

No single therapeutic regimen of choice exists for all persons with PID. Antimicrobial regimens consistent with those recommended by the Centers for

Table 3.43. **Criteria for Clinical Diagnosis of Pelvic Inflammatory Disease*†**

Minimum Criteria

Empirical treatment of PID should be instituted on the basis of the presence of all of the following minimum clinical criteria for pelvic inflammation and in the absence of an established cause other than PID:

- Lower abdominal tenderness
- Adnexal tenderness
- Cervical motion tenderness

Additional Criteria

For women with severe clinical signs, more elaborate diagnostic evaluation is warranted because incorrect diagnosis and management may cause unnecessary morbidity. These additional criteria may be used to increase the specificity of the diagnosis.

Listed below are the **routine** criteria for diagnosing PID:

- Oral temperature >38.3°C
- Abnormal cervical or vaginal discharge
- Elevated erythrocyte sedimentation rate
- Elevated C-reactive protein
- Laboratory documentation of cervical infection with *Neisseria gonorrhoeae* or
- *Chlamydia trachomatis*

Listed below are the **elaborate** criteria for diagnosing PID:

- Histopathologic evidence of endometritis on endometrial biopsy
- Tubo-ovarian abscess on sonography or other radiologic tests
- Laparoscopic abnormalities consistent with PID

---

* Centers for Disease Control and Prevention. 1993 Sexually transmitted diseases treatment guidelines. *MMWR*. 1993;42(No. 44-14):75-81.
† No single history, or physical or laboratory finding is both sensitive and specific for the diagnosis of acute pelvic inflammatory disease. Combinations of findings that improve sensitivity or specificity do so only at the expense of the other.

Disease Control and Prevention are summarized in Table 3.44 (p 393). These empirical regimens provide broad coverage against the etiologic agents of PID. The specific antibiotics listed are examples only. If the patient has an intrauterine device in place, it should be promptly removed. Ambulatory patients should be monitored closely and re-evaluated within 3 days of initiating treatment.

ISOLATION OF THE HOSPITALIZED PATIENT: Standard precautions are recommended.

CONTROL MEASURES:

- Male sexual partners of patients with PID must be examined, cultured when possible, and treated empirically for presumptive gonorrhea and chlamydial infection.
- Patients should be advised to abstain from intercourse until all symptoms have resolved and the patient and her partner(s) have completed treatment. If abstinence is unlikely, the patient and partner must be encouraged to use condoms consistently.

Table 3.44. Recommended Treatment of Pelvic Inflammatory Disease (PID)*

Inpatient	Ambulatory[†]
Regimen A[‡]	**Regimen A**
Cefoxitin, 2 g IV every 6 h (or cefotetan,[§] 2 g every 12 h)	Cefoxitin, 2 g IM, with concurrent administration of probenecid, 1 g orally
plus	**or**
Doxycycline,[‖] 100 mg IV or orally every 12 h	Ceftriaxone, 250 mg IM
plus	**or**
This regimen is continued for at least 48 h after clinical improvement, and followed by doxycycline[‖] 100 mg orally, twice a day, to complete a 14-d total course.	Equivalent parenteral cephalosporin[§]
	plus
	Doxycycline,[‖] 100 mg orally twice a day for 14 d
OR	**OR**
Regimen B[‡]	**Regimen B**
Clindamycin, 900 mg IV every 8 h (15 to 40 mg/kg/d)	Ofloxacin,[¶] 400 mg orally twice a day for 14 d
plus	**plus**
Gentamicin: loading dose, 2.0 mg/kg IV, followed by maintenance, 1.5 mg/kg IV every 8 h	Clindamycin, 600 mg orally 3 times a day for 14 d
plus	**or**
This regimen is continued for at least 48 h after significant clinical improvement is demonstrated and is followed by doxycycline[‖] 100 mg orally twice a day, to complete a 14-d total course, or clindamycin, 600 mg orally 3 times a day, to complete a 14-d total course.	Metronidazole, 500 mg orally twice a day for 14 d[#]

* IV indicates intravenous; IM, intramuscular.
† Patients in whom response to outpatient therapy is inadequate within 48 hours should be hospitalized for parenteral therapy.
‡ When tubo-ovarian abscess is present, many clinicians use clindamycin because it provides more effective anaerobic coverage than does doxycycline. Clindamycin administered intravenously appears to be effective against *C trachomatis* infection; the effectiveness of oral clindamycin against *C trachomatis*, however, has not been determined.
§ The experience with cefotetan is less than that with cefoxitin, although cefotetan provides similar antimicrobial coverage and requires less frequent dosing. Clinical data are limited on other second- and third-generation cephalosporins (ceftizoxime, cefotaxime, ceftriaxone) to replace cefoxitin or cefotetan, although many authorities believe they are also effective therapy for PID.
‖ Doxycycline administered orally has bioavailability similar to that of the IV formulation. Patients who do not tolerate doxycycline should receive erythromycin, 500 mg orally 4 times a day (40 mg/kg/d) for 10 to 14 days, although this recommendation is based on limited clinical data. Use of doxycycline is ordinarily limited to patients 8 years or older because of the potential for dental staining (see Antimicrobials and Related Therapy, p 606). Doxycycline is preferred over tetracycline because of its greater bioavailability and better patient compliance.
¶ Fluoroquinolones are generally contraindicated for children and adolescents younger than 18 years and for pregnant or nursing mothers (see Antimicrobials and Related Therapy, p 605).
# Some experts consider therapy for anaerobic infection with metronidazole to be of major importance in the prevention of sequelae from PID.

- Patients should be tested for other STDs including syphilis, hepatitis B, and HIV infection. Hepatitis B immunization should be initiated in previously unvaccinated persons (see Hepatitis B, p 250). Susceptible women should be immunized for hepatitis B.
- Patients with positive cultures for *N gonorrhoeae* or *C trachomatis* should be recultured 7 to 10 days after completing therapy.
- Because of the high risk of reinfection, some experts recommend that patients with PID should be cultured for *N gonorrhoeae* and *C trachomatis* 4 to 6 weeks after completing treatment.
- The diagnosis of PID provides an opportune time to educate the adolescent about prevention of STDs, including abstinence, consistent use of barrier methods of protection, and the importance of periodic evaluation for STDs.

Pertussis

CLINICAL MANIFESTATIONS: Pertussis begins with mild upper respiratory symptoms (catarrhal stage) and can progress to severe paroxysms of cough (paroxysmal stage), often with a characteristic respiratory whoop, followed by vomiting. Fever is absent or minimal. Symptoms wane gradually (convalescent stage). Disease in infants younger than 6 months may be atypical; apnea is a common manifestation and whoop is often absent. Similarly, older children and adults can have atypical manifestations, with persistent cough and no whoop. The duration of classic pertussis is 6 to 10 weeks; however, more than half of the primary cases last less than 6 weeks and a quarter have cough for 3 weeks or less. Complications include seizures, pneumonia, encephalopathy, and death. Pertussis is most severe when occurring in the first year of life (particularly for preterm infants). According to surveillance data from 1980 to 1989 in the United States, pneumonia, seizures, and encephalopathy occurred in 21.7%, 3.0%, and 0.9%, respectively, of infants with pertussis. The case-fatality rate was 1.3% in children younger than 1 month and 0.3% in those 2 to 11 months of age. Infection in vaccinated children and older persons is often mild. Pertussis does not appear to cause permanent pulmonary sequelae.

ETIOLOGY: *Bordetella pertussis* is a fastidious, Gram-negative, pleomorphic bacilli. A whooping cough syndrome may also be caused by *B parapertussis, Mycoplasma pneumoniae, C trachomatis, C pneumoniae, B bronchiseptica,* and, possibly, certain adenoviruses.

EPIDEMIOLOGY: Humans are the only known hosts of *B pertussis.* Transmission occurs by close contact via respiratory secretions of patients with disease. Asymptomatic infection has been demonstrated but is unlikely to be a major factor in transmission. Pertussis occurs endemically with periodic outbreaks. As many as 90% of nonimmune household contacts acquire the disease. Adolescents and adults recently have been recognized as major sources of pertussis, accounting for as many as 25% of reported cases in recent years; infants and young children are frequently infected by older siblings or adults who often have mild or atypical illness. While pertussis can occur at any age, approximately 35% of reported cases currently occur in infants younger than 6 months, including a substantial proportion in those younger than 3 months, and approximately 60% occur in children younger than 5 years. Infants born prematurely are especially at increased risk of severe pertussis, resulting in hospitalization and including death. Widespread immunization with pertussis vaccine since the 1940s is primarily responsible for the current low morbidity and mortality rates of pertussis in the United States. Patients are most contagious during the cararrhal stage before the onset of paroxysms; communicability then diminishes rapidly but may persist for 3 weeks or more after onset of cough. Erythromycin therapy decreases infectivity and may limit spread. Nasopharyngeal cultures usually become negative for *B pertussis* within 5 days after initiating therapy.

The **incubation period** is 6 to 20 days, usually 7 to 10 days.

DIAGNOSTIC TESTS: Culture of *B pertussis* requires inoculation of nasopharyngeal mucus, obtained by aspiration or with dacron or calcium alginate swab, on special media (such as Regan-Lowe or fresh Bordet-Gengou), with incubation for 10 to 14 days. Because these media may not be routinely available, the laboratory should be informed when *B pertussis* is suspected. Although for optimal results, specimens should be inoculated at the bedside or taken promptly to the laboratory in special transport-media, reasonable rates of positive culture also have been obtained by preincubation in Regan-Lowe transport medium for submission to the laboratory. The organism is most frequently recovered in the catarrhal or early paroxysmal stage and is rarely found after the fourth week of illness. A positive culture is diagnostic. Negative cultures are common, particularly late in the course of the disease, from patients who have been vaccinated previously or who are receiving antibiotics. The direct immunofluorescent assay (DFA) of nasopharyngeal secretions has low sensitivity and variable specificity, requires experienced personnel for interpretation, and is not a reliable criterion for laboratory confirmation of the diagnosis. Since false-positive and false-negative DFA results occur, culture confirmation of all suspected pertussis cases should be attempted. Investigational polymerase chain reaction (PCR) assays of nasopharyngeal specimens for the diagnosis of *B pertussis* infection appear to be more rapid and sensitive than culture. However, as with other PCR assays, laboratory contamination or contamination from the environment at the time of collection may cause false-positive results.

No single serologic test is diagnostic of pertussis. *Bordetella pertussis* infections stimulate a heterogenous antibody response that differs among individuals, depending on age and previous exposure to the organism or to its antigens by immunization. In experienced research laboratories, the serologic diagnosis of pertussis has excellent sensitivity and specificity when acute sera is collected early in the illness and paired acute and convalescent phase sera are tested. Measurement of agglutinating antibodies and use of newer serologic tests, such as enzyme immunoassays for IgG antibody to pertussis toxin and IgA antibody to *B pertussis* filamentous hemagglutinin, are promising diagnostic methods. Efforts to standardize serologic tests for the diagnosis of pertussis and to make these tests more widely available have been initiated.

Although absolute lymphocytosis is often present in patients with classic pertussis, it is a nonspecific finding, especially in infants, who often develop lymphocytosis from other infections. The degree of lymphocytosis usually parallels the severity of the patient's cough.

Because laboratory confirmation of pertussis can be difficult, clinicians often need to make the diagnosis on the basis of characteristic manifestations of prolonged paroxysmal coughing with supportive associated findings, such as inspiratory whoop, post-tussive emesis, and lymphocytosis.

TREATMENT:

- Infants younger than 6 months and other patients with potentially severe disease often require hospitalization for supportive care to manage coughing paroxysms, apnea, cyanosis, feeding difficulties, and other complications. Intensive care facilities may be required for severe cases.
- Antimicrobials given during the catarrhal stage may ameliorate the disease. After paroxysms are established, however, antimicrobials usually have no discernible effect on the course of illness and are recommended primarily to limit the spread of the organisms to others. The drug of choice is erythromycin (40 to 50 mg/kg per day orally in four divided doses; maximum, 2 g/d); some experts prefer the estolate preparation. The recommended duration of therapy to prevent bacteriologic relapse is 14 days. Because of in vitro susceptibilities, clarithromycin (15 mg/kg per day orally in two divided doses; maximum, 1 g/d), and other macrolides also are likely to be effective and, thus, are alternatives for patients who cannot tolerate erythromycin.
- Trimethoprim-sulfamethoxazole (8 to 40 mg/kg per day orally in two divided doses) is another possible alternative, but its efficacy is unproven.
- Erythromycin resistance of *B pertussis* has been rarely reported. Nasopharyngeal cultures should be obtained from persons with pertussis who do not improve with erythromycin therapy and isolates should be tested for in vitro susceptibility.
- Corticosteroids, albuterol (a ß2-adrenergic stimulant), and pertussis-specific immunoglobulin each may be effective in reducing paroxysms of coughing but further evaluation is required before they can be recommended. Pertussis-specific immunoglobulin currently is an investigational product.

ISOLATION OF THE HOSPITALIZED PATIENT*: Droplet precautions are recommended for 5 days after initiation of effective therapy (or until 3 weeks after the onset of paroxysms if appropriate antimicrobial therapy is not given).

CONTROL MEASURES:

Care of Exposed Persons.

Household and Other Close Contacts.
Immunization. Close contacts younger than 7 years who are unimmunized or who have received fewer than four doses of pertussis vaccine (DTP or DTaP) should have pertussis immunization initiated or continued, according to the recommended schedule. Children who received their third dose 6 months or more before exposure should be given a fourth dose at this time. Those who have had at least four doses of pertussis vaccine should receive a booster dose of DTaP (or DTP) unless a dose has been given within the last 3 years or they are more than 6 years old; DTaP is preferred.

---

* In addition to standard precautions.

Chemoprophylaxis. Erythromycin (40 to 50 mg/kg per day orally in four divided doses; maximum, 2 g/d) for 14 days, as tolerated, is recommended for all household contacts and other close contacts, such as those in child care, irrespective of age and vaccination status. Some experts recommend the estolate preparation because it is better tolerated. Prompt use of chemoprophylaxis in household contacts is effective in limiting secondary transmission. The rationale for administering chemoprophylaxis to all household and other close contacts irrespective of age or immunization status is that pertussis immunity is not absolute and may not prevent infection. Persons with mild illness that may not be recognized as pertussis can transmit the infection.

For those who cannot tolerate erythromycin, alternatives are clarithromycin, other macrolides, or trimethoprim-sulfamethoxazole (see Treatment, p 396). However, their efficacies have not been established.

Persons who have been in contact with an infected individual should be monitored closely for respiratory symptoms for 14 days after last contact with the infected individual.

Child Care. Exposed children, especially those incompletely immunized, should be observed for respiratory symptoms for 14 days after contact has been terminated. Pertussis immunization and chemoprophylaxis should be given as recommended for household and other close contacts. Symptomatic children with cough should be excluded from day care, pending physician evaluation. Children with pertussis, if their medical condition allows, may return or enter a child care facility 5 days after initiation of erythromycin therapy. Chemoprophylaxis should be considered for adult staff with close or extensive contact. Staff members should be monitored for respiratory symptoms, cultured for pertussis if symptoms develop, and given chemoprophylaxis if cough develops within 14 days of exposure (see Treatment, p 396).

Schools. Students and staff with pertussis, if their medical condition allows, should be excluded until they have received 5 days of erythromycin (or other recommended drug). Other public health recommendations to control pertussis transmission have not been established. School-wide or classroom chemoprophylaxis has not been generally recommended, usually because of the delay in recognition of outbreaks and difficulties of implementation. The immunization status of children younger than 7 years should be reviewed and vaccine given, if indicated, as for household and other close contacts. Pertussis should be considered in the differential diagnosis of persons with cough illness who may have been exposed. Parents and employees should be notified about possible exposures to pertussis. Exclusion of exposed persons with cough illness, pending physician evaluation, should be considered. The local health department should be consulted about the possible implementation of this and other control measures.

Immunization. Universal immunization with pertussis vaccine of children younger than 7 years is critical for the control of pertussis. The pertussis vaccines available in the United States include whole-cell and acellular vaccines in combination with diphtheria and tetanus toxoids (DTP and DTaP, respectively). They are absorbed onto an aluminum salt, and thus, are administered intramuscularly. Diphtheria-tetanus-pertussis (DTP) vaccine is a suspension of inactivated *B pertussis* cells (whole-cell) and contains multiple antigens. Acellular vaccines (DTaP) contain one or more immunogens derived from *B pertussis* organisms and, unlike whole-cell vaccines, contain minimal or no endotoxin. These antigens include detoxified pertussis toxin (ie, pertussis toxoid [PT]*), filamentous hemagglutinin (FHA), fimbrial proteins (agglutinogens), and pertactin (an outer membrane 69-kd protein). As of December 1996, two acellular pertussis-containing vaccines (DTaP) are licensed in the United States and both were approved in 1996 by the Food and Drug Administration (FDA) for use in infants and for primary immunization (Table 3.45). Licensure of additional products is anticipated.[†] Although licensed vaccines differ in their formulation of pertussis antigens, their efficacy appears similar. All DTaP vaccines, including those that are currently investigational, contain PT. Detailed information on acellular pertussis vaccines, including efficacy, adverse events, and vaccine composition is summarized in a recent Academy statement on DTaP.[‡]

Based on household studies of young children in the United States exposed to pertussis, the efficacy of whole-cell pertussis vaccine for children who received at least three doses is estimated to be 50% to 90% depending upon the case definition. Observed protection varies according to the definition used for pertussis cases and is greatest for culture-confirmed, more severe cases. Vaccine-induced immunity persists for at least 3 years and diminishes thereafter with time. Therefore, 5 to 10 years after immunization, older children and young adults are susceptible to disease due to *B pertussis*. Disease in those previously immunized is usually less severe than primary illness.

Efficacy of acellular pertussis vaccines originally was demonstrated in Japan in children 2 years of age and older. Recently completed trials of several acellular vaccines in Europe have documented comparable efficacies to that of whole-cell pertussis vaccine given to infants as the primary three-dose series. The immunogenicities of the antigens in the acellular vaccines are similar to those of whole-cell DTP vaccine. However, antibody responses do not correlate with protection against disease and, thus, cannot be used to predict efficacy. Duration of protection following immunization with acellular pertussis vaccine has not been established; studies of this question, however, are in progress.

The rates of local reactions (erythema and induration at the injection site), fever, and other common systemic symptoms (drowsiness, fretfulness, and anorexia) are substantially lower after acellular pertussis vaccination than those from whole-cell DTP. Whether the rare, more serious adverse events associated with DTP will occur less frequently after acellular pertussis vaccine is not known (see Adverse Events After Pertussis Vaccination, p 401).

Dose and Route. The dose of DTaP and DTP dose are 0.5 mL, given intramuscularly. The use of reduced volume of individual doses of pertussis vaccines or multiple doses of reduced volume (fractional doses) is not recommended, including for premature or low-birth-weight infants. The effect of such practices on the frequency of serious adverse events and on protection against disease has not been determined.

Interchangeability of Acellular Pertussis Vaccines. When feasible, the same DTaP vaccine product should be used for the first three doses of the pertussis immunization series. No data exist on the safety, immunogenicity, or efficacy of different

---

* Also termed lymphocytosis-promoting factor (LPF).

† On January 29, 1997, the FDA approved another DTaP product, Infanrix (SmithKline Beecham), for immunization of children 6 weeks to 6 years of age. It contains PT, FHA, and pertactin.

‡ See American Academy of Pediatrics, Committee on Infectious Diseases. Acellular pertussis vaccine: recommendations for use as the initial series in infants and children. *Pediatrics.* 1997;99:282-288.

Table 3.45. Licensed Acellular Pertussis-Continuing Vaccines as of December 1996*†

Manufacturer	Antigens	Trade Name	Licensed by FDA	Year Approved
Connaught Laboratories, Inc	PT, FHA	Tripedia	4th and 5th doses	1992
			Initial 4 doses‡	1996 (July)
Wyeth-Lederle Laboratories	PT, FHA, fimbria 2, pertactin	ACEL-IMUNE	4th and 5th doses	1991
			All 5 doses	1996 (December)

* On January 29, 1997, the FDA approved another DTaP product, Infanrix (SmithKline Beecham), for immunization of children 6 weeks to 6 years of age. It contains PT, FHA, and pertactin. Licensure of additional products is anticipated.

† FDA indicates Food and Drug Administration; PT, pertussis toxoid; and FHA, filamentous hemagglutinin.

‡ The FDA has not approved Tripedia for the 5th dose for children who have received only acellular pertussis vaccine for the first four doses in the vaccination series because data concerning the safety of the fifth dose are insufficient. However such data should be available before children who received only acellular products for the first four doses require a fifth dose at 4 to 6 years of age.

DTaP vaccines when administered interchangeably in the primary series. However, in those circumstances in which the type of DTaP product(s) received previously is not known or the previously administered product(s) is not readily available, any of the DTaP vaccines licensed for use in the primary series may be used. These recommendations may change as data become available concerning the response to different DTaP vaccines administered interchangeably in a primary series. For the fourth and fifth dose, any licensed product is acceptable, irrespective of prior vaccines received.

Antipyretic Prophylaxis. Administration of acetaminophen or other appropriate antipyretic at the time of DTP immunization and at 4 and 8 hours after immunization decreases the subsequent incidence of febrile and local reactions. Because DTP-associated convulsions after vaccine are almost always associated with fever, antipyretic prophylaxis every 4 to 6 hours for as long as 24 hours after vaccination may benefit children at increased risk of seizures (see Adverse Events After Pertussis Vaccination, p 401). However, in such circumstances, DTaP is strongly preferred. Caregivers should be aware that antipyretic therapy also could obscure fever caused by concomitant, unrelated infection.

Recommendations for Routine Childhood Immunization. A total of five doses of pertussis vaccine is recommended by school entry, unless contraindicated (see Contraindications and Precautions to Pertussis Immunization, p 404). If the fourth dose of pertussis vaccine is given after the fourth birthday because of delays in completing the immunization schedule, however, the fifth dose is not indicated. The first dose is given at 2 months of age, followed by two additional doses at intervals of approximately 2 months. The fourth dose is recommended at 15 to 18 months of age. The fifth dose is given before school entry (kindergarten or elementary school) at 4 to 6 years of age to protect these children from pertussis in ensuing years and to decrease transmission of the disease to younger children.

In the United States, DTaP is preferred for all doses because of the decreased likelihood of vaccine-associated reactions, such as fever and local reactions. During the transition period from use of DTP to DTaP, DTP is an acceptable alternative. Combination products containing pertussis vaccine (acellular or whole-cell) may be given, provided they are approved by the Food and Drug Administration for the child's current age and administration of the other components of the vaccine also is justified.

Other recommendations are as follows:

- For the fourth dose, DTaP or DTP may be given as early as 12 months of age if the interval between the third and fourth doses is at least 6 months and the child is considered unlikely to return for a visit at the recommended age of 15 to 18 months for this dose.
- Simultaneous administration of DTaP or DTP and other recommended vaccines is acceptable. Vaccines should not be mixed in the same syringe unless the specific combination is approved by the FDA (see Simultaneous Administration of Multiple Vaccines, p 21, and *Haemophilus influenzae* Infections, p 220).
- If pertussis is prevalent in the community, immunization can be started as early as 6 weeks of age, and doses can be given as frequently as 4 weeks apart.
- Pertussis immunization is not routinely indicated at present in persons 7 years or older.
- In children who have begun their primary immunization schedule with DTP, an FDA-approved DTaP vaccine can be used to complete the pertussis immunization schedule.
- For children who have had an adverse reaction to DTP resulting in a precaution for administration of the pertussis immunization (see Contraindications and Precautions to Pertussis Immunization, p 404), DTaP is recommended if the pertussis immunization schedule is to be completed. The risks and benefits of giving additional doses in this circumstance need to be evaluated for each child.
- Children who have a contraindication to pertussis immunization should receive no further doses of pertussis-containing vaccine (see Contraindications and Precautions to Pertussis Immunization, p 404).

Recommendations for Scheduling Pertussis Vaccine in Special Circumstances.

- For the child whose pertussis immunization is resumed after deferral or interruption of the recommended schedule, the next dose in the sequence should be given, irrespective of the interval since the last dose; ie, the schedule is not reinitiated (see Lapsed Immunizations, p 22).
- For children who have received fewer than the recommended number of doses of pertussis vaccine but who have received the recommended number of DT doses for their age (ie, those started on DT, then given DTP or DTaP), dose(s) of DTaP (or DTP) should be given to complete the recommended pertussis immunization schedule. However, the total number of doses of diphtheria and

tetanus toxoids (as DT, DTaP, or DTP) should not exceed six before the fourth birthday. A monovalent pertussis vaccine preparation* may be used instead.

- Children who have had well-documented pertussis should complete the vaccination series with at least DT; some experts recommend including the pertussis component as well, ie, administration of DTaP or DTP. Although well-documented pertussis disease (ie, positive culture for *B pertussis* or epidemiologic linkage to a culture positive case) is likely to confer immunity against pertussis, the duration of such immunity is unknown.

- During pertussis outbreaks, such as in a hospital, pertussis immunization is not usually recommended for adult contacts. Some experts have advised a booster dose of 0.25 mL of monovalent pertussis vaccine in addition to antibiotic prophylaxis for health care and child care center personnel and for close contacts who have chronic pulmonary disease, but the efficacy of immunoprophylaxis and chemoprophylaxis in these circumstances is unproven. Evaluation of acellular pertussis vaccines for use in adults is in progress.

Medical Records. Charts of those children for whom pertussis vaccination has been deferred should be flagged, and the immunization status of these children should be periodically assessed to ensure that they are appropriately immunized.

Adverse Events After Pertussis Vaccination.

- *Local and febrile reactions.* The frequency of fever, common systemic events and local reactions, including erythema, induration, and pain or tenderness following vaccination with acellular pertussis vaccine (given as DTaP) is significantly less than that following administration of DTP. Common reactions to DTP vaccination include redness, edema, induration, and tenderness at the injection site; drowsiness; fretfulness; anorexia; vomiting; crying; and slight-to-moderate fever. These local and systemic manifestations following pertussis vaccination occur within several hours of immunization and subside spontaneously without sequelae. Children with such reactions should receive subsequent doses of pertussis vaccine as scheduled.

  Bacterial or sterile abscesses at the site of the injection are infrequent (six to ten per million injections of DTP). Bacterial abscesses indicate contamination of the product or nonsterile technique and should be reported (see Reporting of Adverse Events, p 27). The causes of sterile abscesses are unknown. Their occurrence usually does not contraindicate further doses of DTaP or DTP.

- *Allergic reactions.* The rate of anaphylaxis to DTP is estimated to be approximately two cases per 100 000 injections; the incidence of allergic reactions following DTaP vaccination is unknown. Severe anaphylactic reactions and resulting deaths, if any, are extremely rare following pertussis immunization. The transient urticarial rashes that occasionally occur after pertussis immunization, unless appearing immediately (ie, within minutes), are unlikely to be anaphylactic (IgE-mediated) in origin. These rashes probably represent a serum sickness-type reaction caused by circulating antigen-antibody complexes due to one of the antigens in pertussis vaccine and corresponding antibody acquired

---

* Distributed by the Division of Biologic Products, Michigan Department of Public Health (see Directory of Telephone Numbers, p 667).

either from an earlier dose or transplacentally. Because formation of such complexes is dependent on a precise balance between concentrations of circulating antigen and antibody, such reactions are unlikely to recur after a subsequent dose and are not contraindications to further doses.

- **Seizures.** The incidence of seizures occurring within 48 hours of administration of whole-cell pertussis (ie, DTP) vaccine has been estimated to be 1:1750 doses administered. In the recently completed field trials in Europe of DTaP vaccine and postlicensure surveillance of adverse events associated with DTaP in the United States, the incidence of seizures has been substantially less than that associated with DTP.

  Most seizures occurring after DTP immunization are brief, self-limited, and generalized, occur in febrile children, and occur after the third and fourth doses of the vaccine series. These characteristics suggest that seizures associated with pertussis vaccine are usually febrile convulsions. These seizures have not been demonstrated to result in the subsequent development of recurrent afebrile seizures (ie, epilepsy) or other neurologic sequelae. Predisposing factors to seizures occurring within 48 hours include underlying convulsive disorder, personal history of convulsions, and family history of convulsions (see Infants and Children With Underlying Neurologic Disorders, p 405, and Children With a Personal or Family History of Seizures, p 58).

- **Hypotonic-hyporesponsive episodes (HHE).** These episodes (also termed "collapse" or "shocklike state") have been reported after DTP vaccination to occur on an incidence of 1:1750 doses administered. However, rates appear to vary widely, ranging from 3.5 to 291 cases per 100 000 immunizations in other observations. They occur less frequently following DTaP vaccination. A follow-up study of a group of children who experienced HHE following DTP demonstrated no evidence of subsequent serious neurologic damage or intellectual impairment.

- **Fever of 40.5°C (104°F) or greater.** Following administration of DTP, approximately 0.3% of recipients have been reported to develop high fever of 40.5°C or greater within 48 hours. The incidence following DTaP is significantly less.

- **Prolonged crying.** Persistent, severe, inconsolable screaming or crying for 3 or more hours is sometimes observed within 48 hours of DTP vaccination (1:100 doses administered). The occurrence of inconsolable crying for 3 or more hours is significantly less following DTaP vaccination. Distinguishing between these features and crying from pain can be difficult and requires close questioning of the patient's caregiver. The significance of persistent crying is unknown. It has been noted after receipt of immunizations other than pertussis vaccine and is not known to be associated with sequelae.

  Frequency of Adverse Events Following DTaP. Moderate to severe systemic events, including fever of 40.5°C (104.9°F) or higher; persistent, inconsolable crying lasting 3 hours or more; and collapse (hypotonic-hyporesponsive episode) rarely have been reported after vaccination with DTaP but each of these events occur rarely and less frequently than after DTP vaccination. When these events occur after the administration of DTP, they appear to be without sequelae; the limited experience with DTaP suggests a similar outcome. Because DTaP causes high fever less frequently than whole-cell DTP, convulsions are anticipated to be much less likely than after receipt of DTaP.

Alleged Reactions to Pertussis Vaccination. The temporal relation of DTP immunization and severe adverse events, such as death, encephalopathy, onset of a seizure disorder, developmental delay, or learning or behavioral problems, does not establish causation by vaccination. Many of the manifestations of alleged vaccine reactions have other causes, such as viral encephalitis, concurrent infections, pre-existing neurologic disorders, and metabolic and other congenital abnormalities. For example, whereas infantile spasms frequently have their onset in the first 6 months of life and, in some cases, have been temporally related to the administration of pertussis vaccine, epidemiologic data demonstrate that the vaccine does not cause infantile spasms. Sudden infant death syndrome (SIDS) has occurred after DTP immunization, but several studies provide evidence that DTP immunization is not associated with SIDS. A large case-control study of SIDS in the United States demonstrated that SIDS victims were no more likely to have recently received DTP vaccination than control children who did not have SIDS. Because SIDS occurs most commonly at the age when DTP immunization is recommended, coincidental, temporal associations between the death and immunization by chance alone are expected.

Evaluation of Adverse Events Temporally Associated With Pertussis Vaccination. Appropriate diagnostic studies should be undertaken to establish an etiology of serious adverse events occurring temporally with immunization rather than assuming that they are caused by the vaccine. However, the cause of events temporally related to immunization cannot always be established even after diagnostic studies.

Severe Acute Neurologic Illness and Permanent Brain Damage. Permanent neurologic disability (brain damage) and even death have previously been considered uncommon sequelae of rare, severe, adverse neurologic events temporally related to whole-cell pertussis vaccine (DTP). Because no specific clinical syndromes or neuropathologic findings have been recognized in these cases, determination of whether pertussis vaccine is the cause of a specific child's deficit is not possible. Such adverse events can occur in both vaccinated and unvaccinated children, particularly in the first year of life. Hence, epidemiologic studies have been necessary to determine the risk of severe sequelae after acute events temporally related to pertussis immunization.

The only case-control study that addresses the issue of whether acute neurologic illness associated with DTP immunization results in permanent brain damage is the National Childhood Encephalopathy Study (NCES) in England, conducted from 1976 to 1979. This study examined the causes and natural history of serious acute neurologic illness in 1182 children aged 2 to 36 months admitted to a hospital and now includes a 10-year follow-up. More than 95% of cases of encephalopathy were unrelated temporally to DTP vaccination. Only 35 of these children had received pertussis vaccine within 7 days, and in many the temporal relation between acute neurologic illness and vaccination may have occurred by chance. Six of these children had infantile spasms, which was demonstrated in a separate analysis not to be attributable to DTP vaccine.

Analysis of the results of the NCES indicated that very rarely whole-cell pertussis vaccine (DTP) may be associated with the development of serious acute neurologic disorders in children who were previously normal. However, the findings of the 10-year follow-up indicate that infants and young children with these disorders are at increased risk of later neurologic impairment or death, irrespective of the initial precipitating event including DTP vaccination. The results do not establish a causal relationship between whole-cell pertussis vaccination and chronic neurological disorders. Other studies also have not provided evidence to support a causal relationship between DTP vaccination and serious acute neurologic illness resulting in permanent neurologic injury.

The Academy concludes, based on currently available data, that pertussis vaccine has not been proven to be a cause of brain damage. Although the data do not prove that pertussis vaccine can never cause brain damage, they do indicate that if it does so, such occurrences must be exceedingly rare. Furthermore, in individual cases, the role of pertussis vaccine is impossible to determine on the basis of clinical or laboratory findings. Limited experience with acellular pertussis vaccine does not allow conclusions concerning the frequency of rare, serious, adverse effects temporally associated with its administration.

Contraindications and Precautions to Pertussis Immunization. Adverse events after pertussis immunization that contraindicate further administration of either DTP or DTaP are as follows:

- *An immediate anaphylactic reaction.* Further immunization with any of the three vaccine components in DTaP or DTP should be deferred because of the uncertainty about which antigen might be responsible. Persons who experience anaphylactic reaction may be referred to an allergist for evaluation and desensitization to tetanus toxoid if a specific allergy can be demonstrated.
- *Encephalopathy within 7 days*, defined as severe, acute, central nervous system disorder unexplained by another cause, which may be manifested by major alterations of consciousness or by generalized or focal seizures that persist for more than a few hours without recovery within 24 hours. Studies indicate that such events associated with DTP are evident within 72 hours of immunization; prudence, however, usually justifies considering such an illness occurring within 7 days of DTP as a possible contraindication to further doses of pertussis vaccine and DT should be substituted for each of the recommended, subsequent doses of diphtheria and tetanus toxoid.

If the following adverse events occur in temporal relation to DTP or DTaP, the decision to administer additional doses of pertussis vaccine should be carefully considered. Although these events were once regarded as contraindications, they are now considered precautions because they have not been proven to cause permanent sequelae:

- A convulsion, with or without fever, occurring within 3 days of DTP or DTaP vaccination.
- Persistent, severe, inconsolable screaming or crying for 3 or more hours within 48 hours.

- Collapse or shocklike state (hypotonic-hyporesponsive episode) within 48 hours.
- Temperature of 40.5°C (104.9°F) or higher, unexplained by another cause, within 48 hours.

Before administration of each dose of pertussis vaccine, the child's parent or guardian should be questioned about possible adverse events after the previous dose.

Although the risks of giving subsequent doses of pertussis vaccine to a child who has had one of these events are not known, the possibility of another reaction of similar or greater severity often may justify discontinuing pertussis immunization. However, in circumstances such as during a community outbreak of pertussis or other circumstances of increased risk, the potential benefit may outweigh the risk of another reaction and justify further immunization. The decision to give or withhold immunization should be based on the clinical assessment of the earlier reaction, the likelihood of pertussis exposure in the child's community, and the potential benefits and risks of pertussis vaccine. If vaccination is undertaken, DTaP is recommended.

Infants and Children With Underlying Neurologic Disorders. The decision to give pertussis vaccine to infants and children with underlying neurologic disorders can be difficult and must be made on an individual basis after careful and continuing consideration of the risks and benefits (see also Children With a Personal or Family History of Seizures, p 58). In some cases, these disorders may constitute a cause for deferring pertussis immunization and, based on the medical history of the child, subsequent administration of pertussis vaccine. Because outbreaks of pertussis continue to occur in the United States, the decision to defer immunization should be reassessed at each subsequent medical visit; and the decision to give pertussis vaccine should be based on the adjudged risks and consequences of seizure after DTP or DTaP vaccination in comparison to the risk of pertussis and its complications. If pertussis immunization is continued, DTaP is recommended. Children with associated neurologic deficits may be at increased risk of complications if they develop pertussis. Children traveling to or residing in areas of endemic or epidemic pertussis are at increased risk of developing pertussis. Efforts should be undertaken to ensure pertussis immunization of children attending child care centers, special clinics, or residential care institutions.

The different circumstances of neurological disorders and relevant recommendations are categorized as follows:

- *A progressive neurologic disorder characterized by developmental delay or neurologic findings.* These conditions are reason for deferral of pertussis immunization often permanently. Administration of DTP (or DTaP) may coincide with or hasten the recognition of inevitable manifestations of the disorder, with resulting confusion about causation. Examples include infantile spasms and other epilepsies beginning in infancy Such disorders should be differentiated from those that are nonprogressive and in which the symptoms may change as the child matures.
- *Infants and children with a personal history of convulsions.* These patients have an increased risk of convulsions after receipt of DTP. A retrospective review of adverse events after the receipt of DTP indicated that children with a personal history of seizure were seven times more likely to have a seizure after DTP vaccination than children who had local or other nonneurologic,

post-DTP adverse events. No evidence indicates that these vaccine-associated seizures induce permanent brain damage, cause epilepsy, aggravate neurologic disorders, or affect the prognosis in children with underlying disorders. However, because the risk of a postvaccination convulsion is increased, pertussis immunization of children with recent seizures should be deferred until a progressive neurologic disorder is excluded. Infants and children with well-controlled seizures or those in whom a seizure is unlikely to recur may be vaccinated. DTaP is recommended because it is less frequently associated with moderate to high fever, and thus, much less likely to precipitate a seizure than is whole-cell pertussis vaccine (ie, DTP). Administration of acetaminophen also should be considered at the time of vaccination and every 4 hours for the ensuing 24 hours.

- *Infants and children known to have, or suspected of having, neurologic conditions that predispose either to seizures or neurologic deterioration.* Such conditions include tuberous sclerosis and certain inherited metabolic or degenerative diseases. Deferral of pertussis immunization should be considered for these patients. Convulsions or encephalopathy can occur in the normal course of these disorders and, thus, may occur after any immunization. DTP (or DTaP) vaccination may be associated with the occurrence of overt manifestations of the disorders with resulting confusion about causation. Hence, children with unstable or evolving neurologic disorders that may predispose to seizures or neurologic deterioration should be observed for a period of time to ascertain the diagnosis and prognosis of the primary neurologic disorder before immunization. Pertussis immunization should be reconsidered at each visit. If the immunization series is completed, DTaP is recommended. Children whose condition is resolved, corrected, or controlled can be vaccinated. No evidence indicates that prematurity in the absence of other factors increases the risk of seizures after immunization and is not a reason to defer vaccination (see Preterm Infants, p 48). Similarly, stable neurologic conditions, such as developmental delay or cerebral palsy, are not contraindications to pertussis immunization.

- *Temporary deferment of pertussis immunization.* Children in the first year of life with neurologic disorders that necessitate temporary deferment of pertussis immunization should not receive either DTP, DTaP, or DT because the risk of acquiring diphtheria or tetanus in children younger than 1 year in this country is remote. At or before the first birthday, however, the decision to give either pertussis vaccine (as DTaP) or DT should be made to ensure that the child is immunized at least against diphtheria and tetanus because as children become ambulatory, their risk of tetanus-prone wounds increases.

Children in whom DTP, DTaP, or DT immunization is deferred may not respond optimally to *Haemophilus influenzae* type b conjugate vaccines that use carrier proteins related to tetanus or diphtheria toxoids, such as HbOC or PRP-T. For such children, vaccination with PRP-OMP may be advantageous (see *Haemophilus influenzae* Infections, p 227).

Children with neurologic disorders that are recognized after the first birthday frequently will have received one or more doses of pertussis-containing vaccine. The physician may temporarily defer additional doses of DTaP in anticipation of stabilization of the child's neurologic status. If the physician determines that the child probably should not receive further pertussis immunizations, DT immunization should be completed according to the recommended schedule (see Diphtheria, p 191, and/or Tetanus, p 518). If pertussis immunization is continued, DTaP is recommended.

Children With a Family History of Convulsions (see also Children With a Personal or Family History of Seizures, p 58). A history of seizure disorders or adverse events after receipt of a pertussis-containing vaccine in a family member is not a contraindication to pertussis immunization. Although the risk of seizures after DTP in children with family history of seizures is increased, these seizures are usually febrile in origin and have a generally benign outcome. In addition, this risk is less with DTaP vaccination and is considerably outweighed by the continuing risk of pertussis in the United States and the substantial number of children with family history of seizures who, if not vaccinated, would remain susceptible to pertussis. DTaP is recommended.

Advice to Parents of Children at Increased Risk of Seizures. Parents of children who may be at increased risk of a seizure after pertussis immunization, such as from personal or family history of convulsions, should be informed of the risks and benefits of pertussis immunization in these circumstances. Advice should be provided about fever, its control (see Antipyretic Prophylaxis, p 399), and appropriate medical care in the unlikely event of a seizure.

Pinworm Infestation
(Enterobius vermicularis)

CLINICAL MANIFESTATIONS: Pinworm infestation (enterobiasis) causes pruritus ani and, rarely, pruritus vulvae. Although pinworms have been found in the lumen of the appendix, most evidence indicates that they are not causally related to acute appendicitis. Many symptoms, such as grinding of the teeth at night and enuresis, have been attributed to pinworm infections, but proof of a relationship has not been established. Urethritis, vaginitis, salpingitis, and pelvic peritonitis can occur because of aberrant migration of the adult worm from the perineum.

ETIOLOGY: *Enterobius vermicularis* is a nematode, or roundworm.

EPIDEMIOLOGY: Enterobiasis occurs worldwide and commonly in family clusters. In the past, 5% to 15% of the population in the United States was estimated to be infected, but the incidence appears to have declined. Prevalence rates are higher in preschool-age and school-age children, in mothers of infected children, and in the institutionalized, where 50% of the population may be infected.

Transmission occurs by multiple routes, the primary of which is fecal-oral, with worm eggs transmitted by fingers and hands and via shared toys, bedding, clothing, toilet seats, and baths. Reinfection by autoinfection or infection acquired from others is necessary to maintain enterobiasis in an individual since female pinworms usually die after depositing eggs on the perianal skin. The period of communicability is as long as the female nematodes are discharging eggs on perianal skin. The eggs remain infective in an indoor environment, usually 2 to 3 weeks. Humans are the only known hosts; dogs and cats do not harbor *E vermicularis*.

The **incubation period** from ingestion of an egg until an adult gravid female migrates to the perianal region is 1 to 2 months or longer.

DIAGNOSTIC TESTS: Diagnosis is usually made when adult worms are visualized in the perianal region, which is best examined 2 to 3 hours after the child is asleep, or in the stool. Alternatively, application of transparent (not translucent) adhesive tape can be applied to the perianal skin to collect any eggs; the tape is then applied to a glass slide and examined under a low-power microscopic lens. Three consecutive specimens should be obtained when the patient first awakens in the morning and before washing.

TREATMENT: The drugs of choice are mebendazole and pyrantel pamoate, given in a single dose and repeated in 2 weeks. Albendazole is also effective. For children younger than 2 years, in whom experience with these drugs is limited, the risks and benefits should be considered before drug administration. Other alternatives include piperazine and pyrvinium pamoate, but they are less effective and cumbersome to use. No unusual cleansing or hygienic measures should be undertaken. Excessive zeal in this regard can induce guilt and is counterproductive. Because of the high frequency of reinfection, families should be informed that recurrence is common. Repeated infections should be treated the same as the first one. Families may need to be treated as a group. Vaginitis is self-limited and does not require separate treatment.

ISOLATION OF THE HOSPITALIZED PATIENT: Standard precautions are indicated.

CONTROL MEASURES: Control is difficult in child care centers and schools because the rate of reinfection is extremely high. In institutions, mass and simultaneous treatment, repeated in 2 weeks, can be effective.

Plague

CLINICAL MANIFESTATIONS: Plague most commonly presents as the bubonic syndrome marked by fever and painful regional lymphadenopathy usually involving inguinal, axillary, or cervical lymph nodes (buboes). Other less common presentations include primary or secondary pneumonic plague (cough, fever, dyspnea, and hemoptysis), primary or secondary septicemic plague (fever, hypotension, and consumption coagulopathy), and rarely meningeal plague. Fever, chills, headaches, and rapidly progressive weakness are characteristic in all cases; occasionally presentations with mild bubonic manifestations or those with prominent gastrointestinal tract symptoms may obscure the correct diagnosis.

ETIOLOGY: Plague is caused by *Yersinia pestis*, a pleomorphic, bipolar staining, Gram-negative coccobacillus.

EPIDEMIOLOGY: Plague is a zoonotic infection of rodents and their fleas that occurs in many areas of the world, including parts of Africa, Asia, South America, and the United States. Plague has been reported throughout the western United

States, but most human cases occur in New Mexico, Arizona, California, and Colorado and arise as isolated cases or in small clusters. In the United States human plague usually is associated with epizootic infections in ground squirrels, prairie dogs, and other wild rodents. Bubonic plague is usually transmitted by the bites of infected fleas and uncommonly by direct contact with infected tissues and fluids. Septicemic plague may result from direct contact with infectious materials or from a flea bite but most often occurs secondary to bubonic plague. Pneumonic plague may be acquired by inhalation of respiratory droplets from a human or cat with respiratory plague or from exposure to aerosols in the laboratory, but most frequently is secondary to plague septicemia. Epidemics of human plague may occur during epizootics in domestic rodents, and when persons are exposed to pneumonic plague. The last epidemics in the United States occurred during the 1920s.

The **incubation period** is 2 to 6 days for bubonic plague and 2 to 4 days for pneumonic plague.

DIAGNOSTIC TESTS: Plague is characterized by massive growth of *Y pestis* in tissues; the organism has a bipolar (safety-pin) appearance in Wayson stain and can be visualized on this and Gram staining of infected tissue. A positive fluorescent antibody test for the presence of *Y pestis* in direct smears or cultures of a bubo aspirate, sputum, cerebrospinal fluid, or blood specimen provides presumptive evidence of *Y pestis* infection. A single positive serologic test by passive hemagglutination assay or enzyme immunoassay in an unvaccinated patient who has not previously had plague also provides presumptive evidence of infection. Seroconversion and/or a fourfold difference in antibody titer between two serum specimens obtained 4 weeks to 3 months apart provides serological confirmation. Culture isolates are confirmed by lysis with a *Y pestis* specific bacteriophage. Isolates suspected as *Y pestis* should be reported to the state health department and submitted to the Plague Section of Centers for Disease Control and Prevention.*

TREATMENT: For children, streptomycin (30 mg/kg per day in two or three divided doses, given intramuscularly) or gentamicin is the treatment of choice in most cases. Tetracycline (25 to 50 mg/kg per day in four divided doses given intravenously) or chloramphenicol (initial dose 25 mg/kg, subsequently 50 mg/kg per day in four divided doses, given intramuscularly until oral antimicrobial therapy is tolerated) also is effective. Tetracycline should not be given to children younger than 8 years of age unless the benefits of its use outweigh the risks of dental staining (see Antimicrobials and Related Therapy, p 606). Treatment with kanamycin or trimethoprim-sulfamethoxazole also is effective. Chloramphenicol, with or without streptomycin, is the treatment of choice for plague meningitis. The usual duration of antimicrobial treatment is 10 days.

Drainage of abscesses may be necessary; drainage material is potentially highly infectious until effective antimicrobial therapy has been given.

ISOLATION OF THE HOSPITALIZED PATIENT†: Droplet precautions are indicated for all patients until pneumonia is excluded and appropriate therapy has been initiated. In patients with pneumonic plague, droplet precautions should be contin-

---

* Foothills Campus, Fort Collins, CO 80521.
† In addition to standard precautions.

ued for 72 hours following initiation of appropriate treatment. For patients with bubonic plague, standard precautions only are recommended.

CONTROL MEASURES:

Care of Exposed Persons. Household members and other persons with intimate exposures to a plague patient should record their temperature twice a day for 7 days and report any fever or other illness to their physician. Persons exposed to a patient with pneumonic plague should receive antimicrobial prophylaxis; for exposed children younger than 8 years, prophylactic trimethoprim-sulfamethoxazole is recommended, whereas for adults and children aged 8 years and older, doxycycline or tetracycline is recommended. Prophylaxis is given for 7 days.

Other Measures. State public health authorities should be notified immediately of any suspect cases of human plague in order to carry out necessary epidemiologic and environmental investigations and to initiate control measures as indicated. The public should be educated about risk factors for plague, measures to prevent the disease, and the signs and symptoms of infection. Persons living in plague-endemic areas should be informed about the role of dogs and cats in bringing plague-infected rodents and their fleas into the peridomestic environment, the need for control of fleas on pets and confinement of pets, and the importance of avoiding contact with sick and dead animals. Other preventive measures include surveillance of rodent populations and the use of insecticides and rodent control measures when surveillance indicates the occurrence of plague epizootics.

Vaccine.* An inactivated whole-cell *Y pestis* vaccine is recommended only for persons whose occupation regularly places them at high risk for exposure to *Y pestis* or plague-infected rodents (eg, some field biologists and laboratory workers) and may be considered for persons traveling to or residing in areas with epizootic or epidemic plague. Primary immunization consists of three intramuscular doses; the second and third doses are given 1 to 3 months and 5 to 6 moths, respectively, after the first dose. Booster doses at 6-month intervals are recommended when vaccinees have continuing risk of exposure and a serum passive hemagglutination *Y pestis* antibody titer of less than 1:128. Since safety and immunogenicity have been evaluated only in persons 18 years of age and older, recommendations for immunization of children have not been established.

Vaccinated persons should take the same preventive measures as unvaccinated persons because the vaccine may not be fully protective. If possible, plague vaccine should not be given simultaneously with other vaccines because data are not available on interactions of plague vaccine with other biologics.

Pneumococcal Infections

CLINICAL MANIFESTATIONS: The pneumococcus is the most common cause of acute otitis media and of invasive bacterial infections in children, including bacteremia, many of whom have no evidence of a primary focus of infection. Pneumococci also are a frequent cause of sinusitis and bacterial pneumonia. Since the introduction

---

* Available from Grear Laboratories, Lenoir, NC.

of widespread *Haemophilus influenzae* type b (Hib) conjugate vaccination, pneumococci have become one of the two most common causes of bacterial meningitis in young children.

ETIOLOGY: *Streptococcus pneumoniae* (pneumococci) are lancet-shaped, Gram-positive diplococci. Ninety pneumococcal serotypes have been identified. Some serotypes are primarily prevalent in adults; others are more prevalent in children. Serotypes in groups 4, 6B, 9V, 14, 18C, 19F, and 23F (Danish serotyping system) cause most invasive childhood pneumococcal infections in the United States. Serotypes 6B, 9V, 14, 19A, 19F, and 23F are the most frequent isolates associated with resistance to penicillin.

EPIDEMIOLOGY: Pneumococci are ubiquitous; many persons have colonization of the upper respiratory tract. Transmission is from person to person, presumably by respiratory droplet contact. Among young children who acquire a new pneumococcal serotype in the nasopharynx, illness (usually otitis media) occurs in 15%, generally within 1 month of acquiring the new serotype. Illness seldom is associated with preceding prolonged carriage. Viral upper respiratory tract viral infections, including influenza, predispose to pneumococcal infections. These infections are most common in infants, young children, and older persons. Disease is increased in occurrence in persons with congenital or acquired immunodeficiency involving humoral immunity (eg, agammaglobulinemia), including HIV infection; those with absent or deficient splenic function, including sickle cell disease, congenital asplenia, and following surgical splenectomy; nephrotic syndrome; chronic renal failure; organ transplantation; diabetes mellitus; chronic pulmonary disease; or congestive heart failure. Patients with cerebrospinal fluid leakage, complicating skull fracture or neurosurgical procedures, can have recurrent pneumococcal meningitis. Invasive pneumococcal disease is often the first clinical manifestation of HIV infection in children, indicating significant humoral immunodeficiency early in the course of infection. Mortality from pneumococcal disease is highest in patients who have meningitis or other bacteremic disease. Pneumococcal infections are most prevalent at the time that respiratory tract viral infections are most common, usually during the winter months. The period of communicability is unknown. It may be as long as the organism is present in respiratory tract secretions, but is probably less than 24 hours after effective antimicrobial therapy is begun.

The **incubation period** varies by type of infection and can be as short as 1 to 3 days.

DIAGNOSTIC TESTS: Material obtained from a suppurative focus should be Gram stained and cultured by appropriate microbiologic techniques. Blood cultures should be obtained in all patients with suspected invasive pneumococcal disease; cultures of cerebrospinal fluid (CSF) and other body fluids (eg, pleural fluid) also are often indicated. The white blood cell (WBC) count may be of assistance in suspected bacteremic disease caused by *S pneumoniae*; young children with high temperatures and leukocytosis (particularly >15 000 cells/μL) have an increased likelihood of bacteremia. Although the predictive value of an elevated WBC count for pneumococcal bacteremia is not high, a normal WBC count is highly predictive of the absence of bacteremia. Recovery of pneumococci from an upper respiratory tract culture is not proof of causation of otitis media, pneumonia, or sinusitis because of the frequent colonization in asymptomatic children. Rapid methods to detect pneumococcal capsular antigen in CSF, pleural and joint fluid, serum, and concentrated urine can facilitate a presumptive diagnosis in suspected invasive disease, particularly in patients who have received antibiotics before the collection of specimens for culture. A negative test does not exclude pneumococcal disease. These tests, however, usually are of limited value in the evaluation of most patients with suspected invasive disease, such as meningitis.

Susceptibility Testing.* All *S pneumoniae* isolates from normally sterile body fluids, such as CSF and blood, should be tested for in vitro antimicrobial quantitative susceptibility to determine the minimum inhibitory concentration (MIC) to penicillin and to cefotaxime or ceftriaxone. *Nonsusceptible* is defined to include both *intermediate resistance* as well as *highly resistant* isolates. Accordingly, current definitions of in vitro susceptibility and nonsusceptibility are as follows:

Drug	Susceptible, µg/mL	Nonsusceptible, µg/mL	
		Intermediate	Resistant
Penicillin	≤ 0.06	0.1–1.0	≥ 2.0
Cefotaxime	≤ 0.5	1.0	≥ 2.0
Ceftriaxone	≤ 0.5	1.0	≥ 2.0

For patients with meningitis whose organism is *nonsusceptible* to penicillin, cefotaxime, and ceftriaxone, testing for vancomycin and rifampin susceptibility should be performed. If the patient has a nonmeningeal infection caused by a *nonsusceptible* isolate to penicillin, cefotaxime, and ceftriaxone, susceptibility testing for vancomycin, rifampin, clindamycin, trimethoprim-sulfamethoxazole, erythromycin, imipenem, meropenem, and chloramphenicol should be considered, depending on the patient's response to antimicrobial therapy.

When quantitative testing methods are not available, the qualitative screening test using a 1-µg oxacillin disk on an agar plate reliably identifies all penicillin-*susceptible* pneumococci based on the criterion of a disk zone diameter of 20 mm or greater. Organisms with an oxacillin disk zone size of less than 20 mm are potentially *nonsusceptible* and require further quantitative susceptibility testing as previously described. The oxacillin disc test, thus, is a screening test for resistance to ß-lactam drugs (ie, penicillins and cephalosporins).

TREATMENT*: *Streptococcus pneumoniae* strains with resistance (ie, *nonsusceptible*) to penicillin G, cefotaxime, ceftriaxone, and other antimicrobial agents have been identified in many regions of the United States as well as worldwide in significantly increasing frequency in recent years. *Nonsusceptible* strains most commonly have *intermediate resistance* to penicillin G (ie, in vitro minimum inhibitory concentrations [MIC] of 0.1 to 1 µg/mL); however, *resistant* strains (ie, MIC of ≥2 µg/mL) are becoming more common. In children in the United States, as many as 40% of isolates from sterile body sites in some geographic areas are *nonsusceptible* to penicillin G, and as many as 50% of these isolates are *resistant.* Approximately 50% of the *nonsusceptible* strains also are *nonsusceptible* to cefotaxime or ceftriaxone. The prevalence

---

* For further information, see American Academy of Pediatrics. Committee on Infectious Diseases. Therapy for children with invasive pneumococcal infection. *Pediatrics.* 1997;99:289-299.

of *nonsusceptible strains* varies geographically but these organisms have appeared unexpectedly in communities that previously had only *susceptible S pneumoniae.*

Vancomycin resistance has not been reported. If a strain with an in vitro MIC greater than 1.0 μg/mL is isolated, the state health department should be notified promptly and arrangements made for confirmatory testing.

Recommendations for treatment of pneumococcal infections are as follows.

Bacterial Meningitis Possibly or Proven To Be Caused By S pneumoniae. Combination therapy with vancomycin and cefotaxime or ceftriaxone should be administered initially to all children older than 1 month with definite or probable bacterial meningitis because of the increased prevalence of penicillin-, cefotaxime-, and ceftriaxone-resistant *S pneumoniae.* Some experts, however, recommend that vancomycin need not be used if compelling evidence indicates that the cause is an organism other than *S pneumoniae* (eg, Gram-negative diplococci on a cerebrospinal fluid [CSF] smear during an outbreak of meningococcal disease).

Because pneumococcal meningitis can occur in infants younger than 1 month, consideration should be given to the addition of vancomycin to the antibiotic regimens for suspected neonatal meningitis, especially if (1) the CSF smear shows Gram-positive diplococci characteristic of pneumococci, and/or (2) bacterial antigen testing supports a diagnosis of pneumococcal meningitis.

For children with severe hypersensitivity to the ß-lactam antibiotics (ie, penicillins and cephalosporins), the combination of vancomycin and rifampin should be considered. Vancomycin should not be given alone as CSF bactericidal concentrations are difficult to sustain and clinical experience to support its use as monotherapy is minimal. Rifampin also should not be given as monotherapy because resistance may develop during therapy. Other possible antimicrobials for the treatment of pneumococcal meningitis include chloramphenicol (which only should be used for pneumococcal meningitis if the in vitro minimal bactericidal concentration [MBC] is 4 μg/mL or less) and meropenem.

A lumbar puncture should be considered after 24 to 48 hours to evaluate therapy if (1) the organism is penicillin-*nonsusceptible* by oxacillin disk or quantitative (MIC) testing, the results from cefotaxime and ceftriaxone quantitative susceptibility testing are not yet available, and the patient's condition has not improved or has worsened; or (2) the child has received dexamethasone, which might interfere with the ability to interpret clinical indications of responses, such as fever.

Based on available results of susceptibility testing of the pneumococcal isolate, therapy should be modified according to the guidelines in Table 3.46, p 414. If the organism is susceptible to penicillin or cefotaxime or ceftriaxone, **vancomycin should be discontinued** and penicillin or cefotaxime or ceftriaxone should be continued. Vancomycin and cefotaxime or ceftriaxone should be continued only if the organism is *nonsusceptible* to penicillin and to cefotaxime or ceftriaxone.

Addition of rifampin or substitution of rifampin for vancomycin after 24 to 48 hours of therapy should be considered if the organism is susceptible to rifampin and (1) after 24 to 48 hours, despite therapy with vancomycin and cefotaxime or ceftriaxone, the clinical condition has worsened; (2) the subsequent Gram-stained smear or culture of CSF indicates failure to eradicate or to reduce substantially the number of organisms; or (3) the organism has an unusually high cefotaxime or cef-

Table 3.46. Antimicrobial Therapy for Bacterial Meningitis Caused By *Streptococcus pneumoniae* Based on Susceptibility Test Results

Susceptibility Test Results*	Antibiotic Management†
Susceptible to penicillin	**Discontinue vancomycin** and Begin penicillin or Continue cefotaxime or ceftriaxone alone‡
Nonsusceptible to penicillin (*intermediate* or *resistant*) **and** *Susceptible* to cefotaxime and ceftriaxone	**Discontinue vancomycin** and Continue cefotaxime or ceftriaxone
Nonsusceptible to penicillin (*intermediate* or *resistant*) **and** *Nonsusceptible* to cefotaxime and ceftriaxone (*intermediate* or *resistant*) **and** *Susceptible* to rifampin	Continue vancomycin and cefotaxime or ceftriaxone. Rifampin may be added or substituted for vancomycin in selected circumstances (see text).

* Based on quantitative susceptibility studies.
† See Table 3.47 for dosage. Some experts recommend the maximum dosages.
‡ Some physicians may choose this alternative for convenience and cost savings.

triaxone MIC (4 µg/mL or greater). Consultation with an infectious disease specialist should be considered in such circumstances.

Dexamethasone. In infants and children 6 weeks of age and older, adjunctive therapy with dexamethasone should be considered after weighing the potential benefits and possible risks (see Dexamethasone Therapy for Bacterial Meningitis in Infants and Children, p 620). The CSF concentrations of vancomycin, ceftriaxone, cefotaxime, and rifampin, when given in the recommended dosages for patients with meningitis (see Table 3.47, p 415) in children treated with dexamethasone are adequate to treat meningitis caused by most *nonsusceptible* strains of *S pneumoniae*. Dexamethasone can lead to decreased fever and a misleading impression of clinical improvement even though CSF sterilization may not have been achieved.

Children With Probable Aseptic Meningitis. During the summer and fall, children will be hospitalized for severe headaches, vomiting, fever, a stiff neck, and CSF pleocytosis caused by enteroviruses. Although antibiotics are not always indicated, some physicians will choose to give antimicrobial therapy to these patients until the CSF and blood cultures are negative. Vancomycin should not be used in these circumstances unless the child appears toxic and/or is hypotensive and pneumococcal infection is suspected.

Nonmeningeal Invasive Pneumococcal Infections Requiring Hospitalization. For nonmeningeal invasive infections in previously well children who are not critically ill, antimicrobials currently in use to treat *S pneumoniae* and other potential pathogens should be initiated at the usually recommended doses (see Table 3.47).

Table 3.47. Doses of Intravenous Antimicrobials for Invasive Pneumococcal Infections*

Antimicrobial	Meningitis		Non-Meningeal Infections	
	Dose, kg/d	Dose Interval	Dose, kg/d	Dose Interval
Penicillin G	250 000–400 000 U†	4–6 h	Same	Same
Cefotaxime	225–300 mg	6–8 h	150–225 mg	Same
Ceftriaxone	100 mg	12–24 h	80–100 mg	Same
Vancomycin	60 mg	6 h	40–60 mg	Same
Rifampin‡	20 mg	12 h	Not indicated	...
Chloramphenicol§	75–100 mg	6 h	Same	Same
Clindamycin§	Not indicated	...	25–40 mg	6–8 h
Meropenem‖	120 mg	8 h	60 mg	8 h
Imipenem-cilastatin¶	...	...	60 mg	6 h

* Doses are for children 1 month of age or older.
† Because 1 unit = 0.6 μg/mL, this range is equal to 150 to 240 mg/kg per day.
‡ Indications for use are not yet completely defined.
§ Drug should be considered only for patients with life-threatening allergic response following administration of ß-lactam antibiotics.
‖ Drug is approved for pediatric patients 3 months of age and older.
¶ Drug is not approved for use in patients younger than 12 years and is not recommended in patients with meningitis because of its potential epileptogenic properties.

For those children with invasive infections potentially due to *S pneumoniae* who are critically ill, additional initial antimicrobial therapy for possible penicillin-, cefotaxime-, or ceftriaxone-*nonsusceptible* strains can be considered. Such patients include those with myopericarditis or severe multilobar pneumonia with hypoxia or hypotension. **If vancomycin is administered, it should be discontinued as soon as antimicrobial susceptibility test results demonstrate effective alternative agents.**

If the organism is highly *resistant* to penicillin, cefotaxime, and ceftriaxone, therapy should be modified based on the clinical response, susceptibilities to other antimicrobials, and results of follow-up cultures of blood and other body fluids. Consultation with an infectious disease specialist should be considered.

For children with severe hypersensitivity to the ß-lactam antibiotics (ie, penicillins and cephalosporins), initial management for a potential pneumococcal infection should include clindamycin or vancomycin, in addition to antimicrobial drugs for other potential pathogens as indicated. Vancomycin should not be continued if the organism is susceptible to other appropriate non-ß-lactam antibiotics. Consultation with an infectious disease specialist should be considered.

Nonmeningeal Invasive Pneumococcal Infections in the Immunocompromised Host. The preceding recommendations for the management of possible pneumococcal infections requiring hospitalization also apply to immunocompromised children, provided they are not critically ill. However, for critically ill patients, consideration should be given to initiating therapy with vancomycin and cefotaxime or ceftriaxone.

Vancomycin should be discontinued as soon as antimicrobial susceptibility test results indicate effective alternative antimicrobials.

Dosages. The recommended doses of intravenous antimicrobials for the treatment of invasive pneumococcal infections are given in Table 3.47.

Otitis Media. Most experts recommend treatment of acute otitis media with oral amoxicillin. Duration of therapy is for 5 to 10 days. In uncomplicated cases, 5 to 7 days is preferred in order to minimize the use of antimicrobials and possible resulting emergence of resistant bacteria in the community. Effective alternative drugs, especially for penicillin-resistant strains of *S pneumoniae* or ampicillin-resistant strains of *H influenzae*, include erythromycin-sulfisoxazole, amoxicillin-clavulanic acid, extended-spectrum cephalosporins, and clarithromycin. Narrow-spectrum drugs, when appropriate, are recommended.

Based on concentrations in middle ear fluid and in vitro activity, no currently available ß-lactam antibiotic, including the oral cephalosporins, has better activity than amoxicillin against penicillin-**susceptible** *S pneumoniae* and against *nonsusceptible* strains of *intermediate resistance*. Cefuroxime axetil, cefpodoxime, and cefprozil are the only orally administered cephalosporins that have activity comparable to but not better than the activity of amoxicillin for highly resistant strains.

For patients who fail standard therapy and are suspected to have penicillin-resistant *S pneumoniae* infection, high-dose amoxicillin, other antibiotics such as clindamycin, a combination of amoxicillin and amoxicillin-clavulanate (to provide higher middle ear fluid concentrations of amoxicillin as well as activity against ß-lactamase-producing organism), and/or myringotomy should be considered. For highly *resistant* strains of *S pneumoniae*, amoxicillin in high dosages of 60 to 80 mg/kg per day should achieve concentrations in middle ear fluid that are likely to be effective. This dose, however, may result in diarrhea and antibiotic discontinuation by parents. Most penicillin-resistant *S pneumoniae* are susceptible to achievable concentrations of clindamycin in middle ear fluid. Clindamycin, however, is not active against *Haemophilus influenzae*.

Sinusitis. Antibiotics effective in the treatment of acute otitis media are also likely to be effective in acute sinusitis and are recommended.

ISOLATION OF THE HOSPITALIZED PATIENT: Standard precautions are recommended, including for patients with infections caused by drug-resistant *S pneumoniae*.

CONTROL MEASURES:

Child Care, Household, and School. No isolation precautions are necessary for children in child care or school who have pneumococcal disease. The need for or benefit of prophylactic antibiotic treatment of contacts of a person with pneumococcal disease has not been demonstrated and chemoprophylaxis is not recommended.

Active Immunization. The 23-valent pneumococcal vaccine is composed of purified capsular polysaccharide antigens of 23 pneumococcal serotypes. It is given subcutaneously or intramuscularly. Each vaccine dose (0.5 mL) contains 25 mg of each polysaccharide antigen. These capsular antigens are those of serotypes causing 88% of cases of bacteremia and meningitis in adults, nearly 100% of cases of bacteremia and meningitis in children, and 85% of cases of acute otitis media. Like other polysaccharide antigens, many of the pneumococcal serotypes in the vaccine have limited immunogenicity in children younger than 2 years. The effectiveness of pneumococcal vaccines in preventing pneumonia has been demonstrated in healthy young adults and older children who have an increased incidence of invasive pneumococcal disease. Vaccinated children with sickle cell disease or those who had undergone splenectomy have experienced significantly less bacteremic pneumococcal disease than nonvaccinated patients.

Investigational multivalent protein-conjugate vaccines that are immunogenic in children younger than 2 years have been developed and currently are under evaluation in field trials.

Adverse Reactions. Mild side effects, such as erythema and pain at the injection site, are common. Fever, myalgia, and severe local reactions are uncommon. Severe systemic reactions, such as anaphylaxis, have been reported rarely.

Recommendations for Immunization.

- Children 2 years and older with increased risk of acquiring systemic pneumococcal infections or of serious disease if they become infected should be immunized. Indications are the following: (1) sickle cell disease; (2) functional or anatomic asplenia; (3) nephrotic syndrome or chronic renal failure; (4) conditions associated with immunosuppression, such as organ transplantation, drug therapy or cytoreduction therapy (including long-term systemic corticosteroid therapy); (5) HIV infection (see HIV Infection, p 279); and (6) CSF leaks.

- Other indications for pneumococcal vaccination that are recommended by the Advisory Committee on Immunization Practices (ACIP) of the Centers for Disease Control and Prevention include persons 2 years of age and older with chronic cardiovascular disease (eg, congestive heart failure or cardiomyopathy), chronic pulmonary disease (eg, emphysema or cystic fibrosis, but not asthma), or chronic liver disease (eg, cirrhosis).

- Pneumococcal vaccination of persons 2 years of age and older living in special environments or social settings in which the risk of invasive pneumococcal disease or its complications is very high (eg, Alaskan Native and certain American Indian populations) is recommended by the ACIP.

- Parents and other caregivers of vaccinated children with functional or anatomic asplena should be informed that vaccination does not guarantee protection from fulminant pneumococcal disease and death. The patients, if old enough to be responsible for their health care (eg, adolescents) also should be informed. Asplenic patients with unexplained fever or manifestations of sepsis should receive prompt medical attention including treatment for suspected bacteremia, the initial signs and symptoms of which may be subtle. Antimicrobial agents selected for initial empiric treatment should be effective against *Neisseria meningitidis,* and ß-lactamase-producing *Haemophilus influenzae* type b as well as *S pneumoniae.*

- When elective splenectomy is to be performed, pneumococcal vaccine should be given approximately 2 weeks or more before the operation, if possible, to increase the likelihood of eliciting a protective antibody response. Similarly, in planning cancer chemotherapy or immunosuppressive therapy for patients with Hodgkin's disease or those who are to undergo bone marrow or solid-organ transplantation, vaccination should precede the initiation of chemotherapy or immunosuppression by approximately 2 weeks or more, if possible.

Immunization during chemotherapy or radiation therapy often results in poor serum antibody responses and immunization is not likely to be effective in preventing pneumococcal infection. Patients who received vaccine during chemotherapy or radiation therapy should be reimmunized 3 months after discontinuation of the therapy.

- Immunization with the pneumococcal vaccine is not recommended for preventing otitis media or any other pneumococcal infection during the first 2 years of life. Data are inadequate to evaluate the effectiveness of pneumococcal vaccine in preventing otitis media in children older than 2 years, although some experts recommend immunization of older children with recurrent otitis media.

- Revaccination after 3 to 5 years is recommended for children 10 years or younger who are at high risk of severe pneumococcal infection. These children include those who (1) have sickle cell disease; (2) are functionally or anatomically asplenic; (3) have conditions associated with a rapid antibody decline after initial immunization, such as from nephrotic syndrome, renal failure, or transplantation; or (4) are at increased risk because of HIV infection or malignancy (eg, leukemia, lymphoma, and Hodgkin's disease). Since most young children who are vaccinated are at continuing high risk of pneumococcal disease, routine vaccinations should be considered for any child who was originally vaccinated before 5 years of age. Reimmunization also is indicated for high-risk, older children and adults who were initially immunized at least 5 years or before. Revaccination once only is recommended.

- Pneumococcal vaccine may be given concurrently with other vaccines (see Simultaneous Administration of Multiple Vaccines, p 21). No data indicate that administration of pneumococcal vaccine with MMR, DTP, poliovirus, *H influenzae* type b, hepatitis B, influenza, or other vaccines increases the severity of reactions or diminishes antibody responses.

Contraindications and Precautions. Immunization generally should be deferred during pregnancy because the effect of the vaccine on the fetus is unknown. However, the risk of severe pneumococcal disease during pregnancy must be weighed against the potential hazards of the vaccine, and in high-risk persons vaccination is justified.

Passive Immunization. Intramuscular or intravenous immunoglobulin administration is recommended for preventing pneumococcal infection in patients with congenital or acquired immunodeficiency diseases, including persons with HIV infection who have recurrent pneumococcal infections (see HIV Infection, p 279).

Chemoprophylaxis. Daily antimicrobial prophylaxis is recommended for children with functional or anatomic asplenia, irrespective of their immunization status, for the prevention of pneumococcal disease (see Asplenic Children, p 56). Oral penicillin G or V (125 mg twice a day for children younger than 5 years; 250 mg twice a day for children 5 years and older) is recommended.

The results of a multicenter study demonstrated that oral penicillin V (125 mg twice a day) given to infants and young children with sickle cell anemia reduces the incidence of severe bacterial infection by 84% compared with the placebo control group. Based on this study, daily penicillin prophylaxis for children with sickle cell anemia beginning before 2 months of age or earlier is recommended.

The number of cases of penicillin-resistant invasive pneumococcal infections and the prevalence of nasopharyngeal carriage of penicillin-resistant strains in patients with sickle cell disease have increased in recent years. Parents, thus, should be informed that penicillin prophylaxis may no longer be as effective at preventing invasive pneumococcal infections as previously.

The age at which to discontinue prophylaxis is often an empirical decision. A recent study has demonstrated that children with sickle cell anemia who are receiving regular medical attention and who have not had a prior severe pneumococcal infection or a surgical splenectomy may safely discontinue prophylactic penicillin at approximately 5 years of age. However, they must be counseled to seek medical attention for all febrile events. The duration of prophylaxis for children with asplenia due to other causes is unknown; however, some experts continue prophylaxis throughout childhood and in adulthood in particularly high-risk patients.

Pneumocystis carinii Infections

CLINICAL MANIFESTATIONS: Infants and children characteristically develop a subacute, diffuse pneumonitis with dyspnea at rest, tachypnea, oxygen desaturation, nonproductive cough, and fever. However, the magnitude of these signs may vary and in some immunocompromised children and adults, the onset can be acute and fulminant. The chest roentgenogram often has bilateral diffuse interstitial or alveolar disease; rarely, lobar, miliary, and nodular lesions occur as well. Occasionally, the chest roentgenogram at the time of diagnosis appears normal. Mortality in immunocompromised patients is high, ranging from 5% to 40% if treated, and close to 100% if untreated.

ETIOLOGY: *Pneumocystis carinii* appears to be an unusual or primitive fungus, based on DNA sequence homologies. It, however, retains several morphologic and biologic similarities to the protozoa, most notably its susceptibility to a number of antiprotozoal agents but resistance to most antifungal agents.

EPIDEMIOLOGY: *Pneumocystis carinii* is ubiquitous in mammals worldwide, particularly rodents. Whether *P carinii* in animals is infectious for humans has not been determined. *Pneumocystis carinii* isolates recovered from mice, rats, and ferrets are genetically diverse from each other and from human *P carinii*, and do not seem to cross-infect other animals. Asymptomatic infection occurs early in life with more than 75% of healthy persons acquiring antibody by 4 years of age. In developing countries and in times of famine in industrialized countries, *P carinii* pneumonia (PCP) has occurred in epidemics, primarily affecting malnourished infants and children. Epidemics also have occurred in premature infants. In industrialized countries today, PCP occurs almost entirely in immunocompromised persons with deficient cell-mediated immunity, particularly those with HIV infection, recipients of immunosuppressive therapy after organ transplantation or treatment for malignancy, and children with congenital immunodeficiency syndromes. *Pneumocystis carinii* pneumonia is the most common serious opportunistic infection in infants and young children with perinatally acquired HIV infection, and is the commonest pediatric

AIDS-defining illness. Although onset of disease can occur at any age, including rare instances in the first month of life, PCP most frequently occurs in HIV-infected children between 3 and 6 months of age. The incidence of PCP is decreasing as chemoprophylaxis is more widely implemented. The mode of transmission is unknown. Proposed hypotheses are (1) person-to-person transmission by the respiratory route (airborne transmission has been demonstrated in experimental animals), and (2) acquisition from the environment. Circumstantial evidence suggests that person-to-person transmission can occur but identifying any contact with an infected person prior to onset is rare. Primary infection probably accounts for disease during infancy whereas either primary infection or reactivation of latent infection from immunosuppression could result in disease after the first 2 years of life. Recurrences in immunocompromised patients, especially those with AIDS, are common. In patients with lymphoma or leukemia, the disease most often occurs during remission or relapse. The period of communicability is unknown.

The **incubation period** is unknown.

DIAGNOSTIC TESTS: A definitive diagnosis of PCP is made by demonstration of organisms in lung tissue or lower respiratory tract secretions. The most sensitive and specific diagnostic procedures have been open-lung biopsy and transbronchial biopsy. However, bronchoscopy with bronchoalveolar lavage, induction of sputum in older children and adolescents, and intubation with deep endotracheal aspiration are less invasive and often diagnostic, and have been sufficiently sensitive in patients with HIV infection (who have an increased number of organisms compared to non-HIV-infected patients with *P carinii* pneumonia). Methenamine silver nitrate and toluidine blue O are the most useful stains for identifying the thick-walled cysts of *P carinii*. Extracystic trophozoites are identified with Giemsa, Wright, and modified Wright-Giemsa stains. Serologic tests and polymerase chain reaction (PCR) assays for detecting *P carinii* infection are experimental and are not recommended for diagnosis. Many children and adults with HIV infection and PCP have elevated serum concentrations of lactate dehydrogenase, but this abnormality is not specific for PCP.

TREATMENT: The drug of choice is trimethoprim-sulfamethoxazole (15 to 20 mg/kg per day of trimethoprim; 75 to 100 mg/kg of sulfamethoxazole daily in divided doses every 6 hours), usually given intravenously. Oral therapy should be reserved for patients with mild disease who do not have malabsorption or diarrhea. The rate of adverse reactions is higher in HIV-infected patients than in patients without HIV infection; the incidence in HIV-infected children treated with trimethoprim-sulfamethoxazole is approximately 15%, but may be as high as 60% in adults with HIV infection. If the adverse reaction is not severe, continuation of therapy is recommended, as 50% of patients with adverse reaction have been subsequently treated successfully with trimethoprim-sulfamethoxazole.

Parenterally administered pentamidine (4 mg/kg per day of salt given once a day) is an alternative drug for children and adults who cannot tolerate trimethoprim-sulfamethoxazole or who have severe disease and who have not responded to trimethoprim-sulfamethoxazole after 5 to 7 days of therapy. The therapeutic efficacy of parenteral pentamidine in adults with PCP has been similar to that of trimethoprim-sulfamethoxazole. However, pentamidine is associated with a high incidence of adverse reactions, including pancreatitis, renal dysfunction, hypoglycemia, hyperglycemia, hypotension, fever, and neutropenia. Pentamidine should not be used concomitantly with didanosine, since both drugs can cause pancreatitis. If a recipient of didanosine develops PCP and requires pentamidine, didanosine should be discontinued until 1 week after the pentamidine therapy has been discontinued.

Atovaquone has been approved for the oral treatment of mild to moderate PCP in adults who are intolerant of trimethoprim-sulfamethoxazone. Experience with the use of atovaquone in children is limited. A dose of 40 mg/kg per day in two divided doses is suggested.

Other potentially useful drugs identified by in vitro studies, animal models, and clinical trials in adults include dapsone with trimethoprim, trimetrexate with leucovorin, and clindamycin with primaquine. Experience with the use of these combinations in children is extremely limited.

A minimal duration of 2 weeks of therapy is recommended; many experts advise 3 weeks of therapy for patients with AIDS. In patients with AIDS, continuous life-long prophylaxis should be initiated at the end of therapy for acute infection.

Corticosteroids appear to be beneficial in the treatment of HIV-infected adults with moderate to severe PCP (as defined by an arterial oxygen pressure [PaO_2] of less than 70 mm Hg, or an arterial-alveolar gradient of more than 35 mm Hg).* For adolescents older than 13 years and adults, 80 mg/d of oral prednisone in two divided doses for the first five days of therapy, 40 mg once a day on days 6 through 10, and 20 mg once a day on days 11 through 21 is recommended. Although no controlled studies of the use of corticosteroids in young children have been performed, most experts would include corticosteroids as part of the therapy for children with moderate to severe PCP. The optimal dose and duration of corticosteroid therapy for children have not been determined, but most experts suggest 2 mg/kg per day of prednisone or its equivalent for 7 to 10 days, followed by a tapering dose during the next 10 to 14 days.

Chemoprophylaxis.† Prophylaxis against a first episode of PCP is indicated for many patients with significant immunocompromise including those with HIV infection and those with primary or acquired immunodeficiency, such as from chemotherapy or other immunosuppressive therapy. Lifelong chemoprophylaxis, regardless of the CD4+ T-lymphocyte count, is strongly recommended for any HIV-infected persons, including children of any age, who already have had an episode of PCP.

Because half of all cases of PCP in children with perinatally acquired HIV occur in infants 3 to 6 months of age, identification as early as possible of infants who have been perinatally exposed to HIV is essential so that prophylaxis can be initiated before they are at risk. The most effective means to implement this recommendation is by diagnosing maternal HIV infection prior to or during pregnancy (see HIV

---

* The National Institutes of Health-University of California Expert Panel for Corticosteroids as Adjunctive Therapy for Pneumocystis Pneumonia. Consensus statement on the use of corticosteroids as adjunctive therapy for pneumocystis pneumonia in the acquired immunodeficiency syndrome. *N Engl J Med.* 1990;323:1500-1504.

† See the following for further information: Centers for Disease Control and Prevention. Recommendations for prophylaxis against *Pneumocystis carinii* pneumonia for adults and adolescents infected with human immunodeficiency virus. *MMWR.* 1992;4(No. RR-4):1-11; and Centers for Disease Control and Prevention. 1995 revised guidelines for prophylaxis against *Pneumocystis carinii* pneumonia for children infected with or perinatally exposed to human immunodeficiency virus. *MMWR.* 1995; 44(No. RR-4):1-11.

Infection, p 279). Prophylaxis for PCP is recommended for all infants born to HIV-infected women beginning at 4 to 6 weeks of age and CD4+ T-lymphocyte counts alone no longer are recommended for determining the need for PCP prophylaxis for infants younger than 1 year (see Table 3.48). Prophylaxis for PCP should be discontinued for children in whom HIV infection has been excluded. Children whose HIV infection status is not yet determined should continue prophylaxis throughout the first year of life.

Prophylaxis should be continued after 1 year of age for HIV-infected children who have had any CD4+ T-lymphocyte determination in the first 12 months of life indicating severe immunosuppression (ie, total count less than 750 cells/μL or a CD4+ percentage of total circulating lymphocytes is less than 15%). Prophylaxis may be discontinued at 1 year of age when CD4+ T-lymphocyte monitoring has been appropriate and counts have remained greater than these threshold values that define immunosuppression (see Table 3.48).

For HIV-infected children 1 to 5 years of age, PCP prophylaxis should be administered if (1) any CD4+ T-lymphocyte count is less than 500 cells/μL or the CD4+ percentage is less than 15%; (2) a rapidly declining CD4+ T-lymphocyte

Table 3.48. Recommendations for *Pneumocystis carinii* Pneumonia (PCP) Prophylaxis for HIV-Exposed Infants and Children, by Age and HIV-Infection Status*

Age and HIV-Infection Status	PCP Prophylaxis[†]
Birth to 4–6 wk, HIV-exposed	No prophylaxis
4–6 wk to 4 mo, HIV-exposed	Prophylaxis
4–12 mo	
HIV-infected or indeterminate	Prophylaxis
HIV-infection excluded[‡]	No prophylaxis
1–5 y, HIV-infected	Prophylaxis if: CD4+ T-lymphocyte count is <500 cells/μL or percentage is <15%[§][‖]
≥5 y, HIV-infected	Prophylaxis if: CD4+ T-lymphocyte count is <200 cells/μL or percentage is <15%[‖]

* Modified from Centers for Disease Control and Prevention. 1995 revised guidelines for prophylaxis against *Pneumocystis carinii* pneumonia for children infected with or perinatally exposed to human immunodeficiency virus. *MMWR.* 1995;44(No. RR-4):1-11.

† Children who have had PCP should receive lifelong PCP prophylaxis.

‡ HIV infection can be reasonably excluded among children who have had two or more negative HIV diagnostic tests (ie, HIV culture or PCR), both of which are performed at ≥ 1 month of age and one of which is performed at ≥4 months of age; or two or more negative HIV IgG antibody tests performed at ≥ 6 months of age among children who have no clinical evidence of HIV disease (see HIV Infection, p 279).

§ Children 1 to 2 years of age who were receiving PCP prophylaxis and had a CD4+ count of less than 750 cells/μL or percentage of less than 15% at less than 12 months of age should continue prophylaxis.

‖ Prophylaxis should be considered on a case-by-case basis for children who might otherwise be at risk for PCP, such as children with rapidly declining CD4+ counts or percentages or children with Category C status of HIV infection.

count occurs; or (3) severely symptomatic HIV disease (category C) is present (see HIV Infection, p 279, and Table 3.48). Criteria are the same for older children and adolescents except for different age-specific definitions of low absolute CD4+ cell counts.

For children 6 years of age or older, any CD4+ count less than 200 cells/µL is an indication for chemoprophylaxis. For adolescents or adults, PCP prophylaxis is indicated if the CD4+ cell counts is less than 200/µL, or the patient has unexplained fever for 2 or more weeks or a history of oropharyngeal candidiasis.

HIV-infected children older than 1 year, not previously receiving PCP prophylaxis (eg, those children not previously identified or whose PCP prophylaxis was discontinued) should begin prophylaxis if at any time their CD4+ cell counts indicate severe immunosuppression (see Table 3.48).

The recommended drug regimen for prophylaxis in all immunocompromised patients (whether from HIV infection, malignancy, or other causes) is trimethoprim-sulfamethoxazole administered for 3 consecutive days each week (see Table 3.49 for dosage). For patients who cannot tolerate the drug, aerosolized pentamidine for those 5 years or older is considered to be an alternative; daily oral dapsone is another alternate drug for prophylaxis in children, especially those younger than 5 years (see Table 3.49). Intravenous pentamidine has also been used, but it appears to be less effective and potentially more toxic than other prophylactic regimens.

Table 3.49. Drug Regimens for *Pneumocystis carinii* Pneumonia Prophylaxis for Children ≥4 Weeks of Age*

Recommended regimen:
Trimethoprim-sulfamethoxazole, 150 mg trimethroprim/M^2/d with 750 mg sulfamethoxozole/M^2/d administered orally in divided doses twice a day 3 times per week on consecutive days (eg, Monday-Tuesday-Wednesday)

Acceptable alternative trimethoprim-sulfamethoxozole dosage schedules:
- 150 mg trimethoprim/M^2/d with 750 mg sulfamethoxazole/M^2/d administered orally **as a single daily dose** 3 times per week on consecutive days (eg, Monday-Tuesday-Wednesday).
- 150 mg trimethoprim/M^2/d with 750 mg sulfamethoxazole/M^2/d administered orally in divided doses twice a day and **administered 7 days per week.**
- 150 mg trimethoprim/M^2/d with 750 mg sulfamethoxazole/M^2/d administered orally in divided doses twice a day and administered 3 times per week on **alternate days** (eg, Monday-Wednesday-Friday).

Alternative regimens if trimethoprim-sulfamethoxazole is not tolerated:
- **Dapsone[†]**
2 mg/kg (not to exceed 100 mg) administered orally once a day.
- **Aerosolized pentamidine[†]** (children ≥5 y old)
300 mg administered via Respirgard II inhaler monthly.

---

* From Centers for Disease Control and Prevention. 1995 revised guidelines for prophylaxis against *Pneumocystis carinii* pneumonia for children infected with or perinatally exposed to human immunodeficiency virus. *MMWR.* 1995;44(No. RR-4):1-11.

[†] If neither dapsone nor aerosolized pentamidine is tolerated, some clinicians use **intravenous pentamidine** (4 mg/kg) administered every 2 or 4 weeks.

Other drugs with potential for prophylaxis include pyrimethamine with dapsone, pyrimethamine-sulfadoxine, and oral atovaquone. Experience with these drugs in both adults and children is very limited. These agents should be considered only in unusual situations in which the recommended regimens are not tolerated or cannot be used.

Although prophylaxis substantially reduces the risk of PCP, pulmonary and extrapulmonary *P carinii* infections have occurred in HIV-infected adults and children receiving prophylaxis.

ISOLATION OF THE HOSPITALIZED PATIENT: Standard precautions are recommended. In addition, patients with PCP should not share a room with immunocompromised patients.

CONTROL MEASURES: Appropriate therapy of infected patients and prophylaxis in immunocompromised patients are the only available means of control. Detailed guidelines have been recently issued by the Centers for Disease Control and Prevention and the Infectious Diseases Society of America, and endorsed by the American Academy of Pediatrics.*

Poliovirus Infections

CLINICAL MANIFESTATIONS: Approximately 90% to 95% of poliovirus infections are asymptomatic. Nonspecific illness with low-grade fever and sore throat (minor illness) occurs in 4% to 8% of infections. Aseptic meningitis, sometimes with paresthesias, occurs in 1% to 5% of patients a few days after the minor illness has resolved. Rapid onset of asymmetric acute flaccid paralysis with areflexia of the involved limb occurs in 0.1% to 2% of infections, and residual paralytic disease involving the motor neurons (paralytic poliomyelitis) occurs in approximately 1 per 250 infections. Cranial nerve involvement and paralysis of respiratory muscles may occur. Findings in the cerebrospinal fluid (CSF) are characteristic of viral meningitis with mild pleocytosis and lymphocytic predominance.

Adults who contracted paralytic poliomyelitis in childhood may develop 30 to 40 years later the post-polio syndrome, which is characterized by muscle pain, exacerbation of weakness, and/or new paralysis or weakness.

ETIOLOGY: Polioviruses are enteroviruses and consist of three serotypes: 1, 2, and 3.

EPIDEMIOLOGY: Poliovirus circulation and resulting infection occur only in humans. Spread is by the fecal-oral and oral-oral (respiratory) routes. Perinatal transmission from mother to newborn infant can occur. Infection is more common in infants and young children, and occurs at an earlier age in living conditions of poor hygiene. The risks of paralytic disease from infection does not appear to be affected significantly by age. In temperate climates, poliovirus infections are most

---

* Centers for Disease Control and Prevention. USPHS/IDSA guidelines for the prevention of opportunistic infections in persons infected with human immunodeficiency virus: a summary. *MMWR.* 1995;44(No. RR-8):5-6, 24-29.

common in the summer and fall; in the tropics, the seasonal pattern is variable, with a less pronounced peak of activity.

Poliomyelitis has become rare in the United States. The last reported case due to indigenously acquired, wild-type poliovirus occurred in 1979 during an epidemic in a religious sect that had refused immunizations. Since then, nearly all cases have been vaccine-associated paralytic poliomyelitis (VAPP) and attributable to oral poliovirus vaccine (OPV). Approximately 8 to 9 cases of VAPP have been reported annually in the United States since 1980. The only other cases have been very rare cases of imported disease, the occurrence of which has continued to decrease in the past decade. No cases of wild-type poliovirus disease have occurred in the Western hemisphere since 1991, resulting in certification in 1994 by an international commission that wild-type poliovirus transmission has been interrupted in this hemisphere. While poliomyelitis continues to occur in some underdeveloped areas of the world, the worldwide incidence of poliomyelitis has decreased by 80% or more since 1988 as the result of the global poliomyelitis eradication initiative of the World Health Organization. These successes are attributable primarily to widespread use of OPV.

Communicability is greatest shortly before and after onset of clinical illness when the virus is present in the throat and excreted in high concentration in the feces. The virus persists in the throat for about 1 week after onset of illness and is excreted in the feces for several weeks and occasionally for months. Patients are potentially contagious as long as fecal excretion persists. In recipients of OPV, the virus persists in the throat for 1 to 2 weeks; it is excreted in the feces for several weeks, although in rare cases it has been excreted for more than 2 months. Immunodeficient patients may excrete virus for prolonged periods.

The **incubation period** of abortive poliomyelitis is 3 to 6 days. For the onset of paralysis in paralytic poliomyelitis, the incubation period is usually 7 to 21 days, but occasionally it is as short as 4 days.

DIAGNOSTIC TESTS: Poliovirus can be recovered from the feces, pharynx, urine, and, rarely, cerebrospinal fluid (CSF) by isolation in cell culture. Two or more stool and throat swab specimens for enterovirus isolation should be obtained at least 24 hours apart from patients with suspected paralytic poliomyelitis as early in the course of the illness as possible, ideally within 14 days of onset of symptoms. Fecal material is most likely to yield virus, but virus also can be recovered from rectal swabs.

If a poliovirus is isolated from a patient with paralysis, the isolate should be sent to the Centers for Disease Control and Prevention through the state health department for testing to distinguish wild-type from vaccine strains. Since infants and children who are immunized with oral poliovirus vaccine (OPV) can excrete vaccine virus in the feces for several weeks, the incidental isolation of poliovirus from enteric sites in healthy young infants should be assumed to be the result of administration of, or exposure to OPV, unless an epidemiological or clinical reason to suspect otherwise exists. Serologic testing of acute and convalescent sera should be performed in patients suspected of having paralytic poliomyelitis, but interpretation of serologic test results can be difficult. Hence, the diagnostic test of choice for confirming poliovirus disease is viral culture of stool specimens and throat swabs obtained as early in the course of the illness as possible (see preceding paragraph).

TREATMENT: Supportive.

ISOLATION OF THE HOSPITALIZED PATIENT: Standard precautions are recommended.

CONTROL MEASURES:

Immunization of Infants and Children.

Vaccines. The two types of poliovirus vaccines are live oral poliovirus vaccine and inactivated poliovirus vaccine given parenterally (subcutaneously). Oral poliovirus vaccine (OPV) contains attenuated poliovirus types 1, 2, and 3, produced in monkey kidney cell cultures. Inactivated poliovirus vaccine (IPV) contains the three types of poliovirus grown in either monkey kidney or human diploid cells and inactivated with formaldehyde. The IPV in use in the United States since the late 1980s is of enhanced potency and is highly immunogenic. Trace amounts of streptomycin, neomycin, and polymyxin B may be present in these IPV formulations; OPV contains trace quantities of streptomycin and neomycin.

Immunogenicity and Efficacy. Both OPV and IPV in their recommended schedules are highly immunogenic and effective in preventing poliomyelitis.

In three-dose series, OPV results in sustained, probably lifelong immunity. Two doses produce a serum antibody response to all three serotypes in more than 90% of recipients. Vaccination with two or more doses of OPV induces excellent intestinal immunity against poliovirus reinfection, which explains its effectiveness in controlling wild-virus circulation.

Administration of IPV results in seroconversion in approximately 95% or more of vaccinees after two doses and in high titers of serum in 99% to 100% after three doses. Immunity, as with OPV vaccination, is prolonged, perhaps lifelong. Mucosal immunity is induced by enhanced-potency IPV but to a lesser extent than that with OPV; IPV inhibits pharyngeal acquisition of poliovirus and, to a lesser extent, intestinal acquisition.

The effectiveness of OPV has been amply demonstrated by its success in the United States and in many other areas of the world in preventing poliomyelitis and in interrupting the circulation of wild-type poliovirus. The effectiveness of IPV has been demonstrated by its use in several countries in Western Europe that have controlled and now eliminated poliomyelitis. These countries include Finland, France, The Netherlands, Norway, and Sweden.

In studies of the immunogenicity of the sequential use of IPV and OPV, seroconversion following two doses of IPV (at 2 and 4 months of age) and a subsequent dose of OPV was 94% or greater to serotypes 1 and 2 and 78% to 100% for serotype 3. Following a second dose of OPV, humoral immunity was greater than 95% to all serotypes. At least two doses of OPV are necessary for optimal intestinal immunity and no additional benefit is gained from a third OPV dose. The rationale of sequential use of IPV and OPV is that two doses of IPV induce sufficient humoral immunity to prevent VAPP in recipients from subsequent administration of OPV, given to induce optimal intestinal immunity as well as to sustain humoral immunity.

Administration With Other Vaccines. Either OPV or IPV may be given concurrently with other routinely recommended childhood vaccines (see Simultaneous Administration of Multiple Vaccines, p 21).

Adverse Reactions. The only well-documented, significant adverse reaction to poliomyelitis vaccination is vaccine-associated paralytic poliomyelitis (VAPP) attributable to OPV. The overall risk of VAPP is approximately one case to 2.4 million doses of OPV distributed. The rate following the first dose is approximately 1 case per 760 000 doses, including recipient and contact cases. The risk of a recipient case following the first OPV dose is estimated to be 1 per 1.5 million doses; for a contact case resulting from exposure to a first-dose recipient it is 1 per 2.2 million doses. For subsequent doses, the risk is substantially lower for both recipients and contacts. For immunodeficient persons, the risk is 3200- to 6800-fold higher than that in immunologically normal recipients.

Of the 124 cases of VAPP reported from 1980 to 1994, 46 (39%) occurred in otherwise healthy recipients, 78% of which were associated with the first dose, and approximately 90% or more occurred in the first year of life. Forty cases occurred in healthy contacts, accounting for 32% of all cases; approximately three-fourths of which were adults. In 30 cases (24%), the patients were immunologically abnormal, the majority of whom had disorders of humoral immunity, ie, antibody-deficiency syndromes. These cases include vaccine recipients and contacts. Six cases from which vaccine-related virus was isolated occurred in community contacts with no history of recent vaccination or contact with a vaccine recipient.

Based on the epidemiology of VAPP, universal application of a sequential schedule is expected to reduce the total number of cases by 50% to 75%. It should eliminate most cases of VAPP in vaccine recipients and reduce the number of cases in unimmunized contacts because IPV provides some degree of mucosal immunity, resulting in reduced excretion of the vaccine virus following OPV administration. Although the use of OPV in a sequential schedule allows continued circulation of vaccine virus and some resulting contact cases of VAPP, this circulation would be reduced by the decreased usage of OPV in the sequential schedule as only two doses rather than four would be given to each child.

Although an Institute of Medicine committee noted an increased risk of Guillian-Barré syndrome (GBS) following OPV administration in two studies in Finland, reanalysis of these data and a subsequent study in the United States indicate that the risk of GBS following OPV administration is not increased.

No serious adverse events have been associated with use of the currently available enhanced-potency IPV products. As with any vaccine, rare adverse reactions cannot be excluded until IPV has been used in large populations. To date, however, data on adverse reactions from France and Canada, which have surveillance systems, and manufacturers' records have demonstrated the safety of IPV.

Since poliovirus vaccines may contain trace amounts of streptomycin, neomycin, and polymyxin B, allergic reactions are possible in recipients with hypersensitivity to one or more of these antibodies.

Schedules.

Oral Poliovirus Vaccine (OPV). For children immunized with OPV only, the first dose is administered when the infant is approximately 2 months old (minimum age of 6 weeks) and a second dose is given when the infant is 4 months old. A third dose is recommended when the child is 6 to 18 months of age to complete the primary series. Administration of the third dose at 6 months of age has the potential advantage of enhancing the likelihood of completion of the primary series and does not compromise seroconversion. An interval of 2 months between doses is recommended. The minimal interval in most circumstances is 6 weeks, but in children in whom accelerated poliomyelitis vaccination is warranted, this interval may be 4 weeks. A supplementary dose of OPV should be given before the child enters school, ie, at 4 to 6 years of age. No evidence for waning immunity exist.

In geographic areas where polio is endemic, a dose may also be given when the newborn infant is discharged from the hospital, and supplemental doses are often administered during mass community-based programs.

Breastfeeding does not affect the overall success of immunization; hence, no interruption of the feeding schedule is necessary.

For children who are not immunized in the first year of life, two doses of OPV should be given approximately 6 to 8 weeks apart, followed by a third dose 2 to 12 months later (see Table 1.3, p 20). If the risk of exposure to polio is substantial, such as for travelers to poliovirus endemic areas or for children whose receipt of vaccines has been delayed, the interval between doses may be 4 to 6 weeks. If the third dose is administered before the fourth birthday, a supplementary (fourth) dose should be given before the child enters school, ie, at 4 to 6 years of age.

Inactivated Poliovirus Vaccine (IPV). For children immunized with IPV only, the primary series consists of three doses. The first two doses should be given at 1- to 2-month (4- to 8-week) intervals beginning at 2 months of age (minimum age of 6 weeks) and a third dose is recommended 6 to 12 months after the second dose. A supplemental dose of IPV should be given before the child enters school, ie, at 4 to 6 years of age.

Sequential Use of IPV Followed by OPV. The recommended schedule for this regimen is two doses of IPV at 2 (minimum age of 6 weeks) and 4 months of age followed by two doses of OPV at 12 to 18 months and 4 to 6 years of age.

To implement these three schedules (for sequential IPV-OPV, OPV-only, and IPV-only), a single schedule for the recommended ages for administration of poliovirus vaccine, irrespective of which vaccine is to be given, has been developed (see Vaccine Recommendations for Children, p 430).

Considerations in the Choice of Vaccine Regimen. The goal of poliomyelitis vaccination programs is the worldwide eradication of both the disease and wild-type poliovirus circulation. In the United States where eradication has been achieved and with certification of the Western hemisphere as free of indigenous wild-type poliovirus in 1994, an additional goal is to reduce and eventually eliminate VAPP by the expanded use of IPV. While prevention of VAPP can be most rapidly achieved by an IPV-only regimen, the number of injections in the current childhood immunization schedule, lack of sufficient combination vaccine products to reduce the number of necessary injections, and local constraints of practice resulting from cost and other factors may prevent the immediate, routine implementation of this option. In addition, the continuing need for optimal intestinal immunity as induced by OPV in order to limit further the circulation of wild-type virus if importation were to occur may be an important public health benefit.

Each of the three poliomyelitis vaccine schedules, ie, OPV-only, IPV-only, and sequential IPV-OPV, is highly effective in protecting against poliomyelitis from wild-type polioviruses and is acceptable. Physicians, thus, have three options for immunizing their patients. Major factors in the selection of the most appropriate options are the following:

- Risk of VAPP.
- Need for optimal intestinal immunity.
- Number of injections required at scheduled visits to administer the recommended vaccines.
- Possible increased number of visits resulting from parental or provider preference to avoid additional injections at one or more visits.
- Possible decreased vaccination rates in infants and young children as a result of the increased number of vaccine injections and visits to complete a sequential or an IPV-only regimen.
- Vaccine costs.
- Parent and/or provider choice.
- Introduction of new combination vaccines.

When these factors are considered, the choice of schedule should be based on the goal of reducing VAPP without compromising poliomyelitis immunity or the delivery of other recommended childhood immunizations in both the public and private sectors. Accordingly, the American Academy of Pediatrics recommends expanded use of IPV, but recognizes that OPV only may be indicated for some children in order to ensure timely completion of the routine childhood immunization schedule against other vaccine-preventable diseases. Once new combination vaccines are widely available, an IPV-only schedule should be feasible for all children in the United States, assuming global progress towards elimination of poliovirus circulation continues. Eventually, assuming successful worldwide eradication, poliovirus vaccination would be discontinued.

These considerations that support expanded use of IPV apply primarily to countries where wild poliovirus transmission has been interrupted for at least several years. Oral poliovirus vaccine remains the vaccine of choice for global eradication in the following: (1) areas where wild poliovirus has recently or is currently circulating; (2) in most developing countries where the higher cost of IPV prohibits its use; and/or (3) areas where inadequate sanitation necessitates an optimal mucosal barrier to wild-type virus circulation.

As the result of these factors, the Academy concludes that regimens of sequential IPV-OPV, IPV-only, or OPV-only are acceptable. In addition to factors previously cited, the choice of schedule for most children will be based on local public health recommendations, practice preference and product availability. Depending on circumstances, the sequential IPV-OPV (ACIP-recommended), IPV-only, or OPV-only regimen may be preferred. In the sequential regimen, two doses of OPV are necessary for optimal intestinal immunity.

Issues in Scheduling IPV Administration. Until appropriate combination vaccines are available, the administration of IPV necessitates additional injections. In scheduling IPV administration, the following options should be considered to decrease the number of injections at the 2- and 4-month visits:

- Hepatitis B vaccine administration at birth and ages 1 and 6 months.
- Additional visits, assuming that the child is likely to return.
- Use of available combination vaccines.

Alternatively, OPV can be given in place of IPV until the appropriate combination vaccines become available.

Vaccine Interchangeability. Completion of poliovirus vaccination with any of the three regimens (sequential IPV-OPV, OPV, or IPV) is preferred. However, four doses of any combination of IPV or OPV by 4 to 6 years of age are considered equivalent to a complete poliovirus vaccination series of one of the three acceptable regimens when administered according to the recommendations for minimum ages and intervals between doses.

Vaccine Recommendations for Children. Expanded use of IPV is indicated during the transition period of global eradication of poliomyelitis to reduce the risk of VAPP and to maintain immunity against wild-type poliovirus infection. The Advisory Committee on Immunization Practices (ACIP) of the Centers for Disease Control and Prevention (CDC) has recommended the sequential use of two doses of IPV followed by two doses of OPV as the current public health strategy for prevention of poliomyelitis. Because logistical problems with the current childhood immunization schedule may make these new recommendations for the use of IPV difficult to implement immediately, their adoption likely will be gradual. Nevertheless, assuming continued progress towards global eradication and the availability of additional combination vaccine products, the routine use of an IPV-only regimen is likely to become more feasible in future years. The Academy recommends the following:

- Poliomyelitis vaccine should be given at 2 months, 4 months, 12 to 18 months, and 4 to 6 years of age for a total of four doses at or before the child enters school. For children who receive OPV only, the third dose may be given as early as 6 months of age in accordance with prior recommendations. An additional dose at school entry is not indicated for children who received the third dose of any vaccine on or after their fourth birthday.
- Physicians have three options for immunizing their patients. Regimens of sequential IPV-OPV, IPV only, or OPV only are acceptable. Each regimen has advantages and disadvantages, and in the circumstances described subsequently, one may be preferred or recommended. Parents or other caregivers should be informed of the advantages and disadvantages of the three acceptable regimens.
- In the following circumstances, immunization with IPV only is recommended:
  — For immunocompromised persons and their household contacts, as OPV is contraindicated (see Precautions and Contraindications to Immunization, p 432).
  — For infants and children in which an adult household member is known to be inadequately vaccinated against poliomyelitis, because unimmunized adults are at increased risk of VAPP.
  — When the number of injections is not likely to decrease compliance and when IPV is preferred by health care providers and parents or other caregivers.
- In the following circumstances, immunization with OPV only is recommended:
  — When parents or providers who prefer not to have the child receive the additional injections needed if IPV were to be used.
  — For infants and children starting vaccination regimens after 6 months of age in whom an accelerated schedule is necessary to complete immunizations, an OPV-only regimen will minimize the number of injections required at each visit. For similar reasons, in populations with low vaccination rates,

OPV may be preferred in order to expedite implementation of the routine childhood immunization schedule.

- The sequential IPV/OPV schedule is recommended to reduce the total number of injections required to reduce the risk of VAPP while maintaining optimal intestinal immunity, especially for travelers to areas where poliovirus is still endemic.
- The Academy supports the World Health Organization recommendation for the use of OPV to achieve global eradication of poliomyelitis, especially for countries with continued or recent circulation of wild-type poliovirus and occurrence of paralytic poliomyelitis, and for those in which the increased cost of IPV and its administration makes its use impractical.

Children Incompletely Immunized. Children who have not received the recommended doses of poliovirus vaccines on schedule should receive sufficient doses of either IPV or OPV to complete the immunization series for their age (see Lapsed Immunizations, p 21). In these circumstances, IPV and OPV are considered interchangeable; the exception is when the sequential IPV-OPV regimen is selected, in which case two doses of OPV are necessary for optimal intestinal immunity. Incompletely immunized children who are at increased risk of exposure to wild poliovirus because of travel to areas where poliovirus is still endemic should be given OPV for the remaining recommended doses. If time does not permit completion of the routine schedule, the intervals between doses can be shortened to 4 weeks; OPV can be administered as long as the child is not immunocompromised or does not live in a household with an immunocompromised member. For children who received one or more doses of OPV and for whom OPV is subsequently contraindicated, the series can be completed with IPV.

Vaccine Recommendations for Adults. Routine primary poliovirus vaccination of previously unvaccinated adults (18 years of age or older) residing in the United States is not indicated. Most adults are immune from their childhood immunization and also have a very small risk of exposure to wild poliovirus in the United States. Immunization is recommended for certain adults who are at a greater risk of exposure to wild polioviruses than the general population, including the following:

- Travelers to areas or countries where poliomyelitis is or may be epidemic or endemic.
- Members of communities or specific population groups with disease caused by wild polioviruses.
- Laboratory workers handling specimens that may contain wild polioviruses.
- Health care workers in close contact with patients who may be excreting wild polioviruses.
- Unvaccinated persons whose children will be receiving OPV.

Immunization of these adults is recommended as follows:

- ***Unvaccinated adults.*** Primary immunization with IPV is recommended. Inactivated poliovirus vaccine is preferred because the risk of vaccine-associated paralytic poliomyelitis (VAPP) after OPV is slightly higher in adults than that in children. Two doses of IPV should be given at intervals of 1 to 2 months (4 to 8 weeks); a third dose is given 6 to 12 months after the second.

If time does not allow three doses of IPV to be given according to the recommended schedule before protection is required, the following alternatives are recommended:

- If protection is not needed until 8 weeks or more, three doses of IPV should be given at least 4 weeks apart.
- If protection is not needed for 4 to 8 weeks, two doses of IPV should be given at least 4 weeks apart.
- If protection is needed in less than 4 weeks, a single dose of either IPV or OPV should be given.

The remaining doses of vaccine to complete the primary immunization should be subsequently given at the recommended intervals if the person remains at an increased risk.

- ***Incompletely immunized adults.*** Those who previously received less than a full primary course of OPV or IPV should be given the remaining required doses of vaccine, either IPV or OPV, regardless of the interval since the last dose and the type of vaccine that was previously received.
- ***Adults who are at an increased risk of exposure to wild poliovirus and who previously completed primary immunization with OPV or IPV.*** These adults should receive a single dose of IPV (or OPV).

Management of Unimmunized or Inadequately Immunized Adults in Households in Which Children (or Close Contacts of Such Children) Are To Be Given OPV. Adults who are known not to have been adequately immunized against poliomyelitis are at a very small risk of developing VAPP when children in the household or child care facility in which they work are given OPV (see Adverse Reactions, p 427). Infants and children in households with adult members known to be inadequately immunized should receive only IPV in order to prevent the occurrence of VAPP from OPV for their household contacts.

Precautions and Contraindications to Immunization.

Immunodeficiency Disorders. Patients with immunodeficiency disorders, including HIV infection, combined immunodeficiency, abnormalities of immunoglobulin synthesis (ie, antibody deficiency syndromes), leukemia, lymphoma, or generalized malignancy, or those being given immunosuppressive therapy with pharmacologic agents (see Immunodeficient and Immunosuppressed Children, p 50) or radiation therapy should not receive OPV because of the theoretical or known risk of paralytic disease. Although a protective immune response to IPV in the immunodeficient patient cannot be ensured, IPV is safe and some protection may result from its administration.

Household Contacts of Persons With Immunodeficiency Disease, Altered Immune States, Immunosuppression Due To Therapy for Other Disease, or Known HIV Infection. Inactivated poliovirus vaccine is recommended for these persons and OPV should not be used. If OPV is inadvertently administered to a household contact of an immunodeficient or HIV-infected person, close contact between the patient and the OPV recipient should be minimized for approximately 4 to 6 weeks after vaccination. Household members should be counseled on practices that will minimize the exposure of the immunodeficient or HIV-infected person to excreted polio vaccine virus. These practices include hand washing after contact with the child and avoidance of diaper changing.

Parents With One or More Immunodeficient Children. Because of the possibility of immunodeficiency in other offspring, OPV should not be given to members of a household with this history until the immune status of the recipient and other family members is documented and immunodeficiency has been excluded.

Pregnancy. Although no convincing evidence indicates that increased rates of adverse effects of either IPV or OPV occur in the pregnant woman or her developing fetus, immunization during pregnancy generally should be avoided for reasons of theoretical risk. If immediate protection against poliomyelitis is needed, IPV or OPV is recommended.

Hypersensitivity or Anaphylactic Reactions Following IPV, OPV, or the Antibiotics Contained in These Vaccines. IPV is contraindicated in persons who have experienced an anaphylactic reaction following a previous dose of IPV or an anaphylactic reaction to the following antibiotics: streptomycin, polymyxin B, and neomycin. OPV is contraindicated in persons who experienced an anaphylactic reaction to a previous dose of OPV.

Other. If a substantial amount of OPV is vomited or regurgitated within 5 to 10 minutes of administration, the dose should be given again. If this repeat dose is not retained, neither dose should be counted and the vaccine should be readministered at a later visit. Breastfeeding and mild diarrhea are not contraindications to either OPV or IPV administration.

Reporting of Adverse Events Following Vaccination. All cases of vaccine-associated paralytic poliomyelitis (VAPP) and other serious adverse events associated temporally with poliomyelitis vaccine should be reported (see Reporting of Adverse Events and Vaccine Injury Compensation, p 27).

Case Reporting and Investigation. Each suspected case of poliomyelitis should be reported promptly to the state health department and prompt an immediate epidemologic investigation. Poliomyelitis should be considered in the differential diagnosis of all cases of acute flaccid paralysis, including Guillain-Barré syndrome and transverse myelitis. If the course is clinically compatible with poliomyelitis, specimens should be obtained for viral studies (see Diagnostic Tests, p 425). If evidence implicates vaccine-derived poliovirus, no vaccination plan is indicated as outbreaks associated with vaccine virus have not been documented. If evidence implicates wild poliovirus and possible transmission, OPV should be provided for all persons within the epidemic area, regardless of prior vaccination status (with the exception of those for whom vaccination is contraindicated, such as HIV-infected persons and others with immunodeficiency, for whom IPV is indicated).

Q Fever

CLINICAL MANIFESTATIONS: Acute Q fever usually is characterized by abrupt onset of fever, chills, weakness, headache, and anorexia, as well as other nonspecific systemic symptoms; chronic Q fever occurs less frequently. Cough and chest pains can signify pneumonia, which occurs in about half the patients. Weight loss and weakness can be pronounced. Hepatosplenomegaly frequently is noted. The illness lasts 1 to 4 weeks and then resolves gradually. Rash is unusual. Endocarditis and hepatitis are the major manifestations of chronic disease. Although the mortality from acute Q fever is less than 1%, mortality among patients with endocarditis is 30% to 60%.

ETIOLOGY: *Coxiella burnetii,* the cause of Q fever, is unique among rickettsiae in that it undergoes a host-dependent phase variation.

EPIDEMIOLOGY: Animal infection is widespread, usually asymptomatic, and primarily involves a large variety of domestic farm animals (especially sheep, goats, and cows), but also cats, rodents, marsupials, and other species. Tick vectors may be important in maintaining animal reservoirs. Infectious organisms can persist in the environment for many years. Human disease is uncommon, but many infections are asymptomatic. The disease occurs endemically throughout the world, typically in areas where cattle are raised and sheep and goats are herded. The disease has been transmitted to humans by inhalation of aerosols spontaneously generated from infected material such as placental tissue from infected cats or animals on farms, and by exposure to infected animals or tissues on farms or ranches or in research facilities. Consumption of raw milk is a risk factor for infection. Some persons who work with animals, ranchers, research laboratory workers, and persons in other occupations or with avocational interests resulting in close contact with infected animals or tissues have a heightened risk of disease. Q fever has occurred among flocks of sheep used as experimental subjects in medical research facilities, and transmission to research investigators and technical personnel has been documented. The handling of animal fetuses and products of conception is a major means of infection. Although seasonal trends are not obvious, in some areas the disease coincides with the lambing season in the early spring. Because the birth of farm animals, such as sheep, goats, and cows, is a somewhat controllable event, the disease can occur throughout the year in areas where planned animal births are permitted. Evidence for human intrauterine infection has been reported. The risk of chronic infection is increased by immunodeficiency and by underlying cardiovascular disease.

The **incubation period** can vary from 14 to 39 days but is usually between 14 and 22 days.

DIAGNOSTIC TESTS: Isolation of C *burnetii* from blood is usually not attempted because of the hazard to laboratory workers. Specific antiphase I and antiphase II immunofluorescent, enzyme immunoassay, complement fixation, and immune adherence hemagglutination antibody tests using paired serum specimens are used diagnostically. Specific IgM, IgG, and IgA tests using immunofluorescence or enzyme immunoassay methods are available in reference and research laboratories. In research laboratories, immunoblotting techniques have been used to diagnose chronic Q fever, polymerase chain reaction can detect small numbers of organisms in tissue, and DNA hybridization in conjunction with polymerase chain reaction can detect small numbers of organisms in blood, urine, and tissue. *Coxiella burnetii* infection does not cause a positive serum Weil-Felix test.

TREATMENT: Tetracycline or doxycycline is the drug of choice. Chloramphenicol is an alternative, but its efficacy has not been proven. Tetracyclines should not be given to children younger than 8 years unless the benefit is greater than the risk of dental staining (see Antimicrobials and Related Therapy, p 606). Therapy should be initiated promptly and continued until the patient has been afebrile for 2 to 3 days. In chronic Q fever, relapses necessitating repeated courses of antimicrobial therapy can occur. The organism can remain latent in tissues for years; treatment of chronic disease is extremely difficult. Treatment of chronic endocarditis is prolonged and appears to be more effective when tetracycline or doxycycline is combined with rifampin, trimethoprim-sulfamethoxazole, or a fluoroquinolone. In patients younger than 18 years of age, fluoroquinolones usually are contraindicated (see Antimicrobials and Related Therapy, p 605). Relapses can occur after discontinuation of treatment.

ISOLATION OF THE HOSPITALIZED PATIENT: Standard precautions are recommended.

CONTROL MEASURES: Experimental vaccines for domestic animals and laboratory workers are promising but not commercially available. Recommendations have been made to reduce the risk of infection in research facilities involving sheep.* Special safety practices are recommended for nonpropagative laboratory procedures involving *C burnetii* and for all propagative procedures, necropsies of infected animals, and manipulation of infected human and animal tissues. Otherwise, no specific management is recommended for persons who have been exposed. Flash pasteurization of milk at 71.6°C (161.1°F) for 15 seconds or 62.9°C (145.2°F) for 30 minutes destroys the organism, but the epidemiologic role of milk in transmission is uncertain.

Rabies

CLINICAL MANIFESTATIONS: Infection with rabies virus characteristically produces an acute illness with rapidly progressive central nervous system manifestations, including anxiety, dysphagia, and convulsions, and almost invariably progresses to death. Some patients may present with paralysis. The differential diagnosis of all acute encephalitic illnesses of unknown etiology with atypical focal neurologic signs or with paralysis should include rabies.

ETIOLOGY: Rabies virus is an RNA virus classified in the rhabdovirus family.

EPIDEMIOLOGY: A large animal reservoir of sylvatic rabies exists in the United States, including raccoons, skunks, foxes, bats, and other species. In some areas, these wild animals infect domestic dogs, cats, and ferrets. From a new focus in Virginia, rabies in raccoons has spread north to Maine and south to North Carolina. Where raccoon rabies is spreading (ie, the mid-Atlantic and northeast states), an increasing number of woodchucks have been found to be rabid. Horses and cows may become infected and secondarily expose humans. Rabies in small rodents, rabbits, and hares is rare. The virus is present in saliva and is transmitted by bites or by lick-

---

* Bernard KW, Parham GL, Winkler WG, Helmick CG. Q fever control measures: Recommendations for research facilities using sheep. *Infect Control.* 1982;3:461-465; and Harrison RJ, Vugia DJ, Ascher MS. Occupational health guidelines for control of Q fever in sheep research. *Ann NY Acad Sci.* 1990;590:283-290.

ing of mucosa or open wounds. Worldwide, most rabies cases in humans result from dog bites in areas in which canine rabies is enzootic. Although experimental evidence has shown that some dogs may harbor the virus in their saliva for as long as 14 days before the appearance of recognizable illness, most dogs and cats become ill within 4 or 5 days of viral shedding, and no case of human rabies in the United States has been attributed to a dog or cat that has remained healthy throughout the standard 10-day period of confinement. In the United States, cases of human rabies have steadily declined since the 1950s, reflecting widespread rabies vaccination of dogs and the availability of effective immunoprophylaxis following exposure to a rabid animal. Despite the epidemic of rabies in raccoons, no human deaths have been attributed to the raccoon rabies virus variant. Of the human cases in recent years, based on the rabies virus isolate, bats have been increasingly implicated as significant wildlife reservoirs. In some of these cases, contact with bats or other rabid animals has not been documented, indicating that insignificant physical contact with a rabid bat may transmit the rabies virus. Airborne transmission has been reported in the laboratory and in bat-infested caves. Transmission has also occurred by transplantation of corneas from patients dying of undiagnosed rabies. Person-to-person transmission by bite has not been documented, although the virus has been isolated from the saliva of patients. The epidemiology of rabies is now aided by strain identification using monoclonal antibodies and nucleotide sequencing.

The **incubation period** in humans averages 4 to 6 weeks, but ranges from 5 days to more than 1 year. Incubation periods of up to 6 years have been confirmed recently by antigenic typing and nucleotide sequencing of strains.

DIAGNOSTIC TESTS: Infection in animals can be diagnosed by demonstration of virus-specific fluorescent antigen in brain tissue. Suspected rabid animals should be euthanized in a manner that preserves brain tissue for appropriate examination. Virus can be isolated from brain, saliva, and other tissues in suckling mice or in tissue culture. Viral isolation takes much longer than fluorescent microscopy of brain tissue. The diagnosis in suspected human cases can be made postmortem and sometimes premortem by fluorescent microscopy of skin biopsies from the nape of the neck, by isolation of the virus from the saliva or cerebrospinal fluid (CSF), or by detection of antibody in the CSF or serum in unvaccinated persons. The laboratory should be consulted before submission of specimens so that appropriate materials can be collected and transport arranged.

TREATMENT: Once symptoms have developed, no drug or vaccine improves the prognosis. Only seven patients with human rabies have survived with intensive, supportive care; all other patients have succumbed despite treatment.

ISOLATION OF THE HOSPITALIZED PATIENT: Standard precautions are recommended for the duration of the illness. If the patient has bitten another person or his or her saliva has contaminated an open wound or mucous membrane, the involved area should be washed thoroughly and immunization of the contact started (see Care of Exposed Persons, p 439).

CONTROL MEASURES:

Education of children by parents, teachers, and medical personnel to avoid contact with stray or wild animals is of primary importance. Children should be cautioned against provoking or attempting to capture stray or wild animals for pets or to touch carcasses. Inadvertent contact of family members and pets with potentially rabid animals, such as raccoons and skunks, may be diminished by securing garbage and other such refuse or materials and not attracting domestic and wild animals. Similarly, chimneys and other potential portals of entry for wild animals, including bats, should be identified and covered.

Exposure Risk and Decisions To Give Immunoprophylaxis. Exposure to rabies results from a break in the skin caused by the teeth of a rabid animal or by the contamination of scratches, abrasions, or mucous membranes with saliva from a rabid animal. The decision to immunize an exposed individual ordinarily should be made in consultation with the local health department, which can provide information on the risk of rabies in a particular area for each species of animal, and in accordance with the guidelines in Table 3.50 (p 438). In the United States, raccoons, skunks, foxes, and bats are more likely to be infected than other animals, but coyotes, cattle, dogs, and cats occasionally are infected. Bites of rodents (such as squirrels and rats) or lagomorphs (rabbits and hares) rarely require specific antirabies prophylaxis. Additional factors must be considered when deciding whether immunoprophylaxis is indicated. An unprovoked attack is more suggestive of a rabid animal than a bite during attempts to feed or handle an animal. Properly immunized dogs and cats have only a minimal chance of developing rabies. However, in rare instances, rabies has developed in properly vaccinated animals.

Rabies postexposure prophylaxis is recommended for all persons bitten by mammalian or carnivorous bats or by domestic animals that may be infected. Exposures other than bites rarely have been demonstrated to result in infection, but seemingly insignificant physical contact with bats may result in viral transmission even without a clear history of a bite. Postexposure prophylaxis, thus, is recommended for persons who report an open wound, scratch, or mucous membrane that has been contaminated with saliva or other potentially infectious material (eg, brain tissue) from a rabid animal. Because the injury inflicted by a bat bite or scratch may be small and not evident or the circumstances of contact may preclude accurate recall (eg, a bat in a room of a sleeping person, previously unattended child, or intoxicated person), prophylaxis is indicated for situations in which a bat is physically present if a bite or mucous membrane exposure cannot be reliably excluded, unless prompt testing of the bat has excluded rabies virus infection. Treatment always should be initiated as soon as possible after bites by known or suspected rabid animals.

Postexposure prophylaxis also is recommended for persons who report a possibly infectious exposure (eg, bite, scratch, or open wound or mucous membrane contaminated with saliva or other infectious material) to a human with rabies. However, exposure to a human with rabies has never been implicated as a means of rabies transmission except after corneal transplantation from donors who died of unsuspected rabies encephalitis. Casual contact with an infected person (eg, by touching a patient) or contact with noninfectious fluids or tissues (eg, urine or feces) alone

Table 3.50. **Rabies Postexposure Prophylaxis Guide**

Animal Type	Evaluation and Disposition of Animal	Postexposure Prophylaxis Recommendations
Dogs and cats	Healthy and available for 10 days of observation	Prophylaxis only if animal develops signs of rabies*
	Rabid or suspected rabid[†]	Immediate vaccination[‡] and RIG
	Unknown (escaped)	Consult public health officials for advice
Skunks, raccoons, bats, foxes, and most other carnivores; woodchucks	Regarded as rabid unless geographic area is known to be free of rabies or until animal proven negative by laboratory tests[†]	Immediate vaccination[‡] and RIG
Livestock, ferrets, rodents, and lagomorphs (rabbits and hares)	Consider individually	Consult public health officials. Bites of squirrels, hamsters, guinea pigs, gerbils, chipmunks, rats, mice, other rodents, rabbits, and hares almost never require antirabies treatment.

* During the 10-day holding period, at the first sign of rabies in the biting dog or cat, treatment with rabies immune globulin (human) (RIG) and vaccine should be initiated. The symptomatic animal should be euthanized immediately and tested.

[†] The animal should be euthanized and tested as soon as possible. Holding for observation is not recommended. Vaccination is discontinued if immunofluorescent test of the animal is negative.

[‡] See text.

does not constitute an exposure and is not an indication for prophylaxis (see Care of Hospital Contacts, p 439).

Handling of Suspect Animals. A suspect dog or cat that has bitten a human should be captured, confined, and observed by a veterinarian for 10 days. Any illness in the animal should be reported immediately to the local health department. If the animal develops signs of rabies, it should be euthanized and its head removed and shipped under refrigeration (iced, not frozen) to a qualified laboratory for examination.

Other biting animals, including ferrets and wild animals, that may have exposed a person to rabies should be reported immediately to the local health department. Management of animals depends on the species, the circumstances of the bite, and the epidemiology of rabies in the area. Prior vaccination of an animal, such as a ferret, may not preclude the necessity for euthanasia and testing if the period of viral shedding is unknown for that species. Because clinical manifestations of rabies in a wild animal cannot be interpreted reliably, a suspect wild mammal should be euthanized at once and its brain examined for evidence of rabies. The exposed person need not be treated if examination of the brain by fluorescent antibody procedures is negative for rabies.

Care of Hospital Contacts. Immunization of hospital contacts of a patient with rabies should be reserved for persons who were bitten or whose mucous membranes or open wounds have come in contact with the saliva, CSF, or brain tissue of a patient with rabies (see Care of Exposed Persons, below). Other hospital contacts of a patient with rabies do not require immunization.

Care of Exposed Persons.

Local Care. The immediate objective of postexposure treatment is to prevent virus from entering neural tissue. Prompt and thorough local treatment of all bites and scratches is essential, as virus may remain localized to the area of the bite for a variable time. All wounds should be flushed thoroughly and cleaned with soap and water. Quaternary ammonium compounds (such as Zephiran), which were recommended in the past, are no longer considered superior to soap. The need for tetanus prophylaxis and measures to control bacterial infection also should be considered. The wound, if possible, should not be sutured.

Immunoprophylaxis. After local care is completed, concurrent use of both passive and active immunoprophylaxis is required for optimal therapy (see Table 3.50, p 348). Prophylaxis should begin as soon as possible after exposure, ideally within 24 hours. However, a delay of several days or more may not compromise effectiveness and prophylaxis should be initiated if otherwise indicated, regardless of interval between exposure and initiation of therapy. In the United States only the human product, rabies immune globulin (RIG), which is preferable to the previously used equine product, is available for passive immunization. Human diploid cell or fetal rhesus lung diploid vaccine should be used for active immunization. Physicians can obtain expert counsel from their local or state health departments.

Active Immunization. Human diploid cell vaccine (HDCV)* or rhesus diploid cell vaccine, rabies vaccine adsorbed (RVA),[†] 1.0 mL, is given intramuscularly in the deltoid area on the first day of treatment, and repeat doses are given on days 3, 7, 14, and 28. A sixth dose is recommended in some European countries but not in the United States, as five doses appear to be equally protective as six doses. The volume of the dose is not reduced for children. Serologic testing after HDCV immunization generally has not been necessary, but has been advised for recipients who may be immunosuppressed.

Care should be taken to ensure that the vaccine is administered intramuscularly. Intradermal vaccine is not advised for postexposure treatment in the United States, although for reasons of cost and availability intradermal regimens are used in some countries. Because antibody responses in adults who received vaccine in the gluteal area sometimes have been less than in those who were injected in the deltoid muscle, the latter site always should be used, except in infants.

---

* Manufactured by Pasteur Merieux Serums and Vaccines and available in the United States from Connaught Laboratories, Swiftwater, Pa.

[†] Manufactured by the Michigan Department of Public Health and available from SmithKline Beecham, Philadelphia, Pa.

- *Adverse reactions and precautions with HDCV.* Reactions, primarily report-ed in adults, after vaccination with HDCV are less common than with previ-ously available vaccines. Reactions are uncommon in children. In a study using five doses of HDCV, local reactions, such as pain, erythema, and swelling or itching at the injection site were reported in approximately 25% of the recipi-ents; mild systemic reactions, such as headache, nausea, abdominal pain, mus-cle aches, and dizziness were reported in approximately 20% of the recipients. Several cases of neurologic illness resembling Guillain-Barré syndrome that resolved without sequelae in 12 weeks and a focal, subacute, central nervous system disorder temporally associated with HDCV have been reported. The rate of neurologic abnormalities after HDCV is approximately 1 in 150 000.

  Immune complex-like reactions in persons receiving booster doses of HDCV have been observed. The reaction, characterized by onset 2 to 21 days postinocculation, presents with a generalized urticaria and can include arthralgia, arthritis, angioedema, nausea, vomiting, fever, and malaise. These illnesses were in no instances life-threatening. Current estimates suggest that this immune complex-like illness can occur in as many as 6% of adults receiving booster doses as part of a pre-exposure immunization regimen. It is rare in persons receiving primary immunization, including most children receiving vaccine in the United States. All serious, systemic, neuroparalytic or anaphylactic reactions to the rabies vaccine should be reported immediately (see Reporting of Adverse Events, p 27).

  If the patient has a serious allergic reaction to HDCV, the RVA vaccine produced in rhesus diploid cells can be given according to the same schedule as HDCV.

  Although the safety of the use of rabies vaccine during pregnancy has not been investigated specifically in the United States, pregnancy should not be considered a contraindication to the use of vaccine after exposure.

- *Nerve tissue vaccines.* Nerve tissue vaccines are not licensed in the United States, but are available in many areas of the world. These preparations induce neuroparalytic reactions in between 1:2000 and 1:8000 recipients, perhaps as a result of sensitization to myelin. Immunization with nerve tissue vaccine should be discontinued if meningeal or neuroparalytic reactions develop. Cor-ticosteroids can be used for treatment of complications, but they should be used only for life-threatening reactions because they definitely increase the risk of rabies in experimentally inoculated animals.

  Passive Immunization. Rabies immune globulin (human) (RIG)* should be used concomitantly with the first dose of vaccine for postexposure prophylaxis to bridge the time between onset of treatment and active antibody production by the vaccinee. The exception to the concomitant use of vaccine and RIG is the patient previously immunized with HDCV or RVA (or another rabies vaccine if the patient is known to have developed serum antibody); these patients should be given two doses of vaccine only, one immediately (day 0) and the other on day 3. If vaccine is not immediately available, RIG should be given alone and vaccination started later. If RIG is not immediately available, vaccine should be given followed by RIG when obtained in the first 7 days after the beginning of treatment. If administration of

---

*Available from Connaught Laboratories, Swiftwater, Pa.

both vaccine and RIG is delayed, both should be used regardless of the interval between exposure and treatment.

The recommended dose of RIG is 20 IU/kg of body weight. Approximately half of the antibody preparation is used to infiltrate the wound(s); the remainder is given intramuscularly. Rabies immune globulin is supplied in 2-mL (300 IU) and 10-mL (1500 IU) vials. Passive antibody can inhibit the response to rabies vaccines; therefore, the recommended dose should not be exceeded. Vaccine never should be administered in the same parts of the body or with the same syringe used to give RIG. Hypersensitivity reactions to RIG rarely, if ever, occur.

Purified equine globulin containing rabies antibodies is available outside of the United States, and generally is accompanied by a low rate of serum sickness (<1%). It is administered at a dose of 40 IU/kg.

Rabies immune globulin (RIG)* is not recommended for the following exposed persons: (1) those who previously received postexposure prophylaxis with HDCV or RVA; (2) those who received a three-dose, intramuscular, pre-exposure regimen of HDCV or RVA; (3) those who received a three-dose, intradermal, preexposure regimen of HDCV with the Merieux product in the United States; and (4) those who have a documented adequate rabies titer after previous vaccination with any other rabies vaccine. These persons should receive two 1.0-mL doses of HDCV or RVA; doses are given on the day of exposure and on day 3.

Pre-exposure Control Measures, Including Immunization. The relatively low frequency of reactions to HDCV and RVA has made the provision of pre-exposure immunization practical for persons in high-risk groups, such as veterinarians, animal handlers, certain laboratory workers, children living in areas where rabies is a constant threat, and persons traveling to live in areas where rabies is common. Others, such as spelunkers, whose vocational or avocational pursuits in exploring caves result in frequent exposures to dogs, cats, foxes, skunks, or bats, also should be considered for pre-exposure prophylaxis.

Rabies vaccine adsorbed is licensed for intramuscular administration only. Both intramuscular (1.0 mL) and intradermal (0.1 mL) dosage formulations of HDCV are available for preexposure use. The preferred site of administration for intradermal vaccine is the skin in the deltoid area. The schedule is the same for both routes of administration; three injections are given on days 0, 7, and 21 or 28. This series of immunizations has resulted in the development of antibodies in all persons properly vaccinated. For this reason, routine serologic testing for rabies antibody is not indicated.

Persons who are taking chloroquine or related antimicrobial drugs, such as mefloquine, should receive HDCV by the intramuscular route. A single case of rabies immunization failure in an individual living in a foreign country who was vaccinated intradermally has been reported, and was probably related to the immunosuppressive effect of chloroquine administered for malaria prophylaxis. Pre-exposure intradermal vaccination should be monitored by serological rabies antibody testing in recipients of concurrent chemoprophylaxis of malaria. Serum antibodies usually will still be present in most American subjects 2 years after the primary series given intramuscularly, but may be less persistent in individuals in other circumstances, as shown by Peace Corps volunteers whose titers may be influenced by antimalarials. Booster vac-

*Available from Connaught Laboratories, Swiftwater, Pa.

cination with HDCV (1.0 mL intramuscularly or 0.1 mL intradermally) or with RVA intramuscularly will produce an effective anamnestic response. Because significant allergic reactions have been associated with HDCV, booster vaccination in approximately 6% of individuals, boosters are not routinely recommended unless the risk of exposure to rabies virus is likely to be continuous or frequent. Such persons include veterinarians, animal handlers, and laboratory workers exposed to high concentrations of rabies virus (eg, in certain research or vaccine production laboratories). Rabies serum antibody titers should be determined at 6-month intervals for those at continuous risk and at intervals up to 2 years for those with risk of frequent exposure. Booster doses of vaccine only should be administered as appropriate to maintain serum antibody concentrations. The Centers for Disease Control and Prevention currently specifies complete viral neutralization at a 1:5 or greater titer by the rapid fluorescent-focus inhibition test as acceptable; the World Health Organization specifies 0.5 IU/mL or more as acceptable.

Public Health. A variety of approved public health measures, including immunization of dogs, cats, and ferrets, and the elimination of stray dogs and selected wildlife, are used to control rabies in animals. Unvaccinated dogs, cats, or other pets bitten by a known rabid animal should be euthanized immediately. If the owner is unwilling to allow the animal to be sacrificed, the animal should be placed in strict isolation for 6 months and vaccinated 1 month prior to release. If the animal has a current vaccination within 1 to 3 years, depending on the vaccine administered and local regulations, it should be revaccinated and observed for 45 days.

Case Reporting. All patients who are suspected of having rabies should be reported promptly to public health authorities.

Rat-Bite Fever

CLINICAL MANIFESTATIONS: Rat-bite fever is caused by either of two organisms and is characterized by fever of abrupt onset, chills, a maculopapular or petechial rash predominantly on the extremities, muscle pain, and headache. Specific clinical manifestations depend on the infecting organism. With *Streptobacillus moniliformis* infection (streptobacillary or Haverhill fever), the bite usually heals promptly, exhibits no or minimal inflammation, and is followed by nonsuppurative migratory polyarthritis or arthralgia in approximately 50% of patients. Complications include soft-tissue and solid-organ abscesses, pneumonia, endocarditis, and pericarditis. With *Spirillum minus* infection, a period of initial apparent healing at the site of the bite usually is followed by ulceration, regional lymphangitis and lymphadenopathy, a distinctive rash of red or purple plaques, and, rarely, arthritic symptoms.

ETIOLOGY: The causes are *Streptobacillus moniliformis*, a microaerophilic, Gram-negative, pleomorphic bacillus; and *Spirillum minus*, a small, Gram-negative, spiral organism with bipolar flagellar tufts.

EPIDEMIOLOGY: Rat-bite fever is a zoonotic illness. *Streptobacillus moniliformis* and *S minus* are found in upper respiratory tract secretions of infected animals. *Streptobacillus moniliformis* is transmitted by the bite of rats, squirrels, mice, cats, and weasels; by ingestion of contaminated food or milk products; and by contact with an infected animal. Haverhill fever refers to infection after ingestion of milk or water contaminated with *S moniliformis*. *Spirillum minus* is transmitted by the bite of rats and mice. On rare occasion, *S moniliformis* and *S minus* have been reported to be transmitted from person to person by a blood transfusion. *Streptobacillus moniliformis* infection accounts for most cases of rat-bite fever in the United States; *S minus* infections occur primarily in Asia. Both diseases are rare.

　　The **incubation period** for *S moniliformis* is usually 3 to 10 days, but can be as long as 3 weeks; for *S minus* it is 7 to 21 days.

DIAGNOSTIC TESTS: *Streptobacillus moniliformis* can be isolated from blood, joint fluid, or material from the bite lesion by inoculation into bacteriologic media enriched with blood, serum, or ascitic fluid. Because it is a fastidious organism, the laboratory should be notified that rat-bite fever is suspected. *Spirillum minus* has not been recovered on artificial media. Organisms can be visualized by use of dark-field microscopy in wet mounts of blood, exudate of the initial lesion, and lymph nodes. Blood specimens also should be stained with Giemsa or Wright stain. *Spirillum minus* can be recovered from blood, lymph nodes, or local lesions by intraperitoneal inoculation of mice or guinea pigs.

TREATMENT: Procaine penicillin should be administered intramuscularly for 7 to 10 days for rat-bite fever caused by either agent. Initial intravenous penicillin G therapy for 5 days followed by oral penicillin V also has been successful. Tetracycline, chloramphenicol, or streptomycin may be substituted in the patient who is allergic to penicillin. Tetracycline should not be given to children younger than 8 years of age unless the benefits of therapy are greater than the risks of dental staining (see Antimicrobials and Related Therapy, p 606). Patients with endocarditis should receive intravenous, high-dose penicillin G for at least 4 weeks. The addition of streptomycin initially may be useful.

ISOLATION OF THE HOSPITALIZED PATIENT: Standard precautions are recommended.

CONTROL MEASURES: Exposed persons should be observed for symptoms. Because the attack rate of rat-bite fever due to *S moniliformis* after a rat bite is 10%, some experts recommend postexposure administration of penicillin. Rat control is important.

Respiratory Syncytial Virus

CLINICAL MANIFESTATIONS: Respiratory syncytial virus (RSV) causes acute respiratory illness in patients of any age. In infants and young children, it is the most important cause of bronchiolitis and pneumonia. During the first few weeks of life, particularly in preterm infants, respiratory signs can be minimal. Lethargy, irritability, and poor feeding, sometimes accompanied by apneic episodes, may be the major manifestations. Most previously healthy infants infected with RSV do not require hospitalization and many who are hospitalized improve within a few days with supportive care and are discharged within less than 5 days. Conditions that increase the risk of severe or fatal RSV infection are cyanotic or complicated congenital heart disease, including those causing pulmonary hypertension; underlying pulmonary disease, especially bronchopulmonary dysplasia; prematurity; and immunodeficiency disease or therapy causing immunosuppression at any age. Long-term sequelae of RSV infection in infants are difficult to assess. Evidence suggests that some infected children develop long-term abnormalities in pulmonary function that may be asymptomatic or manifest as recurrent wheezing.

Infection in older children and adults usually manifests as an upper respiratory tract illness, occasionally with bronchitis. Exacerbation of asthma or other chronic lung conditions is also common.

ETIOLOGY: Respiratory syncytial virus, a large, enveloped RNA virus, is a paramyxovirus. Two major strains (A and B) usually circulate concurrently. The clinical and epidemiologic importance of this strain variation has not been determined.

EPIDEMIOLOGY: Humans are the only source of infection. Transmission is usually by direct or close contact with contaminated secretions, which may involve droplets or fomites. Virus can persist on environmental surfaces for many hours, and for half an hour or more on the hands. Infection among hospital personnel can occur by self-inoculation with contaminated infant secretions. Hospital-acquired infections are frequent among both personnel and infants, and have significant impact on morbidity, mortality, and duration of hospitalization. Initial infection occurs most commonly during the first year of life. Reinfection throughout life is common.

Respiratory syncytial virus usually occurs in annual epidemics during the winter and early spring, and it infects essentially all children during the first 3 years of life. Spread among household and child care contacts, including adults, is common. The period of viral shedding is usually 3 to 8 days, but it may be longer, especially in young infants in whom shedding may continue for as long as 3 to 4 weeks.

The **incubation period** ranges from 2 to 8 days; 4 to 6 days is most common.

DIAGNOSTIC TESTS: Rapid diagnostic procedures, including immunofluorescent and enzyme immunoassay techniques for the direct detection of viral antigen in clinical specimens, are commercially available and generally reliable during RSV outbreaks. The sensitivity of these assays in comparison to culture varies between 53% and 96%, but most are in the range of 80% to 90%. Viral isolation from nasopharyngeal secretions in cell cultures takes 3 to 5 days, but results and sensitivity will vary in different laboratories because methods of isolation are exacting and RSV is a relatively labile virus whose infectivity decreases rapidly at room temperature and after freeze-thawing. The laboratory should be consulted for optimal methods of collection and transport of specimens. Serologic testing of acute and convalescent sera can be used to confirm infection; however, infection may not always be accompanied by detectable seroconversion, especially in young infants.

TREATMENT*: Ribavirin has in vitro antiviral activity against RSV, and has been used to treat hospitalized infants and young children who have or are at high risk for severe RSV infection. It is administered by aerosol by small-particle generator (in order to reach the lower respiratory tract) via an oxygen hood, tent or into ventilator tubing mask for 12 to 20 hours daily for 1 to 7 days.

Ribavirin treatment for RSV infections has been controversial because of the cost, aerosol route of administration, concern for potential toxicity for exposed persons, and conflicting results of efficacy trials. Initial randomized, water placebo-controlled clinical trials and concurrent cohort trials demonstrated more rapid improvement in respiratory signs and symptoms scores, increase in oxygenation, and decrease in RSV titers in ribavirin-treated infants. A small, randomized, water placebo-controlled trial in patients receiving mechanical ventilation demonstrated a significant reduction in the number of days of ventilation, need for supplemental oxygen therapy, and hospital stay in patients treated with ribavirin. In addition, hospital costs also were reduced. These studies indicating beneficial results from ribavirin treatment led to earlier recommendations for ribavirin therapy for selected high-risk infants. In recent studies, however, ribavirin therapy was not effective in reducing the severity of RSV disease and could have prolonged illness in comparison to untreated controls or patients receiving saline placebo by aerosol.

Because of concerns about cost, benefit, safety, and variable clinical efficacy, definitive indications for ribavirin therapy are not possible at this time. Decisions about whether to give ribavirin should be based on the particular clinical circumstances and physicians' preferences. Ribavirin aerosol therapy is a consideration for the following selected infants and young children at high risk for serious RSV disease:

- Those with complicated congenital heart disease (including pulmonary hypertension) and those with bronchopulmonary dysplasia, cystic fibrosis, and other chronic lung disease. Previously healthy premature infants (less than 37 weeks' gestational age) and those less than 6 weeks of age also are at greater risk for severe RSV illness.
- Those with underlying immunosuppressive diseases or therapy (eg, those with acquired immunodeficiency syndrome, severe combined immunodeficiency disease, or organ transplantation) who have high mortality with RSV infection or prolonged RSV illness.
- Those who are severely ill, with or without mechanical ventilation. Severity of illness is often difficult to judge clinically in infants with RSV infection and useful criteria include blood gas determinations and the clinical response to other therapies.
- Hospitalized patients who may be at increased risk of progressing from a mild to a more complicated course because they are younger than 6 weeks or they have an underlying condition, such as multiple congenital anomalies or certain neurologic or metabolic diseases (eg, cerebral palsy or myasthenia gravis).

---

* For further information on the safety and efficacy of ribavirin aerosol therapy, see the following: American Academy of Pediatrics, Committee on Infectious Diseases. Use of ribavirin in the treatment of respiratory syncytial virus infection. *Pediatrics.* 1993;92:501-504; and American Academy of Pediatrics, Committee on Infectious Diseases. Reassessment of indications for ribavirin therapy. *Pediatrics.* 1996;97:137-140.

Corticosteroids. In previously healthy infants with RSV bronchiolitis, corticosteroids are not effective and thus, are not indicated.

Immunoprophylaxis. * Respiratory syncytial virus immune globulin intravenous (RSV-IGIV)[†] has been approved for prevention of RSV disease in children less than 24 months of age with bronchopulmonary dysplasia (BPD) or with a history of premature birth (less than 35 weeks' gestation). RSV-IGIV is prepared from donors selected for high serum titers of RSV neutralizing antibody. It is given once per month just prior to and during the RSV season at a dose of 15 mL/kg (750 mg/kg).

Recommendations by the Academy for the use of RSV-IGIV are as follows:

- RSV-IGIV prophylaxis should be considered for infants and children younger than 2 years with BPD who are currently receiving or have received oxygen therapy within the 6 months prior to the anticipated RSV season. Patients with BPD with more severe underlying lung disease may benefit clinically from prophylaxis for two RSV seasons, whereas those with less severe underlying disease may benefit only for the first year. Decisions regarding individual patients may necessitate consultation with neonatologists, intensivists, and/or pulmonologists.

- Infants with a gestational age of 32 weeks or less at birth who do not have BPD also may benefit from RSV-IGIV prophylaxis. The major risk factors to consider are gestational age and chronologic age at the beginning of the RSV season. Infants with a gestational age of 28 weeks or less may benefit from prophylaxis until 12 months of age. Infants 29 to 32 weeks of gestational age may benefit from prophylaxis until 6 months of age. Decisions regarding each patient should be individualized. Regional data on hospitalization rates for RSV infection may assist in the decision-making process.

- RSV-IGIV is not approved by the Food and Drug Administration for patients with congenital heart disease (CHD). Available data indicate that RSV-IGIV should not be used in those with cyanotic CHD. However, patients with BPD and/or prematurity who meet the criteria in preceding recommendations and who also have asymptomatic acyanotic CHD (eg, patent ductus arteriosus or ventricular septal defect) may benefit from prophylaxis.

- RSV-IGIV use, either prophylactically or therapeutically, has not been evaluated in randomized trials in immunocompromised infants and children. Although specific recommendations for all immunocompromised patients cannot be made, children with severe immunodeficiencies (eg, severe combined immunodeficiency or severe HIV infection) may benefit from RSV-IGIV. If these infants and children are receiving monthly infusions of intravenous immunoglobulin, physicians may consider substituting RSV-IGIV during the RSV season.

- The need for and efficacy of RSV-IGIV prophylaxis in an RSV outbreak in a high-risk hospital unit (eg, pediatric intensive care unit) has not been documented. The major means of prevention is appropriate infection control practices (see Control Measures, p 447).

---

* For additional information, see American Academy of Pediatrics, Committee on Infectious Diseases, Committee on Fetus and Newborn. Respiratory syncytial virus immune globulin intravenous: indications for use. *Pediatrics.* 1997;99:645-650.

[†] RespiGam, Medimmune Inc, Gaithersburg, Md.

- When RSV-IGIV prophylaxis is given, it should be initiated before the onset of the RSV season and terminated at the end of the season. In most areas of the United States, the usual time for the beginning of RSV outbreaks is between October and December and termination is between March and May, but regional differences occur. The onset of RSV occurs earlier in southern states than in northern states. Physicians should consult with health departments and/or diagnostic virology laboratories in their area to determine the optimal schedule.
- In infants and children receiving RSV-IGIV prophylaxis, immunization with MMR and varicella vaccines should be deferred for 9 months after the last dose. RSV-IGIV use should not alter the primary immunization schedule for other routinely recommended vaccines. The manufacturer of RSV-IGIV has suggested that an additional dose of vaccine might be needed to assure an adequate immune response to DTP, DTaP, *Haemophilus* conjugate, and OPV, but more information is needed before recommendations can be made. The available data at this time do not support the need for supplemental doses of any of these routinely administered vaccines.

ISOLATION OF THE HOSPITALIZED PATIENT*: Contact precautions are recommended for the duration of the illness, including for patients treated with ribavirin. The effectiveness of these precautions is dependent on compliance and necessitates that the requirements for use of gloves and gown when entering the patient's room and for good hand washing practices should be scrupulously implemented. Patients with laboratory-documented RSV infection can be cohorted in the same room.

CONTROL MEASURES: The control of nosocomial RSV is complicated by the continuing chance for introduction through infected patients, staff, and visitors. During the peak RSV season, many infants and children hospitalized with respiratory symptoms will be infected with RSV and should be managed with contact precautions (see Isolation of the Hospitalized Patient, above). Early identification of RSV-infected patients (see Diagnostic Tests, p 444) is important so that appropriate precautions can be instituted promptly. During large outbreaks, a variety of measures have been demonstrated to be effective, including (1) laboratory screening of patients for RSV infection, (2) cohorting infected patients and staff, (3) excluding visitors with respiratory infections, and (4) excluding staff with respiratory illness or RSV infection from caring for susceptible infants. These additional measures may be most important in preventing transmission to patients with compromised cardiac, pulmonary, or immune systems.

A critical aspect of RSV prevention in high-risk infants is education of parents and other caregivers about the importance of reducing exposure to and transmission of RSV. Preventive measures include limiting, where feasible, exposure to contagious settings (eg, child care centers) and emphasis on hand washing in all settings including the home, especially during periods when contacts of high-risk children have respiratory infections.

---

* In addition to standard precautions.

Rhinovirus Infections

CLINICAL MANIFESTATIONS: Rhinovirus infections are the most frequent causes of the common cold. Rhinoviruses can also be involved in bronchitis, sinusitis, otitis media, and lower respiratory tract disease in young children. Rhinoviruses can precipitate asthmatic attacks.

ETIOLOGY: Rhinoviruses are RNA viruses classified as picornaviruses. At least 100 antigenic serotypes have been identified by neutralizing antibodies. Infection with one type confers relative type-specific immunity, but offers little protection against other types.

EPIDEMIOLOGY: Humans are the only known hosts. Transmission occurs predominately by person-to-person contact through self-inoculation by contaminated secretions on the hands, but in some circumstances transmission may occur by aerosol. Infections occur throughout the year, but peak activity is most frequent in the fall and spring. Several serotypes usually circulate simultaneously, but the prevalent types in a population tend to change during a period of years. By adulthood, antibodies to many serotypes have developed. Household spread is common. The period of communicability is variable, but it correlates with the shedding of virus in nasopharyngeal secretions which is for 7 to 10 days in most instances, but may be for as long as 3 weeks.

The **incubation period** is approximately 2 to 3 days.

DIAGNOSTIC TESTS: Inoculation of nasal secretions in appropriate cell cultures for viral isolation is the best means of making a specific diagnosis. The large number of antigenic types and the need to perform a neutralization assay make serologic testing impractical.

TREATMENT: Only symptomatic treatment is given. Placebo-controlled studies indicate that over-the-counter antihistamine/decongestant cold medications are ineffective, especially in children younger than 5 years.

ISOLATION OF THE HOSPITALIZED PATIENT*: Contact precautions are recommended for hospitalized young children and infants for the duration of the illness.

CONTROL MEASURES: Frequent hand washing and hygienic measures in schools, households, and other settings where transmission is common may help reduce the spread of rhinoviruses.

---

* In addition to standard precautions.

Rickettsial Diseases

The rickettsiae are pleomorphic bacteria, and most have arthropod vectors. Humans are incidental hosts and are not useful in propagating the organism in nature except for louse-borne typhus, for which humans are the principal reservoir and the human body louse is the vector. Rickettsiae are obligate intracellular parasites and cannot be grown in cell-free media. They have typical bacterial cell walls and cytoplasmic membranes and divide by binary fission. Their natural life cycles usually involve lower mammalian species as reservoirs, with the exception of *Rickettsia prowazekii*, the cause of louse-borne typhus, and animal-to-human or vector-to-human transmission occurs as a result of environmental or occupational exposure.

Ticks are the vector for many of these diseases. Thus, control measures involve prevention of tick transmission of rickettsial agents to humans (see Control Measures for Prevention of Tick-Borne Infections, p 126).

Rickettsial infections have many features in common, including the following:

- Multiplication of the organism in an arthropod host.
- Intracellular replication.
- Limited geographic and seasonal occurrence related to arthropod life cycles, activity, and distribution.
- Zoonotic diseases.
- Humans are incidental hosts (except for louse-borne typhus).
- Local, primary lesions occur with some rickettsial diseases.
- Fever, rash (except in Q fever and in most cases of ehrlichiosis), headache, myalgias, and respiratory tract symptoms are prominent features.
- Generalized capillary and small-vessel endothelial damage, thrombus formation, and tissue necrosis are common pathologic features.
- With the exception of Q fever, rickettsialpox, and ehrlichiosis, nonspecific serum *Proteus vulgaris* agglutinins (Weil-Felix test) develop during infection. However, their presence frequently is unreliable in diagnosis, because false-positive and false-negative test results can occur. In addition, specific serologic assays are available and, if available, should replace the nonspecific Weil-Felix test.
- Group-specific serum antibodies are detectable in convalescence.
- Various serologic tests for detecting these antibodies, including indirect immunofluorescence, complement fixation, microagglutination, indirect hemagglutination, latex fixation, enzyme immunoassay, radioisotope precipitation, and radioimmunoassay, are available or in development in reference and research laboratories. The immunofluorescent test is recommended in most cases because of its relative simplicity, sensitivity, and specificity.
- The polymerase chain reaction (PCR) to detect rickettsiae in blood or tissue provides promise for early diagnosis of many rickettsial diseases.
- In experienced laboratories, immunohistologic or polymerase chain reaction testing of skin biopsy specimens can be used to diagnose rickettsial infections in patients with rash.
- Treatment early in the course of illness can blunt serologic responses.

- Rickettsial diseases can be fulminant, so prompt and specific therapy is important. Appropriate antimicrobial treatment usually is effective in patients who are treated during the first week of illness. If the disease remains untreated in the second week, even optimal therapy is less effective.
- Infections usually respond to tetracyclines or chloramphenicol if given early and in an adequate dosage, although these drugs are rickettsiostatic and not rickettsicidal. Repeated doses of tetracycline drugs should not be given to children younger than 8 years unless the benefits of therapy are greater than the risks of dental staining (see Antimicrobials and Related Therapy, p 606).
- Immunity against reinfection by the same agent after natural infection is usually of long duration, except in the case of scrub typhus caused by *Rickettsia tsutsugamushi*. Among the four different groups of rickettsial diseases, generally partial or complete cross-immunity is conferred by infections with rickettsiae within groups but not among groups.
- Many rickettsial diseases, especially Rocky Mountain spotted fever and Q fever, are reportable to state and local health departments.
- For details, the following chapters on rickettsial diseases should be consulted:
  - Ehrlichiosis
  - Q fever
  - Rickettsialpox
  - Rocky Mountain spotted fever
  - Flea-borne typhus
  - Louse-borne typhus

A number of other epidemiologically distinct but clinically similar tick-borne spotted fever infections caused by rickettsiae have been recognized. The etiologic agents of some of these infections share the same group antigen as *Rickettsia rickettsii*; these include *R conorii*, the etiologic agent of boutonneuse fever (also known as Kenya tick-bite fever, African tick typhus, Mediterranean spotted fever, India tick typhus, and Marseille fever) that is endemic in southern Europe, Africa, and the Middle East; *R sibirica*, the etiologic agent of Siberian tick typhus endemic in central Asia; *R australis*, the etiologic agent of North Queensland tick typhus endemic in eastern Australia; and *R japonica*, the etiologic agent of a spotted fever rickettsiosis endemic in Japan. All of these infections have clinical, pathologic, and epidemiologic features similar to those of Rocky Mountain spotted fever and are treated similarly, but they usually are milder and associated with a small indurated lesion that develops at the site of the tick bite (tache noire), with resultant eschar and regional lymph node enlargement. The specific diagnosis is confirmed serologically. These conditions are of importance among persons traveling to endemic areas.

Rickettsialpox

CLINICAL MANIFESTATIONS: Rickettsialpox is characterized by generalized erythematous papulovesicular eruptions on the trunk, extremities (including face, palms, and soles), and mucous membranes after the appearance of a primary lesion at the site of the bite of the mouse mite vector. A black scab or eschar develops at the site about the time of onset of fever. Regional lymph nodes in the area of the primary eschar typically become enlarged. Systemic disease lasts about 1 week; manifestations can include chills, fever, headache, drenching sweats, myalgias, anorexia, photophobia, and regional lymphadenopathy. The disease is self-limited, and rarely associated with complications.

ETIOLOGY: Rickettsialpox is caused by *Rickettsia akari,* which is classified with the spotted-fever–group rickettsiae and antigenically is related to *Rickettsia rickettsii.*

EPIDEMIOLOGY: The natural host for *R akari* in the United States is *Mus musculus,* the common house mouse. The disease is transmitted by a mouse mite. Disease risk is heightened in areas infested with mice. The disease was first recognized in apartment house dwellers in New York City and was found in large urban settings, paralleling the distribution of mice. The disease also has been recognized in the northeastern United States, Ohio, Utah, Croatia, Ukraine, Russia, Korea, and South Africa. All age groups can be affected. No seasonal pattern of disease occurs. The disease is not communicable among humans and currently is rare in the United States.

The **incubation period** is 9 to 14 days.

DIAGNOSTIC TESTS: *Rickettsia akari* can be isolated from blood during the acute stage of disease, but culture is not attempted routinely and only should be done in specialized laboratories. The Weil-Felix test for all *Proteus vulgaris* Ox agglutinins is negative. An indirect fluorescent antibody or complement fixation test for *R rickettsii* (the cause of Rocky Mountain spotted fever) will demonstrate fourfold change in antibody titers between acute and convalescent sera, because antibodies to *R akari* have extensive cross-reactivity with those against *R rickettsii.* Direct fluorescent antibody testing of paraffin-embedded eschars and histopathologic examination of papulovesicles for distinctive features are useful diagnostic techniques.

TREATMENT: Tetracycline or chloramphenicol will shorten the course of the disease; symptoms resolve within 48 hours after initiation of doxycycline therapy. Tetracyclines should not be given to children younger than 8 years of age unless the benefits of therapy are greater than the risks of dental staining (see Antimicrobials and Related Therapy, p 606). Treatment is effective when given for 3 to 5 days; relapse is rare.

ISOLATION OF THE HOSPITALIZED PATIENT: Standard precautions are recommended.

CONTROL MEASURES: Disinfestation with residual insecticides and rodent control measures limit or eliminate the vector. No specific management of exposed persons is necessary.

Rocky Mountain Spotted Fever

CLINICAL MANIFESTATIONS: Rocky Mountain spotted fever (RMSF) is a systemic, febrile illness with a characteristic rash usually occurring before the sixth day of illness. Fever, headache, myalgia, toxicity, confusion, nausea, vomiting, and anorexia are major clinical features. Abdominal pain, diarrhea, and cough are noted less frequently. The rash initially is erythematous and macular, and later can become maculopapular and frequently petechial. Rash first appears on the wrists and ankles, spreading within hours proximally to the trunk. The palms and soles typically are involved. Although early development of a rash is a useful diagnostic sign, in some cases the rash fails to develop or only does so late in the illness. Thrombocytopenia of varying severity develops in most cases, and anemia has been noted in approximately 30% of patients as a result of endothelial and microvascular damage. Leukopenia is noted less frequently. The illness can last as long as 3 weeks and can be severe with prominent central nervous system disease; involvement of cardiac, pulmonary, gastrointestinal tract, renal, and/or other organs; disseminated intravascular coagulation; and shock leading to death. Significant long-term sequelae, particularly neurologic, are common in patients with severe RMSF.

ETIOLOGY: *Rickettsia rickettsii* is an obligate intracellular pathogen and a member of the spotted fever group of rickettsiae.

EPIDEMIOLOGY: The disease is transmitted to humans by the bite of ticks. Many small wild animals and dogs have antibodies to *R rickettsii*, but their role as natural hosts is not clear since ticks are both reservoirs and vectors of *R rickettsii*. In ticks, the agent is transmitted transovarially and between stages. Persons with occupational or recreational exposure to the tick vector (eg, pet owners, animal handlers, and outdoor persons) are at an increased risk of acquiring the organism. Persons of all ages, races, socioeconomic status, and both sexes can be infected, but most cases occur in those younger than 15 years, probably because they are most frequently in tick habitats. Laboratory-acquired infection has resulted from accidental inoculation and aerosol contamination. Transmission has occurred on rare occasion by blood transfusion. Mortality is highest in males, in persons older than 30 years, in nonwhites, and in persons with no known tick bite or attachment. Delay in disease recognition (or its possibility) and resulting late initiation of appropriate antimicrobial therapy increases the risk of death; factors include absence of rash, initial presentation before the fourth day of illness, and presentation in months other than May through July.

The disease is widespread in the United States. Most cases are reported in the south Atlantic, southeastern, and south central states. Focal sites in an affected area can account for much of the morbidity in an area. The dog tick (*Dermacentor variabilis*) primarily is responsible for transmission in these geographic areas and some areas of western United States. Summer is the season of highest prevalence. In the western United States, the upper Rocky Mountain states have the highest incidence; the vector is usually the wood tick (*Dermacentor andersoni*). The Lone Star tick (*Amblyomma americanum*) is a vector of *R rickettsii* in south central United States. Transmission parallels the tick season in a given geographic area. April through

October are the months of highest prevalence. The disease also occurs in Canada, Mexico, and Central and South America.

The **incubation period** is usually about 1 week but ranges from 2 to 14 days. It appears to be related to the size of the rickettsial inoculum.

DIAGNOSTIC TESTS: Culture of *R rickettsii* usually is not attempted because of the danger of transmission to laboratory personnel; only those laboratories with adequate biohazard containment equipment should attempt isolation of rickettsiae. The diagnosis can be established retrospectively by one of the multiple rickettsial group-specific serologic tests in which a fourfold increase or decrease in antibody titer between acute and convalescent sera is demonstrated, as determined by indirect immunofluorescence, complement fixation (CF), latex agglutination, indirect hemagglutination, or microagglutination tests. Criteria for diagnosis with single convalescent serum specimens also have been established. The indirect fluorescent antibody (IFA) and indirect hemagglutination (IHA) are the most sensitive and specific tests. Antibodies are detected by IFA 7 to 10 days after onset of illness. A microtiter enzyme immunoassay has been developed to determine the IgM and IgG responses to *R rickettsii.* The CF and microagglutination tests are highly specific for this disease, but they lack sensitivity, particularly if the patient has received early antibiotic treatment. The nonspecific and insensitive Weil-Felix serologic test (Proteus Ox-19 and Ox-2 agglutinins) becomes positive 10 to 14 days after onset of the illness but its use is not recommended due to availability of specific assays. No microbiologic test is readily available for rapid diagnosis early in the illness. However, *R rickettsii* have been identified by immunofluorescent staining of skin biopsy specimens obtained from the site of the rash. With adequate specimens, this method can be 70% sensitive and 100% specific, but it is not widely available.

In reference laboratories, polymerase chain reaction (PCR) tests have been developed for the detection of *R rickettsii* in blood and biopsy specimens during the acute phase of the illness. Polymerase chain reaction is a specific but insensitive test. Because fewer organisms are present in blood than in lesion-related endothelial cells, the sensitivity of testing skin biopsy specimens by PCR is likely to be greater than that of testing blood.

TREATMENT: Early initiation of treatment based on clinical manifestations and epidemiologic considerations affords the highest likelihood of success in patients with suspected RMSF. Chloramphenicol or doxycycline is the drug of choice. Tetracycline drugs should not be given routinely to children younger than 8 years of age (see Antimicrobials and Related Therapy, p 606). However, when comparing the benefits and risks of doxycycline and chloramphenicol in children younger than 8 years, some experts consider doxycycline to be the drug of choice for children of any age with presumed or proven RMSF for the following reasons: tetracycline staining of teeth is dose-related; doxycycline is less likely to stain developing teeth than other tetracyclines; and whereas clinical manifestations of ehrlichiosis and RMSF overlap, tetracyclines are effective against both infections but chloramphenicol may not be (see Ehrlichiosis, p 196). Therapy is continued until the patient has been afebrile for at least 2 or 3 days. The usual duration is 7 to 10 days.

ISOLATION OF THE HOSPITALIZED PATIENT: Standard precautions are recommended.

CONTROL MEASURES: Control of ticks in their natural habitat is not practical. Avoidance of tick-infested areas is the best preventive measure. If a tick-infested area is entered, persons should wear protective clothing and apply tick/insect repellents to clothes and exposed body parts for added protection. They should be taught to thoroughly inspect themselves, their children (bodies and clothing), and pets for ticks after spending time outdoors during the tick season, and to remove ticks promptly (see Control Measures for Prevention of Tick-Borne Infections, p 126).

No licensed *R rickettsii* vaccine is currently available in the United States.

Rotavirus Infections

CLINICAL MANIFESTATIONS: Infection can result in diarrhea, usually preceded or accompanied by emesis and low-grade fever. In severe cases, dehydration, electrolyte abnormalities, and acidosis may occur and result in neurologic signs. In immunocompromised children, including those with HIV infection, persistent infection with manifestations of multisystem involvement can develop.

ETIOLOGY: Rotaviruses are RNA viruses belonging to the family *Reoviridae*, with at least 7 distinct antigenic groups (A to G). Group A viruses are the major causes of rotavirus diarrhea in the United States. Groups B and C viruses also have been identified as causes of gastroenteritis. Serotyping is based on the VP7 glycoprotein (G) and VP4 protease-cleaved hemagglutinin (P); G types 1 to 4 and P types 1A and 1B most commonly are associated with disease.

EPIDEMIOLOGY: Most human infections result from contact with infected persons. Rotavirus (RV) infections occur in many animal species, but transmission from animals to humans has not been documented. However, reassortment between human and animal rotaviruses have occurred and can generate new serotypes. Rotavirus in infected patients is present in high titer in stools, which is the only body specimen consistently positive for the virus. It is present in stool before the onset of diarrhea, and can persist for as long as 10 days after the onset of symptoms in normal hosts. Transmission is presumed to be by the fecal-oral route. Rotavirus can be found on toys and hard surfaces in child care centers, indicating that fomites may serve as a mechanism of transmission. Respiratory transmission also may have a role in disease transmission. Spread within families and institutions is common. Rotavirus is the most common cause of nosocomially acquired diarrhea in children and is an important cause of acute gastroenteritis in children attending child care. Common-source outbreaks have been reported.

Human RV infections occur throughout the world and may be more frequent in lower socioeconomic areas. In developed countries RVs are the single most common agent of diarrhea in infants younger than 2 years who require medical attention. Death from dehydration is a major cause of mortality in developing countries but is unusual in developed countries. Disease is most prevalent during the cooler months of the year in temperate climates. In North America, the annual epidemic peak characteristically starts in the fall in Mexico and the southwest United States, moving sequentially to reach the northeast areas and maritime Canada by spring. Specific seasonal patterns in tropical climates are less pronounced. Virtually all children are infected by 3 years of age. The rate of hospitalization from RV diarrhea in infected children can be as high as 2.5%. Although clinically apparent cases of gastroenteritis most commonly occur in infants between 4 and 24 months of age, serologic assays have demonstrated infection in other age groups and multiple infections may occur. Reinfection has been demonstrated serologically in 30% to 50% of adult contacts of infected infants, though only a minority manifest symptoms. Infections in neonates are often asymptomatic. Breastfeeding has not been proven to prevent infection, but may be associated with milder disease.

The **incubation period** is usually from 1 to 3 days.

DIAGNOSTIC TESTS: Enzyme immunoassay (EIA) and latex agglutination assays for group A RV antigen detection in stool are commercially available. Both types of assays are useful for the detection of RV antigens during diarrhea. However, EIAs are more sensitive for the detection of antigen late in the course of illness. Both assays have high specificity, but false-positive and nonspecific reactions can occur in neonates and in persons with underlying intestinal disease. These nonspecific reactions can be distinguished from true positive ones by the performance of confirmatory assays. In research laboratories, virus also can be identified in stool by electron microscopy and nucleic acid amplification techniques. Characterization of strains is possible by determination of the viral RNA migration patterns on polyacrylamide gel electrophoresis. Strains can be characterized further for antigenic and subgroup analysis by other research techniques.

TREATMENT: No specific antiviral therapy is available. Oral or parenteral fluids are given to prevent and correct dehydration.* Orally administered human immunoglobulins given as an investigational therapy in immunocompromised patients with prolonged infections has reduced viral shedding and shortened the duration of diarrhea.

ISOLATION OF THE HOSPITALIZED PATIENT†: Strict adherence to contact precautions is indicated for the duration of the illness. In view of the prolonged fecal shedding of low concentration of virus after recovery, continuation of contact precautions for the duration of hospitalization can be justified, particularly if transmission can occur to immunocompromised and other high-risk infants.

CONTROL MEASURES:

Child Care. General measures for interrupting enteric transmission in child care centers are recommended (see Children in Out-of-Home Child Care, p 80). Specific and effective control measures have not been established. Children with RV diarrhea in whom stool cannot be contained by diapers or toilet use should be excluded until

---

* For further information and detailed recommendations, see Duggan C, Santosham M, Glass RI. The management of acute diarrhea in children: oral rehydration, maintenance, and nutritional therapy. *MMWR.* 1992;41(No. RR-16):1-20.
† In addition to standard precautions.

the diarrhea ceases. Surfaces should be washed with soap and water. Chlorine-based disinfectants will inactivate RV and may help prevent disease transmission resulting from contact with environmental surfaces.

Vaccines. Several efficacy trials of multivalent live-attenuated, orally administered group A RV vaccines have been completed and others are in progress. The results of these field trials may lead to licensure of one or more RV vaccine(s) within the next several years.

Rubella

CLINICAL MANIFESTATIONS:

Postnatal Rubella. Rubella is usually a mild disease characterized by an erythematous, maculopapular, discrete rash, generalized lymphadenopathy (most commonly suboccipital, postauricular, and cervical), and slight fever. Transient polyarthralgia and polyarthritis occasionally occur in children and are common in adolescents and adults, especially females. Encephalitis and thrombocytopenia are rare complications.

Congenital Rubella. The most commonly described anomalies associated with the congenital rubella syndrome are ophthalmologic (cataracts and retinopathy), cardiac (patent ductus arteriosus, pulmonary artery stenosis), auditory (sensorineural deafness), and neurologic (behavioral disorders, meningoencephalitis, and mental retardation). In addition, infants with congenital rubella are frequently growth-retarded and may have radiolucent bone disease, hepatosplenomegaly, thrombocytopenia, and purple skin lesions (giving a "blueberry muffin" appearance). Mild forms of the disease can be associated with few or no obvious clinical manifestations at birth.

ETIOLOGY: Rubella virus is an RNA virus classified as a rubivirus in the Togaviridae family.

EPIDEMIOLOGY: Humans are the only source of infection. Postnatal rubella is transmitted primarily through direct or droplet contact from nasopharyngeal secretions. The peak incidence of infection is in the late winter and early spring. Approximately 25% to 50% of infections are asymptomatic. Immunity from either wild-type or vaccine virus is usually prolonged, but reinfection on rare occasions has been demonstrated and very rarely has resulted in the congenital rubella. The period of maximal communicability appears to be the few days before and 5 to 7 days after the onset of the rash. Volunteer studies have demonstrated the presence of rubella virus in nasopharyngeal secretions from 7 days before to 14 days after the onset of the rash. A small number of infants with congenital rubella continue to shed virus in nasopharyngeal secretions and urine for 1 year or more and can transmit infection to susceptible contacts. In approximately 10% to 20% of these patients, virus can be isolated from the nasopharynx when the infant is 6 months old.

Before the widespread use of rubella vaccine, rubella was an epidemic disease, occurring in 6- to 9-year cycles, and most cases occurred in children. The incidence of rubella in the United States has declined by approximately 99% from the prevaccine era. The risk of acquiring rubella has declined sharply in all age groups, including adolescents and young adults. In the vaccine era, most cases have occurred in young, unvaccinated adults in outbreaks in colleges and occupational settings. Although the number of susceptible individuals has decreased since the introduction and widespread use of rubella vaccine, recent serologic surveys have indicated that approximately 10% of young adults are susceptible to rubella. This degree of susceptibility in young adults is primarily the result of lack of vaccination.

The **incubation period** for postnatally acquired rubella ranges from 14 to 21 days, usually 16 to 18 days.

DIAGNOSTIC TESTS: Rubella virus most consistently can be isolated from nasal specimens by inoculation of appropriate cell culture. The laboratory should be notified that rubella is suspected since additional testing is required to detect the virus. Throat swabs, blood, urine, and cerebrospinal fluid also can yield virus, particularly in congenitally infected infants. Serologic testing also is useful for confirming the presence of infection, especially in the absence of typical clinical manifestations. Acute and convalescent sera should be tested; a fourfold or greater rise in antibody titer or seroconversion is indicative of infection. Many virology laboratories can detect rubella-specific IgM antibody, the presence of which usually indicates recent postnatal infection or congenital infection in a newborn infant, but false-positive results occur. Congenital infection also can be confirmed by stable or increasing serum concentrations of rubella-specific IgG during a period of several months. Every effort should be made to establish a laboratory diagnosis when rubella infection is suspected in pregnant women or newborn infants. The diagnosis of congenital rubella infection in children older than 1 year is difficult; serology usually is not diagnostic and viral isolation, while confirmatory, is possible in only a small proportion of congenitally infected children of this age. The hemagglutination inhibition (HAI) rubella antibody test, which previously was the most frequently used method of serologic screening, generally has been supplanted by a number of equally or more sensitive assays for determining rubella immunity, including latex agglutination, fluorescence immunoassay, passive hemagglutination, hemolysis-in-gel, and enzyme immunoassay tests. Some persons in whom antibody has been absent by HAI testing have been found to be immune when their sera is tested by more sensitive assays.

TREATMENT: Supportive.

ISOLATION OF THE HOSPITALIZED PATIENT*: For postnatal rubella, droplet precautions are recommended 7 days after the onset of the rash. Contact isolation is indicated for proven or suspected congenital rubella. Children with congenital rubella should be considered contagious until they are at least 1 year old, unless nasopharyngeal and urine cultures after 3 months of age are repeatedly negative for rubella virus.

CONTROL MEASURES:

School and Child Care. Children with postnatal rubella should be excluded from school or child care for 7 days after the onset of the rash. Patients with congenital rubella in child care should be considered contagious until they are at least 1 year

---

* In addition to standard precautions.

old, unless nasopharyngeal and urine cultures are repeatedly negative for rubella. Mothers of these infants should be made aware of the potential hazard of their infants to susceptible, pregnant contacts.

Care of Exposed Persons. When a pregnant woman is exposed to rubella, a blood specimen should be obtained as soon as possible and tested for rubella antibody. An aliquot of frozen sera should be stored for possible repeat testing at a later time. The presence of rubella-specific IgG antibody in a properly performed test at the time of exposure indicates that the individual is most likely immune. If antibody is not detectable, a second blood specimen should be obtained 3 to 4 weeks later and tested concurrently with the first specimen. If antibody is present in the second but not the first specimen, infection is assumed to have occurred. If the second test is negative, another blood specimen should be obtained 6 weeks after the exposure and also tested concurrently with the first specimen; a negative test result in both specimens indicates that infection has not occurred, and a positive test in the second but not the first (seroconversion) indicates recent infection.

Immune Globulin (IG). The routine use of IG for postexposure prophylaxis of rubella in early pregnancy is not recommended. Administration of IG should be considered only if termination of the pregnancy is not an option. Limited data indicate that IG in a dose of 0.55 mL/kg may prevent or modify infection in an exposed, susceptible person. In one study, the attack rate of clinically apparent infection was reduced from 87% in control subjects to 18% in recipients of IG. However, the absence of clinical signs in a woman who has received IG does not guarantee that fetal infection has been prevented. In this study, 44% of the IG recipients were infected. Infants with congenital rubella are known to have been born to mothers who were given IG shortly after exposure.

Vaccine. Live-virus rubella vaccine given after exposure does not prevent illness. However, immunization of exposed, nonpregnant persons may be indicated because if the exposure did not result in infection, immunization will protect the individual in the future. Immunization of a person who is incubating natural rubella or who is already immune is not deleterious.

Rubella Vaccine. The live-virus rubella vaccine currently distributed in the United States is the RA 27/3 strain grown in human diploid cell cultures. Vaccine is administered by subcutaneous injection of 0.5 mL, either alone or preferably as the combined vaccine containing measles and mumps vaccines (MMR). Vaccine can be given simultaneously with other vaccines (see Simultaneous Administration of Multiple Vaccines, p 21). Serum antibody to rubella is induced in at least 95% of the recipients following a single dose at 12 months of age or older. Clinical efficacy and challenge studies have demonstrated that one dose confers long-term, probably lifelong, immunity against both clinical and asymptomatic infection in more than 90% of vaccinees. Asymptomatic reinfection, on rare occasions, has occurred.

Two doses of rubella vaccine given as MMR are now recommended in accordance with the routine two-dose measles immunization schedule (see Measles, p 344). Although primary rubella vaccine failures have not been a major problem, the potential consequences of rubella vaccine failure are substantial (ie, congenital rubella), and the second dose of rubella vaccine provides an added safeguard against such failures.

Vaccine Recommendations (see Table 3.51, p 460, for a summary). Rubella vaccine is currently recommended to be administered in combination with measles and mumps vaccine (MMR) when a child is 12 to 15 months of age and at school entry at 4 to 6 years, according to recommendations for routine measles vaccination; those who have not received this dose at school entry should be given their second dose at 11 to 12 years or before (see Measles, p 344).

Special emphasis must continue to be placed on the immunization of postpubertal males and females, especially college students, military recruits, and health care workers. Those who have not received at least one dose of vaccine or who have no serologic evidence of immunity to rubella are considered susceptible and should be immunized with MMR vaccine. Clinical diagnosis of infection is usually unreliable and should not be accepted as evidence of immunity. Women should be informed of the theoretical risk to the fetus if they are pregnant or become pregnant within 3 months of vaccination (see Precautions and Contraindications, p 461, for further discussion). Specific recommendations are as follows:
- Postpubertal females without documentation of presumptive evidence of rubella immunity should be immunized, unless they are known to be pregnant. Postpubertal females should be warned not to become pregnant for 3 months after receiving rubella vaccine.
- During annual health care examinations, premarital and family planning visits, and sexually transmitted clinic visits, postpubertal females should be assessed for rubella susceptibility and, if deemed susceptible, should be immunized with MMR vaccine. Serological screening is only indicated if aggressive follow-up and immunization are implemented.
- Routine prenatal screening for rubella immunity should be undertaken and rubella vaccine, given as MMR vaccine, should be administered to susceptible women in the immediate postpartum period before discharge. Physicians can help ensure immunization of susceptible women by inquiring about the immune status of the mothers of their patients during medical visits for well-child care of newborn infants.
- Previous or simultaneous administration of Rho (D) immune globulin (human) or blood products is not a contraindication to vaccination, but serologic testing should be done at least 8 weeks after vaccination in these cases in order to ascertain that seroconversion has occurred.
- Breastfeeding is not a contraindication to postpartum immunization (for additional information, see Human Milk, p 73).
- Special efforts should be made to be certain that all individuals are protected who plan to attend or work in educational institutions, child care centers, or other places where they are likely to be exposed to, or spread, rubella.
- All susceptible health care personnel who may be exposed to patients with rubella should be immunized for the prevention or transmission of rubella to pregnant patients as well as for their own health.

Adverse Reactions.
- Five percent to 15% of susceptible children who receive MMR vaccine develop fever 5 to 12 days after vaccination. Rash occurs in approximately 5% of vaccinees. Lymphadenopathy occurs less commonly.

Table 3.51. Indications and Contraindications for Rubella Vaccination

Indications	Contraindications
Children ≥12 mo (with measles and mumps vaccines [as MMR]) in a 2-dose schedule*	Pregnancy
	Immunodeficiency or immuno-compromised condition[†]
Susceptible individuals in the following groups:	Recipient of immune globulin or blood in past 3 mo[‡]
Prepubertal girls and boys	
Adults, especially premarital or postpartum women	
College students	
Child care personnel	
Health care personnel	
Military personnel	

* See Measles, p 344.
† Exception is HIV infection (see text for further discussion).
‡ Rubella vaccine may be given postpartum concurrently or after the administration of anti-Rho (D) immune globulin or blood products (see text for indications for subsequent testing for seroconversion). If rubella vaccine is given as MMR, longer intervals may be necessary (see p 458 and Table 3.37, p 353).

- Joint pain, usually in small peripheral joints, has been reported in approximately 0.5% of children. Arthralgia and transient arthritis tend to be more frequent in susceptible postpubertal females, occurring in approximately 25% and 10%, respectively, of vaccine recipient. Joint involvement usually begins 7 to 21 days after vaccination and is generally transient. Persistent or recurrent joint symptoms have been reported in adult women by one group of investigators from Canada, but data from the United States and other countries suggest that this adverse event is uncommon. An Institute of Medicine Committee concluded that the available evidence was consistent with a causal relationship between rubella vaccination and persistent arthritis, although the available data on current vaccine strains are limited*; subsequent studies, however, have not supported this relationship.
- The incidence of joint manifestations after vaccination is lower than that after natural infection at the corresponding age. In addition, in those reimmunized, the likelihood of these manifestations can be expected to be considerably less than that in previously immunized individuals, most of whom are already immune.
- Transient peripheral neuritic complaints, such as paresthesia and pain in the arms and legs, also have been reported, although rarely.
- Central nervous system manifestations have been reported, but no causal relationship with rubella vaccine has been established.

* Howson CP, Katz M, Johnston RB Jr, Fineberg HV. Chronic arthritis after rubella vaccination. *Clin Infect Dis.* 1992;15:307-312.

- Thrombocytopenia can occur following rubella vaccination with MMR (see Measles, p 344).

Precautions and Contraindications.

- ***Pregnancy.*** Rubella vaccine should not be given to pregnant women. If vaccine is inadvertently given or if pregnancy occurs within 3 months of immunization, the patient should be counseled on the theoretic risks to the fetus. The maximal theoretic risk for the occurrence of congenital rubella is estimated to be 1.6%, based on data accumulated by the Centers for Disease Control and Prevention (CDC) from 226 susceptible women who received the current rubella vaccine (the RA27/3 strain) during the first trimester. Of the offspring, 2% had asymptomatic infection but none had congenital defects. In view of these observations, receipt of rubella vaccine in pregnancy is not an indication for interruption of pregnancy.

    Routine serologic testing of postpubertal women before immunization is not necessary. Serologic testing is a potential impediment to protection of these women against rubella because it requires two visits, one to identify susceptibles and one to administer vaccine. However, a sample of blood may be obtained before vaccination and stored for at least 3 months. If a woman becomes pregnant or has become pregnant after vaccination, the prevaccination specimen can be tested. Demonstration of rubella antibody in the pre-vaccine specimen indicates immunity and eliminates anxiety about fetal injury from rubella vaccine virus.

    Vaccinating susceptible children whose mothers or other household contacts are pregnant does not cause a risk. Most vaccinees intermittently shed small amounts of virus from the pharynx 7 to 28 days after vaccination, but no evidence of transmission of the vaccine virus has been found in studies of more than 1200 susceptible household contacts. Susceptible children, thus, should receive the vaccine.

- ***Febrile illness.*** Children with minor illnesses with or without fever, such as upper respiratory tract infection, may be vaccinated (see Vaccine Safety and Contraindications, p 26). Fever per se is not a contraindication to immunization. However, if other manifestations suggest a more serious illness, the child should not be vaccinated until recovery has occurred.

- ***Recent administration of immune globulin.*** Rubella vaccine should not be given in the 2 weeks before or the 3 months after the administration of immunoglobulin or blood transfusion because of the possibility that antibody will neutralize vaccine virus and prevent successful immunization. Since rubella vaccine is usually given as MMR and high doses of IG (such as those given for the treatment of Kawasaki disease) can inhibit the response to the measles vaccine for longer intervals, rubella vaccination with MMR necessitates deferral for longer periods in such circumstances (see Measles, p 344, and Table 3.37, p 353). Rubella vaccine may be given to postpartum women at the same time as anti-Rho (D) IG (Rhogam) or after blood products are given, but these women should be tested 8 or more weeks later to determine if they have developed an active antibody response.

- ***Altered immunity.*** Patients with immunodeficiency diseases and those receiving immunosuppressive therapy (eg, patients with leukemia, lymphoma, or generalized malignancy), including large, systemic doses of corticosteroids, alkylating agents, antimetabolites, or radiation; or who are otherwise immunocompromised should not receive live-virus rubella vaccine (see Immunodeficient and Immunosuppressed Children, p 50). The exceptions are patients with symptomatic HIV infection who are not severely immunocompromised; these patients may be vaccinated against rubella with MMR (see HIV Infection, p 279). The risk of rubella exposure for patients with altered immunity can be reduced by vaccinating their close, susceptible contacts. Vaccinated persons do not transmit rubella vaccine virus.

  After cessation of immunosuppressive therapy, rubella vaccine is in most circumstances withheld for an interval of not less than 3 months (with the exception of corticosteroid recipients, see below). This interval is based on the assumption that immunologic responsiveness will have been restored in 3 months and the underlying disease for which immunosuppressive therapy was prescribed is in remission or under control. However, because the interval can vary with the intensity and type of immunosuppressive therapy, radiation therapy, underlying disease, and other factors, a definitive recommendation for an interval after cessation of immunosuppressive therapy when rubella vaccine can be safely and effectively administered often is not possible.

  Corticosteroids. For patients who have received high doses of corticosteroids for 14 days or more, and who are not otherwise immunocompromised, the recommended interval is at least 1 month (see Immunodeficient and Immunosuppressed Children, p 51).

Surveillance for Congenital Infections. Accurate diagnosis and reporting of the congenital rubella syndrome and vaccine complications are extremely important in assessing the control of rubella. All birth defects in which rubella infection is etiologically suspected should be thoroughly investigated and reported to the Centers for Disease Control and Prevention through local or state health departments.

Salmonella Infections

CLINICAL MANIFESTATIONS: *Salmonella* infections cause asymptomatic carriage, gastroenteritis, enteric fever, bacteremia, and focal infections (such as meningitis, osteomyelitis, and abscesses). These diseases are not mutually exclusive categories but represent the broad spectrum of illness caused by *Salmonella.* For example, gastroenteritis may be complicated by bacteremia and/or a metastatic focal infection. The most commonly recognized illness is gastroenteritis, in which diarrhea, abdominal cramps and tenderness, and fever are common manifestations. The site of infection is usually the small intestine, but colitis can occur.

Enteric fever is caused by *Salmonella typhi* and several other *Salmonella* serotypes. The onset of illness typically is gradual, with manifestations such as fever, constitutional symptoms (eg, headache, malaise, anorexia, and lethargy), abdominal pain and tenderness, hepatomegaly, splenomegaly, rose spots, and/or changes in mental status. Constipation may be an early feature. Diarrhea can occur later, usually in the second week of illness, and may not be a prominent symptom. Sustained or intermittent bacteremia can occur in both enteric fever and nontyphoidal *Salmonella* bacteremia. Recognizable focal infections ultimately may occur in as many as 10% of patients with *Salmonella* bacteremia.

ETIOLOGY: *Salmonella* organisms are Gram-negative bacilli in the family Enterobacteriaceae. *Salmonella* can be classified into one of the following three species: *S typhi* (one serotype), *Salmonella choleraesuis* (one serotype), and *Salmonella enteritidis* (>2000 serotypes). A second method of classification is based on somatic antigens and subdivides *Salmonella* organisms into multiple serogroups. Most serotypes that cause human disease are in serogroups A-E. The H (flagellar) antigen further delineates these groups into serotypes. The serotype designation conventionally is used as a species designation. The most frequently reported human isolates in the United States in recent years have been *S typhimurium* (serogroup B), *Salmonella heidelberg* (B), *S enteritidis* (D), *Salmonella newport* (C2), *Salmonella infantis* (C1), *Salmonella agona* (B), *Salmonella hadar* (C2), and *Salmonella saint-paul* (B); *S typhi* is classified in serogroup D.

EPIDEMIOLOGY: The principal reservoirs for nontyphoidal *Salmonella* serotypes are animals, including poultry, livestock, reptiles, and pets. The major vehicles of transmission are foods of animal origin, including poultry, red meat, eggs, and unpasteurized milk. Many other food vehicles, such as fruits, vegetables, and rice, have been implicated. These vehicles are usually contaminated by contact with animal products or an infected human. Other modes of transmission include ingestion of contaminated water (primary route); contact with infected animals (eg, pet turtles, iguanas, and other reptiles); direct person-to-person transmission via the fecal-oral route; and contact with contaminated medications, dyes, and medical instruments. Ingestion of raw or improperly cooked eggs or raw milk, which may be contaminated even though certified, can produce severe disease. Unlike nontyphoidal *Salmonella* serotypes, *S typhi* is found only in humans. Cases of typhoid fever in the United States usually are acquired during foreign travel, or by consumption of food contaminated by a chronic carrier.

Age-specific attack rates for *Salmonella* infection are highest in those younger than 5 years and older than 70 years, and peak early in the first year of life. Invasive infections and mortality are more frequent in infants, the elderly, and those with an underlying disease, particularly hemoglobinopathies (including sickle cell disease), malignancy, acquired immune deficiency, and other immunosuppressive conditions. Most reported cases are sporadic in occurrence, but outbreaks in the home and in institutions are common. Nosocomial epidemics, including outbreaks of meningitis in newborn nurseries, have been reported. Typhoid fever, while uncommon in the United States, is endemic in many developing areas of the world.

The risk of transmission exists throughout the duration of fecal excretion. This period is variable. The median duration of excretion after infection with nontyphoidal *Salmonella* is longer in younger children than in older children or adults. Twelve weeks after infection, 45% of children younger than 5 years excrete *Salmonella* compared with 5% of older children and adults. The duration of excretion can be prolonged by antimicrobial therapy. Approximately 1% of patients continue to excrete *Salmonella* for more than 1 year.

The **incubation period** for gastroenteritis is from 6 to 72 hours. For enteric fever, the incubation period is from 3 to 60 days, but is usually 7 to 14 days.

DIAGNOSTIC TESTS: Cultures of stool, blood, urine, and material from foci of infection, as indicated by the suspected *Salmonella* syndrome, should be obtained. Culture of a bone marrow aspirate may allow recovery of the organism causing enteric fever. Serologic tests for *Salmonella* agglutinins ("febrile agglutinins," the Widal's test) may suggest the diagnosis of *S typhi* infection, but because of false-positive and false-negative results, these tests are not reliable.

TREATMENT:
- Antimicrobial therapy usually is not indicated for patients with uncomplicated (noninvasive) gastroenteritis caused by nontyphoidal *Salmonella* species, because therapy does not shorten the duration of disease and can prolong the duration of excretion of *Salmonella* organisms. Although of unproven benefit, antimicrobial therapy is recommended for Salmonella gastroenteritis occurring in patients with an increased risk of invasive disease and other complications, including infants younger than 3 months and persons with malignancies, hemoglobinopathies, HIV infection or other immunosuppressive illnesses, recipients of immunosuppressive therapy, persons with chronic gastrointestinal tract disease, and patients with severe colitis.
- Ampicillin, amoxicillin, trimethoprim-sulfamethoxazole, cefotaxime, or cef-triaxone is recommended for susceptible strains in patients for whom therapy is indicated. Strains acquired in developing countries often exhibit resistance to many antibiotics but usually are susceptible to ceftriaxone or cefotaxime, and to fluoroquinolones (eg, ciprofloxacin or ofloxacin). However, the fluoro-quinolones are not recommended for use in patients younger than 18 years of age unless the benefits of therapy outweigh the potential risks for use of the drug (see Antimicrobials and Related Therapy, p 605).
- In invasive *Salmonella* disease (such as typhoid, non-*S typhi* bacteremia, or osteomyelitis), appropriate drugs are chloramphenicol, ampicillin, amoxicillin, and trimethoprim-sulfamethoxazole, cefotaxime, ceftriaxone, or a fluoro-quinolone (see Antimicrobials and Related Therapy, p 605). Drug choice, route of administration, and duration are based on susceptibility of the organism, site of infection, host, and clinical response. For susceptible *S typhi*, administration of ampicillin, chloramphenicol, ceftriaxone, or cefotaxime for at least 14 days is recommended. Relapse is common after completion of therapy; retreatment is indicated. In other invasive infections in immunocom-petent hosts without localization, such as bacteremia or enteric fever, patients also should be treated for 14 days; whereas those with localized infection, such as osteomyelitis or abscess, and patients with bacteremia and AIDS should receive 4 to 6 weeks of therapy to prevent relapse. For *Salmonella* meningitis, ceftriaxone or cefotaxime is recommended, often for 4 weeks or longer.

- Chronic (1 year or more) *S typhi* carriage may be eradicated in some patients by high-dose parenteral ampicillin, high-dose oral amoxicillin, ciprofloxacin (see Antimicrobials and Related Therapy, p 605), or cholecystectomy.
- Antipyretics can cause precipitous declines in temperature and shock, and should be avoided in patients with enteric fever syndromes.
- Heparin should not be used to treat patients with asymptomatic, disseminated intravascular coagulation that occurs in many patients with enteric fever.
- Corticosteroids may be beneficial to patients with severe enteric fever, which is characterized by delirium, obtundation, stupor, coma, or shock. These drugs, however, should be reserved for critically ill patients in whom relief of the manifestations of toxemia may be life saving. The usual regimen is high-dose dexamethasone given intravenously at an initial dose of 3 mg/kg, followed by 1 mg/kg every 6 hours for a total course of 48 hours.

ISOLATION OF THE HOSPITALIZED PATIENT*: Contact precautions should be used for diapered and/or incontinent children for the duration of illness. In children with typhoid fever, precautions should be continued until cultures of three consecutive stool specimens obtained after cessation of antimicrobial therapy are negative for *S typhi*.

CONTROL MEASURES: Important measures include proper sanitation methods for food processing and preparation, sanitary water supplies, proper hand washing and personal hygiene, sanitary sewage disposal, exclusion of infected persons from handling food, prohibiting the sale of turtles for pets, reporting cases to appropriate health authorities, and investigating outbreaks. Eggs and other foods of animal origin should be cooked thoroughly. Raw eggs and food containing raw eggs should not be eaten. Notification of public health authorities and determination of serotype are of primary importance in detection and investigation of outbreaks.

Child Care. Outbreaks of *Salmonella* infection are unusual in child care programs, and specific strategies for controlling infection in out-of-home child care have not been evaluated. General measures for interrupting enteric transmission in child care centers are recommended (see Children in Out-of-Home Child Care, p 80).

When *S typhi* disease is identified in a symptomatic child care attendee or staff member, stool specimens from other attendees and staff members should be cultured, and all infected persons should be excluded until three consecutive stool cultures are negative.

When species other than *S typhi* are identified in a symptomatic child care attendee or staff member with enterocolitis, older children and staff do not need to be excluded once they are asymptomatic. Asymptomatic contacts need not be cultured. If multiple symptomatic infected persons are identified, the decision to exclude these persons or cohort them in the program should be made in consultation with public health authorities. Antimicrobial therapy is not recommended for asymptomatically infected individuals, persons with uncomplicated diarrhea, or those exposed to an infected individual.

---

* In addition to standard precautions.

Typhoid Vaccine. Resistance to infection with *S typhi* is enhanced by typhoid vaccination, but the degree of protection with currently available vaccines is limited and can be overcome by ingestion of a large bacterial inoculum. Three typhoid vaccines are available for use in the United States (see Table 3.52); a fourth, an acetone-inactivated parenterally administered vaccine, is available only to the military in the United States.

The three vaccines currently available to civilians in the United States are (1) an orally administered, live-attenuated vaccine prepared from the Ty21a strain of *S typhi*, (2) a capsular polysaccharide vaccine purified Vi (virulence) antigen for parenteral use, and (3) a parenteral heat-phenol-inactivated vaccine that has been used widely for many years. Although no prospective, randomized trials comparing any of the three US-licensed typhoid vaccines have been conducted, several field trials of differing design and age groups have demonstrated the efficacy of each vaccine which has ranged from 17% to 66%. The oral Ty21a vaccine is not approved for use for children younger than 6 years of age, the Vi capsular polysaccharide vaccine (Vi CPS) is not approved for children younger than 2 years; and the parenteral inactivated vaccine is not approved for infants younger than 6 months.

Selection of vaccine is based on the age of the child, need for boosters, possible contraindications (see Contraindications and Precautions, p 468), and reactions (see Adverse Events, p 467). In most circumstances, either the oral Ty21a or Vi CPS is the vaccine of choice, unless contraindicated, because the parenteral inactivated vaccine causes substantially more adverse reactions and is no more effective than the Ty21a or Vi CPS vaccines.

Indications. In the United States, vaccination is recommended only for the following:
- ***Travelers to areas where a risk of exposure to*** S typhi ***is recognized.*** Risk is greatest for travelers to developing countries, especially Latin American, Asia, and Africa, who have prolonged exposure to contaminated food and drink. Such travelers need to be cautioned that typhoid vaccine is not a substitute for careful selection of food and drink.
- ***Persons with intimate exposure to a documented typhoid fever carrier,*** such as occurs with continued household contact.
- ***Laboratory workers with frequent contact with*** S typhi. The vaccine is not recommended for persons attending rural summer camps, those in areas of natural disaster (eg, floods), control of common-source outbreaks, or for sewage sanitation workers in the United States. Worldwide, it is indicated only for persons living in typhoid-endemic areas.

Dosages. For primary vaccination, the following for each vaccine is recommended:
- ***Oral Ty21a vaccine.*** Children (6 years of age and older) and adults should take one enteric-coated capsule every 2 days for a total of four capsules. Each capsule should be taken with cool liquid, no warmer than 37°C, approximately 1 hour before meals. The capsules must be kept refrigerated and all four doses must be taken to achieve maximal efficacy.
- ***Vi capsular polysaccharide vaccine.*** Primary vaccination of persons 2 years of age and older with Vi CPS consists of one 0.5 mL (25 µg) dose administered intramuscularly.

Table 3.52. Commercially Available Typhoid Vaccines Available in the United States

Typhoid	Type	Route	Minimum Age of Receipt, y	No. of Doses*	Booster Frequency, y	Side Effects (Incidence)
Ty21a	Live-attenuated	Oral	6	4	5	<5%
Vi CPS	Polysaccharide	Intramuscular	2	1	2	<7%
Heat-phenol inactivated	Killed whole-cell	Subcutaneous	0.5	2	3	<35%

* Primary vaccination. For further information on dosage, schedules, and adverse events, see text.

- *Parenteral inactivated vaccine.* Vaccination consists of two doses given subcutaneously at an interval of 4 weeks or longer. For those 10 years of age and older, the dose is 0.5 mL; for those less than 10 years of age, it is 0.25 mL. If time is insufficient for administration of two doses of vaccine at an interval of 4 weeks or longer, three doses of the parenteral vaccine at weekly intervals are given. However, this schedule may be less effective.

Booster Doses. In circumstances of continued or repeated exposure to *S typhi*, booster doses are recommended to maintain immunity after primary vaccination.

The optimal booster schedule for persons who have received the oral Ty21a vaccine has not been determined. Continued efficacy for 5 years after vaccination has been demonstrated; however, the manufacturer of Ty21a vaccine recommends revaccination with the entire four-dose series every 5 years if continued or renewed exposure to *S typhi* is expected. This recommendation may change as more data become available on the duration of protection from the Ty21a vaccination.

The manufacturer of Vi CPS recommends a booster dose every 2 years after the primary dose if continued or renewed exposure is expected.

If the parenteral inactivated vaccine is used initially, booster doses should be administered every 3 years if continued or renewed exposure is expected. A single booster dose of parenteral inactivated vaccine is sufficient, even if more than 3 years have elapsed since the prior vaccination.

No data have been reported concerning the use of one vaccine as a booster after primary vaccination with a different vaccine. However, using the primary series of four doses of the oral Ty21a vaccine or one dose of Vi CPS as a booster for persons previously vaccinated with parenteral vaccine is a reasonable alternative to administration of a parenteral booster dose.

Adverse Events. Ty21a produces minimal, if any, adverse reactions. In placebo-controlled trials, adverse reactions occurred with equal frequency among groups receiving vaccine and placebo. Reported side effects have included abdominal discomfort, nausea, vomiting, fever, headache, and rash or urticaria.

Reported adverse events from Vi CPS also are minimal; they include fever (0% to 1%), headache (1.5% to 3%), and local reaction of erythema or induration of 1 cm or greater (7%).

Parenteral, inactivated vaccines can produce several systemic and local adverse reactions, including fever (7% to 24%), headache (9% to 10%), and severe local pain and/or swelling (3% to 35%). Because of adverse reactions, 21% to 23% of those vaccinated missed school or work. More severe reactions have been reported sporadically, including hypotension, chest pain, and shock.

Contraindications and Precautions. The only contraindication to administration of one of the parenteral typhoid vaccinations is a history of severe local or systemic reactions after a previous dose. No data have been reported for any of the three typhoid vaccines in pregnant women. Since oral vaccine is a live-attenuated vaccine, it should not be administered to immunocompromised persons, including those known to be infected with HIV. Because the antimalarial drug mefloquine can inhibit the growth of the live Ty21a strain in vitro, vaccination with Ty21a vaccine should be delayed for at least 24 hours before or after a dose of this drug. The vaccine manufacturer advises that Ty21a vaccine should not be administered to persons receiving sulfonamides or other antimicrobial agents until 24 hours or more after a dose.

No data exist on the immunogenicity of Ty21a vaccine when administered concurrently or within 4 weeks of other vaccines. In the absence of such data, if typhoid vaccination is warranted, it should not be delayed because of the administration of other vaccines.

Scabies

CLINICAL MANIFESTATIONS: The disease manifests as an intensely pruritic, erythematous, papular eruption caused by burrowing of adult female mites in the epidermis. Itching is most intense at night. In older children and adults, the sites of predilection are the interdigital folds, flexor aspects of the wrists, extensor surfaces of the elbows, anterior axillary folds, belt line, thighs, navel, penis, areolae, abdomen, intergluteal cleft, and buttocks. In infants younger than 2 years, the eruption is often vesicular and is likely to occur on the head, neck, palms, and soles, but these areas are usually spared in older children and adults. The eruption is caused by the immature stages of the mite and a hypersensitivity reaction to the proteins of the parasite which form a short distance behind the location of the burrowing mite.

The characteristic scabietic burrow appears as a gray or white, tortuous, threadlike line. Most burrows are obliterated by scratching long before a patient is seen by a physician. Excoriations are common. Occasionally, 2- to 5-mm red-brown nodules are present, particularly on covered parts of the body such as the genitalia, groin, and axilla. These scabietic nodules are a granulomatous response to the dead mite antigens and feces, and can persist for weeks and even months after effective treatment. Cutaneous secondary bacterial infection can occur, caused most commonly by *Streptococcus pyogenes* and *Staphylococcus aureus*.

Norwegian scabies is an uncommon form of infestation characterized by intense infestation and widespread crusted hyperkeratotic lesions. It occurs usually in debilitated, developmentally disabled, or immunologically impaired persons.

ETIOLOGY: The mite *Sarcoptes scabiei* subsp *hominis* is the cause of the disease. *Sarcoptes scabiei* subsp *canis*, acquired from dogs, can cause a self-limited and mild infestation, usually in the area in direct contact with the infested animal.

EPIDEMIOLOGY: Humans are the source of the infection. Transmission occurs most often by close personal contact. Infection acquired from dogs and other animals is uncommon. Minimum contact with a patient with crusted scabies (Norwegian) can result in transmission because of the large number of mites in the exfoliating scales. Scabies can be transmitted as long as the patient remains infected and untreated, including the interval before symptoms develop. Scabies occurs worldwide in cycles thought to be 15 to 30 years long. Scabies affects persons from all socioeconomic levels without regard to age, sex, or standards of personal hygiene. Scabies is endemic in many countries.

The **incubation period** in persons without previous exposure is usually 4 to 6 weeks. Persons who were previously infested and are already sensitized develop symptoms 1 to 4 days after repeat exposure to the mite, but these reinfestations are usually milder.

DIAGNOSTIC TESTS: Diagnosis is confirmed by identification of the mite, the mites' eggs or scybala (feces) from skin scrapings of intact burrows, or papules from sites of predilection. Mineral oil, microscope immersion oil, or water applied to the skin facilitates collection of scrapings. A No. 15 scalpel is used to scrape along the entire length of the burrow (the mite is often found at one end of the burrow), and the scrapings and oil are placed on a slide under a cover slip and examined microscopically under low power.

TREATMENT: Infested children and adults should apply lotion or cream containing a scabicide over the entire body below the head. Because scabies can affect the head, scalp, and neck in infants and young toddlers, treatment of the entire head, neck, and body in this age group is required. The drug of choice, particularly for infants, young children, and pregnant or nursing women, is 5% permethrin, a synthetic pyrethroid (Elimite). Alternative drugs are lindane (Kwell, Scabene) and 10% crotamiton (Eurax). Permethrin should be removed by bathing after 8 to 14 hours, lindane after 8 to 12 hours, and crotamiton after 48 hours. Crotamiton is applied once a day for 2 to 5 days, but it is associated with frequent treatment failures. Ivermectin in a single dose administered orally is effective in the treatment of severe or Norwegian scabies and should be considered for patients whose infection is refractory to topical therapy. The drug is not approved for use by the Food and Drug Administration, but can be obtained from the manufacturer.*

The frequency of lindane applications should not exceed that recommended in order to avoid the possibility of neurologic toxicity from absorption through the skin. Lindane should be used cautiously in young infants and pregnant women.

Because scabietic lesions are the result of a hypersensitivity reaction to the mite, itching may not subside for several weeks despite successful treatment. The use of oral antihistamines and topical corticosteroids can help relieve symptoms.

Antibacterial therapy is indicated for secondary bacterial infections of the excoriated lesions.

* Merck and Co, West Point, Pa.

ISOLATION OF THE HOSPITALIZED PATIENT*: Contact precautions are recommended until the patient has been treated with an appropriate scabicide.

CONTROL MEASURES:
- Prophylactic therapy is recommended for household members. Manifestations of scabies infestation can appear as late as 2 months after exposure, during which time patients can transmit scabies. All members of the household should be treated at the same time to prevent reinfection. Bedding and clothing worn next to the skin during the 4 days before initiation of therapy should be laundered in a washer with hot water and dried using a hot drying cycle. The parasites do not survive more than 3 to 4 days without skin contact. Clothing that cannot be laundered should be removed from the patient and stored for several days to a week to avoid reinfestation.
- Children should be allowed to return to child care or school after treatment has been completed.
- Epidemics and localized outbreaks may require stringent and consistent measures to treat contacts. Caretakers who have had prolonged skin-to-skin contact with infested patients may benefit from prophylactic treatment.
- Environmental disinfestation is unnecessary and unwarranted. Thorough vacuuming of environmental surfaces, however, is recommended following use of a room by a patient with Norwegian scabies.
- Persons with crusted scabies and their close contacts must be treated promptly and aggressively to avoid outbreaks.

Schistosomiasis

CLINICAL MANIFESTATIONS: Initial entry of the infecting larvae (cercariae) through the skin is frequently accompanied by a transient, pruritic papular rash (cercarial dermatitis). After penetration, the organism enters the bloodstream, migrates through the lungs, and ultimately lodges in the venous plexus, draining either the intestines or the bladder (depending on the *Schistosoma* species). Four to 8 weeks after exposure, an acute illness can develop, manifested by fever, malaise, cough, rash, abdominal pain, diarrhea, nausea, lymphadenopathy, and eosinophilia (Katayama fever). In acute infections with heavy infestation due to *S mansoni* or *S japonicum*, a mucoid, bloody diarrhea accompanied by tender hepatomegaly occurs. The severity of symptoms associated with chronic disease is related to the worm burden. Individuals with low to moderate worm burdens can be asymptomatic; heavily infected individuals can have a range of symptoms caused primarily by inflammation and fibrosis triggered by eggs produced by adult worms. Portal hypertension can develop and cause hepatosplenomegaly, ascites, and esophageal varices. Chronic involvement of the colon produces abdominal pain and bloody diarrhea. Other organ systems can be involved from eggs embolized, eg, to the lungs causing pulmonary hypertension or to the central nervous system, notably the spinal cord in *S mansoni* or *S haematobium* infections. In *S haematobium* infections, the bladder becomes

---

* In addition to standard precautions.

inflamed and fibrotic. Symptoms include dysuria, urgency, terminal microscopic and gross hematuria, secondary urinary tract infections, and nonspecific pelvic pain.

Swimmer's itch (cercarial dermatitis) is caused by the larvae of other avian and mammalian schistosome species that penetrate human skin but do not complete the life cycle and do not cause chronic fibrotic disease. Manifestations include mild to moderate pruritus at the penetration site a few hours after exposure, followed in 5 to 14 days by an intermittent pruritic, sometimes papular, eruption. In previously sensitized individuals, more intense papular eruptions may occur for 7 to 10 days after exposure.

ETIOLOGY: The trematodes (flukes) *Schistosoma mansoni, S japonicum, S haematobium,* and, rarely, *S mekongi* and *S intercalatum* cause the disease. All species have similar life cycles. Swimmer's itch is caused by multiple avian and mammalian species of *S bilharziella.*

EPIDEMIOLOGY: Humans are the principal hosts for the major species. Persistence of schistosomiasis depends on the presence of an appropriate snail as an intermediate host. Eggs excreted in stool (*S mansoni* and *S japonicum*) or urine (*S haematobium*) into fresh water hatch into motile miracidia, which infect snails. After development in the snails, cercariae emerge and penetrate the skin of humans encountered in the water. Children are frequently infected after infancy when they begin to explore the environment.

Schistosoma mansoni occurs throughout tropical Africa, in several Caribbean islands including Puerto Rico, and in Venezuela, Brazil, Suriname, and the Arabian peninsula. *Schistosoma japonicum* is found in China, the Philippines, and Indonesia. *Schistosoma haematobium* occurs in Africa and the eastern Mediterranean region. *Schistosoma mekongi* is limited to a small area of the Mekong delta in southeast Asia (Kampuchea and Laos). *Schistosoma intercalatum* is found in Central Africa. Children are frequently involved in transmission because of habits of uncontrolled defecation, urination, and frequent wading in infected waters. Communicability lasts as long as live eggs are excreted in the urine and feces. Adult worms of the *S mansoni* species have been documented to live as long as 26 years in the human host. Thus, schistosomiasis can be diagnosed in patients many years after they have left the endemic areas.

Swimmer's itch occurs in all regions of the world after exposure to fresh, brackish, or salt water.

The **incubation period** is unknown.

DIAGNOSTIC TESTS: Infection with *S mansoni* and other species (except *S haematobium*) is determined by microscopic examination of concentrated stool specimens to detect characteristic eggs. In light infections, several specimens may have to be examined before eggs are found and a biopsy of the rectal mucosa may be necessary. The fresh tissue obtained should be compressed between two glass slides and examined under low power (unstained) for eggs. *Schistosoma haematobium* is diagnosed by examining filtered urine for eggs. Egg excretion peaks often between noon and 3 pm. Biopsy of the bladder mucosa may be necessary. Serologic tests are available through the Centers for Disease Control and Prevention and some commercial laboratories, and may be particularly helpful in detecting light infections.

Swimmer's itch can be difficult to differentiate from other causes of dermatitis. A skin biopsy may demonstrate larvae but their absence does not exclude the diagnosis.

TREATMENT: The drug of choice for schistosomiasis caused by any species is praziquantel; the alternative drug for *S mansoni* is oxamniquine.* No satisfactory alternative drug for *S japonicum* is available.

Swimmer's itch is a self-limited disease that requires only symptomatic treatment of the urticarial rash.

ISOLATION OF THE HOSPITALIZED PATIENT: Standard precautions are recommended.

CONTROL MEASURES: Elimination of the intermediate snail host is difficult to achieve in most areas. Thus, treatment of infected populations, sanitary disposal of human waste, and education about the source of infection are the key elements of current control measures. Travelers to endemic areas should be advised to avoid contact with freshwater streams and lakes.

Shigella Infections

CLINICAL MANIFESTATIONS: In mild infections, manifestations consist of watery or loose stools for several days, with minimal or no constitutional symptoms. Abrupt onset of fever, systemic toxic effects, headache, and profuse watery diarrhea occur in patients with small-bowel infection. Convulsions can occur. Abdominal cramps, tenderness, tenesmus, and mucoid stools with or without blood characterize large-bowel disease (bacillary dysentery). Rare sequelae include bacteremia, Reiter's syndrome (after *Shigella flexneri* infection), hemolytic-uremic syndrome (from *Shigella dysenteriae* type 1 infection), colonic perforation, and fulminant toxic encephalopathy (ekiri) which can be lethal within 4 to 48 hours of onset.

ETIOLOGY: *Shigella* organisms are Gram-negative bacilli in the family Enterobacteriaceae. Four species (of more than 40 serotypes) have been identified. *S sonnei* currently accounts for more than half the cases in the United States and *S flexneri* accounts for a large percentage of the remainder. *S dysenteriae* type 1 (the Shiga bacillus) is rare in the United States but widespread in rural Africa and the Indian subcontinent. *S boydii* is uncommon in the United States.

EPIDEMIOLOGY: Feces of infected humans are the source of infection. No animal reservoir is known. Predisposing factors include crowded living conditions, low hygienic standards, closed population groups with substandard environmental sanitation (eg, residential homes for retarded children), and travel to countries with low standards of food sanitation. Because transmission of *Shigella* can occur following ingestion of a small inoculum, fecal-oral transmission from person-to-person contact is the common route by which children are infected. Other modes of transmission include ingestion of contaminated food or water, homosexual activity, and contact with a contaminated, inanimate object. Houseflies are also vectors, causing physical transport of infected feces. Infection is most common in children 1 to 4 years of age

---

* Available from Pfizer, Inc, New York, NY.

and is an important problem in child care centers in the United States. Communicability exists until the organism is no longer present in feces. Even without antimicrobial therapy, the convalescent carrier state usually ceases within 4 weeks of the onset of illness. A chronic carrier state (>1 year) is rare.

The **incubation period** varies from 1 to 7 days but is usually 2 to 4 days.

DIAGNOSTIC TESTS: Cultures of feces or rectal swab specimens containing feces should be performed. Blood should be cultured only in severely ill, immunocompromised or malnourished patients, because bacteremia is rare. A stool smear stained with methylene blue may disclose polymorphonuclear leukocytes and/or erythrocytes, a finding indicative of enterocolitis, which is consistent with but not specific for *Shigella* infection.

TREATMENT:
- Antimicrobial therapy is effective in shortening the duration of diarrhea and eliminating organisms from feces and is recommended for all patients with bacillary dysentery. Small-bowel disease is often self-limited, lasting 48 to 72 hours, but may progress to dysentery. In cases of mild illness, the primary indication for treatment is to prevent further spread of the organism.
- Antimicrobial susceptibility testing of clinical isolates is indicated because resistance to antimicrobial agents is common. Plasmid-mediated, multiple antimicrobial resistance has been identified in all *Shigella* species.
- For cases in which susceptibility is unknown or an ampicillin-resistant strain is isolated, the drug of choice is trimethoprim-sulfamethoxazole. Patients infected with strains that are resistant to trimethoprim-sulfamethoxazole should be treated with cefixime, ceftriaxone, cefotaxime, ciprofloxacin, or ofloxacin. The latter two are not recommended for use in persons younger than 18 years (see Antimicrobials and Related Therapy, p 605). For susceptible strains, ampicillin is effective; amoxicillin is less effective for treatment of *Shigella* infections. The oral route of therapy is acceptable except in seriously ill patients.
- Antimicrobial therapy should be administered for 5 days.
- Antidiarrheal compounds that inhibit intestinal peristalsis are contraindicated because they may prolong the clinical and bacteriologic course of disease.

ISOLATION OF THE HOSPITALIZED PATIENT*: Contact precautions are indicated in diapered and/or incontinent children for the duration of illness.

CONTROL MEASURES:

Child Care. General measures for interrupting enteric transmission (especially hand washing) in child care centers are recommended (see Children in Out-of-Home Child Care, p 80). Hand washing is the single most important measure to decrease transmission rates.

When *Shigella* infection is identified in a child care attendee or staff member, stool specimens from other symptomatic attendees and staff members should be cultured. Stool specimens from household contacts who have diarrhea also should

---

* In addition to standard precautions.

be cultured. All symptomatic persons in whom *Shigella* organisms are isolated from stool should receive antimicrobial therapy (see Treatment, p 473) and should not be permitted to reenter the program until the diarrhea has ceased. If several persons are infected, a cohort system should be considered until stool cultures are negative. To prevent spread of the infection, efforts should be made to prevent the transfer of children to other child care centers.

General Control Measures. Strict attention to hand washing is essential to limit spread. Other important control measures include sanitary water supply, food processing, and sewage disposal; exclusion of infected persons as food handlers; prevention of contamination of food by flies; and case reporting to appropriate health authorities (eg, hospital infection control officer and public health department).

Vaccination. No vaccine currently is available commercially.

Sporotrichosis

CLINICAL MANIFESTATIONS: Sporotrichosis presents most commonly as a cutaneous infection. Skin infection usually occurs at a site of minor trauma, causing an ulcerative subcutaneous nodule that is firm and slightly tender. Although infection can remain localized, the primary infection in most cases spreads along local lymphatic channels to form multiple nodules that ulcerate and suppurate (lymphocutaneous sporotrichosis).

Extracutaneous sporotrichosis most commonly affects the bones and joints, particularly those of the hand, elbow, ankle, and knee. Pulmonary sporotrichosis clinically resembles tuberculosis. It can occur in healthy persons, usually in middle-aged men who are either alcoholic, receiving prolonged corticosteroid therapy, or have an underlying medical condition such as tuberculosis, diabetes mellitus, or sarcoidosis. Disseminated sporotrichosis has been reported to involve a variety of organ systems (eg, ocular, genitourinary, or central nervous system) and occurs predominantly in immunocompromised patients.

ETIOLOGY: *Sporothrix schenckii* is a dimorphic fungus that grows as an oval- or cigar-shaped yeast at 37°C.

EPIDEMIOLOGY: *Sporothrix schenckii* is a ubiquitous organism that is most common in tropical and subtropical regions of Central and South America. In the United States, it is found predominantly in the Midwest. The fungus is isolated from soil and plants, including hay, straw, thorny plants (especially roses), and sphagnum moss. Cutaneous disease generally occurs secondary to inoculation of debris into a wound. As a result, persons engaging in occupations such as gardening or farming are at increased risk for infection. Inhalation of spores can lead to pulmonary disease. Rarely, transmission from infected cats has lead to cutaneous disease.

The **incubation period** is 7 to 30 days after cutaneous inoculation, but has been reported to be as long as 6 months.

DIAGNOSTIC TESTS: A positive culture from tissue, wound drainage, or sputum is usually diagnostic of infection. Histopathology can be helpful; however, the organism is difficult to detect in biopsy samples. No standardized serologic test is available.

TREATMENT: Sporotrichosis can resolve spontaneously in several months to years, but treatment is usually indicated. The treatment of choice for cutaneous disease is a saturated solution of potassium iodide (SSKI) given orally until several weeks after all lesions are healed. Significant side effects include gastrointestinal symptoms, rhinorrhea, and rash and are common. Amphotericin B has been recommended for patients who are intolerant of SSKI, have iodide sensitivity, fail therapy with SSKI, or have extracutaneous disease. A satisfactory rate of clinical responses and a low incidence of side effects has led some experts to recommend itraconazole as the drug of choice for both cutaneous and extracutaneous disease; however, no controlled studies to document its efficacy have been reported and safety of this drug in children has not been established. Osteoarticular, pulmonary, or disseminated infection responds less well than cutaneous infection to either amphotericin B or itraconazole, despite prolonged therapy. Surgical therapy may be necessary to achieve resolution of skeletal and cavitary pulmonary disease.

ISOLATION OF HOSPITALIZED PATIENTS: Standard precautions are indicated.

CONTROL MEASURES: Eliminating exposure to the organism through the use of protective gloves and clothing in occupational and avocational activities associated with infection can reduce the risk of disease.

Staphylococcal Food Poisoning

CLINICAL MANIFESTATIONS: Staphylococcal food poisoning is characterized by the abrupt onset of severe abdominal cramps, nausea and vomiting, diarrhea, and, occasionally, low-grade fever. The short incubation period, brevity of illness, and usual lack of fever help distinguish staphylococcal food poisoning from other types of food poisoning, except that caused by *Bacillus cereus*. Chemical food poisoning usually has a shorter incubation period. *Clostridium perfringens* food poisoning usually has a longer incubation period and infrequently is accompanied by vomiting, which is common in staphylococcal and B cereus food poisoning. Patients with food-borne *Salmonella* or *Shigella* infection often have fever, and a longer incubation period.

ETIOLOGY: The cause of staphylococcal food poisoning is enterotoxins produced by strains of *Staphylococcus aureus* and, rarely, *Staphylococcus epidermidis*. Of the eight immunologically distinct heat-stable enterotoxins (A, B, C1-3, D, E, and F), enterotoxins A and D are the most common in the United States. Enterotoxin F is identical with the toxin associated with toxic shock syndrome (TSST-1) and has not been implicated in outbreaks of food poisoning.

EPIDEMIOLOGY: Illness is caused by preformed toxin present in food containing enterotoxicogenic staphylococci. Contamination is usually by food handlers who may be healthy but colonized with this organism. Food products most commonly involved include ham, poultry, filled pastries, and egg and potato salads. The disease is not transmissible from person to person.

The **incubation period** is from 30 minutes to 6 hours.

DIAGNOSTIC TESTS: Diagnosis in an outbreak is made by isolation of the same phage types or pulsed-field gel electrophoresis types of *S aureus* from stools or vomitus of affected persons, the implicated food, and the food handler responsible for contaminating the food. Lesions on the hands of food handlers may be the source of contamination and should be cultured. Other possible sources that should be cultured include nose, throat, and rectum. The vomitus and stools of patients may contain the offending *S aureus* species and also should be cultured. Identification of enterotoxin or staphylococcal organisms in incriminated foods can be performed by the Food and Drug Administration. Pulsed-field gel electrophoresis and subtyping of staphylococcal isolates can be performed by the Centers for Disease Control and Prevention.

TREATMENT: Antibiotics are not indicated.

ISOLATION OF THE HOSPITALIZED PATIENT: Standard precautions are recommended.

CONTROL MEASURES: Optimum cooking and refrigeration of foods, particularly meat, dairy, and bakery products, will help to prevent the disease. Cooked foods should be immediately cooled and refrigerated at temperatures less than 5°C (41°F). Food handlers with staphylococcal infections should be excluded from food preparation and food handling.

Staphylococcal Infections

CLINICAL MANIFESTATIONS: *Staphylococcus aureus* causes a wide variety of suppurative infections, ranging from localized to invasive diseases. Localized diseases include furuncles, impetigo (bullous and nonbullous), and wound infections. *Staphylococcus aureus* is a leading cause of impetigo. Suppurative and/or invasive infections include septicemia, osteomyelitis, arthritis, endocarditis, and pneumonia. Meningitis is rare. *Staphylococcus aureus* also causes toxin-mediated diseases, such as toxic shock syndrome (see Staphylococcal Toxic Shock Syndrome, p 481), scalded skin syndrome, and food poisoning (see Staphylococcal Food Poisoning, p 475). Most staphylococcal abscesses and toxin-related diseases are caused by *S aureus*. Methicillin-resistant *S aureus* strains are not more virulent than methicillin-susceptible *S aureus* strains, but the former may be more difficult to treat because of multiple antimicrobial resistance and resulting limited therapeutic drug choices.

Coagulase-negative staphylococci, primarily *Staphylococcus epidermidis*, cause bacteremia in premature infants and immunocompromised patients and frequently cause infections of vascular access devices, cerebrospinal fluid shunts, and prosthetic heart valves. Coagulase-negative staphylococci also can cause urinary tract infections, especially in adolescent females.

ETIOLOGY: Staphylococci are Gram-positive cocci that appear microscopically as grapelike clusters. Staphylococci multiply aerobically and anaerobically; they are resistant to temperatures as high as 50°C (122°F), to high salt concentrations, and to drying; and they can survive on clothing and in dust.

Coagulase-negative staphylococci are classified in 11 species. Most infections are caused by *S epidermidis*. Slime production by *S epidermidis* is associated with invasiveness. *Staphylococcus saprophyticus* causes urinary tract infections.

EPIDEMIOLOGY: *Staphylococcus aureus* is ubiquitous. Strains can be part of the normal human flora, and they colonize the anterior nares and moist body areas in approximately 30% of humans. Persons who have skin or draining staphylococcal lesions are contagious. Carriers also can transmit staphylococci. Infants who have been colonized while in the nursery can be the source of disease spread in the family. The recent increase in community-acquired methicillin-resistant *S aureus* (MRSA) is most likely the result of transmission from persons who acquired MRSA while in the hospital. Person-to-person transmission is the usual mode of spread, occurring via the hands, nasal discharge or droplets. Communicability occurs for as long as lesions or the carrier state persist.

Coagulase-negative staphylococci are ubiquitous on skin and mucosal surfaces. Person-to-person spread is the common mode of transmission. Infection usually is the result of invasion by a person's endogenous strain. Foreign bodies, such as shunts, intravascular catheters, or prosthetic heart valves, predispose to infection with coagulase-negative staphylococci and with *S aureus*.

For bullous impetigo and the scalded skin syndrome, the **incubation period** is usually 1 to 10 days. For other staphylococcal infections, the incubation period is extremely variable. A long delay can occur between acquisition of the organism and the onset of disease.

DIAGNOSTIC TESTS: Gram-stained smears of material from lesions can provide presumptive evidence of infection. Isolation of organisms by culture of blood, tissue, pleural fluid, bone, or lesions is definitive. The positive coagulase test or mannitol fermentation differentiates *S aureus* from coagulase-negative staphylococci. When clusters of infections occur, examination of antimicrobial susceptibility, plasmid typing, phage-type patterns, or pulsed-field gel electrophoresis (PFGE) of the isolated strains may help determine the source of the outbreak. The PFGE is the most reliable method to detect identical strains. Antimicrobial susceptibility tests of isolates always should be performed.

TREATMENT:

Staphylococcus aureus.

- Serious infections require intravenous therapy with a penicillinase-resistant penicillin, such as nafcillin or oxacillin, because most *S aureus* strains either in the community or in hospitals produce penicillinase and are resistant to penicillin and ampicillin. First- or second-generation cephalosporins (eg, cephalothin or cefuroxime) and clindamycin also are effective. The expanded spectrum (third-generation) cephalosporins usually are not as active in vitro against *S aureus*, and some may be ineffective in some infections. Patients who are allergic to penicillin can be treated with a cephalosporin (if the patient is not also allergic to cephalosporin, which is the case in 5% to 10% of patients), clindamycin or vancomycin. For *S aureus* strains resistant to the penicillinase-resistant penicillins (ie, MRSA), intravenous vancomycin is indicated. Although all *S aureus* strains are susceptible to vancomycin, a penicillinase-resistant penicillin (methicillin or oxacillin) should be used for susceptible strains rather than vancomycin to minimize the emergence of vancomycin-resistant strains.
- Duration of therapy for serious, invasive infections depends upon the site of infection and is usually 3 weeks or more. After the initial parenteral therapy and clinical response of the patient, completion of the recommended antimicrobial course with an oral drug can be considered if good compliance and therapeutic blood concentrations of the antimicrobial agent can be assured. **The exception to this recommendation is endocarditis.**
- Drainage of abscesses is desirable and usually required.
- Skin and soft-tissue infections, such as impetigo or cellulitis due to *S aureus*, usually can be treated with oral penicillinase-resistant ß-lactam drugs, such as cloxacillin, dicloxacillin, or a first- or second-generation cephalosporin. For localized, superficial skin lesions, topical antibacterial therapy with mupirocin or bacitracin and local hygiene may be sufficient. When a patient or health care worker is found to be a chronic carrier of *S aureus*, including MRSA, topical mupirocin therapy may be effective in eradicating carriage. Although an increasing number of MRSA strains are resistant in vitro to mupirocin, concentrations used topically (2% or 20 000 µg/mL) are high enough to be effective even for these strains.

Coagulase-Negative Staphylococci.

- Serious infections require intravenous therapy with an antimicrobial agent. Almost all strains that cause infections are resistant to penicillin, and methicillin-resistant strains are common, especially in nosocomial infections. If the strain is susceptible to methicillin, a semisynthetic penicillinase-resistant penicillin, such as nafcillin or oxacillin, should be used. If the strain is resistant to methicillin, vancomycin is indicated. Rifampin and gentamicin also are effective, but rapid emergence of resistance necessitates that they always be used in combination with a penicillinase-resistant penicillin or vancomycin. Use of either gentamicin or rifampin in combination with vancomycin may increase antibacterial activity (ie, synergy). Intravenous vancomycin should be considered for the initial treatment of all severe infections caused by coagulase-negative staphylococci.

- Removal of associated foreign bodies and drainage of abscesses is desirable and usually required.

Endocarditis can be caused by either *S aureus* or, in patients with prosthetic cardiac valves, coagulase-negative staphylococci. Guidelines for antimicrobial therapy of endocarditis in adults caused by either *S aureus* or coagulase-negative staphylococci have been formulated by the American Heart Association and should be consulted for regimens that may be appropriate for children.*

ISOLATION OF THE HOSPITALIZED PATIENT: For patients with exposed lesions (eg, draining wounds, scalded skin syndrome, bullous impetigo, and abscesses), contact precautions should be implemented for the duration of illness.[†] Standard precautions are recommended for patients with staphylococcal bacteremia and meningitis. For patients with *S aureus* pneumonia, droplet precautions are recommended for the first 24 hours of antimicrobial therapy.[†]

Patients infected or colonized with MRSA should be managed with contact precautions for the duration of illness because the carriage usually persists for weeks to months.[†]

CONTROL MEASURES:
- Maximum precautions to avoid transmission of staphylococci via hands and clothing of personnel should be routine in hospitals. Because the most important route of staphylococcal transmission is the hands of hospital personnel, **careful hand washing before and after every patient contact is mandatory.**
- Routinely obtaining specimens for culture from hospital personnel is not recommended. However, identification of carriers who disseminate a strain that has been implicated in epidemic disease in a closed population is helpful. Consideration should be given to removing carriers from areas of patient contact and treating them with topical intranasal antimicrobial agents, such as mupirocin and, in some instances, with appropriate orally administered antimicrobial agents. The goal of therapy in this instance is to eliminate carriage of an epidemiologically virulent strain. The carrier state can be difficult to eradicate.
- Infection control measures for the prevention of neonatal *S aureus* disease and outbreak include the following:
  — Application of triple dye or bacitracin ointment to the umbilical stump of all infants as soon as possible after delivery or immediately after umbilical vessel catheterization can also be helpful. Many years of experience support the routine use of triple dye in term infants. In unusual circumstances, treatment with oral antistaphylococcal agents of all infants and personnel who are carriers may be neccessary.
  — Hexachlorophene should not be used for routine bathing because systemic absorption can result in adverse central nervous system reactions. Endemic MRSA strains have been eradicated without the use of hexachlorophene.

---

* Wilson WR, Karchmer AW, Dajani AS, et al. Antibiotic treatment of adults with infective endocarditis due to streptococci, enterococci, and staphylococci. *JAMA*. 1995;274:1706-1713.
[†] In addition to standard precautions.

— Surveillance of recently discharged infants for infections should be performed, because observation for disease in neonates, both in the nursery and at home for several weeks, is the most reliable indicator of *S aureus* outbreaks. Infections with *S aureus* that occur within the first two weeks after discharge from the nursery should be reported to the nursery and infection control staff.

• Epidemic *S aureus* disease in newborn nurseries presents special problems. Recommendations include the following:

— Overcrowding and understaffing should be alleviated because these conditions perpetuate *S aureus* transmission.

— Contact precautions should be used in the care of infants with definite or suspected staphylococcal disease. Cohorting of infants and staff should be instituted in the affected nursery so nursery personnel are not in contact with both colonized and noncolonized infants during any one work shift. In addition, all colonized or exposed infants in a room should be discharged and the room carefully cleaned before new infants are admitted to that room. Staff, especially nursing staff, caring for one cohort should not care for another cohort when more than one patient cohort is present. Visiting staff (eg, radiology personnel, laboratory technicians, and consulting physicians) should be instructed to start their tasks or examinations with uninfected infants and finish their activities with infected infants to minimize transmission.

— Meticulous infection control techniques for patient contact, including careful hand washing by personnel, should be reemphasized. During an outbreak, hand-washing soaps containing antimicrobial agents are preferred.

— During outbreaks, specimens for culture should be obtained from the umbilicus and anterior nares of infants and the nares and hands of personnel to determine the prevalence of colonization and to identify the staphylococcal strains involved in the outbreak. These strains should be tested to determine if they are the same strain (see Diagnostic Tests, p 477). If the strains are identical, measures to find a common source should be instituted. If the strains are different, measures to prevent importation of pathogens should be considered.

— Occasionally, personnel colonized with the outbreak strain will need to be removed from patient contact until carriage has been eliminated.

— Surveillance in the nursery should be continued after the epidemic has terminated.

— Persons involved in hospital outbreaks should be observed and warned of the possibility of delayed disease and the potential for spread to family members.

• To minimize the risk of emergence of vancomycin-resistant enterococci, routine use of low-dose vancomycin infusions for prevention of vascular catheter infections caused by coagulase-negative staphylococcus is **not** recommended.

Staphylococcal Toxic Shock Syndrome

CLINICAL MANIFESTATIONS: Toxic shock syndrome (TSS) is an acute febrile illness characterized by fever, hypotension, a diffuse macular erythroderma that desquamates, mucous membrane hyperemia, myalgia, and multiorgan system involvement, and can be fatal. The erythematous, sunburn-like rash occurs during the acute phase, with desquamation of the skin, especially of the palms and soles, 7 to 10 days later. Other organ systems that can be affected include renal (abnormal urinalysis and renal function tests), hepatic (elevated serum transaminase and bilirubin concentrations), hematologic (thrombocytopenia and preponderance of immature and mature neutrophils in peripheral blood), and central nervous system (disorientation or alterations in consciousness without focal neurologic signs).

The case definition established by the Centers for Disease Control and Prevention is based on the following five major diagnostic criteria:
- Fever of 38.9°C (102°F) or higher
- Presence of a diffuse macular erythroderma
- Desquamation 1 to 2 weeks after the onset of illness, particularly of the palms and soles
- Hypotension, defined as a systolic blood pressure of 90 mm Hg or less for adults and less than the fifth percentile for children younger than 16 years; an orthostatic decrease in diastolic blood pressure of 15 mm Hg or more with a position change from lying to sitting; orthostatic syncope; or orthostatic dizziness
- Involvement of three or more of the following organ systems: gastrointestinal tract, muscular, mucous membrane, renal, hepatic, hematologic, and central nervous system.

In addition, if blood and cerebrospinal fluid cultures are obtained, they must be sterile, with the only exception that blood cultures may be positive for *Staphylococcus aureus*. Serologic tests for Rocky Mountain spotted fever, ehrlichiosis, leptospirosis, and measles also, when obtained, must be negative.

Toxic shock syndrome is probable when at least four of the five major criteria are fulfilled. Patients who die before desquamation would have occurred but whose illness is otherwise compatible with TSS are considered definite cases. The syndrome can be confused with Kawasaki disease, scarlet fever, Rocky Mountain spotted fever, ehrlichiosis, meningococcemia, measles, leptospirosis, and other febrile diseases with mucocutaneous manifestation and/or hypotension. Telogen effluvium, including hair thinning or patchy hair loss, and nail splitting, ridging, or loss, frequently occur 1 to 2 months after onset. Neuropsychologic sequelae can occur but appear to be infrequent.

ETIOLOGY: In most patients, the etiologic agent is a TSS toxin-1–producing strain of *S aureus;* however, TSS toxin-1–negative strains of *S aureus* also have been implicated.

EPIDEMIOLOGY: Toxic shock syndrome became widely recognized in 1980, with the documentation of an increased risk of illness among menstruating women who used tampons. Since then, the incidence of cases associated with menstruation and the proportion of TSS associated with menstruation has decreased. Disease occurs in males as well as females. Cases of nonmenstrual TSS have been associated with cutaneous or subcutaneous lesions, childbirth or abortion, surgical wound infections, vaginal infections occurring at times other than during menstruation or the post-partum period, and other sources of focal staphylococcal infection, including sinusitis and pneumonia. The source of infection in some cases may be unknown. Patients considered at risk for TSS include (1) menstruating women using tampons or other inserted vaginal devices; (2) persons (male and female) with focal *S aureus* infection; and (3) women using diaphragms or contraceptive sponges. The case-fatality rate with treatment is 2% to 4%. No evidence of person-to-person transmission or identified common exposures has been found.

The median **incubation period** in cases of postsurgical TSS is 2 days.

DIAGNOSTIC TESTS: Because *S aureus* may be isolated from the anterior nares and vagina of 10% to 30% of healthy persons, and approximately 30% of such strains can produce TSS toxin-1, identification of TSS toxin-1–producing *S aureus* is only presumptive evidence. The diagnosis is made on the basis of clinical criteria (see Clinical Manifestations, p 481).

TREATMENT:
- Management of the hypotensive patient depends on the severity of the illness and its complications. Aggressive intravenous fluid replacement for hypovolemic shock is necessary; in some cases vasopressor agents are required.
- Antistaphylococcal antibiotics are recommended to eradicate the focus of toxin-producing *S aureus* and reduce the risk of a recurrent episode. Antibiotic therapy, however, does not necessarily affect the outcome of the acute illness.
- Any vaginal foreign bodies (eg, tampons and contraceptive sponges) or incision and wound packing (nonmenstrual) should be removed. Infected wounds should be explored and drained, even if the wound does not show prominent signs of inflammation.
- Additional modalities of therapy have been necessary in some patients to correct electrolyte and acid-base imbalance and to manage complications of prolonged shock, acute renal failure, adult respiratory distress syndrome, myocardial failure, and disseminated intravascular coagulation with thrombocytopenia. The use of corticosteroid therapy or intravenous immune globulin in severe cases is of unknown benefit.
- To decrease the risk of recurrence, menstruating patients should not use tampons during subsequent menstrual periods.

ISOLATION OF THE HOSPITALIZED PATIENT: Standard precautions are recommended.

CONTROL MEASURES: None.

Group A Streptococcal Infections

CLINICAL MANIFESTATIONS: The most common clinical illness produced by group A streptococcal (GAS) infection is acute pharyngitis or tonsillitis. Some patients, usually untreated, develop purulent complications, including otitis media, sinusitis, peritonsillar and retropharyngeal abscesses, and suppurative cervical adenitis. The significance of streptococcal upper respiratory tract disease is its acute morbidity and nonsuppurative sequelae, ie, rheumatic fever and acute glomerulo-nephritis. Scarlet fever occurs most commonly in association with pharyngitis, and, rarely, with pyoderma or an infected surgical or traumatic wound. Scarlet fever has a characteristic sandpaper-like rash, which is caused by one or more of the several erythrogenic exotoxins produced by GAS strains. Although rare today, severe scarlet fever with systemic toxicity does occur. Other than the occurrence of rash, the epidemiology, symptoms, sequelae and treatment of scarlet fever are no different from those of streptococcal pharyngitis.

Toddlers (1 to 3 years old) with GAS respiratory tract infection frequently present with moderate fever and seromucoid rhinitis, and may have a protracted illness with fever, irritability, and anorexia. The classic clinical presentation of streptococcal upper respiratory tract infection as pharyngitis is uncommon in children younger than 3 years. Rheumatic fever also is uncommon at this age.

The second most common site of GAS infection is the skin. Streptococcal skin infections (ie, pyoderma or impetigo) can result in glomerulonephritis, which occasionally can occur in epidemics, but rheumatic fever is not a sequela of strep-tococcal pyoderma.

Other infections that GAS can cause include erysipelas, perianal cellulitis, vaginitis, bacteremia, pneumonia, endocarditis, pericarditis, septic arthritis, cellulitis, necrotizing fasciitis, osteomyelitis, myositis, puerperal sepsis, surgical wound infection, and neonatal omphalitis. Necrotizing fasciitis in children most often occurs as a complication of varicella. Bacteremic GAS infections can be severe, with or without an identified focus of local infection, and can be associated with streptococcal toxic shock syndrome. The portal of entry of severe and/or invasive infections is often the skin or soft tissue such as in minor or unrecognized trauma.

The toxic shock syndrome caused by GAS infection is associated with hypotension (shock), renal impairment, coagulopathy (disseminated intravascular coagulation or thrombocytopenia), adult acute respiratory distress syndrome, rash and local tissue destruction, and a fatality rate as high as 70%. The occurrence of shock and multiorgan failure early in the course characterizes streptococcal toxic shock syndrome and helps differentiate it from other invasive GAS infections. A consensus case definition has been proposed by a working group of the Centers for Disease Control and Prevention (CDC) (see Table 3.53, p 484).

ETIOLOGY: More than 80 distinct M-protein types of group A ß-hemolytic strep-tococci (*Streptococcus pyogenes*) have been identified. Epidemiologic studies suggest an association between certain serotypes (eg, types 1, 3, 5, 6, 18, 19, and 24) and rheumatic fever, but a specific "rheumatogenic" factor has not been identified. Several serotypes (eg, 49, 55, and 57) clearly are associated with pyoderma and acute glomerulonephritis. Pharyngitis-associated nephritis is often associated with

Table 3.53. Proposed Case Definition for the Streptococcal Toxic Shock Syndrome*

1. Isolation of group A streptococci
   A) From a normally sterile site (eg, blood, cerebrospinal fluid, peritoneal fluid, tissue biopsy, surgical wound, etc)
   B) From a nonsterile site (eg, throat, superficial skin lesion, etc)
2. Clinical signs of severity
   A) Hypotension: systolic blood pressure ≤90 mm Hg in adults or <5th percentile for age in children

   and

   B) 2 or more of the following signs:
   - Renal impairment: creatinine ≥2 mg/dL for adults or greater than or equal to twice the upper limit of normal for age
   - Coagulopathy: platelets ≤100 000/mm³ or disseminated intravascular coagulation
   - Liver involvement: serum alanine aminotransferase (SGOT), aspartate aminotransferase (SGPT), or total bilirubin concentrations greater than or equal to twice the upper limit of normal for age
   - Adult respiratory distress syndrome
   - A generalized erythematous macular rash that may desquamate
   - Soft-tissue necrosis, including necrotizing fasciitis or myositis, or gangrene

An illness fulfilling criteria 1A and 2 (A and B) can be defined as a *definite* case. An illness fulfilling criteria 1B and 2 (A and B) can be defined as a *probable* case if no other etiology for the illness is identified.

---

* Modified from the Centers for Disease Control and Prevention. The Working Group on Severe Streptococcal Infection. Defining the group A streptococcal toxic shock syndrome: rationale and consensus definition. *JAMA.* 1993;269:390-391.

other serotypes (eg, type 12). Groups C and G streptococci have been associated with pharyngitis, and occasionally nephritis, but do not cause rheumatic fever. The GAS toxic shock syndrome is believed to be a toxin-mediated disease.

EPIDEMIOLOGY: Pharyngitis usually results from contact with a person who has streptococcal pharyngitis. Fomites and household pets such as dogs are not vectors of GAS infection. Transmission of GAS infection, including outbreaks of pharyngitis that occur in schools, almost always follows contact with respiratory secretions. Pharyngitis and impetigo (and as a result their nonsuppurative complications) may be associated with crowding, which is often present in socioeconomically disadvantaged populations. The close contact that occurs in schools, child care and military installations can facilitate transmission. Food-borne outbreaks have occurred and are a consequence of human contamination of food in conjunction with improper preparation or refrigeration procedures.

Streptococcal pharyngitis can occur at any age but it is most common among school-age children. Group A streptococcal pharyngitis and pyoderma are less common in adults than in children except during epidemics.

Geographically, both streptococcal pharyngitis and impetigo are ubiquitous. Impetigo is more common in tropical climates and in warm seasons, presumably in part because of antecedent insect bites and other minor skin trauma. However, impetigo occurs in all climates. Streptococcal pharyngitis occurs more frequently in the late fall, winter, and spring in temperate climates, presumably because of close person-to-person contact indoors that occurs in schools. Communicability of patients with streptococcal pharyngitis is highest during the acute infection, and in untreated individuals gradually diminishes during a period of weeks. Patients are not contagious within 24 hours of the initiation of appropriate antimicrobial therapy.

Throat culture surveys of asymptomatic children during school outbreaks of pharyngitis have yielded streptococcal prevalence rates as high as 15% to 30%. These children include persons with asymptomatic infections and pharyngeal carriers with no immune response to GAS cellular and extracellular antigens. In carriers, the organism may persist for several months but the risk of transmission to others is not appreciable, perhaps because of diminished numbers of organisms in the pharynx or the disappearance of bacteria from nasal secretions.

Incidence rates of rheumatic fever in the United States have decreased for several decades, but outbreaks of rheumatic fever in the 1980s in both school-age children and military personnel in different geographic areas demonstrated that acute rheumatic fever still can occur. Although the reason(s) for these local outbreaks is not clear, their occurrence re-emphasizes the importance of diagnosing GAS pharyngitis and of compliance with the recommended duration of antibiotic therapy.

In streptococcal impetigo, the organism usually is acquired from others with impetigo, possibly by physical contact. Colonization of healthy skin by GAS usually precedes the development of skin infection. Impetiginous lesions occur at the site of open (eg, insect bites or burns) lesions since GAS does not penetrate intact skin. In addition, persons with streptococcal pharyngitis or upper respiratory tract carriage can infect their open lesions or those of others. Following the development of impetiginous lesions, usually the upper respiratory tract becomes colonized. Infections of surgical wounds and postpartum (puerperal) sepsis usually result from contact transmission via hand carriage. At times, anal or vaginal carriers and persons with pyoderma or local suppurative infections can transmit GAS to surgical and obstetrical patients resulting in nosocomial outbreaks. Infections in neonates can result from intrapartum or contact transmission; in the latter situation, infection often begins with omphalitis.

In recent years, the incidence of severe, invasive GAS infections, including bacteremia, streptococcal toxic shock syndrome, and necrotizing fasciitis, has increased. The incidence appears to be highest in the very young and in older persons. Varicella is a significant risk factor in children. Other risk factors include intravenous drug use, HIV infection, diabetes mellitus, and chronic cardiac or pulmonary disease. A causal relationship between the preceding use of nonsteroidal anti-inflammatory drugs and these severe GAS infections has not been established. The portal of entry is unknown in nearly 50% of cases; in most cases, it is believed to be skin or mucous membrane. Infection rarely follows GAS pharyngitis.

The **incubation period** of streptococcal pharyngitis is 2 to 5 days. For impetigo, a 7- to 10-day period between the acquisition of GAS on healthy skin and development of lesions has been demonstrated.

DIAGNOSTIC TESTS: The throat culture remains the test of choice for children with pharyngitis because the clinical differentiation of viral and GAS pharyngitis usually is impossible. A specimen, properly obtained by vigorous swabbing of the tonsils and posterior pharynx, should be cultured on sheep blood agar to confirm GAS infection. Latex agglutination, fluorescent antibody, coagglutination, and precipitation techniques performed on colonies growing on the agar are accurate in differentiating group A from other ß-hemolytic streptococci. Appropriate use of bacitracin-susceptibility disks (containing 0.04 units) allows presumptive identification of GAS but is a less accurate method of diagnosis. False-negative cultures occur in less than 10% of symptomatic patients when the throat swab specimen is properly obtained and cultured. Recovery of GAS from the pharynx does not distinguish patients with streptococcal infection (defined by a serologic antibody response) from streptococcal carriers who have pharyngitis caused by a different organism (ie, a virus). The number of colonies of GAS on the agar culture plate does not accurately differentiate infection from carriage. Cultures that are negative for GAS infection after 24 hours should be incubated for a second day to optimize isolation of GAS.

Several rapid diagnostic tests for GAS pharyngitis are available. Most of these tests are based on acid extraction of group A carbohydrate antigen from organisms obtained by throat swab. Although these tests vary in methodology, their sensitivities and specificities in general are similar when carefully performed, including rigorous attention to technique and use of controls. The specificities of these tests generally are high, but the reported sensitivities vary considerably. As with throat cultures, the accuracy of these tests is most dependent on the quality of the throat swab specimen, which must contain pharyngeal and tonsillar secretions, and on the experience of the person who is performing the test. Therefore, when a patient suspected of having GAS pharyngitis has a negative rapid streptococcal test, a throat culture should be obtained to ensure that the patient does not have GAS infection. Because of the high specificity of these rapid tests, a positive test does not require throat culture confirmation.

Rapid diagnostic tests using new techniques, such as optical immunoassay and chemiluminescent DNA probes, have been developed recently. Available data suggest that these tests are as sensitive as standard throat cultures on sheep blood agar and more sensitive than other rapid tests for GAS. However, additional corroborative information is needed before these tests can be recommended for routine use without a confirmatory throat culture in patients with negative test results.

Indications for Throat Cultures. Factors to be considered in the decision to obtain a throat culture in children with pharyngitis are the patient's age, clinical signs and symptoms, the season and the family and community epidemiology, including contact with a case of GAS infection, presence in the family of a person with acute rheumatic fever or history thereof, or poststreptococcal glomerulonephritis. Group A streptococcal infection is less common in children younger than 3 years, but outbreaks of streptococcal pharyngitis have been reported in young children in child care settings. Children with manifestations highly suggestive of viral infection, such as coryza, conjunctivitis, hoarseness, cough, anterior stomatitis, discrete ulcerative lesions, or diarrhea, are unlikely to have GAS as the cause of their pharyngitis and should not be cultured. Children with the acute onset of sore throat, fever, headache, pain on swallowing, abdominal pain, nausea, vomiting, and cervical adenitis are much more likely to have GAS as the cause of their pharyngitis.

Indications for culturing contacts vary according to circumstances. Culturing asymptomatic household contacts usually is not recommended except during outbreaks or when contacts are at increased risk for developing sequelae of GAS infection. Siblings and all other household contacts of a child who has acute rheumatic fever or poststreptococcal glomerulonephritis should have throat cultures taken and, if positive, should be treated regardless of whether the contact is currently or recently symptomatic. Household contacts of an index case with streptococcal pharyngitis who have recent or current symptoms suggestive of streptococcal infection also should be cultured. Pyoderma lesions should be cultured in families with one or more cases of acute nephritis or streptococcal toxic shock syndrome in order that antibiotic therapy can be administered for eradicating GAS.

Posttreatment throat cultures usually are indicated only in patients who are at high risk for rheumatic fever or who are symptomatic. Repeated courses of antibiotic therapy are not usually indicated in asymptomatic patients whose throat cultures continue to be positive for GAS after appropriate antibiotic therapy; the exceptions are those who have or have had, or whose family members have or have had, rheumatic fever or rheumatic heart disease or in other unique epidemiologic circumstances, such as outbreaks of rheumatic fever or acute poststreptococcal glomerulonephritis.

Children in whom repeated episodes of pharyngitis occur at short intervals with GAS documented by culture or antigen detection test present a special problem. Often these persons are chronic GAS carriers who are experiencing frequent viral illnesses. In assessing such children, poor compliance with oral treatment also should be excluded. In some areas, erythromycin resistance may occur, resulting in treatment failures. These strains also are resistant to other macrolides, such as clarithromycin and azithromycin. Culturing asymptomatic household members usually is not helpful. However, if multiple household members have symptomatic pharyngitis or other GAS infection, such as impetigo or pyoderma, simultaneous cultures of all household members and treatment of all persons with positive cultures may be of value.

In schools, child care centers, or other environments where large numbers of persons are in close contact, the prevalence of GAS upper respiratory tract carriage in healthy children can be as high as 5% to 15% in the absence of an outbreak of streptococcal disease. Therefore, classroom or more widespread culture surveys are not indicated routinely and should be considered only if one or more cases of rheumatic fever, glomerulonephritis or severe invasive GAS disease occurred.

Cultures of impetiginous lesions are not indicated routinely since they often yield both streptococci and staphylococci, and determination of the primary pathogen from culture results may not be possible.

In suspected invasive GAS infections, cultures of blood and focal sites of possible infection are indicated. In necrotizing fasciitis, magnetic resonance imaging can be helpful in confirming the anatomical diagnosis.

TREATMENT:

Pharyngitis.

- Penicillin V is the drug of choice for the treatment of GAS pharyngitis, except in penicillin-allergic individuals. Group A streptococci resistant to penicillin have not been documented. Ampicillin or amoxicillin are often used in place of penicillin V, but have no microbiologic advantage over penicillin. Penicillin therapy prevents rheumatic fever even when therapy is started as long as 9 days after the onset of the acute illness, shortens the clinical course, reduces the risk of transmission, and decreases the risk of suppurative sequelae. For patients seen early in their illness, a brief delay for processing of the throat culture before therapy is started does not increase the risk of rheumatic fever. In all patients with acute rheumatic fever, a complete course of penicillin or other appropriate antibiotic for GAS pharyngitis should be given to eradicate GAS from the throat, even though the organism may not be recovered in the initial throat culture.

  The dose of orally administered penicillin V is 400 000 U (250 mg), two to three times a day for 10 days for children and 500 mg two to three times a day for adolescents and adults. To prevent rheumatic fever, oral treatment with penicillin should be given for at least 10 days, regardless of the promptness of clinical recovery. Although different preparations of oral penicillin vary in absorption, their clinical efficacy is similar. Treatment failures may occur more frequently with oral penicillin than with intramuscularly administered benzathine penicillin G as a result of poor compliance with oral therapy.

- Intramuscular benzathine penicillin G (BPG) is appropriate therapy. It ensures adequate blood concentrations and avoids the problem of compliance, but is painful. For children who weigh less than 60 lb (27.3 kg) BPG is given in a single dose of 600 000 U; for larger children and adults, the dose is 1 200 000 U. Mixtures containing shorter-acting penicillins (eg, procaine penicillin) in addition to BPG have not been demonstrated to be superior to BPG alone, except in reducing discomfort from the injection. Although supporting data are limited, the combination of 900 000 U of BPG and 300 000 U of procaine penicillin G is satisfactory therapy for most children; however, the efficacy of this combination for heavier patients, such as adolescents and adults, has not been demonstrated. Discomfort is less if the preparation of benzathine penicillin G is brought to room temperature before intramuscular injection.

- Orally administered erythromycin is indicated for patients allergic to penicillin. Treatment should be given for 10 days. Erythromycin estolate (20 to 40 mg/kg per day in two to four divided doses) or erythromycin ethyl succinate (40 mg/kg per day in two to four divided doses) is effective in treating streptococcal pharyngitis; the maximal dose is 1 g/d. Other macrolides, such as clarithromycin for 10 days or azithromycin for 5 days (a regimen approved by the Food and Drug Administration) can be used in place of erythromycin. Although GAS strains resistant to erythromycin have been prevalent in some areas of the world (eg, Japan and Finland) and have resulted in treatment failures, they remain uncommon in most areas of the United States. Erythromycin-resistant strains also are resistant to other macrolide drugs.

- A 10-day course of a narrow-spectrum (first-generation), oral cephalosporin is an acceptable alternative, particularly for individuals allergic to penicillin. However, as many as 15% of penicillin-allergic persons also are allergic to cephalosporins. Patients with immediate, anaphylactic-type hypersensitivity to penicillin should not be treated with a cephalosporin. Reports have suggested that a 5-day course of certain oral cephalosporins is similar to a 10-day course of oral penicillin in eradicating GAS from the upper respiratory tract. However, additional studies are warranted to expand and confirm these observations before these regimens can be recommended. The additional cost of cephalosporins and their wider range of antibacterial activity compared with penicillin preclude recommending them for routine use in persons with GAS pharyngitis who are not allergic to penicillin.
- Tetracyclines and sulfonamides should **not** be used for treating GAS pharyngitis. Many strains are resistant to tetracycline and sulfonamides do not eradicate GAS, although sulfonamides are effective for continuous prophylaxis in preventing recurrent rheumatic fever (see Secondary Prophylaxis of Rheumatic Fever, p 492).

Children who have a recurrence of GAS pharyngitis shortly after completing a 10-day course of recommended oral antimicrobials can be retreated with that antimicrobial; given an alternative oral drug; or administered an intramuscular dose of benzathine penicillin G, especially if poor compliance with oral therapy is likely. Alternative drugs include cephalosporin, amoxicillin-clavulanate, dicloxacillin, erythromycin, or other macrolides. Expert opinions concerning the most appropriate therapy in this circumstance differ.

Management of the patient who has repeated and frequent episodes of acute pharyngitis associated with a positive throat culture for GAS is problematic. To determine whether the patient is a chronic streptococcal pharyngeal carrier experiencing repeated episodes of intercurrent viral pharyngitis (which is the case in the majority of cases), the following needs to be determined: (1) whether the clinical findings are suggestive of GAS or viral etiology; (2) whether epidemiologic factors in the community are suggestive of GAS or viral etiology; (3) the nature of the clinical response to the antimicrobial therapy (which in bona fide GAS pharyngitis is usually rapid with or without therapy); (4) whether throat cultures are positive for GAS between episodes of acute pharyngitis; and (5) whether a serologic response to GAS extracellular antigens (eg, anti-streptolysin 0) has occurred. Serotyping of GAS isolates is usually only available in research laboratories, but if performed, homogeneity of the isolates suggests carriage while heterogeneity suggests repeated infections.

Pharyngeal carriers. Antimicrobial therapy is not indicated for most GAS pharyngeal carriers. Exceptions, ie, specific situations in which eradication of carriage is indicated, include the following: (1) during outbreaks of acute rheumatic fever or poststreptococcal glomerulonephritis; (2) during an outbreak of GAS pharyngitis in a closed or semi-closed community; (3) when a family history of rheumatic fever exists; (4) when multiple episodes of documented, symptomatic GAS pharyngitis continue to occur within a family during a period of many weeks despite appropriate therapy; (5) when a family has an excessive anxiety about GAS infections; and (6) when tonsillectomy is considered only because of chronic GAS carriage.

Streptococcal carriage can be difficult to eradicate with conventional penicillin therapy. A number of antimicrobial agents including clindamycin, amoxicillin-clavulanate, narrow-spectrum cephalosporins, dicloxacillin, and a combination of rifampin and penicillin have been demonstrated to be more effective than penicillin in eliminating chronic streptococcal carriage. Of these drugs, oral clindamycin given as 20 mg/kg per day in three doses (maximum, 1.8 g/d) for 10 days has been reported recently to be the most effective. Proven eradication of the carrier state is helpful in the evaluation of subsequent episodes of acute pharyngitis; however, chronic carriage may recur because of reacquisition of GAS.

Streptococcal Impetigo.

- Local antibacterial preparations, such as bacitracin or mupirocin ointment, may be useful in limiting person-to-person spread of GAS impetigo and in eradicating localized disease. With multiple lesions or impetigo in multiple family members, child care groups, or athletic teams, GAS impetigo should be treated systemically with antibiotic regimens, as recommended for pharyngitis. However, since episodes of impetigo frequently are caused by *Staphylococcus aureus*, children with impetigo usually should be treated with an antibiotic active against both GAS and *S aureus* infections.

Other Infections.

- High-dose, parenteral antimicrobial therapy is required for infections such as endocarditis, pneumonia, septicemia, meningitis, arthritis, osteomyelitis, and streptococcal toxic shock syndrome. Treatment is often prolonged (2 to 6 weeks).
- The drug of choice for severe, invasive GAS infection is penicillin G. Clindamycin, given intravenously, may be particularly beneficial in the treatment of some of these infections, such as necrotizing fasciitis and toxic shock syndrome, and is recommended by some experts in addition to penicillin G. Since clindamycin-resistant strains of GAS have been reported, clindamycin should not be given alone until the infecting organism is demonstrated by in vitro testing to be susceptible.
- The use of intravenous immune globulin in persons with invasive GAS infections, such as toxic shock syndrome, may be beneficial when given in conjunction with appropriate antimicrobial therapy and currently is under investigation. Since effectiveness in controlled studies has not been demonstrated, however, immune globulin is not routinely recommended at this time.
- Hyperbaric oxygen has been used in the treatment of necrotizing fasciitis and myositis due to GAS, but its benefit has not been established.

Prevention of Sequelae.
Acute rheumatic fever and acute glomerulonephritis are serious nonsuppurative sequelae of GAS infections. During epidemics, rheumatic fever may develop in as many as 3% of untreated patients with acute streptococcal pharyngitis. With endemic infections, the attack rates are lower. The risk of rheumatic fever virtually can be eliminated by adequate treatment of the antecedent GAS infection; however, cases of rheumatic fever have occurred even after alleged appropriate therapy. The effectiveness of antimicrobial therapy to prevent acute poststreptococcal glomerulonephritis, especially following pyoderma, is less certain. Suppurative

sequelae, such as peritonsillar abscesses and cervical adenitis, usually are prevented by prompt therapy of the primary infection. Severe infections, such as streptococcal toxic shock syndrome, are most commonly associated with skin and soft-tissue infections, and occasionally may follow an upper respiratory tract infection, but whether severe infection can be prevented by early therapy is unknown.

ISOLATION OF THE HOSPITALIZED PATIENT*: Droplet precautions are recommended for children with pharyngitis or pneumonia until 24 hours after initiation of effective therapy. For burns with secondary GAS infections and extensive or draining cutaneous infections that cannot be covered or contained adequately by dressings, contact precautions should be used for at least 24 hours after the start of effective therapy.

CONTROL MEASURES: The most important means of controlling GAS disease and its sequelae is prompt identification and treatment of infections.

School and Child Care. Children with streptococcal pharyngitis or skin infections should not return to school or child care until at least 24 hours after beginning antimicrobial therapy. Close contact with other children during this time should be avoided, if possible.

Care of Exposed Persons. Contacts of documented cases of streptococcal infection who have recent or current clinical evidence of a streptococcal infection should have appropriate cultures obtained and should be treated if the culture is positive. Rates of GAS acquisition are higher among sibling contacts (25%) than among parent contacts in nonepidemic settings; rates as high as 50% for sibling contacts and 20% for parent contacts have been reported during epidemics. More than half of those contacts who acquire the organism will become ill. Asymptomatic acquisition of GAS may pose some risk of nonsuppurative complications; studies indicate that as many as one third of patients with rheumatic fever had no history of recent streptococcal infection and another third had minor respiratory tract infections that were not brought to medical attention. However, cultures of asymptomatic household contacts usually are not indicated except during outbreaks or when the contacts are at increased risk for developing sequelae of infection (see Indications for Throat Cultures, p 486). Short courses (fewer than 10 days) of antibiotics for contacts are inappropriate. In some circumstances, such as a large family with documented, repeated intrafamily transmission resulting in frequent episodes of GAS pharyngitis during a prolonged period, physicians may elect to treat all family members. Throat cultures should be obtained in these circumstances to identify those individuals harboring the organism. However, these circumstances arise infrequently.

Chemoprophylaxis. For children with repeated episodes of documented GAS pharyngitis occurring at short intervals, some experts recommend oral penicillin prophylaxis during the seasons of the year of greatest risk. The dosage is the same as for secondary prophylaxis of rheumatic fever (see Table 3.54).

Limited data suggest that household contacts of patients with severe, invasive GAS disease, including streptococcal toxic shock syndrome, are at substantially increased risk for the development of severe, invasive GAS disease compared with the general population. However, additional studies are needed to define further

---

* In addition to standard precautions.

Table 3.54. **Chemoprophylaxis of Recurrences of Rheumatic Fever***

Drug	Dose	Route
Benzathine penicillin G	1 200 000 U every 4 wk[†]	Intramuscular
or		
Penicillin V	250 mg twice a day	Oral
or		
Sulfadiazine or sulfisoxazole	0.5 g once a day for patients ≤27 kg (60 lb)	Oral
	1.0 g once a day for patients >27 kg (60 lb)	
For individuals allergic to penicillin and sulfonamide drugs		
Erythromycin	250 mg twice a day	Oral

* Modified from Dajani A, Taubert K, Ferrieri P, et al. Treatment of acute streptococcal pharyngitis and prevention of rheumatic fever: a statement for health professionals. *Pediatrics.* 1995;96:758-764.
† In high-risk situations, administration every 3 weeks is recommended.

the magnitude of the risk, the potential effectiveness of prophylactic antimicrobial agents, and the settings in which chemoprophylaxis would be cost-beneficial. As a result, no recommendations for chemoprophylaxis for these household contacts can be made at this time.

Secondary Prophylaxis of Rheumatic Fever. Patients who have a well-documented history of rheumatic fever (including cases manifested solely by Sydenham's chorea) and those who have documented evidence of rheumatic heart disease should be given continuous antibiotic prophylaxis to prevent recurrent attacks (secondary prophylaxis) because asymptomatic and symptomatic GAS infections can result in a rheumatic recurrence. Continuous prophylaxis should be initiated as soon as the diagnosis of rheumatic fever or rheumatic heart disease is made.

Duration. Secondary prophylaxis should be long-term, perhaps for life, in patients with rheumatic heart disease (even after prosthetic valve replacement because these patients remain at risk for recurrence of rheumatic fever). The risk of recurrence declines as the interval from the most recent episode lengthens, and patients without rheumatic heart disease are at a lower risk of recurrence than those with cardiac involvement. Duration depends on whether residual heart damage (valvular disease) is present or absent. These considerations influence the duration of secondary prophylaxis in adults, but should not alter the practice of secondary prophylaxis in children and adolescents. Secondary prophylaxis in all patients who have had rheumatic fever should be continued for at least 5 or more years or until the individual is 21 years of age, whichever is longer (see Table 3.55). Prophylaxis also should be continued if the risk of contact with persons with GAS infection is high, such as for parents with school-age children and teachers.

When streptococcal infections occur in family members of rheumatic fever patients, infected persons should be treated promptly with an appropriate antibiotic (see Indications for Throat Cultures, p 486, and Treatment, p 488).

The drug regimens in Table 3.55 are effective for secondary prophylaxis. The intramuscular regimen has been proven to be the most reliable because the success

Table 3.55. Duration of Prophylaxis for Persons Who Have Had Rheumatic Fever: Recommendations of the American Heart Association*

Category	Duration
Rheumatic fever without carditis	5 y or until age 21 y, whichever is longer
Rheumatic fever with carditis but no residual heart disease (no valvar disease[†])	10 y or well into adulthood, whichever is longer
Rheumatic fever with carditis and residual heart disease (persistent valvar disease[†])	At least 10 y since last episode and at least until age 40 y; sometimes lifelong prophylaxis

* Dajani A, Taubert K, Ferrieri P, et al. Treatment of acute streptococcal pharyngitis and prevention of rheumatic fever: a statement for health professionals. *Pediatrics*. 1995;96:758-764.
† Clinical or echocardiographic evidence.

of oral prophylaxis depends primarily on patient compliance, although inconvenience and the pain of injection may cause some patients to discontinue intramuscular prophylaxis. In some countries and in situations where the risk of GAS infection is high, benzathine penicillin G is given every 3 weeks because of greater effectiveness. In the United States, administration every 4 weeks appears adequate in most patients. Oral sulfadiazine is as effective as oral penicillin for secondary prophylaxis, but may not be readily available in the United States. Based on extrapolation from data demonstrating effectiveness of sulfadiazine, sulfisoxazole is an appropriate alternative.

Allergic reactions to oral penicillin are similar to those with intramuscular penicillin, but they usually are less severe and occur less frequently. These reactions also occur less often in children than in adults. Anaphylaxis is extremely rare in patients receiving oral penicillin. Severe allergic reactions in patients receiving continuous benzathine penicillin G prophylaxis also are rare. Anaphylaxis and death have been reported but usually in patients older than 12 years with severe rheumatic heart disease. Most of these severe reactions may result from vasovagal responses rather than anaphylaxis. Reactions include a serum sickness-like reaction, characterized by fever and joint pains, which can be mistaken for an acute rheumatic fever recurrence.

Reactions to sulfadiazine or sulfisoxazole are infrequent and usually minor; obtaining blood counts may be advisable after 2 weeks of prophylaxis, since leukopenia has been reported. Prophylaxis with a sulfonamide in late pregnancy is contraindicated because of interference with fetal bilirubin metabolism. Febrile mucocutaneous syndromes (erythema multiforme, Stevens-Johnson syndrome, or epidermal necrolysis) have been associated with penicillin as well as with sulfonamides. When an adverse event occurs with any of these therapeutic regimens, the drug should be stopped immediately and an alternative drug selected. For the rare patient allergic to both penicillins and sulfonamides, erythromycin is recommended.

Poststreptococcal Reactive Arthritis. Following an episode of acute GAS pharyngitis, a reactive arthritis may develop in the absence of clinical manifestations and laboratory findings that would fulfill the Jones criteria for the diagnosis of acute rheumatic fever. This syndrome has been termed poststreptococcal reactive arthritis (PSRA). In contrast to the arthritis of acute rheumatic fever, the arthritis of PSRA does not respond dramatically to anti-inflammatory agents. Because some patients with PSRA apparently may have silent or delayed-onset carditis, these patients should be observed carefully for several months for the subsequent development of carditis. Some experts recommend prophylaxis for these patients for several months to a year if carditis does not develop; if carditis occurs, the patient should be considered to have rheumatic fever and prophylaxis should be continued (see Secondary Prophylaxis of Rheumatic Fever, p 492).

Bacterial Endocarditis Prophylaxis. Patients with rheumatic valvular heart disease also require additional short-term antibiotic prophylaxis at the time of certain procedures (including dental and surgical procedures) to prevent the possible development of bacterial endocarditis (see Prevention of Bacterial Endocarditis, p 601). Patients who have had rheumatic fever without evidence of valvular heart disease do not need prophylaxis for prevention of endocarditis. Penicillin, ampicillin or amoxicillin should not be used for endocarditis prophylaxis in patients who are receiving oral penicillin for secondary rheumatic fever prophylaxis because of relative resistance to penicillins and aminopenicillins of viridans streptococci in the oral cavity in such patients. Erythromycin is the alternative antibiotic recommended for such patients.

Group B Streptococcal Infections

CLINICAL MANIFESTATIONS: Group B streptococci are a major cause of perinatal bacterial infections, including endometritis, amnionitis, and urinary tract infections in parturient women and systemic and focal infections in infants from birth until 3 or more months of age. Invasive disease in neonates is categorized into two entities based on time of onset after birth. Early-onset disease usually occurs within the first 24 hours of life (range, 0 to 6 days) and is characterized by respiratory distress, apnea, shock, pneumonia, and, occasionally, meningitis. Late-onset disease, which typically occurs at 3 to 4 weeks of age (range, 7 days to 3 months), frequently is manifested as occult bacteremia or meningitis; other focal infections, such as osteomyelitis, septic arthritis, and cellulitis, also can occur. Group B streptococci also cause chorioamnionitis and postpartum endometritis, as well as other infections in adults, particularly those with diabetes mellitus, malignancy, or other immunocompromising conditions.

ETIOLOGY: Group B streptococci (*Streptococcus agalactiae*) are divided into the following serotypes: Ia, Ib/c, Ia/c, II, III, IV, V, VI and VII. All serotypes may cause infections in newborn infants and in adults. Serotype III is the predominant cause of early-onset meningitis and late-onset infections in newborns.

EPIDEMIOLOGY: Group B streptococci (GBS) are common inhabitants of the gastrointestinal and the genitourinary tracts. Less commonly, they colonize the pharynx. The colonization rate in pregnant women and newborn infants ranges from 5% to 35%. Colonization during pregnancy usually is constant but can be intermittent. Neonatal GBS disease has an incidence of one to four cases per 1000 live births; the incidence varies considerably among hospitals. Early-onset disease accounts for approximately three fourths of neonatal disease and occurs in approximately one infant per 100 to 200 colonized women. Transmission from mother to infant occurs in utero shortly before or during delivery. After delivery, person-to-person transmission can occur. Although uncommon, GBS can be acquired in the nursery from colonized infants or hospital personnel (probably via hand contamination), or in the community. The risk of early-onset disease is increased in preterm infants born at less than 37 weeks of gestation, those born after the amniotic membranes have been ruptured for more than 18 hours, and in infants born of women with intrapartum fever, chorioamnionitis, or GBS bacteriuria. Low or an absent concentration of type-specific serum antibody also is a predisposing factor. Other risk factors are maternal age younger than 20 years and African-American ethnicity. The period of communicability is unknown, but may extend throughout the duration of colonization or of disease. Infants can remain colonized for several months after birth and after treatment for symptomatic infection.

The **incubation period** of early-onset disease is less than 6 days. In late-onset disease the incubation period from GBS acquisition to disease is unknown. Onset usually occurs from 7 days to 3 months of age.

DIAGNOSTIC TESTS: Gram-positive cocci in fluids that ordinarily are sterile (such as cerebrospinal, pleural, joint fluid, or urine) provide presumptive evidence of infection. Cultures of blood or body fluids are necessary to establish the diagnosis. Serotype identification by type-specific antisera is available in reference laboratories. Group B streptococcal antigen may be detected in serum, cerebrospinal fluid (CSF), or urine by latex particle agglutination or other rapid tests; positive tests in symptomatic infants constitute presumptive evidence of infection. The sensitivity and specificity of rapid diagnostic tests are variable, and false-positive results occur in a minimum of 5% to 8% of urine samples, especially bagged urine specimens that become contaminated during collection. A positive test in an asymptomatic infant, thus, is not diagnostic of invasive infection, and testing of urine by this method is not recommended.

TREATMENT:
- Penicillin G or ampicillin plus an aminoglycoside is the initial treatment of choice for a newborn infant with presumptive, invasive, life-threatening group B streptococcal (GBS) infection.
- Penicillin G alone can be given when GBS has been identified as the course of the infection and when clinical and microbiologic responses have been documented. Some experts advise determination of the susceptibility of the organism to penicillin or ampicillin, especially for CSF isolates.
- For infants with GBS meningitis, the recommended dosage of penicillin G for infants 7 days or younger is 250 000 to 450 000 U/kg per day intravenously, in three divided doses; for infants more than 7 days old, 450 000 U/kg per day intravenously, in four divided doses, is recommended. For ampicillin, the recommended dosage for infants with meningitis age 7 days or younger is 200 mg/kg per day intravenously in three divided doses; for infants more than 7 days old, 300 mg/kg per day in four to six divided doses is recommended. The optimal dose, however, is unknown.

- For meningitis, some experts believe that a second lumbar puncture at approximately 24 hours after initiation of therapy to document bacteriologic cure has prognostic importance. Additional lumbar punctures and other studies are often indicated if response to therapy is in doubt after 36 to 72 hours of treatment. Consultation with a specialist in infectious diseases may be useful.
- For infants with bacteremia without a defined focus, treatment should be continued for at least 10 days. For infants with uncomplicated meningitis, 14 to 21 days of treatment usually is satisfactory, but longer periods of treatment may be necessary for infants with prolonged or complicated courses. Osteomyelitis requires treatment for 4 weeks or more, depending on the severity of infection, response to treatment, and complications. Treatment duration in all cases should be guided by the patient's clinical and bacteriologic responses.
- Because of the high frequency of coinfection, the twin of an index case with early-onset disease should be carefully observed and empirically treated for suspected septicemia if any manifestations of illness occur.

ISOLATION OF THE HOSPITALIZED PATIENT: Standard precautions are recommended except during a nursery outbreak of GBS disease (see Control Measures).

CONTROL MEASURES:

Chemoprophylaxis. Recommendations for prevention of early onset neonatal GBS infection are as follows:
- Obstetric care practitioners should adopt a strategy for prevention of early onset GBS disease. Patients should be informed regarding the available strategies for its prevention. Individual patient requests regarding GBS cultures should be honored.
- Regardless of the prevention strategy used, women should be managed as follows:
  — Women found to have symptomatic or asymptomatic GBS bacteriuria during pregnancy at the time of diagnosis should be treated. Because such women usually have heavy GBS colonization, they also should receive intrapartum chemoprophylaxis.
  — Intrapartum chemoprophylaxis should be administered to women who have previously given birth to an infant with GBS disease; prenatal culture screening is not necessary.
- Until further data become available to define the most effective prevention strategy, either one of the two following strategies is appropriate:
  1. All pregnant women at 35 to 37 weeks of gestation should be screened for anogenital GBS colonization. All women identified as GBS carriers by culture should be offered intrapartum chemoprophylaxis even if a risk factor is not present.
     — If the results of GBS cultures are not known at the onset of labor or rupture of membranes, intrapartum antimicrobial prophylaxis should be administered if one of the following is present: gestation of less than 37 weeks, rupture of membranes for 18 hours or longer, or a temperature of 38°C (100.4°F) or greater.

— Culture techniques that maximize the likelihood of GBS recovery should be utilized. The optimal method for GBS screening is collection of a single swab or two separate swabs of the distal vagina and anorectum followed by inoculation into selective broth medium, overnight incubation, and then subculture onto solid blood agar medium.

— Oral antimicrobial agents should not be used to treat women who are found to have GBS colonization during prenatal screening. Such treatment is not effective in eliminating carriage or preventing neonatal disease.

These recommendations are summarized in Fig 3.1.

2. A prevention strategy based on the presence of intrapartum risk factors without culture screening (eg, gestation of less than 37 weeks, duration of membrane rupture more than 18 hours, or temperature greater than 38°C) is an acceptable alternative.

These recommendations are summarized in Fig 3.2.

- For intrapartum chemoprophylaxis, intravenous penicillin G (5 million units initially and then 2.5 million units every 4 hours) is the drug of choice. Intravenous ampicillin (2 g initially and then 1 g every 4 hours until delivery) is an acceptable alternative, but penicillin G is preferred because it has a narrow spectrum and is therefore less likely to select for antibiotic-resistant organisms. Intravenous clindamycin or erythromycin may be used for women allergic to penicillin. The number of doses of antibiotics received and the duration of intrapartum chemoprophylaxis are considered important factors in the prevention of early-onset infection.

- Routine use of prophylactic antimicrobial agents for infants born to mothers who have received intrapartum chemoprophylaxis is not recommended. However, therapeutic use of these agents is appropriate for those infants with clinically suspected septicemia. The duration of therapy in symptomatic infants varies depending on the results of blood culture, cerebrospinal fluid findings (if determined), and clinical course. If the laboratory evaluation and clinical course are inconsistent with a diagnosis of invasive infection, the duration of empiric therapy should be as short as 48 to 72 hours.

- Guidelines regarding management of asymptomatic infants born to women given intrapartum chemoprophylaxis are empiric. The following, suggested approach is not an exclusive course of management. Other treatment modalities taking into account individual circumstances and individual physician or institutional preferences may be appropriate.

— For asymptomatic infants whose mothers have received intrapartum prophylaxis, those with gestations of less than 35 weeks should have a limited diagnostic evaluation (complete blood count [and differential] and blood culture) and should be observed without antimicrobial therapy in the hospital for at least 48 hours. If during observation, signs of systemic infection develop, a complete diagnostic evaluation should be performed and antimicrobial therapy should be initiated.

Fig 3.1. **Prevention strategy for early-onset group B streptococcal (GBS) disease using prenatal culture screening at 35 to 37 weeks of gestation.**

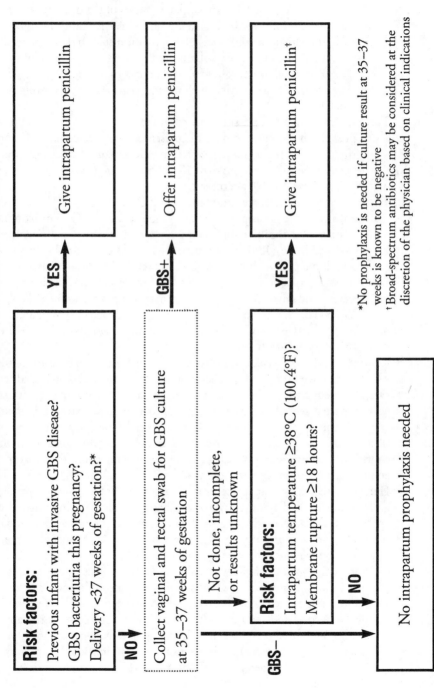

Risk factors:
Previous infant with invasive GBS disease?
GBS bacteriuria this pregnancy?
Delivery <37 weeks of gestation?*

NO → Collect vaginal and rectal swab for GBS culture at 35–37 weeks of gestation

YES → Give intrapartum penicillin

Not done, incomplete, or results unknown → **Risk factors:**
Intrapartum temperature ≥38°C (100.4°F)?
Membrane rupture ≥18 hours?

GBS+ → Offer intrapartum penicillin

YES → Give intrapartum penicillin†

GBS−

NO → No intrapartum prophylaxis needed

*No prophylaxis is needed if culture result at 35–37 weeks is known to be negative
†Broad-spectrum antibiotics may be considered at the discretion of the physician based on clinical indications

Fig 3.2. **Prevention strategy for early-onset group B streptococcal (GBS) disease using risk factors without prenatal culture screening.**

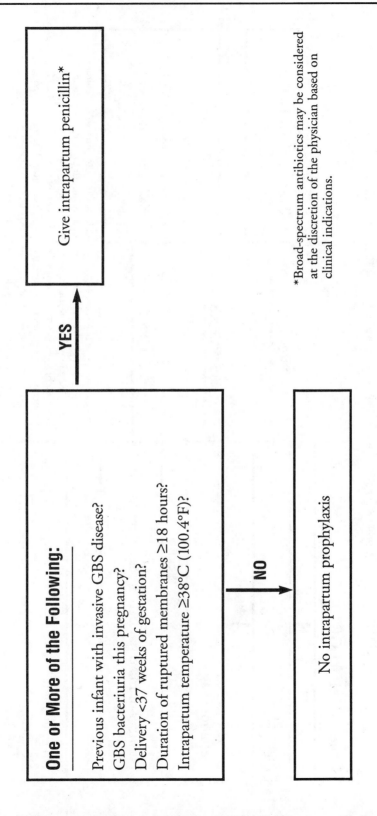

One or More of the Following:

Previous infant with invasive GBS disease?
GBS bacteriuria this pregnancy?
Delivery <37 weeks of gestation?
Duration of ruptured membranes ≥18 hours?
Intrapartum temperature ≥38°C (100.4°F)?

YES → Give intrapartum penicillin*

NO → No intrapartum prophylaxis

*Broad-spectrum antibiotics may be considered at the discretion of the physician based on clinical indications.

Fig 3.3. **Empiric management of neonate born to a mother who received intrapartum antimicrobial prophylaxis (IAP) for prevention of early onset group B streptococcal (GBS) disease.**

This algorithm is suggested but is not an exclusive approach of management.

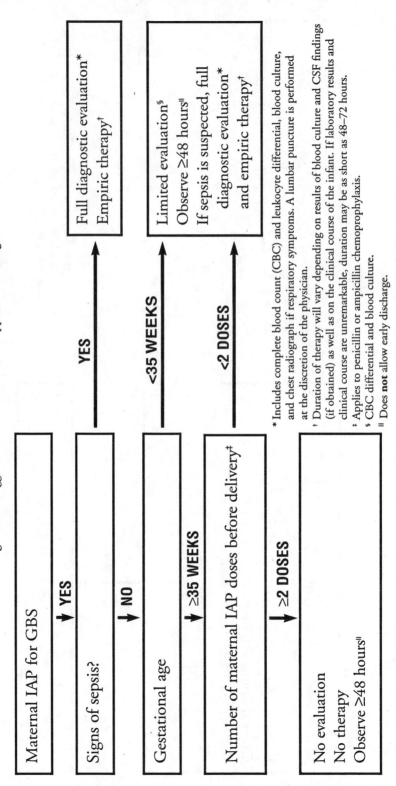

* Includes complete blood count (CBC) and leukocyte differential, blood culture, and chest radiograph if respiratory symptoms. A lumbar puncture is performed at the discretion of the physician.

† Duration of therapy will vary depending on results of blood culture and CSF findings (if obtained) as well as on the clinical course of the infant. If laboratory results and clinical course are unremarkable, duration may be as short as 48–72 hours.

‡ Applies to penicillin or ampicillin chemoprophylaxis.

§ CBC differential and blood culture.

‖ Does **not** allow early discharge.

— In asymptomatic infants with a gestational age of 35 weeks or longer, the duration of intrapartum prophylaxis before delivery determines subsequent management. If two or more doses of maternal prophylaxis were given before delivery, no laboratory evaluation or antimicrobial therapy is recommended. These infants should be observed in the hospital for at least 48 hours (ie, does not allow for early discharge). If only one dose of maternal prophylaxis was given before delivery, infants should have a limited evaluation and at least 48 hours of observation before hospital discharge.

These recommendations are summarized in the algorithm in Fig 3.3.

Investigations designed to evaluate and compare these and other strategies are needed urgently to assess outcomes, including the incidence of neonatal GBS disease, occurrence of adverse reactions to antimicrobial prophylaxis, and the emergence of perinatal infections due to penicillin-resistant organisms. Characterization of prevention failures also is important.

Neonatal Infection Control. Routine cultures of infants to determine GBS colonization are not recommended. Epidemiologic evaluation of late-onset cases in a special care nursery may be required to exclude a nosocomial source.

Nursery Outbreak. Cohorting of ill and colonized infants and the use of a gown and gloves during an outbreak are recommended. Other methods of control (eg, treatment of asymptomatic carriers with penicillin or treatment of the umbilical cord with triple dye or hexachlorophene) are impractical or ineffective. Routine hand washing by personnel caring for infants colonized or infected with GBS is the best way to prevent spread to other infants.

Non-Group A or B Streptococcal and Enterococcal Infections

CLINICAL MANIFESTATIONS: Streptococci of groups other than A or B may be associated with invasive disease in newborn infants, older children, and adults. Urinary tract infection, endocarditis, upper and lower respiratory tract infections, and meningitis are the principal clinical syndromes.

ETIOLOGY: Streptococci of groups C and G and *Enterococcus* species are common pathogens. The two most common enterococcal species are *E faecalis* and *E faecium*. Streptococci belonging to groups D, F, H, and K also can be pathogens. Nongroupable streptococci, such as viridans and anaerobic streptococci (peptostreptococci) also can cause infections.

EPIDEMIOLOGY: The common habitats in humans of these streptococcal groups are skin (C, F, and G), oropharynx (C, F, G, H, and K), gastrointestinal tract (D, F, G, and *Enterococcus*), and vagina (C, D, F, G, and *Enterococcus*). The normal habitats of different species of viridans streptococci include the oropharynx, dental surfaces, skin, and genitourinary tract. Intrapartum transmission probably is responsible for most cases of early-onset neonatal infection. Environmental contamination or transmission via the hands of health care workers can lead to colonization of patients.

The **incubation period** and the period of communicability are unknown.

DIAGNOSTIC TESTS: Microscopic examination of fluids that are ordinarily sterile can yield presumptive evidence of infections by Gram-positive cocci. The diagnosis is established by culture and serogrouping of the isolate, using group-specific antisera. Identification of the species of enterococci may be useful to predict antimicrobial susceptibility. In addition, in some circumstances biochemical testing may be necessary to accurately identify the organism. Antibiotic susceptibility testing of enterococci from sterile sites is important to determine ampicillin and vancomycin susceptibility. Some automated methods may not detect vancomycin resistance.

TREATMENT: Enterococci and occasional streptococcal strains (eg, some types of *S viridans*) are less susceptible to penicillin than are most streptococcal isolates. Enterococci are not susceptible to cephalosporins, and strains resistant to ampicillin or vancomycin have been identified. In invasive enterococcal infections, including endocarditis and meningitis, ampicillin or vancomycin in combination with an aminoglycoside (usually gentamicin), for possible synergy and for bactericidal activity, should be administered until in vitro susceptibility is known and appropriate combination therapy can be selected. Combination therapy with ampicillin and gentamicin may be required for optimum treatment of severe infections due to groups C, F, and G. In other infections, penicillin G or ampicillin alone is sufficient.

Endocarditis. Guidelines for antimicrobial therapy in adults have been formulated by the American Heart Association and should be consulted for regimens that may be appropriate for children and adolescents.*

ISOLATION OF THE HOSPITALIZED PATIENT: Standard precautions are recommended. The exception is for patients with vancomycin-resistant enterococcal infection or colonization, for whom contact precautions are indicated until the patient is culture-negative and no longer receiving antibiotics.†

CONTROL MEASURES: Patients with valvular or congenital heart disease should receive antimicrobial prophylaxis to prevent streptococcal and enterococcal endocarditis at the time of dental and selected other surgical procedures (see Prevention of Bacterial Endocarditis, p 601).

---

* Wilson WR, Karchmer AW, Dajani AS, et al. Treatment of adults with infective endocarditis due to streptococci, enterococci, staphylococci, and HACEK microorganisms. *JAMA.* 1995;274:1706-1713.
† In addition to standard precautions.

Strongyloidiasis
(Strongyloides stercoralis)

CLINICAL MANIFESTATIONS: Infection can be manifested by eosinophilia only. Hence, strongyloidiasis warrants consideration whenever eosinophilia (>500/μL), without an obvious clinical correlation, is found in a patient who has resided in an endemic area. Infective larvae first entering the body can produce transient pruritic papules at the site of penetration of the skin, usually on the feet. Larval migration through the lungs can cause pneumonitis with coughing productive of blood-streaked sputum. The intestinal phase of infection can be accompanied by vague abdominal pain, distention, vomiting, and diarrhea that consists of mucoid, voluminous stools. Malabsorption has been reported. Larval migration from defecated stool can result in pruritic skin lesions in the perianal area, buttocks, and upper thighs. The lesions may present as migrating, pruritic, serpiginous, erythematous tracks called "cutaneous larva currens." In immunocompromised patients or those receiving corticosteroids, complications include disseminated strongyloidiasis (caused by hyperinfection), diffuse pulmonary infiltrates, and septicemia from Gram-negative bacilli.

ETIOLOGY: *Strongyloides stercoralis* is a nematode (roundworm).

EPIDEMIOLOGY: Strongyloidiasis is endemic in the tropics and subtropics, including the southern and southwestern United States, wherever suitable moist soil and improper disposal of human waste coexist. Humans are the principal hosts. Dogs, cats, and other animals also can be reservoirs. Transmission involves penetration of the skin by infective larvae, either from autoinfection or contact with infected soil. Infections rarely can be acquired from intimate skin contact or from inadvertent coprophagia, such as from ingestion of contaminated food scavenged from garbage. Because some larvae mature into the infective forms in the colon, autoinfection is common. Asymptomatic infection, especially in healthy hosts, is common. In immunocompromised patients, autoinfection is more frequent and causes hyperinfection with resulting disseminated strongyloidiasis wherein the patient's organs and tissues are suffused with larvae and the number of adult worms in the small intestine is extraordinarily high. In addition, because these larvae penetrate the wall of the colon, bacteremia and meningitis caused by enteric flora can occur. Even mild immunosuppression caused by treatment with corticosteroids can precipitate hyperinfection. The period of communicability lasts as long as the patient is infected, which can be several decades.

The **incubation period** is not known.

DIAGNOSTIC TESTS: Stool examination discloses the characteristic larvae, but several specimens may have to be examined before a positive one is found. Examination of duodenal contents obtained by a commercially available string test (Enterotest*) or direct aspirate is more likely to demonstrate larvae. Serodiagnosis can be helpful but is only available in a few reference laboratories, and false-negative results do occur. The enzyme immunoassay test for antibodies is positive in approximately 85% of cases; however, cross-reaction with the antigens of filarial worms also occurs

---

* HDC Corp, San Jose, Calif.

and limits the specificity of serodiagnosis. Eosinophilia (>500/µL) is common. In disseminated strongyloidiasis, larvae can be found in the sputum.

TREATMENT: Thiabendazole* is curative in most patients. Side effects of nausea, vomiting, and malaise are common. Treatment may have to be repeated or prolonged in the hyperinfection syndrome. Relapses occur and should be treated. Albendazole is widely used in countries other than the United States because the drug is highly efficacious in the treatment of strongyloidiasis. Thiabendazole and albendazole are contraindicated in pregnancy. Ivermectin,[†] in a single dose, has been reported to be effective, but is not approved for use by the Food and Drug Administration except as an investigational drug.

ISOLATION OF THE HOSPITALIZED PATIENT: Standard precautions are recommended.

CONTROL MEASURES: Sanitary disposal measures for human waste should be followed. Education about the risk of infection through bare skin is important.

For the patient who has an immunologic defect or who requires immunosuppressive therapy and is from an endemic region, examination of the stool and, possibly, duodenal fluid and respiratory secretions for *S stercoralis* should be considered before immunosuppressive therapy is started. Serologic tests seem to be the most sensitive for diagnosis, but they do not distinguish between past and current infection, and results from a reference laboratory may not be immediately available. If a patient's status requires the initiation of immunosuppressive therapy before the results of diagnostic tests can be obtained, the risks of empiric antiparasitic therapy for strongyloidiasis must be weighed against the risks of a disseminated infection.

Syphilis

CLINICAL MANIFESTATIONS:

Congenital Syphilis. Infection can result in stillbirth, hydrops fetalis, or prematurity. It can be asymptomatic, especially in the first weeks of life, or it may have multisystem manifestations, including hepatosplenomegaly, lymphadenopathy, mucocutaneous lesions, osteochondritis, hemolytic anemia and thrombocytopenia. Late manifestations of congenital syphilis, usually appearing after 2 years of age, can involve the central nervous system, bones and joints, teeth, eyes, and skin. Some consequences of intrauterine infection may not become apparent until many years after birth, such as interstitial keratitis (5 to 20 years) and eighth nerve deafness (10 to 40 years).

Acquired Syphilis. Infection can be divided into three stages. The primary stage appears as one or more painless, indurated ulcers (chancre) of the skin and mucous membranes at the site of inoculation, most commonly on the genitalia. The secondary stage, beginning 1 to 2 months later, is characterized by a polymorphic rash which is most frequently maculopapular and generalized, and classically involves the

---

* Available from Merck and Co, West Point, Pa.

palms and soles. In moist areas around the vulva or anus, hypertrophic papular lesions (condyloma latum) can occur. Generalized lymphadenopathy, fever, malaise, splenomegaly, sore throat, headache, and arthralgia can be present. A variable latent period follows, but sometimes is interrupted in the first few years by recurrences of symptoms of secondary syphilis. The tertiary stage can be marked by aortitis, various manifestations of neurosyphilis, or gummatous changes of the skin, bone, or viscera, occurring from several years to decades after the primary infection.

ETIOLOGY: *Treponema pallidum* is a thin, motile spirochete that is extremely fragile, surviving only very briefly outside the host. The organism has not been cultivated successfully on artificial media.

EPIDEMIOLOGY: Syphilis occurs throughout the world but is most frequent in large urban areas. The incidence of both acquired and congenital syphilis increased dramatically in the United States in the late 1980s and early 1990s but subsequently declined in all but large urban areas and the rural South. In the pediatric population, the disease is most common in adolescents. In adults in the United States, infection in males is twice as common as infection in females, but the difference is diminishing. In HIV-infected adults, syphilis is common and the risk of neurologic complications may be increased.

Congenital syphilis is contracted from an infected mother via transplacental transmission of *T pallidum* at any time during pregnancy or at birth. In women with untreated early syphilis, 40% of pregnancies result in spontaneous abortion, stillbirths, or perinatal deaths. Infection can be transmitted to the fetus at any stage of the disease; the rate of transmission is almost 100% during the secondary stage and slowly decreases with time. The moist secretions of congenital syphilis are highly infectious. Organisms rarely are found in lesions more than 24 hours after treatment has begun.

Acquired syphilis is contracted almost always through direct sexual contact with ulcerative lesions of the skin or mucous membranes of infected persons. Sexual abuse must be suspected in any young child with acquired syphilis. Open, moist lesions of the primary or secondary stages teem with spirochetes. Infectious lesions usually do not occur more than 1 year after infection, but relapses with infectious secondary lesions have occurred as many as 4 years later.

The **incubation period** for acquired primary syphilis is typically about 3 weeks, but ranges from 10 to 90 days, after exposure.

DIAGNOSTIC TESTS: Definitive diagnosis is achieved by identifying spirochetes by microscopic darkfield examination or direct fluorescent antibody tests of lesion exudate or tissue. Specimens should be scraped from moist, mucocutaneous lesions or aspirated from a regional lymph node. Since false-negative microscopic results are common, serologic testing, follow-up, and often repeated testing are necessary. Specimens from mouth lesions require direct fluorescent antibody techniques to distinguish *T pallidum* from nonpathogenic treponemes. Polymerase chain reaction (PCR) tests have been developed but are not yet commercially available.

Presumptive diagnosis is possible using two types of serologic tests, ie, (1) nontreponemal tests and (2) treponemal tests. Neither type of test alone is sufficient for diagnosis.

The standard nontreponemal tests for syphilis include the VDRL slide test, the rapid plasma reagin (RPR), and the automated reagin test (ART). These tests measure antibody directed against lipoidal antigen from *T pallidum* and/or its interaction with host tissues. They are inexpensive and rapidly performed, and provide quantitative results, which are helpful indicators of disease activity and useful for follow-up after treatment. Nontreponemal tests may be falsely negative, ie, nonreactive, in early primary syphilis, latent acquired syphilis of long duration, and late congenital syphilis. Occasionally, a nontreponemal test on sera with high concentrations of antibody against *T pallidum* will be weakly reactive or falsely negative, a reaction termed the "prozone" phenomenon. This reaction usually can be detected by experienced laboratory technicians and diluting the serum will result in a positive test.

A reactive nontreponemal test from a patient with typical lesions usually indicates the need for treatment. However, any reactive nontreponemal test should be confirmed by one of the specific treponemal tests to exclude a false-positive test, which can be caused occasionally by Wharton's jelly contamination of cord blood, certain viral infections (eg, infectious mononucleosis, hepatitis, varicella, and measles), lymphoma, tuberculosis, malaria, endocarditis, connective tissue disease, pregnancy, abuse of injection drugs, and laboratory or technical error. Treatment should not be delayed pending the treponemal test results in symptomatic patients or patients at high risk of infection. A sustained fourfold decrease in titer of the nontreponemal test following treatment demonstrates adequate therapy; a similar titer increase after treatment suggests reinfection or relapse. The quantitative nontreponemal test usually becomes nonreactive after successful therapy within 1 year in primary syphilis and within 2 years in secondary and congenital syphilis, but may remain positive despite treatment in late latent (1 year or more) or tertiary syphilis.

Treponemal tests currently in use are the fluorescent treponemal antibody absorption (FTA-ABS) test and the microhemagglutination test for *T pallidum* (MHA-TP). Positive FTA-ABS and MHA-TP tests usually remain reactive for life, even with successful therapy.

Treponemal tests also are not 100% specific for syphilis; positive reactions occur in patients with other spirochetal diseases such as yaws, pinta, leptospirosis, rat-bite fever, and Lyme disease. Nontreponemal tests can be used to differentiate Lyme disease from syphilis, as the VDRL is uniformly nonreactive in Lyme disease.

Usually a serum nontreponemal test is obtained initially and if it is reactive, a treponemal test is performed. The probability of syphilis is high in a sexually active patient whose serum is reactive on both a nontreponemal and a treponemal test.

In summary, the nontreponemal antibody tests (VDRL, RPR, and ART) are useful for screening; the treponemal tests (FTA-ABS and MHA-TP) are used to establish a provisional diagnosis. Quantitative nontreponemal antibody tests are used to assess the adequacy of therapy and to detect reinfection and relapse.

Cerebrospinal Fluid Tests (CSF). For evaluation of possible neurosyphilis, the VDRL test should be performed. The RPR, FTA-ABS, and MHA-TP tests should not be used for CSF evaluation. VDRL test results should be interpreted cautiously because a negative CSF VDRL does not exclude a diagnosis of neurosyphilis and the CSF VDRL can be positive in an uninfected newborn with a transplacentally acquired, high serum VDRL titer.

Testing During Pregnancy. All women should be screened serologically for syphilis early in pregnancy with a nontreponemal test (eg, VDRL or RPR) and preferably again at delivery. In areas of high prevalence and in patients considered at high risk for syphilis, a nontreponemal serum test at the beginning of the third trimester (28 weeks) also is indicated. For those treated during pregnancy, follow-up serology is necessary to assess the efficacy of therapy. Occasional, low-titer nontreponemal antibody test results that are false-positive occur in pregnancy; they should be confirmed as false-positive with an FTA-ABS or MHA-TP test and a repeat nontreponemal test in 4 to 6 weeks.

Evaluation of Newborn Infants for Congenital Infection. **No newborn should be discharged from the hospital without determination of the mother's serologic status for syphilis. Testing of cord blood or infant sera is not adequate for screening because these tests can be nonreactive when the mother is positive.**

An infant should be evaluated for congenital syphilis if he or she is born to a mother with positive nontreponemal tests confirmed by a positive treponemal test and who has one or more of the following conditions:

- Syphilis untreated or inadequately treated (see Treatment, p 509).
- Syphilis during pregnancy treated with a nonpenicillin regimen, such as erythromycin.
- Syphilis during pregnancy treated with an appropriate penicillin regimen, but the expected decrease in nontreponemal antibody titer after therapy did not occur.
- Syphilis treated less than 1 month before delivery (since treatment failures occur and the efficacy of treatment cannot be assumed).
- Syphilis treatment not documented.
- Syphilis treated before pregnancy, but with insufficient serologic follow-up to assess the response to treatment and current infection status.

Evaluation of syphilis of infants born to women with any of the preceding conditions should include the following:

- Physical examination.
- Quantitative nontreponemal serologic test for syphilis on the infant's sera (not on cord blood because false-positive and false-negative results can occur).
- If available, determination of antitreponemal IgM antibody by a testing method recognized by the Centers for Disease Control and Prevention (CDC) either as a standard or provisional method.
- Cerebrospinal fluid VDRL, analysis for cells, and protein concentration.
- Long-bone roentgenograms (unless the diagnosis has been otherwise established).
- Other clinically indicated tests (eg, chest roentgenogram, complete blood cell count, and liver function tests).

Pathologic examination of the placenta or umbilical cord using specific fluorescent antitreponemal antibody staining, if available, also is recommended.

A guide for interpretation of the results of nontreponemal and treponemal serologic tests for syphilis in mothers and their infants is given in Table 3.56 (p 508). A nonreactive nontreponemal test in both the infected mother and infant can occur in a neonate with congenital syphilis if the mother acquired the disease late in pregnancy or in the case of a prozone phenomenon. In addition, the mother's test can be reac-

Table 3.56. Guide for Interpretation of the Syphilis Serology of Mothers and Their Infants

Nontreponemal Test (eg, VDRL, RPR, ART)		Treponemal Test (eg, MHA-TP, FTA-ABS)		Interpretation*
Mother	Infant	Mother	Infant	
–	–	–	–	No syphilis or incubating syphilis in the mother and infant
+	+	–	–	No syphilis in mother (false-positive nontreponemal test with passive transfer to infant)
+	+ or –	+	+	Maternal syphilis with possible infant infection; or mother treated for syphilis during pregnancy; or mother with latent syphilis and possible infection of infant[†]
+	+	+	+	Recent or previous syphilis in the mother; possible infection in infant
–	–	+	+	Mother successfully treated for syphilis before or early in pregnancy; or mother with Lyme disease, yaws, or pinta (ie, false-positive serology)

* Table presents a guide and not the definitive interpretation of serologic tests for syphilis in mothers and their newborn infants. Other factors that should be considered include the timing of maternal infection, the nature and timing of maternal treatment, quantitative maternal and infant titers, and serial determination of nontreponemal test titers in both mother and infant.
[†] Mothers with latent syphilis may have nonreactive nontreponemal tests.

tive and the infected infant's test nonreactive, depending on the timing of maternal and fetal infection. Transplacental transmission of both nontreponemal and treponemal antibodies to the fetus can occur in a mother who has been treated appropriately for syphilis during pregnancy, resulting in positive tests in the uninfected newborn infant. The neonate's nontreponemal test titer in these circumstances is usually less than or equal to the mother's titer and reverts to negative in 4 to 6 months, whereas a positive FTA-ABS or MHA-TP test from passively acquired antibody may not become negative for 1 year or longer. A reactive antitreponemal IgM antibody test on the infant's serum by a method considered reliable by the CDC is specific for congenital syphilis and, thus, can be useful. The frequency of false-negative test results has not been well documented. However, as of December 1996, no IgM tests are commercially available in the United States. Thus, in an infant asymptomatic at birth, distinguishing between early infection and passive transfer of antibody from a previously treated mother remains difficult or impossible.

In an infant with clinical or roentgenographic findings (eg, metaphysitis of the long bones) suggestive of congenital syphilis, a positive nontreponemal and/or treponemal test in serum strongly supports the diagnosis regardless of the therapy the mother received during the pregnancy.

Cerebrospinal Fluid (CSF) Testing. Cerebrospinal fluid should be examined in all infants who are evaluated for congenital syphilis (see Evaluation of Newborn Infants for Congenital Infection, p 507), and in all patients with suspected neurosyphilis or with acquired, untreated syphilis of more than 1 year's duration. The CSF abnormalities in patients with neurosyphilis include increased protein concentration and leukocyte cell count and a reactive VDRL. However, because of the wide range of normal values for CSF cell counts and protein concentrations in the newborn, interpretation is often difficult. A negative CSF VDRL test does not exclude neurosyphilis; conversely, the test can be positive in an uninfected newborn with a transplacentally acquired high serum VDRL titer. If CSF test results cannot exclude infection in an infant evaluated for congenital syphilis, the infant should be treated. In patients beyond the neonatal period, normal CSF findings differentiate latent syphilis from asymptomatic neurosyphilis in individuals with acquired, untreated syphilis of more than 1 year's duration.

TREATMENT: Parenteral penicillin G remains the preferred drug for treatment of syphilis at any stage. Recommendations for penicillin G and duration of therapy vary, depending on the stage of the disease and its clinical manifestations. Parenteral penicillin G is the only documented effective therapy for patients who have neurosyphilis, congenital syphilis, or syphilis during pregnancy, and it is strongly recommended for HIV-infected patients. Such patients should always be treated with penicillin, after desensitization for penicillin allergy if necessary, or should be managed in consultation with a specialist.

Penicillin Allergy. Skin testing for penicillin hypersensitivity with the major and minor determinants can identify reliably individuals at high risk for reacting to penicillin; currently, only the major determinant (penicilloyl-poly-L-lysine) and penicillin G are available commercially. Testing with the major determinant of penicillin G is estimated to miss 3% to 6% of penicillin-allergic patients who are at risk for serious or fatal reactions. Thus, a cautious approach to penicillin therapy is advised when the patient cannot be tested with all of the penicillin skin test reagents. An oral desensitization protocol for patients with a positive skin test is available.*

Congenital Syphilis: Newborn Infants (see also Table 3.57, p 510). Infants should be treated for congenital syphilis if they have proven or probable disease, as is demonstrated if (1) they have physical or roentgenographic evidence of active disease; (2) their serum quantitative nontreponemal titer is at least four times higher than the mother's titer; (3) their CSF VDRL is reactive or the CSF cell count and/or protein concentration is abnormal; (4) they have a positive antitreponemal IgM

---

* Centers for Disease Control and Prevention. 1993 sexually transmitted diseases treatment guidelines. *MMWR.* 1993;42(No. RR-14):44-46.

Table 3.57. Recommended Treatment of Neonates (≤4 Weeks of Age) With Proven or Possible Congenital Syphilis

Clinical Status	Antimicrobial Therapy*
Proven or highly probable disease	Aqueous crystalline penicillin G, for 10 to 14 d[†]
Asymptomatic, normal CSF and radiographic examination—maternal treatment history:	
None, inadequate penicillin treatment,[‡] undocumented, failed, or reinfected	Aqueous crystalline penicillin G, IV, for 10 to 14 d[†] **or** Clinical, serologic follow-up, and benzathine penicillin G, IM, single dose[§]
Adequate therapy but given less than 1 month before delivery, mother's response to treatment is not demonstrated by a four-fold decrease in titer of a nontreponemal serologic test, or erythromycin therapy	Clinical, serologic follow-up, and benzathine penicillin G, IM, single dose[§]

* See text for drug dosage and details. IV indicates intravenously, and IM indicates intramuscularly.
† If more than 1 day of therapy is missed, the entire course should be restarted.
‡ See text for definition (includes those in whom sequential serologic tests on the mother do not demonstrate a fourfold or greater decrease in a nontreponemal antibody titer).
§ Some experts recommend aqueous crystalline penicillin G as for proven or highly probable disease (see text below). Other experts would follow the infant without giving antibiotic therapy if both clinical and serologic follow-up can be assured.

antibody test performed by a test method deemed reliable by the CDC; or (5) the placenta or umbilical cord is positive for treponemes using specific fluorescent antibody staining. If an asymptomatic infant has a nontreponemal titer that is higher than but less than four times that of the mother, some experts recommend treatment if follow-up cannot be assured. When an infant warrants evaluation for congenital syphilis (see Evaluation of Newborn Infants for Congenital Infection, p 507), the infant should be treated if test results cannot exclude infection, if the infant cannot be fully evaluated, or if adequate follow-up cannot be assured.

In infants with proven or probable disease, aqueous crystalline penicillin G is preferred. The dosage should be based on chronologic, not gestational, age. The recommended dosage is 100 000 to 150 000 U/kg per day (given every 8 to 12 hours), intravenously, to complete a 10- to 14-day course. Alternatively, some experts recommend procaine penicillin G (50 000 U/kg per day intramuscularly) for treatment of congenital syphilis; however, adequate CSF concentrations may not always be achieved by this regimen. If more than 1 day of therapy is missed, the entire course should be restarted.

Asymptomatic infants born to mothers who received appropriate penicillin treatment for syphilis during pregnancy and responded with a documented fourfold decrease in their VDRL, RPR, or ART titer are at minimal risk for congenital syphilis. However, these infants should be examined carefully, preferably monthly, until their nontreponemal serologic test results are negative.

Infants whose mothers received inadequate treatment for syphilis during pregnancy require special consideration. Maternal treatment for syphilis during pregnancy is deemed inadequate for this purpose in the following circumstances: (1) the mother's penicillin dose is unknown, undocumented, or inadequate; (2) the mother received erythromycin for syphilis; (3) treatment was given within 30 days of the infant's birth; or (4) the mother's response to treatment has not been established by demonstrating a fourfold fall in titer by nontreponemal serologic testing for syphilis.

Asymptomatic infants born to mothers whose treatment for syphilis may have been inadequate, as defined by one or more of these criteria, should be fully evaluated, including CSF examination (see Evaluation of Newborn Infants for Congenital Infection, p 507). Some experts would treat all such infants with aqueous crystalline penicillin G (or aqueous procaine penicillin G) for 10 days. However, if the infant's physical examination, CSF findings, roentgenograms of long bones, platelet counts, and liver function studies are normal, many experts would treat infants in the specific circumstances given in Table 3.57 (p 510) with a single dose of 50 000 U/kg of benzathine penicillin G intramuscularly. In the case in which maternal response to treatment has not been demonstrated but the mother received an appropriate regimen of penicillin therapy more than 1 month before delivery, the infant's evaluation is normal, and both clinical and serologic follow-up can be ensured, some experts would follow the infant without giving antibiotic therapy.

Congenital Syphilis: Older Infants and Children. Because of the difficulty in establishing the diagnosis of neurosyphilis, infants diagnosed after 4 weeks of age should be treated with aqueous crystalline penicillin, 200 000 to 300 000 U/kg per day intravenously (administered every 6 hours) for 10 to 14 days. This regimen should also be used to treat children older than 1 year who have late and previously untreated congenital syphilis. Some experts also suggest giving such patients benzathine penicillin G, 50 000 U/kg intramuscularly, in three weekly doses following the 10 to 14-day course of intravenous aqueous penicillin. If the patient has minimal clinical manifestations of disease, the CSF examination is normal, and the CSF VDRL is negative, some experts would treat with three doses of benzathine penicillin G, 50 000 U/kg intramuscularly, only.

Syphilis in Pregnancy. Regardless of the stage of pregnancy, patients should be treated with penicillin according to the dosage schedules appropriate for the stage of syphilis as recommended for nonpregnant patients. For women with early acquired syphilis, some experts recommend two doses of benzathine penicillin (2.4 million units intramuscularly) given 1 week apart, rather than one dose. For penicillin-allergic patients, no proven alternative therapy has been established. A pregnant woman with a history of penicillin allergy should be treated with penicillin after desensitization. In some patients, skin testing may be helpful. Desensitization should be performed in consultation with a specialist and only in facilities where emergency assistance is available (see Penicillin Allergy, p 509).

Erythromycin treatment of syphilis during pregnancy cannot be considered reliable to cure infection in the fetus. Tetracycline is not recommended for pregnant women because of potential adverse effects on the fetus.

Early Acquired Syphilis (primary, secondary, latent syphilis of less than 1 year's duration). A single dose of benzathine penicillin G intramuscularly, in a total dose of 50 000 U/kg (not to exceed 2.4 million units), is the preferred treatment. All children should have a CSF examination before treatment to exclude a diagnosis of neurosyphilis. Evaluation of CSF in adolescents and adults is necessary only if clinical signs or symptoms of neurologic involvement are present.

For nonpregnant patients allergic to penicillin, tetracycline (adult dose, 500 mg orally four times a day) or doxycycline (adult dose 100 mg orally twice a day) should be given for 2 weeks. The clinical experience with doxycycline is less, but patient adherence to a regimen requiring twice a day doses is likely to be better. Tetracycline or doxycycline should not be given to children younger than 8 years unless the benefits of therapy are greater than the risks of dental staining (see Antimicrobials and Related Therapy, p 606). Drugs other than penicillin and tetracycline do not have proven efficacy in the treatment of syphilis. Single-dose therapy with ceftriaxone is not effective. For nonpregnant, penicillin-allergic patients, if follow-up can be ensured, erythromycin (500 mg orally four times a day) for 14 days, or ceftriaxone regimens of 8 to 10 days, in consultation with an expert, can be given. When follow-up cannot be ensured, especially for children younger than 8 years of age, consideration must be given to hospitalization and desensitization followed by administration of penicillin G (see Penicillin Allergy, p 509).

Syphilis of More Than 1 Year's Duration (except neurosyphilis). Benzathine penicillin G, at a dose of 50 000 U/kg (not to exceed 2.4 million units) should be given intramuscularly, weekly for 3 successive weeks. In patients who are allergic to penicillin, either tetracycline (adult dose, 500 mg orally four times a day) or doxycycline (adult dose, 100 mg orally twice a day) for 4 weeks should be given only if a CSF examination has excluded neurosyphilis. Tetracycline or doxycycline ordinarily should not be given to children younger than 8 years of age unless the benefits of therapy are greater than the risks of dental staining (see Antimicrobials and Related Therapy, p 606). Testing of the CSF VDRL, protein concentration, and cell count is mandatory for those with suspected or symptomatic neurosyphilis, those who have concurrent HIV infection, those who have failed treatment, and those receiving antibiotics other than penicillin. Cerebrospinal fluid examination is recommended for all patients with syphilis for more than 1 year to exclude asymptomatic neurosyphilis.

Neurosyphilis. The recommended regimen for adults is aqueous crystalline penicillin G, 12 to 24 million units a day (2 to 4 million units every 4 hours) intravenously for 10 to 14 days. If compliance with therapy can be assured, patients may be treated with an alternative regimen of 2.4 million units of procaine penicillin intramuscularly daily (single dose) plus probenecid, 2.0 g per day orally in four divided doses, both for 10 to 14 days. Some experts recommend following this regimen with a single dose of benzathine penicillin G, 2.4 million units intramuscularly. In children, aqueous crystalline penicillin G, 200 000 to 300 000 U/kg per day (50 000 U/kg every 4 to 6 hours) for 10 to 14 days, in doses not to exceed the adult dose, is recommended, possibly followed by a single dose of benzathine penicillin, 50 000 U/kg per dose (not to exceed 2.4 million units) in three weekly doses.

If the patient has a history of allergy to penicillin, consideration should be given to desensitization, and the patient should be managed in consultation with a specialist (see Penicillin Allergy, p 509).

Other Considerations.

- Mothers of infants with congenital syphilis should be tested for other sexually transmitted diseases (STDs) including gonorrhea, *Chlamydia trachomatis*, HIV, and hepatitis B infection.
- All recent sexual contacts of persons with acquired syphilis should be evaluated for other STDs as well as for syphilis. (see Control Measures, p 514).
- All patients with syphilis should be tested for other STDs.
- For HIV-infected patients with syphilis, careful follow-up is essential. Patients infected with HIV who have early syphilis may be at increased risk for neurologic complications and higher rates of treatment failure with the currently recommended regimens. Nevertheless, such risk, although not precisely defined, is probably small. No therapy, however, has been demonstrated to be more effective in preventing the development of neurosyphilis than that recommended for patients without HIV infection.

Follow-up and Retreatment.

Congenital Syphilis. Treated infants should have careful follow-up evaluations at 1, 2, 4, 6, and 12 months of age. Serologic nontreponemal tests should be performed 3, 6, and 12 months after the conclusion of treatment, or until they become nonreactive. Nontreponemal antibody titers should decline by 3 months of age and should be nonreactive by 6 months of age if the infant was not infected and the initially positive serologic test reflected transplacentally acquired maternal antibody. Patients with persistent, stable titers, including those with low titers, should be considered for retreatment.

Treated infants with congenital neurosyphilis and initially positive CSF VDRL tests or abnormal or uninterpretable CSF cell counts and/or protein concentrations should undergo repeat clinical evaluation and CSF examination at 6-month intervals until their CSF examination is normal. A reactive CSF VDRL at 6 months is an indication for retreatment. If cell counts are still abnormal at 2 years or are not decreasing at each examination, retreatment is indicated.

Early Acquired Syphilis. Treated, pregnant women with syphilis should have quantitative nontreponemal serologic tests performed monthly for the remainder of their pregnancy. Other patients with early acquired syphilis should return for repeat quantitative nontreponemal tests at 3, 6, and 12 months after the conclusion of treatment. Patients with syphilis for more than 1 year should also undergo serologic testing 24 months after treatment. Careful follow-up serologic testing is particularly important in patients treated with antibiotics other than penicillin.

Retreatment. In the following circumstances, retreatment is indicated:
- The clinical signs or symptoms of syphilis persist or recur.
- A sustained, fourfold increase in the titer of a nontreponemal test occurs; in a pregnant woman, a fourfold increase in titer alone is an indication for retreatment.

- An initially high-titer nontreponemal test fails to decrease fourfold within a year; in a pregnant woman with primary or secondary syphilis, it fails to decrease fourfold within a 3-month period; or in a pregnant woman with latent syphilis, it fails to decrease fourfold within 6 months.

Retreated patients should be treated with the schedules recommended for patients with syphilis for more than 1 year. In general, only one retreatment course is indicated. The possibility of reinfection or concurrent HIV infection should always be considered when retreating patients with early syphilis.

The CSF should be examined before retreatment unless evidence indicates that the patient has been reinfected and again requires treatment for early syphilis. Patients with neurosyphilis must have periodic serologic testing in follow-up, clinical evaluation at 6-month intervals, and repeat CSF examinations for at least 3 years or until CSF examination is normal.

ISOLATION OF THE HOSPITALIZED PATIENT: Standard precautions are recommended for all patients, including infants with suspected or proven congenital syphilis. However, in addition, for infants with suspected or proven congenital syphilis, parents, visitors, and medical staff should use gloves when handling the infant until therapy has been administered for at least 24 hours. Because moist, open lesions and possibly blood are contagious in all patients with syphilis, these precautions are also required for primary and secondary syphilis with skin and mucous membrane lesions.

CONTROL MEASURES:
- All women should be screened for syphilis early in pregnancy and preferably at delivery. Women at high risk for syphilis also should be screened at 28 weeks (see p 507).
- Education about STDs, treatment of sexual contacts, reporting of each case to local public health authorities for contact investigation and appropriate follow-up, and serologic screening of high-risk populations are indicated.
- All recent sexual contacts of a person with acquired syphilis should be identified, examined, serologically tested, and treated appropriately. Sexual contacts within the last 3 months who are seronegative are at high risk for early syphilis and should be treated for early acquired syphilis. Every effort, including physical examination and serologic testing, should be made to establish a diagnosis in these patients.
- All individuals, including hospital personnel, who have had close, unprotected contact with a patient with early congenital syphilis before identification of the disease or during the first 24 hours of therapy should be examined clinically for the presence of lesions 2 to 3 weeks after contact. Serologic testing should be performed and repeated 3 months after contact, or sooner if symptoms occur.

Tapeworm Diseases
(Taeniasis and Cysticercosis)

CLINICAL MANIFESTATIONS:

Taeniasis. Mild gastrointestinal symptoms, such as nausea, diarrhea, and pain, can occur. Tapeworm segments can be seen migrating from the anus or feces.

Cysticercosis. Manifestations depend on the location and numbers of cysts of the pork tapeworm and the host response. Cysts may be found anywhere in the body. The most common and serious manifestations usually are caused by those in the central nervous system. Cysts in the brain (neurocysticercosis) can cause seizures, behavioral disturbances, obstructive hydrocephalus and other neurologic symptoms. Neurocysticercosis can be a leading cause of epilepsy, depending on epidemiological circumstances. The host reaction to degenerating cysts can produce signs and symptoms of meningitis. Cysts in the spinal column can cause gait disturbance, pain or transverse myelitis. Subcutaneous cysts produce palpable nodules, and ocular involvement can cause visual impairment.

ETIOLOGY: Taeniasis is caused by intestinal infection by the adult tapeworm, *Taenia saginata* (beef tapeworm) or *Taenia solium* (pork tapeworm). Usually only one adult worm is present in the intestine. Cysticercosis is caused by the larvae of *T solium (Cysticercus cellulosae)*.

EPIDEMIOLOGY: These tapeworm diseases have worldwide distribution, and prevalence rates are high in areas with poor sanitation and human fecal contamination where cattle graze or swine are fed. Most cases in the United States are imported from Mexico, Central and South America, Africa, Asia, Spain, and Portugal. Taeniasis is acquired by eating undercooked beef (*T saginata*) or pork (*T solium*) that contains encysted larvae. Infection is often asymptomatic.

Cysticercosis is transmitted by fecal-oral contact by ingesting the eggs of the pork tapeworm, *T solium,* either by heteroinfection from a contact harboring the adult tapeworm or by autoinfection. The eggs are found in human feces only, since humans are the only definitive host. The eggs liberate oncospheres in the intestine which migrate to tissues throughout the body, including the central nervous system where cysts form. Although most cases of cysticercosis in the United States have been imported from Mexico and Central and South America, cysticercosis in this country can be acquired from index cases who recently immigrated from an endemic area and still have *T solium* infection.

The **incubation period** for taeniasis, the time from ingestion of the larvae until segments are passed in the feces, is 2 to 3 months. For cysticercosis, it is months to years.

DIAGNOSIS: Diagnosis of taeniasis (adult tapeworm infection) is based on demonstration of the proglottids or ova in feces or the perianal region. Species identification of the parasite is based on the different structures of the terminal gravid segments. Diagnosis of neurocysticercosis is based primarily on computed tomography (CT) or magnetic resonance imaging (MRI). Enhanced CT may be helpful in identifying spinal and intraventricular lesions. The enzyme-linked immunotransfer blot assay to detect serum and cerebrospinal fluid (CSF) antibody to *T solium* is the antibody test of choice and is available through the Centers for Disease Control and Prevention. The test is more sensitive with serum samples than with CSF specimens. The serum antibody assays are often negative in children with solitary parenchymal lesions but are usually positive in patients with multiple, inflamed lesions.

TREATMENT:

Taeniasis. Praziquantel is highly effective in eradicating infection with the adult tapeworm.

Cysticercosis. Treatment of neurocysticercosis is based on the number of lesions and presence or absence of inflammation as determined by CT or MRI of the brain. Acutely inflamed, single, intraparenchymal cysts involute rapidly (8 to 12 weeks) and, thus, rarely require therapy. Single, uninflamed lesions often follow the same course if untreated. Multiple, uninflamed cysts require antihelmintic therapy because they may persist and cause progressive neurologic symptoms. Praziquantel given for 15 days, in one or more courses, is effective. It may be given with dexamethasone for 2 or 3 days to minimize the inflammatory response resulting from larvicidal antihelminthics, and is indicated if neurologic symptoms develop during therapy. Albendazole given for 8 days or longer may be slightly more effective than praziquantel and has recently been approved by the Food and Drug Administration for this indication. Whereas dexamethasone lowers the serum concentration of praziquantel, it increases the concentration of albendazole.

Intraventricular cysts and hydrocephalus may require surgical intervention. Seizures may recur for months and will require anticonvulsant medication until patients have been seizure-free for 1 to 2 years.

Ocular cysticercosis is usually treated by surgical excision of cysts and not with antihelmintic drugs because of the inflammatory reaction that might occur; studies of the effectiveness of albendazole are in progress.

ISOLATION OF THE HOSPITALIZED PATIENT: Standard precautions are recommended.

CONTROL MEASURES: Eating raw or undercooked beef or pork should be avoided. Persons known to harbor the adult tapeworms of *T solium* should be treated immediately and use careful hand washing and care in the disposal of fecal material until the infection is eradicated.

Stool examination of food handlers who have recently emigrated from endemic countries for detection of eggs and/or proglottids is advisable.

Persons traveling to developing countries with high endemic rates of cysticergosis should avoid eating uncooked vegetables and/or fruits that have not been peeled.

Other Tapeworm Infections
(Including Hydatid Disease)

Most infections are asymptomatic, but nausea, abdominal pain, and diarrhea have been observed in persons who are heavily infested.

Hymenolepis nana. This tapeworm, also called dwarf tapeworm, has its entire cycle within humans. Therefore, person-to-person transmission is possible. More problematic is autoinfection, which tends to perpetuate the infection in the host because the eggs can hatch within the intestine and reinitiate the cycle, leading to the development of new worms. This cycle makes eradicating the infection with praziquantel difficult. If infection persists after treatment, retreatment with this drug is indicated.

Dipylidium caninum. This tapeworm, with the dog or cat flea as its intermediate host, infects children when they inadvertently swallow a flea while playing with a pet. Diagnosis is made by finding the characteristic eggs or tapeworm segments in the stool.

Diphyllobothrium latum *(and related species).* This tapeworm, also called fish tapeworm, has fish as one of its intermediate hosts. Consumption of infected raw, freshwater fish (including salmon) leads to the infection. The worm sometimes causes megaloblastic anemia secondary to vitamin B12 deficiency. The diagnosis is made by recognition of the characteristic eggs or proglottids passed in the stool. Therapy with praziquantel is effective. Hydroxocobalamin injections and folic acid supplements may be required.

Echinococcus granulosus *and* E multilocularis. These tapeworms are the causes of hydatid disease. The distribution of *E granulosus* is related to sheep or cattle herding. Countries with the highest prevalence include Argentina, Greece, Italy, Lebanon, Romania, South Africa, Spain, Syria, Turkey, and the countries in the former Soviet Union. In the United States, small endemic foci exist in Arizona, California, New Mexico, and Utah. Dogs, coyotes, wolves, dingos, and jackals can become infected by swallowing protoscolices of the parasite within hydatid cysts in the organs of sheep or other intermediate hosts. Dogs pass embryonated eggs in their stools, and the sheep become infected by swallowing the eggs. If humans swallow *Echinococcus* eggs, they can become inadvertent intermediate hosts and develop cysts in various organs, such as the liver, lungs, kidney, and spleen. These cysts grow slowly (1 cm in diameter per year) and eventually can contain several liters of fluid. If a cyst ruptures, anaphylaxis and multiple secondary cysts from seeding of protoscolices can result. Clinical diagnosis is frequently difficult. A history of contact with dogs in an endemic area is helpful. Space-occupying lesions can be demonstrated by roentgenograms or computed tomography of various organs. Serologic tests, available at the Centers for Disease Control and Prevention, are helpful, but false-negative results can occur. Surgical treatment is indicated in some patients and requires meticulous care to prevent spillage of the cyst contents. Injection of a 0.1% cetrimide solution or 95% ethanol into the cyst before attempted removal can minimize the risk of dissemination if spillage occurs. Treatment with albendazole for several months is of benefit in many cases.

Echinococcus multilocularis, a species whose life cycle involves foxes and rodents, causes the alveolar form of hydatid disease, which is characterized by invasive growth of the larvae in the liver with occasional metastatic spread. The alveolar form of hydatid disease is limited to the Northern hemisphere and is diagnosed usually in persons 50 years or older. The preferred treatment is surgical extirpation of the entire larval mass. In nonresectable cases, continuous treatment with mebendazole or albendazole has been associated with clinical improvement.

Tetanus
(Lockjaw)

CLINICAL MANIFESTATIONS: Generalized tetanus (lockjaw) is a neurologic disease manifest by trismus and severe muscular spasms. It is caused by the neurotoxin produced by the anaerobic bacterium *Clostridium tetani* in a contaminated wound. Onset is gradual, occurring over 1 to 7 days, and progresses to severe generalized muscle spasms, which frequently are aggravated by any external stimulus. Severe spasms persist for 1 week or more and subside in a period of weeks in those who recover. Neonatal tetanus, a common cause of neonatal mortality in developing countries but rare in the United States, arises from contamination of the umbilical stump.

Localized tetanus is manifested by local muscle spasms in areas contiguous to a wound. Cephalic tetanus is a dysfunction of the cranial nerves associated with infected wounds on the head and neck. Both conditions may precede generalized tetanus.

ETIOLOGY: *Clostridium tetani*, the tetanus bacillus, is a spore-forming, anaerobic, Gram-positive bacillus. It produces a potent exotoxin (tetanospasmin), which acts at the myoneural junction of skeletal muscle and on neuronal membranes in the spinal cord, blocking inhibitory pulses to motor neurons. The action of tetanus toxin on the brain and sympathetic nervous system is less well documented. *Clostridium tetani* is a wound contaminant; it causes neither tissue destruction nor an inflammatory response.

EPIDEMIOLOGY: Tetanus occurs worldwide and is more frequent in warmer climates and months, in part because of the frequency of contaminated wounds. The organism, a normal inhabitant of soil and of animal and human intestines, is ubiquitous in the environment, especially where contamination by excreta is frequent. Wounds, recognized or unrecognized, are the sites at which the organism multiplies and elaborates toxin. Contaminated wounds, those with devitalized tissue and deep-puncture trauma, are at greatest risk. Neonatal tetanus is common in many developing countries where women are not immunized appropriately against tetanus. Widespread active immunization against tetanus has vastly modified the epidemiology of the disease in the United States. Tetanus is not transmissible from person to person.

The **incubation period** is 2 days to 2 months, averaging 10 days, and most cases occur within 14 days. In neonates it is usually 5 to 14 days. Shorter incubation periods have been associated with more heavily contaminated wounds, more severe disease, and a worse prognosis.

DIAGNOSTIC TESTS: The offending wound should be cultured. However, confirmation of the causative organism is made infrequently by culture. The diagnosis is made clinically by excluding other possibilities such as hypocalcemic tetany, phenothiazine reaction, strychnine poisoning, and hysteria.

TREATMENT:
- Tetanus immune globulin (TIG) (human) is recommended for treatment. A single dose of 3000 to 6000 U is recommended for children and adults; the optimum therapeutic dose, however, has not yet been established. Doses as small as 500 U have been demonstrated to be effective in the treatment of tetanus neonatorum. Preparations currently available must be given intramuscularly. Part of the dose should infiltrate locally around the wound, although the efficacy of this approach has not been proven. The result of studies on the benefit from intrathecal TIG are conflicting. The TIG formulation in use in the United States is not licensed or appropriate for intrathecal or intravenous use.
- In countries where TIG is not available, equine tetanus antitoxin (TAT) should be used. This product is no longer available in the United States. Tetanus antitoxin is administered as a single dose of 50 000 to 100 000 U after appropriate testing for sensitivity and desensitization if necessary (see Sensitivity Tests for Reactions to Animal Sera, p 42, and Desensitization to Animal Sera, p 43). Part of this dose (20 000 U) should be given intravenously. Doses as small as 10 000 U may be as effective as larger doses. Serum sickness occurs in 10% to 20% of recipients of products prepared from equine serum.
- Intravenous immune globulin (IGIV) contains antibodies to tetanus and can be considered for treatment if TIG is not available. Approval by the Food and Drug Administration has not been given for this use and the dosage has not been determined.
- All wounds should be properly cleaned and débrided, especially if extensive necrosis is present. In neonatal tetanus, wide excision of the umbilical stump is not indicated.
- Supportive care and pharmacotherapy to control tetanic spasms are of major importance.
- Oral (or intravenous) metronidazole (30 mg/kg per day, given at 6-hour intervals) is effective in reducing the number of vegetative forms of *C tetani* and is the antibiotic of choice. Parenteral penicillin G (100 000 U/kg per day, given at 4- to 6-hour intervals) is an alternative treatment. Therapy for 10 to 14 days is recommended.

ISOLATION OF THE HOSPITALIZED PATIENT: Standard precautions are recommended.

CONTROL MEASURES:

Care of Exposed Persons (see Table 3.58, p 520). Less than 1% of the recently reported cases of tetanus in the United States have occurred in individuals with adequate, up-to-date immunization. After primary immunization with tetanus toxoid, antitoxin persists at protective levels in most persons for at least 10 years and for a longer time after a booster immunization.

Table 3.58. Guide to Tetanus Prophylaxis in Routine Wound Management

History of Absorbed Tetanus Toxoid (Doses)	Clean, Minor Wounds		All Other Wounds*	
	Td[†]	TIG[‡]	Td[†]	TIG[‡]
Unknown or <3	Yes	No	Yes	Yes
≥3[§]	No[‖]	No	No[¶]	No

* Such as, but not limited to, wounds contaminated with dirt, feces, soil, and saliva; puncture wounds; avulsions; and wounds resulting from missiles, crushing, burns, and frostbite.
† For children <7 years old, DTaP (or DTP) is recommended; if pertussis vaccine is contraindicated, DT is given. For persons ≥7 years of age, Td is recommended. Td indicates adult-use tetanus and diphtheria toxoids; TIG, tetanus immune globulin (human).
‡ Equine tetanus antitoxin should be used when TIG is not available.
§ If only 3 doses of fluid toxoid have been received, a fourth dose of toxoid, preferably an adsorbed toxoid, should be given.
‖ Yes, if more than 10 years since last dose.
¶ Yes, if more than 5 years since last dose. (More frequent boosters are not needed and can accentuate side effects.)

- In the management of clean, minor wounds in those who have completed a primary series, ie, three doses of tetanus toxoid or receipt of a booster dose within 10 years, an additional dose of tetanus toxoid is not necessary.
- For other, more serious wounds, if indicated according to the guidelines in Table 3.58, a dose of tetanus toxoid should be given as soon as possible after the injury. While any open wound is a potential source of tetanus, those contaminated with dirt, feces, soil, and/or saliva are at increased risk. Wounds containing devitalized tissue, including necrotic or gangrenous wounds, frostbite, crush and avulsion injuries, and burns, are particularly prone to contamination with *C tetani*. Indications for TIG or antitoxin in partially immunized persons with more serious wounds also are listed in Table 3.58. If tetanus immunization is incomplete at the time of wound treatment, a dose should be given, and the series should be completed according to the primary immunization schedule. Tetanus immune globulin should be administered for tetanus-prone wounds in HIV-infected patients, regardless of the history of tetanus immunizations.
- In usual practice, when tetanus toxoid is required for wound prophylaxis in a child 7 years or older, the use of Td instead of tetanus toxoid alone is advisable so that adequate concentrations of diphtheria immunity also are maintained. When a booster injection is indicated for wound prophylaxis in a child younger than 7 years, DTaP (or DTP) should be used unless pertussis vaccine is contraindicated (see Pertussis, p 394), in which case immunization with DT is recommended.
- Passive protection with TIG or antitoxin is not indicated for patients with clean, minor wounds, regardless of immunization status, or for patients with other wounds who have had three or more previous injections of tetanus toxoid. Patients with more serious wounds who have had fewer than three previous injections of tetanus vaccine should receive TIG or antitoxin, as well as an additional dose of tetanus toxoid within 3 days. Intramuscular TIG is recom-

mended in a dose of 250 U. Tetanus antitoxin is used if TIG is unavailable; the dose is 3000 to 5000 U intramuscularly, after appropriate testing of the patient for sensitivity (see Sensitivity Tests for Reactions to Animal Sera, p 42). If tetanus toxoid and TIG or TAT are given concurrently, separate syringes and sites should be used. Administration of TIG or TAT does not preclude initiation of active immunization with tetanus toxoid. Efforts should be made to initiate immunization and arrange for its completion.

- Regardless of immunization status, dirty wounds should be properly cleaned and débrided if dirt and/or necrotic tissue are present. Wounds should receive prompt surgical treatment to remove all devitalized tissue and foreign material as an essential part of tetanus prophylaxis. It is not necessary or appropriate to extensively débride puncture wounds.

Immunization: Active immunization with tetanus toxoid is indicated for all persons. Adsorbed tetanus toxoid is preferred to fluid toxoid because immunity lasts longer. Vaccine is given intramuscularly and may be given concurrently with other vaccines (see Simultaneous Administration of Multiple Vaccines, p 21). *Haemophilus influenzae* conjugate vaccines containing tetanus toxoid (PRP-T) are not substitutes for tetanus toxoid immunization. Recommendations for use of tetanus toxoid-containing vaccines are summarized in Fig 1.1 (p 18) and Table 1.3 (p 20) are as follows:

- Immunization for children from 2 months to the seventh birthday (see Fig 1.1 and Table 1.3, p 18 and p 20) should consist of five doses of tetanus toxoid-containing vaccine. The initial three doses are given as DTaP (or DTP) vaccine, administered intramuscularly at 2-month intervals beginning at approximately 2 months of age (see Pertussis, p 399). A fourth dose is recommended 6 to 12 months after the third dose, usually at 15 to 18 months of age. A fifth dose of DTaP (or DTP) is given before school entry (kindergarten or elementary school) at 4 to 6 years of age, unless the fourth dose was given after the fourth birthday.

- Children younger than 1 year in whom pertussis immunization is deferred or contraindicated (see Pertussis, p 400) should be immunized with DT in a three-dose schedule in which doses are given at 2-month intervals. A fourth dose of DT should be given approximately 6 to 12 months after the third dose and the fifth dose given before school entry at 4 to 6 years of age. Children who have not received previous doses of DT, DTP, or DTaP and who are 1 year or older should receive two doses of DT approximately 2 months apart, followed by a third dose 6 to 12 months after the second dose to complete the initial series. An additional dose is necessary before school entry when the child is 4 to 6 years old, unless the fourth dose was given after the fourth birthday.

- Children who have received one or two doses of DTP, DTaP, or DT in the first year of life and for whom further pertussis vaccination is contraindicated should receive additional doses of DT until a total of five doses of diphtheria and tetanus toxoids are received by the time of school entry. The fourth dose is administered 6 to 12 months after the third dose. The preschool (fifth) dose is omitted if the fourth dose was given after the fourth birthday.

---

* Vaccines containing both tetanus and diphtheria toxoids in use in the United States, including DTaP, DTP, DT and Td, are adsorbed to aluminum salts.

- Children who have received fewer than the recommended number of doses of pertussis vaccine but who have received the recommended number of DT doses for their age (ie, those in whom vaccination was started with DT and who were then given DTaP [or DTP]), dose(s) of DTaP (or DTP) should be given to complete the recommended pertussis immunization schedule (see Pertussis, p 399). However the total number of doses of diphtheria and tetanus toxoids (as DT, DTaP, or DTP) should not exceed six before the fourth birthday.
- Children 7 years and older and adults not previously immunized should receive Td (ie, adult-type tetanus and diphtheria toxoids, see Table 1.3, p 20). The Td preparation contains not more than 2 Lf (limes flocculating) units of diphtheria toxoid, as compared with 6.7 to 25 Lf units in the DTaP, DTP and DT preparations for use in infants and younger children. Because of the lower dose of diphtheria toxoid, Td is less likely than DT to produce reactions in older children and adults. Two doses of Td are given 1 to 2 months apart; a third dose should be given 6 to 12 months after the second.
- After the initial immunization series is completed at 4 to 6 years, a booster dose of tetanus toxoid (given as Td) is recommended at 11 to 12 years of age (and should be given no later than by 16 years of age) and every 10 years thereafter. This 10-year period is determined from the last dose administered, irrespective of whether it was given during routine childhood immunization or as part of wound management. Because the immunity conferred by adsorbed preparations of tetanus toxoid has proved to be of long duration, routine boosters more frequently than every 10 years are not indicated and may be associated with an increased incidence and severity of reactions.
- If more than 5 years have elapsed since the last dose, a booster of Td should be considered for persons who are going to wilderness expeditions where tetanus boosters may not be readily available.
- Prevention of neonatal tetanus can be accomplished by prenatal immunization of the previously unimmunized mother. Two doses should be administered at least 4 weeks apart and the second dose should be given at least 2 weeks before delivery. Pregnant women who have not completed their primary series should receive a second dose of Td as soon as possible. Tetanus toxoid immunization is not contraindicated during pregnancy.
- Active immunization against tetanus should always be undertaken during convalescence from tetanus because this exotoxin-mediated disease usually does not confer immunity.

Adverse Events, Precautions, and Contraindications. Severe anaphylactic reactions, Guillain-Barré syndrome (GBS), and brachial neuritis attributable to tetanus toxoid have been reported but are extremely rare. No increased risk of GBS has been observed with use of DTP or DTaP vaccine in children. When immunizing children in whom GBS developed within 6 weeks after receipt of tetanus toxoid-containing vaccine (ie, DTP, DTaP, DT, or Td), the risks and benefits of additional doses should be considered. Such children who have not previously completed the primary series should do so, as the potential benefits outweigh the possible risks. Children who have already received three or more doses should not be given additional routine tetanus toxoid immunizations.

An immediate anaphylactic reaction to tetanus toxoid-containing vaccine (ie, DTaP, DTP, DT, or Td) is a contraindication to further doses unless the patient can be desensitized to the toxoid (see Pertussis, p 394). Because of uncertainty about which vaccine component (ie, diphtheria, tetanus or pertussis) might be responsible and the importance of tetanus vaccination, persons who experience anaphylactic reactions may be referred to an allergist for evaluation and possible desensitization.

Other Control Measures. Sterilization of hospital supplies will prevent the infrequent instances of tetanus that may occur in a hospital from contaminated sutures, instruments, or plaster casts.

For the prevention of neonatal tetanus, preventive measures (in addition to maternal immunization) include community immunization programs for adolescent girls and women of childbearing age and appropriate training of midwives in recommendations for immunization and sterile technique.

Tinea Capitis
(Ringworm of the Scalp)

CLINICAL MANIFESTATIONS: Fungal infection of the scalp can present with one of the following distinct clinical syndromes:
- Patchy areas of dandruff-like scaling, with subtle or extensive hair loss. This form is easily confused with dandruff, seborrheic dermatitis, or atopic dermatitis.
- Discrete areas of hair loss studded by the stubs of broken hairs—so-called black dot ringworm.
- Numerous discrete pustules or excoriations with little hair loss or scaling.
- Kerion, which is a boggy, inflammatory mass surrounded by follicular pustules. Kerion may be accompanied by fever and local lymphadenopathy and is frequently misdiagnosed as impetigo, cellulitis, or an abscess of the scalp.

A pruritic fine papulovesicular eruption (dermatophytid, "id" reaction) involving the trunk, hands or face, caused by a hypersensitivity response to the infecting fungus, may accompany the scalp lesions.

Tinea capitis can be confused with many other diseases, including seborrheic dermatitis, psoriasis, alopecia areata, trichotillomania, folliculitis, impetigo, and lupus erythematosus.

ETIOLOGY: *Trichophyton tonsurans* is currently the cause of tinea capitis in more than 90% of cases in North and Central America. *Microsporum canis, M audouinii,* and *T mentagrophytes* are now less common. The causative agents may vary in different geographic areas, but in general are adapted to infecting humans or animals.

EPIDEMIOLOGY: Infection of the scalp with *T tonsurans* is the result of person-to-person transmission. This organism remains viable on combs, brushes, couches, and sheets for long periods. Occasionally, *T tonsurans* is cultured from the scalps of asymptomatic children, and it is readily cultured from asymptomatic family members of infected individuals. Persons who harbor the organism are thought to have a significant role as reservoirs for infection and reinfection within families, schools, and communities. Tinea capitis due to *T tonsurans* occurs most commonly in children between the ages of 3 and 9 years, and it appears to be more common in black children.

Microsporum canis infection results from transmission from animals to humans. It is frequently the result of contact with household pets.

The **incubation period** is unknown.

DIAGNOSTIC TESTS: Hairs for potassium hydroxide wet mount examination and for culture may be obtained by gentle scraping of a moistened area of the scalp with a curved scalpel. Broken hairs in black dot ringworm should be obtained when possible. In cases of *T tonsurans* infection, microscopic examination of a potassium hydroxide wet mount preparation discloses numerous arthroconidia within the hair shaft. In *Microsporum* infection, spores surround the hair shaft. Use of dermatophyte test medium (DTM) is a reliable, simple, and inexpensive method of diagnosing tinea capitus. Skin scrapings or hairs from lesions are inoculated directly onto the culture medium and incubated at room temperature. After 1 to 2 weeks, a phenol red indicator in the agar will turn from yellow to red in the area surrounding a dermatophyte colony. When necessary, the diagnosis can be confirmed by culture on Sabouraud's dextrose agar.

Wood's light examination of the hair of patients with *Microsporum* infection results in brilliant green fluorescence. However, because *T tonsurans* does not fluoresce under Wood's light, this diagnostic test is not helpful in most cases of tinea capitis.

TREATMENT: Tinea capitis requires systemic antifungal therapy. Microsize griseofulvin is given orally, 10 to 20 mg/kg per day, maximum 1 g, in a single dose. The dose of ultramicrosize griseofulvin is 5 to 10 mg/kg per day, maximum 750 mg, also in a single dose. Optimally, griseofulvin is given after a meal containing fat (eg, peanut butter or ice cream). Treatment for 4 to 6 weeks is usually required, and it should be continued 2 weeks beyond clinical resolution. Some children may require higher doses of microsize griseofulvin (20 to 25 mg/kg per day) or the ultramicrosize drug formulation to achieve clinical cure. Treatment with either oral itraconazole or oral terbinafine also is effective for tinea capitis, but these products have not been approved by the Food and Drug Administration for this indication and they are much more expensive than griseofulvin.

Topical antifungal medications are not effective in the treatment of tinea capitis. Selenium sulfide shampoo, 2.5%, used twice a week, decreases fungal shedding and may help curb the spread of infection. Selenium sulfide shampoo, 1%, also appears effective.

Kerion, caused by a hypersensitivity reaction to the fungal infection, can be treated with corticosteroid therapy in addition to griseofulvin. Prednisone or prednisolone given orally in doses of 1.5 to 2 mg/kg per day usually effect a rapid response. Treatment with corticosteroids should be continued for approximately 2 weeks, with tapering doses toward the end of therapy. Antibiotics and/or surgery are not indicated.

ISOLATION OF THE HOSPITALIZED PATIENT: Standard precautions are recommended.

CONTROL MEASURES: Early treatment of infected persons is indicated, as is examination of siblings and other household contacts for evidence of tinea capitis. Ribbons, combs, and brushes should not be shared by family members. Barber tools should be cleaned and sterilized.

Children receiving treatment for tinea capitis may attend school. Hair cuts, shaving of the head, or wearing a cap during treatment are not necessary.

Tinea Corporis
(Ringworm of the Body)

CLINICAL MANIFESTATIONS: Superficial tinea infections of the nonhairy (glabrous) skin involve the face, trunk, and limbs, but not the scalp, beard, groin, hands, and feet. The lesion is generally circular (hence, the term "ringworm"), slightly erythematous, and well demarcated with a scaly, vesicular, or pustular border. Pruritis is common. Lesions are often mistaken for atopic dermatitis, seborrheic dermatitis or contact dermatitis. Consequently, a frequent source of confusion in diagnosis is an alteration in the appearance of lesions resulting from topical corticosteroid application. This atypical presentation has been termed "tinea incognita." In patients with diminished T-lymphocyte function (eg, HIV infection), the rash may appear as grouped papules or pustules unaccompanied by scaling and erythema.

A pruritic fine papulovesicular eruption (dermatophytid or "id" reaction) involving the trunk, hands, or face, caused by a hypersensitivity response to the infecting fungus, may accompany the rash.

ETIOLOGY: The prime causes of the disease are fungi of the genera *Trichophyton,* especially *T rubrum* and *T mentagrophytes; Microsporum,* especially *M canis*; and *Epidermophyton floccosum.*

EPIDEMIOLOGY: The fungi occur worldwide and are transmissible by direct contact with infected humans, animals, or fomites. Fungi in the lesions are communicable.

The **incubation period** is unknown.

DIAGNOSIS: Use of dermatophyte test medium (DTM) is a reliable, simple, and inexpensive method of diagnosis. Skin scrapings from lesions are inoculated directly onto the culture medium and incubated at room temperature. After 1 to 2 weeks, a phenol red indicator in the agar will turn from yellow to red in the area surrounding a dermatophyte colony. When necessary, the diagnosis can be confirmed by culture on Sabouraud's dextrose agar. The organisms also can be identified by microscopic examination of a potassium hydroxide wet mount of skin scrapings.

TREATMENT: Topical application of miconazole, clotrimazole, terbinafine, econazole, tolnaftate, naftifine, or ciclopirox preparation twice a day, or of econazole, ketoconazole, oxiconazole, or sulconazole preparation once a day, is recommended (see Topical Drugs for Superficial Fungal Infections, p 632). Although clinical resolution may be evident within 2 weeks of therapy, a minimum duration of 4 weeks is generally indicated. Topical preparations of antifungal medication mixed with high-potency corticosteroids should not be used because corticosteroids can cause striae and atrophy of the skin.

If the lesions are extensive or unresponsive to topical therapy, griseofulvin is administered orally for 4 weeks (see Tinea Capitis, p 523). Oral itraconazole and oral terbinafine are effective alternative therapies for tinea corporis, but these products are not approved by the Food and Drug Administration for treatment of tinea corporis in children.

ISOLATION OF THE HOSPITALIZED PATIENT: Standard precautions are recommended.

CONTROL MEASURES: Direct contact with known or suspected sources of infection should be avoided. Periodic inspections of contacts for early lesions and prompt therapy are recommended.

Tinea Cruris
(Jock Itch)

CLINICAL MANIFESTATIONS: Tinea cruris is an extremely common superficial fungal disorder of the groin and upper thighs. The eruption is sharply marginated and usually is bilaterally symmetric. Involved skin is erythematous and scaly and varies in color from red to brown; occasionally, it is accompanied by central clearing and a vesiculopapular border. In chronic infections, the margin can be subtle, and lichenification can be present. Tinea cruris may be extremely pruritic. It should be differentiated from intertrigo, seborrheic dermatitis, psoriasis, primary irritant dermatitis, allergic contact dermatitis (generally caused by the therapeutic agents applied to the area), or erythrasma (a superficial bacterial infection of the skin caused by *Corynebacterium minutissimum*).

ETIOLOGY: The fungi *Epidermophyton floccosum, Trichophyton rubrum,* and *T mentagrophytes* are the most common causes. This infection is commonly seen in association with tinea pedis.

EPIDEMIOLOGY: Tinea cruris occurs predominantly in adolescent and adult males. Moisture, close-fitting garments, friction, and obesity are predisposing factors. Direct or indirect person-to-person transmission may occur.

The **incubation period** is unknown.

DIAGNOSTIC TESTS: The fungi responsible for tinea cruris may be detected by microscopic examination of a potassium hydroxide wet mount of scales. Use of dermatophyte test medium (DTM) is a reliable, simple, and inexpensive method of diagnosing tinea. Skin scrapings from lesions are inoculated directly onto the culture medium and incubated at room temperature. After 1 to 2 weeks, a phenol red indicator in the agar will turn from yellow to red in the area surrounding a dermatophyte colony. When necessary, the diagnosis can be confirmed by culture on Sabouraud's dextrose agar. A characteristic, coral-red fluorescence under Wood's light can identify the presence of erythrasma and, thus, exclude tinea cruris.

TREATMENT: Topical application for 4 to 6 weeks of clotrimazole, haloprogin, miconazole, terbinafine, tolnaftate, or ciclopirox preparation gently rubbed into the affected areas and surrounding skin twice daily, or topical econazole, ketoconazole, naftifine, oxiconazole, or sulconazole preparation once daily is effective (see Topical Drugs for Superficial Fungal Infections, p 632). Tinea pedis, if present, should be treated concurrently (see Tinea Pedis).

Topical preparations of antifungal medication mixed with high-potency corticosteroids should not be used because the corticosteroids can cause striae and atrophy of the skin. Loose-fitting, washed, cotton underclothes to reduce chafing, as well as the use of a bland, absorbent powder can be helpful adjuvants to therapy. Griseofulvin orally for 2 to 6 weeks may be effective in unresponsive cases (see Tinea Capitis, p 523). Oral itraconazole and oral terbinafine are effective alternative therapies for tinea corporis, but these products are not approved by the Food and Drug Administration for treatment of tinea cruris and they are usually not necessary.

ISOLATION OF THE HOSPITALIZED PATIENT: Standard precautions are recommended.

CONTROL MEASURES: Infections should be treated promptly. Potentially involved areas should be kept dry, and loose undergarments should be recommended. Patients should be advised to dry the groin area before drying their feet to avoid inoculating dermatophytes of tinea pedis into the groin area.

Tinea Pedis
(Athlete's Foot, Ringworm of the Feet)

CLINICAL MANIFESTATIONS: Tinea pedis consists of fine vesiculopustular or scaly lesions that are frequently pruritic. The lesions can involve all areas of the foot, but usually they are patchy in distribution, with a predisposition to fissures and scaling between the toes, particularly in the third and fourth interdigital spaces. Toenails may be infected and can be dystrophic (tinea unguium). This condition must be differentiated from dyshidrotic eczema, atopic dermatitis, contact dermatitis, juvenile plantar dermatosis and erythrasma (a superficial bacterial infection caused by *Corynebacterium minutissimum*).

Tinea pedis (and many other fungal infections) can be accompanied by a hypersensitivity reaction to the fungi (the dermatophytid or "id" reaction), with resulting vesicular eruptions on the palms and the sides of the fingers, and, occasionally, by an erythematous vesicular eruption on the extremities and trunk.

ETIOLOGY: The fungi *Trichophyton rubrum, T mentagrophytes,* and *Epidermophyton floccosum* are the most common causes.

EPIDEMIOLOGY: Tinea pedis is a common infection in adolescents and adults but is relatively uncommon in young children. It occurs worldwide. The fungi are acquired by contact with skin scales containing fungi or with fungi in damp areas, such as swimming pools, locker rooms, and shower rooms. Tinea pedis in a family

member tends to spread throughout the household. It is communicable for as long
as the infection is present. The rapid growth of fingernails and toenails makes fungal
infection of the nail plate rare in children.

The **incubation period** is unknown.

DIAGNOSIS: Tinea pedis is usually diagnosed by the clinical manifestations and may
be corroborated by microscopic examination of a potassium hydroxide wet mount
of the cutaneous scrapings. Use of dermatophyte test medium (DTM) is a reliable,
simple, and inexpensive method of diagnosis for use in complicated or unresponsive
cases. Skin scraping or nail clippings are inoculated directly onto the culture medium
and incubated at room temperature. After 1 to 2 weeks, a phenol red indicator in the
agar will turn from yellow to red in the area surrounding a dermatophyte colony.
When necessary, the diagnosis can be confirmed by culture on Sabouraud's dextrose
agar. Infection of the nail can be verified by fungal culture of desquamated subungual material.

TREATMENT: Topical application of miconazole, haloprogin, clotrimazole,
ciclopirox, terbinafine, or tolnaftate preparation twice a day, or of econazole, ketoconazole, naftifine, oxiconazole, or sulconazole preparation once a day, can be used
for active infections (see Topical Drugs for Superficial Fungal Infections, p 632).
Acute vesicular lesions may be treated with intermittent use of open, wet compresses
(eg, with Burrow's solution, 1:80).

Griseofulvin administered orally for 6 to 8 weeks may be necessary for the
treatment of severe, chronic, and recalcitrant tinea pedis. Oral itraconazole and
oral terbinafine also are effective alternative therapies for tinea pedis unresponsive to
topical therapy, but these products have not been approved by the Food and Drug
Administration for this purpose in children. Id reactions are treated by wet compresses, topical corticosteroids, occasionally systemic corticosteroids, and eradication
of the primary source of infection.

Recurrence is prevented by proper foot hygiene, which includes keeping the feet
dry and cool, gentle cleaning, drying between the toes, the use of absorbent antifungal foot powder, frequent airing of affected areas, and avoidance of occlusive foot-
wear and nylon socks or other fabrics that interfere with dissipation of moisture.

In the past, most nail infections, particularly toenail infections, have been
highly resistant to oral griseofulvin therapy. Recent studies in adult patients, however,
have demonstrated a high cure rate following therapy with oral itraconazole or oral
terbinafine. Further studies on the safety and efficacy of these drugs in children
are necessary before either drug can be recommended. Recurrences are common.
Removal of the nail plate with use of oral therapy during the period of regrowth
can help to effect a cure in resistant cases.

ISOLATION OF THE HOSPITALIZED PATIENT: Standard precautions are
recommended.

CONTROL MEASURES: Treatment of patients with active infections should reduce
transmission. Public areas conducive to transmission (eg, swimming pools) should
not be used by those with active infection. Chemical foot baths are of no value and
can facilitate spread of infection. Because recurrence after treatment is common,

proper foot hygiene is important (as described in Treatment). Patients should be advised to dry the groin area before drying their feet to avoid inoculating tinea pedis dermatophytes into the groin area.

Tinea Versicolor
(Pityriasis Versicolor)

CLINICAL MANIFESTATIONS: Tinea (pityriasis) versicolor is a common, superficial disorder of the skin characterized by multiple scaling and oval macular and patchy lesions, usually distributed over the upper portions of the trunk, proximal areas of the arms, and neck. Facial involvement is particularly common in children. The lesions can be hypopigmented or hyperpigmented (fawn colored or brown) and can be somewhat lighter than the surrounding skin. The lesions fail to tan during the summer and during the winter are relatively darker, hence the term "versicolor." Common conditions confused with this disorder include pityriasis alba, postinflammatory hypopigmentation, vitiligo, melasma, seborrheic dermatitis, pityriasis rosea, and secondary syphilis.

ETIOLOGY: *Malassezia furfur* is the cause. This dimorphic lipid-dependent fungus exists on normal skin in the yeast phase and causes clinical lesions only when substantial growth of hyphae occurs. Moist heat encourages rapid overgrowth.

EPIDEMIOLOGY: Tinea versicolor occurs worldwide, but is more common in tropical areas. Although primarily a disorder of adolescents and young adults 15 to 30 years, it also can occur in prepubertal children and, at times, infants. The fungus is transmitted by personal contact during periods of scaling.

The **incubation period** is unknown.

DIAGNOSIS: The clinical appearance is usually diagnostic. Involved areas are yellow fluorescent under Wood's light. Scale scrapings examined microscopically in a potassium hydroxide wet mount preparation or stained with methylene blue or May-Grünwald-Giemsa stain disclose the pathognomonic clusters of yeast cells and hyphae ("spaghetti and meatball" appearance). Growth of this yeast on culture requires a source of long-chain fatty acids, which may be accomplished by overlaying Sabouraud's dextrose agar medium with sterile olive oil.

TREATMENT: Topical treatment with 2.5% selenium sulfide lotion or 1% shampoo usually is recommended, but oral antifungal drugs have distinct advantages in ease of administration and shorter courses of treatment.

Topical preparations are applied in a thin layer covering the body surface from the face to the knees daily for 30 minutes for a week, followed by monthly applications for 3 months (to help prevent recurrences). Other topical preparations with therapeutic efficacy include sodium hyposulfite or thiosulfate in 15% to 25% concentrations (eg, Tinver lotion) applied twice a day for 2 to 4 weeks, or antifungal agents such as clotrimazole, econazole, haloprogin, ketoconazole, miconazole, or naftifine (see Topical Drugs for Superficial Fungal Infections, p 632).

A single dose of ketoconazole (400 mg orally) or 5-day course of itraconazole (200 mg orally once a day) has been effective in adults. These drugs, however, have not been tested extensively in children for this disorder and are not yet approved by the Food and Drug Administration for this indication. Some experts recommend for children that the duration of ketoconazole should be three days rather than the single dose given adults (for pediatric dosage recommendations for ketoconazole and itraconazole, see Recommended Doses of Parenteral and Oral Antifungal Drugs, p 628). Exercise to increase sweating and skin concentrations of medication may enhance the effectiveness of systemic therapy. Patients should be warned that repigmentation may not occur for several months after successful treatment.

ISOLATION OF THE HOSPITALIZED PATIENT: Standard precautions are recommended.

CONTROL MEASURES: Infected individuals should be treated.

Toxocariasis
(Visceral Larva Migrans, Ocular Larva Migrans)

CLINICAL MANIFESTATIONS: The severity of the symptoms depends on the number of larvae ingested and the degree of allergic response. Most persons who are lightly infected are asymptomatic. Visceral larva migrans typically occurs in children 1 to 4 years old with history of pica but can occur in older children. Characteristic manifestations include fever, leukocytosis, persistent eosinophilia, hypergammaglobulinemia, and hepatomegaly. Other manifestations include malaise, anemia, cough, and, in rare instances, pneumonia, myocarditis, and encephalitis. When ocular invasion (endophthalmitis or retinal granulomas) occurs, other evidence of infection usually is lacking, suggesting that the visceral and ocular manifestations are distinct syndromes. Atypical forms of presentation include hemorrhagic rash and convulsions.

ETIOLOGY: Toxocariasis is caused by *Toxocara* species, which are common roundworms of dogs and cats (especially puppies or kittens), specifically *T canis* an *T cati* in the United States; most cases are caused by *T canis*. Other nematodes of animals can also cause this syndrome, although rarely.

EPIDEMIOLOGY: Humans are infected by the ingestion of eggs in soil containing infective larvae. A history of pica, particularly the eating of soil, is common. Direct contact with dogs is of secondary importance as eggs are not infective immediately when shed in the feces. Most reported cases are from North America and other developed countries, and involve children. Puppies in the household are the apparent source for most cases, but the eggs are found wherever dogs and cats defecate, such as parks and other public places.

The **incubation period** is unknown.

DIAGNOSTIC TESTS: Hypereosinophilia and hypergammaglobulinemia associated with elevated titers of isohemagglutinins to the A and B blood group antigens are presumptive evidence of infection. Microscopic identification of the larvae in a liver biopsy specimen is diagnostic but this finding is infrequent. A negative liver biopsy for larvae, therefore, does not exclude the diagnosis. An enzyme immunoassay for *Toxocara* antibodies in serum, available at the Centers for Disease Control and Prevention and some private laboratories, can provide presumptive evidence of toxocariasis. It is both specific and sensitive for the diagnosis of visceral larva migrans, but is less sensitive for the diagnosis of ocular larva migrans.

TREATMENT: Mebendazole, thiabendazole, albenzadole, and diethylcarbamazine appear to reduce symptoms of visceral larva migrans. Mebendazole may have less toxicity than thiabendazole or diethylcarbamazine. Albendazole has recently been approved by the Food and Drug Administration, but not for this indication. In severe cases with myocarditis or involvement of the central nervous system, corticosteroid therapy is indicated. Correcting the underlying causes of pica will help prevent reinfection.

Antihelmintic treatment of ocular larva migrans is not effective. Inflammation may be reduced by injection of corticosteroids and secondary damage aided by surgery.

ISOLATION OF THE HOSPITALIZED PATIENT: Standard precautions are recommended.

CONTROL MEASURES: Proper disposal of cat and dog feces is essential. Treatment of puppies and kittens with antihelmintics at 2, 4, 6, and 8 weeks of age prevents excretion of eggs by worms acquired transplacentally or through mother's milk. Covering sandboxes when not in use is helpful. No specific management of exposed persons is recommended.

Toxoplasma gondii Infections
(Toxoplasmosis)

CLINICAL MANIFESTATIONS: Infants with congenital infection are asymptomatic at birth in 70% to 90% of cases, although visual impairment, learning disabilities, or mental retardation will become apparent in a large percentage of children months to several years later. Symptoms of congenital toxoplasmosis present at birth can include a maculopapular rash, generalized lymphadenopathy, hepatomegaly, splenomegaly, jaundice, and/or thrombocytopenia. As a consequence of intrauterine meningoencephalitis, the infant can develop cerebrospinal fluid abnormalities, hydrocephalus, microcephaly, chorioretinitis, and/or convulsions. Cerebral calcifications may be demonstrated on a roentgenogram or by computed tomography of the head. Some severely affected infants die in utero or within a few days of birth.

Isolated ocular toxoplasmosis most often occurs as a result of congenital infection but can result from acquired infection. Ocular disease can become reactivated years after the initial infection, both in healthy and immunocompromised individuals.

Toxoplasma infection acquired after birth is usually asymptomatic. When symptoms do develop, they are nonspecific and include malaise, fever, sore throat, and myalgia. Lymphadenopathy, frequently cervical, is the most common sign. Occasionally, patients may present with a mononucleosis-like illness associated with a macular rash and hepatosplenomegaly. The clinical course is usually benign and self-limited. Myocarditis, pericarditis, and pneumonitis are rare complications.

Chronically infected immunodeficient patients, such as those with HIV infection, can develop encephalitis from reactivated infection, or less commonly, systemic toxoplasmosis. Although rare, infants who are born to HIV-infected mothers or mothers immunosuppressed for other reasons, and who are chronically infected with *Toxoplasma*, may acquire congenital toxoplasmosis as a result of reactivated maternal parasitemia.

Infants with both perinatally acquired HIV infection and congenital toxoplasmosis who are not treated early appear to have a more fulminant HIV disease course.

ETIOLOGY: *Toxoplasma gondii*, a protozoan parasite, is the only known species of *Toxoplasma* that is pathogenic for humans.

EPIDEMIOLOGY: *Toxoplasma gondii* is worldwide in distribution and infects most species of warm-blooded animals. Members of the cat family are the definitive hosts. Cats acquire the infection when they are exposed to feces from an infected cat or when they feed on infected animals, such as mice or uncooked household meats. The parasite replicates sexually in the feline small intestine. For 2 to 4 weeks after primary infection, cats excrete the oocysts in their stools. After excretion, oocysts require a maturation phase (sporulation) of 24 to 48 hours in temperate climates before they are infective by the oral route. Intermediate hosts (including sheep, pigs, and cattle) can have tissue cysts in their brain, myocardium, skeletal muscle, and other organs. These cysts remain viable for the lifetime of the host. Humans become infected primarily either by consumption of poorly cooked meat or by accidental ingestion of sporulated oocysts from soil or in contaminated food. Transmission of *T gondii* has been documented to result from blood or blood product transfusion and organ (ie, heart) or bone marrow transplantation from a seropositive donor with latent infection. Congenital transmission in the overwhelming majority of cases occurs as a result of primary maternal infection during gestation. The frequency of congenital toxoplasmosis in the United States has been estimated to be 1 in 1000 to 1 in 10 000 live births. Rarely, infection has occurred as a result of a laboratory accident.

The **incubation period** of the acquired infection, based on a well-studied outbreak, is estimated to be approximately 7 days, with a range of 4 to 21 days.

DIAGNOSTIC TESTS: Serologic tests are the primary means of diagnosis, but results must be interpreted carefully. IgG-specific antibodies are measured commonly by an indirect immunofluorescence test or enzyme immunoassay (EIA) in most clinical laboratories. IgG-specific antibodies peak in concentration 1 to 2 months after infection and remain positive indefinitely. For determination of acute infection, the Centers for Disease Control and Prevention recommends a capture-EIA for IgM antibodies. IgM-specific antibodies can be detected 2 weeks after the infection, reach peak concentrations in 1 month, decline thereafter, and usually become undetectable within 6 to 9 months. On rare occasions, IgM-specific antibodies are detectable for as long as 2 years following acute infection. Tests to detect IgA antibodies, which fall to undetectable concentrations sooner than IgM antibodies, are useful in the diagnosis of congenital infections and other patients for whom more precise information about the duration of infection is needed. These tests are available only in reference laboratories. Tests for specific IgM antibodies should be performed by an experienced laboratory; test kits used by some laboratories can give false-positive and false-negative results.

Seroconversion or a fourfold rise in specific IgG antibody titer suggests recently acquired infection, but the results can be misleading if serum specimens are not tested concurrently to control for day-to-day laboratory variability. Patients with seroconversion or a fourfold rise in IgG antibody titer should have specific IgM antibody determinations performed by a reference laboratory.

Prenatal. A definitive diagnosis of congenital toxoplasmosis can be made prenatally by (1) detecting the parasite in fetal blood or amniotic fluid or (2) documenting the presence of *Toxoplasma* IgM and IgA antibodies in fetal blood. The parasite can be isolated by mouse inoculation or its genomic material can be detected by the polymerase chain reaction (PCR) in a reference laboratory. Serial fetal ultrasounds should be performed in cases of suspected congenital infection to detect any increase in size of the lateral ventricles of the central nervous system or other signs of fetal infection.

Postnatal. If the diagnosis is unconfirmed at the time of delivery in an infant with suspected toxoplasmosis, ophthalmologic, auditory, and neurologic examinations and computed tomography of the head should be performed. An attempt should be made to isolate *T gondii* from the placenta, cord, and/or the infant's peripheral blood by mouse inoculation. Alternatively, the buffy coat from 1 mL of blood or the cell pellet from the cerebrospinal fluid may be tested by PCR for genetic evidence of the parasite. Congenital toxoplasmosis also can be diagnosed serologically by the detection of *Toxoplasma*-specific IgM or IgA or the persistence of *Toxoplasma* IgG beyond 12 months of age. Blood should be sent to a reference laboratory that performs the mouse inoculation and the *Toxoplasma* IgM and IgA assays by the double-sandwich IgM EIA (DS-IgM EIA) or IgM immunosorbent agglutination assay (ISAGA). The DS-IgM EIA and the ISAGA detect *Toxoplasma* IgM in approximately 75% to 80% of infants with congenital infection. The sensitivity of both the immunofluorescent and capture-EIA assays for *Toxoplasma* IgM are significantly less than that of the DS-IgM, IgA EIA or ISAGA assays, and negative results with these assays do not exclude congenital infection. Circulating maternal *Toxoplasma* IgG antibodies in an uninfected infant usually become undetectable by 6 to 12 months of age.

Infants should be evaluated for congenital toxoplasmosis if they are born to women who are infected concurrently with HIV and *Toxoplasma* or to women who have evidence of primary *Toxoplasma* infection during gestation.

HIV Infection. Patients with HIV infection latently infected with *Toxoplasma* have variable titers of IgG antibody to *Toxoplasma* but rarely have IgM antibody. While seroconversion and fourfold rises in IgG antibody titers may occur, the ability to diagnose active disease in AIDS patients commonly is impaired by immunosuppression in these patients. In many cases, a presumptive diagnosis of *Toxoplasma* encephalitis is based on the presence of the characteristic clinical and roentgeno-graphic findings in an HIV-infected patient who is seropositive for *Toxoplasma* IgG. If the patient does not respond to an empiric trial of anti-*Toxoplasma* therapy, demonstration of *T gondii* organisms, antigen, or DNA in biopsied tissue, blood, and/or cerebrospinal fluid may be necessary to confirm the diagnosis.

Infants born to women who are dually infected with both HIV and *Toxoplasma* or to women who have evidence of primary *Toxoplasma* infection during gestation should be evaluated for congenital toxoplasmosis.

Diagnosis of ocular toxoplasmosis is based on observation of characteristic retinal lesions in conjunction with serum *Toxoplasma*-specific IgG or IgM antibodies.

TREATMENT: Most cases of acquired infection do not require specific antimicrobial therapy. When indicated, the combination of pyrimethamine and sulfadiazine,* which is synergistic against *Toxoplasma,* is the most widely accepted regimen for children and adults with acute, symptomatic disease. Pyrimethamine, 1 mg/kg per day (maximum daily dose, 25 mg) orally once a day in combination with sulfadiazine, 85 to 100 mg/kg per day in four divided doses (maximum daily dose 8 g) should be given for 3 to 6 weeks. Supplemental folinic acid (calcium leucovorin) must be administered concurrently (5 to 10 mg every 3 days orally or parenterally) to prevent hematologic toxic effects. Alternatively, pyrimethamine can be used in combination with clindamycin if the patient does not tolerate sulfadiazine. The use of corticosteroids in the management of ocular complication and of central nervous system disease is controversial.

Patients infected with HIV who have had toxoplasmic encephalitis should receive suppressive therapy. Regimens for primary treatment also are effective for suppressive therapy.

For HIV-infected adults, primary chemoprophylaxis against toxoplasmosis has been recommended for those who are *Toxoplasma*-seropositive and have low CD4+ T-lymphocyte counts by the US Public Health Services (USPHS) and Infectious Diseases Society of America (IDSA) Prevention of Opportunistic Infections Working Group.* The recommended drug is trimethoprim-sulfamethoxazole. Current data are insufficient for formulation of specific guidelines for children. Based on recommendations for adults, chemoprophylaxis in some circumstances should be considered and is recommended by some experts.

Detailed recommendations on the treatment and prevention of toxoplasmosis in HIV-infected persons are available in the guidelines issued by the USPHS/IDSA[†] (also see HIV Infection, p 279).

For both symptomatic and asymptomatic congenital infection, pyrimethamine combined with sulfadiazine (supplemented with folinic acid) also is recommended as initial therapy. Duration of therapy is prolonged and often is one year. However, the optimal dosage and duration are not definitely established and should be decided in consultation with appropriate specialists.

---

* Available from Eon Labs, Laurelton, NY (800-525-0225).
[†] Centers for Disease Control and Prevention. USPHS/IDSA guidelines for the prevention of opportunistic infections in persons infected with human immunodeficiency virus: a summary. *MMWR.* 1995;44 (No. RR-8):6-8.

Treatment of primary *Toxoplasma* infection in pregnant women, including those with HIV infection, also should be decided in consultation with appropriate specialists. Spiramycin treatment of primary infection during gestation reduces the frequency of congenital infection, but maternal therapy will not prevent sequelae in the fetus once congenital toxoplasmosis has occurred. Spiramycin is only available as an investigational drug in the United States on request from the Food and Drug Administration.

ISOLATION OF THE HOSPITALIZED PATIENT: Standard precautions are recommended.

CONTROL MEASURES: Pregnant women whose *Toxoplasma* serostatus is negative or unknown should avoid activities that potentially expose them to cat feces (such as changing litter boxes, gardening, and landscaping), or they should wear gloves if such activities are unavoidable. Daily changing of cat litter will reduce the chance of infection as oocysts are not infective during the first 1 to 2 days after passage. Infectivity is destroyed by use of near-boiling water for 5 minutes. Domestic cats can be protected from infection by feeding commercially prepared cat food and preventing them from eating undercooked kitchen scraps and hunting wild rodents.

Oral ingestion of *Toxoplasma* oocysts can be avoided by (1) cooking meat to 150°F (66°C) before consumption (smoked meat and meat cured in brine are considered safe), (2) washing fruits and vegetables, and (3) cleaning kitchen surfaces after handling fruits, vegetables, and/or raw meat, and (4) preventing contamination of food by flies and cockroaches.

Trichinosis
(Trichinella spiralis)

CLINICAL MANIFESTATIONS: The clinical spectrum of infection ranges from inapparent infection to fulminating, fatal illness, but most infections are inapparent. The severity of the disease is proportional to the infective dose. During the first week after ingesting infected meat, the patient may experience abdominal discomfort, nausea, vomiting, and/or diarrhea. Two to 8 weeks later, as larvae migrate into tissues, fever, myalgia, periorbital edema, urticarial rash, and conjunctival and subungual hemorrhages may develop. Larvae may remain viable in tissues for years; calcification of larvae in skeletal muscle usually occurs within 6 to 24 months and may be detected on roentgenograms. In severe infections, myocardial failure, neurologic involvement, and pneumonitis can follow in 1 or 2 months.

ETIOLOGY: Infection is caused by nematodes of *Trichinella*. Five species capable of infecting only warm-blooded animals have been identified. *Trichinella spiralis* is the most common cause of human infection.

EPIDEMIOLOGY: The infection is enzootic worldwide in many carnivores, especially scavengers. Infection occurs as a result of ingestion of raw or insufficiently cooked meat containing encysted larvae of *T spiralis*. The usual source of human infections is pork, but horse meat and wild carnivorous game, such as bear and walrus meat in North America, can be sources. Feeding pigs uncooked garbage perpetuates the cycle of infection. In the United States, the incidence of the infection in humans has declined considerably, but infection occurs sporadically, often within a family or among friends who have prepared uncooked sausage from fresh pork. The disease is not transmitted from person to person.

The **incubation period** is usually 1 to 2 weeks.

DIAGNOSTIC TESTS: Eosinophilia approaching 70%, in conjunction with compatible symptoms and dietary history, suggests the diagnosis. Serologic tests are available through state laboratories at the Centers for Disease Control and Prevention. Serum antibody titers rarely become positive before the third week of illness. Testing paired acute and convalescent sera is usually diagnostic. Larvae in a muscle biopsy can be visualized microscopically, beginning 2 weeks after infection. The tissue is best examined fresh, compressed between two microscope slides. Identification of larvae in suspect meat can be the most rapid source of diagnostic information.

TREATMENT: Mebendazole for 10 days is recommended. Thiabendazole for 7 days is an alternative drug. Corticosteroids alleviate symptoms of the inflammatory reaction and can be lifesaving when the central nervous system or heart is involved.

ISOLATION OF THE HOSPITALIZED PATIENT: Standard precautions are recommended.

CONTROL MEASURES: Transmission to pigs can be reduced by not feeding them garbage and by active rat control. Persons should be educated about the necessity of cooking pork thoroughly (until the meat is no longer pink). Freezing of pork at −23.3°C (−10°F) for 10 days kills the larvae. However, *Trichinella* organisms in Arctic wild animals can survive this procedure. Individuals known to have recently ingested contaminated meat should be treated with mebendazole (or thiabendazole).

Trichomonas vaginalis Infections
(Trichomoniasis)

CLINICAL MANIFESTATIONS: Infection with *Trichomonas* is frequently asymptomatic. The usual clinical picture in symptomatic postmenarcheal female patients consists of a frothy vaginal discharge and mild vulvovaginal itching. Dysuria and lower abdominal pain can occur. The vaginal discharge is usually pale yellow to gray-green and has a musty odor. Symptoms frequently are more severe just before or after menstruation. The vaginal mucosa is often deeply erythematous and the cervix is friable and diffusely inflamed, sometimes covered with numerous petechiae ("strawberry cervix"). Infected males can develop urethritis, epididymitis, or prostatitis, but the majority are asymptomatic. Recurrence or reinfection is common.

ETIOLOGY: *Trichomonas vaginalis* is a flagellated protozoan, slightly larger in size than a granulocyte.

EPIDEMIOLOGY: *Trichomonas* infection is primarily sexually transmitted and frequently coexists with other such infections, particularly gonococcal infections. Although *T vaginalis* can be acquired without direct sexual contact, no well-documented cases have been reported, and its presence in a prepubertal child should raise strong suspicion of sexual abuse. *Trichomonas vaginalis* acquired during birth by newborns can cause a vaginal discharge in the first weeks of life.

The **incubation period** averages 1 week, but may vary from 4 to 28 days.

DIAGNOSTIC TESTS: Diagnosis is usually made by examination of a wet mount preparation of the vaginal discharge. The lashing of the flagella and the jerky motility of the organism are distinctive. Positive preparations are more frequent in women who have symptoms and are directly related to the number of organisms, but are found in only 40% to 80% of cases. Culture of the organism and antibody tests using an enzyme immunoassay, or direct or indirect immunofluorescence techniques for demonstration of the organism, are more sensitive than wet mounts but are not generally required for diagnosis. Culture for *T vaginalis* is positive in more than 95% of cases.

TREATMENT: Metronidazole is the treatment of choice, resulting in cure rates of approximately 95%. For prepubertal girls, 15 mg/kg per day in three divided doses (maximum daily dose, 2 g for 7 days), 500 mg twice a day for 7 days, or 40 mg/kg (maximum, 2 g) in a single dose is recommended. In adolescents and adults, treatment is a single dose of 2 g. The sexual partner should be treated concurrently, even if asymptomatic. Patients should abstain from alcohol for 48 hours because of the disulfiramlike effects of the drug. Metronidazole should not be used in the first trimester of pregnancy, but may be used thereafter.

Treatment failures should be retreated with metronidazole (1 g in two divided doses for adolescents and adults) for 7 days. Repeated failure should be treated with metronidazole, 2 g once a day for 3 to 5 days. *Trichomonas* strains with reduced susceptibility to metronidazole have been reported; however, effective alternatives to metronidazole therapy are not available.

Persons infected with *Trichomonas* should be evaluated for the presence of other sexually transmitted diseases, including syphilis, *Neisseria gonorrhoeae*, *Chlamydia trachomatis*, hepatitis B, and HIV infection.

ISOLATION OF THE HOSPITALIZED PATIENT: Standard precautions are recommended.

CONTROL MEASURES: Measures to prevent sexually transmitted diseases, particularly the consistent use of condoms, are indicated.

Trichuriasis
(Whipworm Infection)

CLINICAL MANIFESTATIONS: Abdominal pain, tenesmus, and bloody diarrhea with mucous can occur. Chronic infection associated with heavy infestation can be associated with rectal prolapse.

ETIOLOGY: *Trichuris trichiura*, the whipworm, is the agent. Adult worms are 30 to 50 mm in length, with a large threadlike anterior end that is embedded in the mucosa of the large intestine.

EPIDEMIOLOGY: The parasite has a worldwide distribution but is more common in the tropics and in areas of poor sanitation. In some areas of Asia, the prevalence is 50%. In the United States, trichuriasis generally has been limited to rural areas of the southeast and to migrants from tropical areas. Infections are usually asymptomatic. Eggs require a minimum of 10 days of incubation in the soil before they are infectious. The disease is not communicable from person to person.

The **incubation period** is not known.

DIAGNOSTIC TESTS: Eggs may be found on direct examination of the stool or using concentration techniques.

TREATMENT: Mebendazole for 3 days is usually effective in eradicating most of the worms. Albendazole also is effective.

ISOLATION OF THE HOSPITALIZED PATIENT: Standard precautions are recommended.

CONTROL MEASURES: Proper disposal of fecal material is indicated.

African Trypanosomiasis
(African Sleeping Sickness)

CLINICAL MANIFESTATIONS: The rapidity and severity of clinical manifestations vary with the infecting species. With *Trypanosoma brucei gambiense* (West African) infection, a cutaneous nodule or chancre may appear at the site of parasite inoculation within a few days of a bite by an infected tsetse fly. Systemic illness, however, occurs months to years later and is characterized by intermittent fever, posterior cervical lymphadenopathy ("Winterbottom's sign") and multiple nonspecific complaints, including malaise, weight loss, arthralgia, rash, pruritus, and edema. Months to years later, the central nervous system (CNS) can be invaded, producing a chronic meningoencephalitis characterized by behavioral changes, cachexia, headache, hallucinations, delusions, and somnolence. In contrast, in *Trypanosoma brucei rhodesiense* (East African) infection, generalized illness develops days to weeks after parasite inoculation. Acute manifestations include high fever, cutaneous chancre, myocarditis, hepatitis, anemia, thrombocytopenia, and laboratory evidence of disseminated intravascular coagulation. Clinical meningoencephalitis can develop as early as 3 weeks after the onset of the untreated systemic illness. *Trypanosoma brucei rhodesiense* infection has a high fatality rate; without treatment, infected patients usually die within days to months of the clinical onset of disease.

ETIOLOGY: African trypanosomiasis is caused by subspecies of the *T brucei* complex (see Clinical Manifestations), which are extracellular protozoan hemoflagellates.

EPIDEMIOLOGY: Approximately 20 000 human cases occur annually worldwide, although only one or two cases, acquired in Africa, are reported every year in the United States. Transmission is confined to an area in Africa between the latitudes of 15° north and 20° south, corresponding precisely with the distribution of the tsetse fly vector (*Glossina* species). In East Africa, wild animals such as antelope, bushbuck and hartebeest constitute the major reservoir of *T brucei rhodesiense.* Domestic pigs and dogs have been found as incidental reservoirs. Humans are the only important reservoir of *T brucei gambiense* in West and Central Africa.

The **incubation period** in *T brucei rhodesiense* infection is 3 to 21 days, usually 5 to 14 days; in *T brucei gambiense* infection, it is usually longer and extremely variable, ranging from several months to years.

DIAGNOSTIC TESTS: Diagnosis is made by identification of trypomastigotes in the blood, cerebrospinal fluid (CSF), or fluid aspirated from a chancre or lymph node. Examination of the CSF is critical to management and should be performed using the double-centrifugation technique. Concentration and Giemsa staining of the buffy coat layer of peripheral blood also can be helpful. *Trypanosoma brucei gambiense* is more likely to be found in lymph node aspirates. Although an increased concentration of IgM in either serum or CSF is considered characteristic of African trypanosomiasis, polyclonal hyperglobulinemia is common.

TREATMENT: When no evidence of CNS involvement is present (including absence of trypanosomes and CSF pleocytosis), the drug of choice for the acute hemolymphatic stage of infection due to either subspecies of *T brucei* is suramin* or eflornithine.[†] Pentamidine is an alternative drug. Some experts recommend the combination of suramin and pentamidine for *T brucei gambiense.* Until recently, melarsoprol,* a toxic parenteral arsenical compound, was the drug of choice for CNS involvement with both species of *T brucei.* However, eflornithine[†] has been demonstrated to be effective for CNS disease caused by *T brucei gambiense.* Melarsoprol* is still the drug of choice for CNS disease caused by *T brucei rhodesiense.* Because of the risk of relapse, patients should be followed with repeated CSF examinations for 2 years.

ISOLATION OF THE HOSPITALIZED PATIENT: Standard precautions are recommended.

CONTROL MEASURES: Travelers to endemic areas should avoid known foci of sleeping sickness and/or tsetse fly infestation and minimize fly bites by use of protective clothing, bed netting, and insect repellents. Infected patients should not breastfeed or donate blood.

---

* Available from the Drug Service, Centers for Disease Control and Prevention (see Directory of Telephone Numbers, p 667).
† Available from Marion Merrell Dow, Inc, Cincinnati, OH.

American Trypanosomiasis
(Chagas' Disease)

CLINICAL MANIFESTATIONS: The early phase of this disease is frequently asymptomatic. However, children are more likely to exhibit symptoms than adults. In some patients, a red nodule known as a chagoma develops at the site of the original inoculation, usually on the face or arms. The surrounding skin becomes indurated and later hypopigmented. Unilateral, firm edema of the eyelids, known as Romaña's sign, is the earliest indication of the infection, but is present in less than 50% of patients with signs of acute Chagas' disease. The edematous skin is violaceous, with conjunctivitis and enlargement of the ipsilateral preauricular lymph node. A few days after the appearance of Romaña's sign, fever, generalized lymphadenopathy, and malaise develop. Acute myocarditis, hepatosplenomegaly, edema, and meningoencephalitis can follow. Serious sequelae consisting of cardiomyopathy and heart failure (the major cause of death), megaesophagus, and/or megacolon can develop many years after the initial manifestations. Congenital disease is characterized by low birth weight, hepatomegaly, and meningoencephalitis, with convulsions and tremors.

ETIOLOGY: *Trypanosoma cruzi*, a protozoan hemoflagellate, is the cause.

EPIDEMIOLOGY: The parasites are transmitted through the feces of the insects of the triatomid family, usually of an infected reduviid (conenose or "kissing") bug. These insects defecate while taking blood. The bitten person is inoculated by inadvertently rubbing the insect feces containing the parasite into the site of the bite or mucous membranes of the eye or the mouth. The parasite also can be transmitted congenitally, during organ transplantation, and through blood transfusion. Accidental laboratory infections can result from the handling of blood from infected persons or laboratory animals, the vectors, and vector excreta. The disease is limited to the Western hemisphere, predominantly Mexico and Central and South America. Although small mammals in the southern and southwestern United States harbor *T cruzi*, vector-borne transmission to humans is extremely rare in the United States. Several transfusion-associated cases have been documented in the United States. Infection is common in immigrants from Central and South America. The disease is a leading cause of death in South America, where between 7 and 15 million people are infected.

The **incubation period** for the acute disease is 1 to 2 weeks. The chronic manifestations do not appear for years to decades.

DIAGNOSTIC TESTS: During the acute disease, the parasite is demonstrable in blood, either by Giemsa staining or by direct wet-mount preparation. In chronic infections, which are characterized by low-level parasitemia, recovery or identification of the parasite by culture on special media or by xenodiagnosis, respectively, should be undertaken. Serologic tests include complement fixation, indirect hemagglutination, indirect immunofluorescence, and enzyme-linked immunoassay.

TREATMENT: The acute phase of Chagas' disease is treated with nifurtimox* or benznidazole.† These drugs are not effective against the forms of the parasite usually found in the chronic phase of the disease.

ISOLATION OF THE HOSPITALIZED PATIENT: Standard precautions should be followed.

CONTROL MEASURES: Education about the mode of spread and the methods of prevention is warranted in endemic areas. Homes should be examined for the presence of the vectors and if found, thorough disinfection is indicated. Vector control is recommended through the use of effective control of the rodent population on which the vectors feed, insecticides, elimination of habitats of the vectors, and screens on windows and doors to exclude the insect vectors. Travelers to endemic areas should avoid contact with reduviid insects by avoiding habitation in buildings that do not have control measures for these insects and in those constructed of mud, palm thatch, or adobe brick, especially those with cracks in the walls or roof. The use of bed netting may also be beneficial, especially for those traveling to highly endemic areas who plan to camp or sleep outdoors.

Blood donors in endemic areas must be screened by serologic tests, and infected patients should not donate blood. Blood recipients can be protected in endemic areas by treatment of the donated blood with gentian violet at a dilution of 1:4000.

Blood and serologic examinations should be performed on members of households with an infected patient if they have had a similar exposure to the vector as the patient. Serologic testing before and after travel should be considered for those visiting highly endemic areas with poor control measures and where contact with vectors may be unavoidable.

Tuberculosis

CLINICAL MANIFESTATIONS: Most infected children and adolescents are asymptomatic when the tuberculin skin test is found to be positive. The primary complex of infection is usually not evident on chest roentgenogram, and primary infection in most immunologically normal children does not rapidly progress to disease. Early clinical manifestations occurring 1 to 6 months after initial infection can include one or more of the following nonspecific findings: fever, weight loss, cough, night sweats, and chills. Pulmonary roentgenographic findings include lymphadenopathy of the hilar, mediastinal, cervical, or other nodes; involvement of a segment or lobe, occasionally with atelectasis or consolidation; pleural effusion; cavitary lesions; and miliary disease. Meningitis also can occur. Extrapulmonary manifestations that can occur 12 months or more after the initial infection include disease of the middle ear and mastoid, bones, joints, and skin. In approximately 25% of children younger than 15 years who are not treated in the early stages of infection, extrapulmonary

---

* Available from the Drug Service, Centers for Disease Control and Prevention (see Directory of Telephone Numbers, p 667).
† Available from Roche, Nutley, NJ.

disease occurs. Tuberculosis of the kidney and reactivation or adult-type pulmonary tuberculosis are rare in young children but can occur in adolescents. The majority of adults have reactivation disease and were initially infected years before. The manifestations in patients with drug-resistant tuberculosis are indistinguishable from those in patients with drug-resistant disease.

ETIOLOGY: The agent is *Mycobacterium tuberculosis*, an acid-fast bacillus (AFB). Human pulmonary disease caused by *M bovis*, the cause of bovine tuberculosis, occurs occasionally in the United States, while *M africanum* is rare. Other mycobacteria rarely cause pulmonary disease in immunocompetent children but may cause lymphadenopathy (see Diseases Caused By Nontuberculous Mycobacteria, p 563).

DEFINITIONS: Exposure to tuberculosis refers to a patient that has had recent contact with a person with suspected or confirmed, contagious pulmonary tuberculosis whose tuberculin skin test is negative, and who has a normal physical examination and chest roentgenogram. Some exposed persons have early infection (and will develop subsequent skin test reactivity) and some do not; the two groups at this stage cannot be distinguished. **Tuberculosis infection** is defined by a positive tuberculin skin test in a person who has no physical findings of disease and the chest roentgenogram is either normal or reveals only granulomas or calcification in the lung and/or regional lymph nodes. **Tuberculosis disease** is defined as a person with infection in whom signs, symptoms, and/or roentgenographic manifestations caused by *M tuberculosis* are apparent; disease may be pulmonary and/or extrapulmonary. In adults, the distinction between infection and disease is usually clear, but in young children the two stages are often less distinct.

EPIDEMIOLOGY: Case rates of tuberculosis for all ages are highest in urban, low-income areas, and in nonwhite racial and ethnic groups, among whom more than two thirds of reported cases in the United States now occur. Some rural areas also have high rates. Foreign-born children in recent years have accounted for nearly one quarter of newly diagnosed pediatric cases. More than 35% of those 5 to 14 years are foreign-born in comparison to approximately 15% of those younger than 5 years. Specific groups with the highest rates of infection and disease include first-generation immigrants from high-risk countries (eg, Asia); Native Americans, including Alaskan natives; the homeless; and residents of correctional facilities.

Infants and postpubertal adolescents are at increased risk of progression of infection to disease. Other predictive factors for development of disease include tuberculin skin test conversion; immunodeficiency, particularly that caused by HIV infection; intravenous drug use; and certain diseases or medical conditions, specifically Hodgkin's disease, lymphoma, diabetes mellitus, chronic renal failure, malnutrition, and immunosuppression induced by drugs (such as prolonged or high-dose corticosteroid therapy).

A diagnosis of tuberculosis infection or disease in a child is a sentinel event representing recent transmission of *M tuberculosis* in the community. Transmission of *M tuberculosis* is usually airborne, with inhalation of droplet nuclei produced by an adult or adolescent with infectious pulmonary tuberculosis. The duration of infectivity of an adult receiving effective treatment depends on the drug susceptibilities of the organism, the number of organisms in the sputum (as determined by microscopic examination of stained smears), and cough frequency. Although infectivity usually lasts only a few weeks after initiation of effective drug therapy, it may last longer, especially when the adult patient is nonadherent with medical therapy or is infected with a resistant strain. If the sputum is negative for organisms on three smears and if the cough has disappeared, the person is considered noncontagious. The majority of adult and adolescent patients are noncontagious within a few weeks of starting appropriate therapy (ie, drugs to which the infecting organism is susceptible). Children younger than 12 years with primary pulmonary tuberculosis usually are not contagious because their pulmonary lesions are small, cough is minimal or nonexistent, and the resulting expulsion of bacilli is minimal.

The portal of entry is usually the respiratory tract; skin, gastrointestinal tract, and mucous membranes have been rarely implicated. On rare occasions, *M tuberculosis* is transmitted from mother to fetus transplacentally or by infected amniotic fluid.

The **incubation period** from infection (ie, acquisition of *M tuberculosis*) to development of a positive reaction to a tuberculin skin test is 2 to 12 weeks (usually within 10 weeks); the median is 3 to 4 weeks. The risk of developing disease is highest during the 6 months after infection and remains high for 2 years; however, years may elapse between infection and development of disease. In most instances, untreated infection becomes dormant and never progresses to clinical disease in the healthy host.

DIAGNOSTIC TESTS: Isolation of tubercle bacilli by culture from early morning gastric aspirates, or from sputum, pleural fluid, cerebrospinal fluid (CSF), urine, other body fluids, or biopsy material establishes the diagnosis. In a young child (or when the cough is nonproductive or may be absent), the best culture material for the diagnosis of pulmonary tuberculosis usually is an early morning gastric aspirate. Gastric aspirates should be obtained with a nasogastric tube upon awakening the child and prior to ambulation or feeding. Specimens from three aspirates should be submitted unless a stained smear (or polymerase chain reaction test) of the first aspirate is positive. Regardless of the results of the AFB smears (which are rarely positive), each specimen should be cultured.

Because *M tuberculosis* is slow-growing, its detection may take as long as 10 weeks on solid culture methods and 2 to 6 weeks by the radiometric method. Even with optimal culture techniques, the organism is isolated from fewer than 50% of children and 75% of infants with pulmonary tuberculosis. Identification of isolates on culture can be more rapid if a DNA probe is used. Attempts should be made to demonstrate acid-fast bacilli (AFB) in sputum and/or body fluids by the Ziehl-Neelsen method or by auramine-rhodamine staining and fluorescence microscopy. Auramine-rhodamine staining is superior and, if available, preferred. Histologic examination for and demonstration of AFB in biopsies from lymph node, pleura, liver, bone marrow, or other tissues can be valuable for diagnosis, but *M tuberculosis* cannot be distinguished from other mycobacteria in stained specimens.

Polymerase chain reaction (PCR) tests for rapid diagnosis and restriction fragment length polymorphism analysis (DNA fingerprinting) for epidemiologic evaluation are of limited availability and are expensive. Polymerase chain reaction tests are approved only for smear-positive respiratory tract specimens. DNA fingerprinting currently is only available in research and reference laboratories. Both tests should be ordered in consultation with or by a specialist in tuberculosis.

Identification of a source case should be very actively pursued to support the diagnosis, determine possible drug resistance (which will affect the choice of drugs for the pediatric patient), and identify all persons with infection or disease.

Culture material should be obtained from children with evidence of active disease, whenever possible, but especially when (1) an isolate is not available from a source case; (2) the isolate from the source case is drug-resistant; (3) the child is immunocompromised (especially if HIV-infected); or (4) the child has extrapulmonary disease.

Tuberculin Testing.* The skin test is the only practical tool for diagnosing tuberculous infection in asymptomatic individuals. The Mantoux test containing 5 tuberculin units (TU) of purified protein derivative (PPD), administered intradermally, is preferred. Other strengths of Mantoux PPD skin tests (1 or 250 TU) should not be used because the interpretation of the reaction is not standardized.

Several problems with multiple puncture tests (MPTs) severely limit their use, including lack of antigen standardization, false-positive and false-negative results when compared to the results of Mantoux tests, variable sensitivity and specificity depending on the local incidence of infection and disease, and the possibility of the booster phenomenon in subsequent Mantoux skin testing.

Positive Mantoux test results (see Table 3.59, p 545) indicate likely infection with *M tuberculosis*. Tuberculin reactivity appears 2 to 12 weeks after initial infection. Tuberculin reactivity caused by *M tuberculosis* infection usually continues for the individual's lifetime, despite appropriate chemotherapy.

The American Academy of Pediatrics recommends focusing tuberculin skin testing on children who are at increased risk of acquiring tuberculous infection and disease (see Recommendations for Skin Testing, p 546). Routine tuberculin testing, including school-based programs that include populations at low risk, has either a low yield of positive results or a larger number of false-positive results, and represents an inefficient use of health care resources. Therefore, children without risk factors who reside in low-prevalence regions, including those who are 1 year of age, do not need to have routine tuberculin skin testing.

Tuberculin skin testing can be administered during the same visit that vaccinations are given, including MMR and varicella vaccine. Previous BCG vaccination is not a contraindication to skin testing. Other strengths of PPD skin test antigens (1 or 250 TU) should not be used because the interpretation of the reaction is not standardized.

Mantoux skin test results should be read by experienced health care professionals who have been trained in the proper means to do so because of lack of reliability of interpretations by non-health care professionals. When a primary care physician is unavailable to read the test, it can be read by the specifically trained staff of an after-hours clinic or local public health clinic, school-based nurses, home health care staff, or emergency department personnel, and the primary care physician should be notified promptly of the result.

---

* For further information see American Academy of Pediatrics, Committee on Infectious Diseases. Screening for tuberculosis in infants and children. *Pediatrics*. 1994;93:131-134; and American Academy of Pediatrics, Committee on Infectious Diseases. Update on tuberculosis skin testing of children. *Pediatrics*. 1996;97:282-284.

Table 3.59. Definitions of Positive Mantoux Skin Test (5 TU of PPD) Results in Children*
Tests should be read at 48 to 72 hours after PPD placement

Induration ≥5 mm

Children in close contact with known or suspected infectious cases of tuberculosis:
- Households with active or previously active cases if treatment cannot be verified as adequate before exposure, treatment was initiated after the child's contact, or reactivation is suspected

Children suspected to have tuberculosis:
- Chest roentgenogram consistent with active or previously active tuberculosis
- Clinical evidence of tuberculosis[†]

Children receiving immunosuppressive therapy[‡] or with immunosuppressive conditions, including HIV infection

Induration ≥10 mm

Children at increased risk of disseminated disease:
- Young age: <4 y of age
- Other medical risk factors, including Hodgkin's disease, lymphoma, diabetes mellitus, chronic renal failure, or malnutrition (see Table 3.60, p 548)

Children with increased environmental exposure to tuberculosis:
- Born, or whose parents were born, in high-prevalence regions of the world
- Frequently exposed to adults who are HIV-infected, homeless, users of illicit drugs, residents of nursing homes, incarcerated or institutionalized persons, and migrant farm workers
- Travel and exposure to high prevalence regions of the world

Induration ≥15 mm

Children ≥4 y of age without any risk factors

---

* These definitions apply regardless of previous BCG vaccination (see also Interpretation of Mantoux Skin Tests in Persons Who Received BCG, p 561).
† Evidence on physical examination or laboratory assessment that would include tuberculosis in the working diagnosis (eg, meningitis).
‡ Including immunosuppressive doses of corticosteroids.

The recommended time for assessing the result of the Mantoux test (ie, measurement of the size of induration) is 48 to 72 hours after placement. Positive tests, as defined in Table 3.59, may persist for longer than 72 hours.

A negative Mantoux skin test never excludes tuberculous infection or disease. Approximately 10% of immunocompetent children with culture-documented disease do not react initially to the standard Mantoux test (5 TU of PPD). Host-related factors, such as young age, poor nutrition, immunosuppression, other viral infections (especially measles, varicella, and influenza), and severe, disseminated tuberculosis can decrease tuberculin skin test reactivity. Many adults coinfected with HIV and *M tuberculosis* do not react to tuberculin on skin testing. Coinfected children also are frequently anergic.

Control skin tests to assess cutaneous anergy are indicated only in patients with suspected or proven immunosuppression and in those with possible severe, disseminated disease. Their use in otherwise healthy children with pulmonary disease and in tuberculin skin testing of high-risk children is unwarranted. In addition, standardized and reliable skin tests for assessing anergy in infants and children are generally not available.

Interpretation of the Mantoux Test Results (see Table 3.59, p 545). The interpretation of the skin test reaction depends on the purpose for which the test was given and on the consequences of incorrect classification. The classification of test responses is based on epidemiologic and clinical factors. The appropriate cutoff size of induration for a positive result varies with the person tested and the related epidemiologic factors. In areas of the United States where nontuberculous mycobacteria are common, only 5% of children in the general population who have a 5- to 9-mm area of induration to a Mantoux tuberculin skin test are infected with *M tuberculosis*. However, a child with the same reaction who is in contact with an adult with infectious tuberculosis has an almost 50% chance of infection. Whether the child is likely to have been exposed to an adult with tuberculosis is critical information.

Current guidelines from the Centers for Disease Control and Prevention (CDC), American Thoracic Society (ATS), and the American Academy of Pediatrics accept 15 mm or greater of induration as a positive result for any person. Induration of 5 mm or greater is interpreted as a positive result for the following groups: (1) persons who have had close recent contact with individuals who have contagious tuberculosis; (2) persons who have chest roentgenograms consistent with old healed tuberculosis; and (3) persons with HIV infection or with risk factors for HIV infection whose HIV status is unknown. The Academy also includes in this category (ie, ≥ 5-mm induration) those children with clinical evidence of tuberculosis and those with immunosuppression from causes other than HIV infection. Induration of 10 mm or greater is considered a positive result in other groups at high risk of disseminated infection or likelihood of exposure to tuberculosis.

Applying these definitions in clinical practice necessitates detailed evaluation and special considerations. First, classifying children by risk group requires the willingness and ability of medical personnel to obtain a thorough history of the child and of adults caring for the child. Second, children with identical reactions may be evaluated differently, depending on the risk factors for tuberculosis. Third, the physician is greatly aided by knowledge of the tuberculosis case rates and characteristics of tuberculosis within his or her community.

Interpretation of Mantoux test results in prior recipients of BCG vaccine can be difficult (see Interpretation of Mantoux Skin Tests in Persons Who Received BCG, p 561). Since reliable criteria for distinguishing a positive skin test result caused by BCG from that caused by *M tuberculosis* infection are lacking, recommendations for interpreting Mantoux skin test results are generally the same as for those who have not received BCG.

Recommendations for Skin Testing. The most reliable control programs for tuberculosis are based on aggressive, expedient contact investigations rather than routine skin test screening of large populations. Specific recommendations are as follows:

- All children need routine health care evaluations that include assessment of their risk of exposure to tuberculosis. Only children deemed to have increased risk of exposure to persons with tuberculosis should be considered for tuberculin (Mantoux) skin testing. The frequency of such skin testing should be according to the degree of risk of acquiring tuberculosis infection as detailed in Table 3.60, p 548.

- Routine tuberculin skin testing of children with no risk factors residing in low-prevalence communities is not indicated.
- Children who have no risk factors, but who reside in high-prevalence regions, and children whose histories for risk factors are incomplete or unreliable, should be considered for tuberculin (Mantoux) skin testing at 4 to 6 and 11 to 16 years of age. The decision to test should be based on the local epidemiology of tuberculosis in conjunction with advice from regional tuberculosis control officials.
- Family investigation is indicated whenever a tuberculin skin test result of a parent or child converts from negative to positive (indicating recent infection). Children of health care workers are not at increased risk of acquiring tuberculosis infection unless the workers' tuberculin skin test results convert to positive or the workers have diagnoses of tuberculosis.
- Children with HIV infection and those living in households with HIV-infected persons should receive annual tuberculin (Mantoux) skin testing. Skin testing can begin at 3 months of age and should be performed annually thereafter.
- Tuberculin skin testing can be done at the same time that measles-containing vaccine (ie, usually MMR) and other vaccines are given. If testing is indicated in a child who does not have clinical or roentgenographic manifestations suggestive of tuberculosis and cannot be performed concurrently with measles vaccination, testing should be postponed for 4 to 6 weeks (see Tuberculin Testing, p 544). The effect of live-virus varicella vaccine on tuberculin skin test is not known.

HIV Testing. Persons with tuberculosis disease should be tested for HIV infection, including counseling before and after testing.

TREATMENT (SEE TABLE 3.61, P 549):

Specific Drugs. Antituberculous drugs kill *M tuberculosis* or inhibit its multiplication, thereby arresting progression of tuberculosis and preventing most complications of early, primary disease. Chemotherapy does not cause rapid disappearance of already caseous or granulomatous lesions (eg, mediastinal lymphadenitis with endobronchial breakthrough). Dosage recommendations and possible adverse reactions of major antituberculous drugs are summarized in Tables 3.61 and 3.62, p 549 and p 550).

Isoniazid is bactericidal and rapidly absorbed, and penetrates well into body fluids, including cerebrospinal fluid (CSF). It is metabolized in the liver and excreted primarily through the kidneys. The drug is well tolerated. The incidence of hepatitis in children and adolescents is low (see Evaluation and Monitoring of Therapy in Children and Adolescents, p 556). In children given recommended doses, peripheral neuritis or convulsions caused by inhibition of pyridoxine metabolism is rare. Children receiving isoniazid, therefore, usually do not need pyridoxine supplements unless they have nutritional deficiencies. Hence, pyridoxine is recommended for children and adolescents on meat- and milk-deficient diets, those with nutritional deficiencies (including all symptomatic HIV-infected children), breastfeeding infants and their mothers, and pregnant women.

Table 3.60. **Tuberculin Skin Test Recommendations***

Children for whom immediate skin testing is indicated:
- Contacts of persons with confirmed or suspected infectious tuberculosis (contact investigation); this includes children identified as contacts of family members or associates in jail or prison in the last five years
- Children with radiographic or clinical findings suggesting tuberculosis
- Children immigrating from endemic countries (eg, Asia, Middle East, Africa, Latin America)
- Children with travel histories to endemic countries and/or significant contact with indigenous persons from such countries

Children who should be tested annually for tuberculosis[†]:
- Children infected with HIV or living in household with HIV-infected persons.
- Incarcerated adolescents

Children who should be tested every 2–3 years[†]:
- Children exposed to the following individuals: HIV infected, homeless, residents of nursing homes, institutionalized adolescents or adults, users of illicit drugs, incarcerated adolescents or adults and migrant farm workers. Foster children with exposure to adults in the preceding high-risk groups are included

Children who should be considered for tuberculin skin testing at ages 4–6 and 11–16 years:
- Children whose parents immigrated (with unknown tuberculin skin test status) from regions of the world with high prevalence of tuberculosis; continued potential exposure by travel to the endemic areas and/or household contact with persons from the endemic areas (with unknown tuberculin skin test status) should be an indication for repeat tuberculin skin testing
- Children without specific risk factors who reside in high-prevalence areas; in general, a high-risk neighborhood or community does not mean an entire city is at high risk; rates in any area of the city may vary by neighborhood, or even from block to block; physicians should be aware of these patterns in determining the likelihood of exposure; public health officials or local tuberculosis experts should help clinicians identify areas that have appreciable tuberculosis rates

Children at increased risk of progression of infection to disease: Those with other medical risk factors, including diabetes mellitus, chronic renal failure, malnutrition, and congenital or acquired immunodeficiencies deserve special consideration. Without recent exposure, these persons are not at increased risk of acquiring tuberculosis infection. Underlying immune deficiencies associated with these conditions theoretically would enhance the possibility for progression to severe disease. Initial histories of potential exposure to tuberculosis should be included on all of these patients. If these histories or local epidemiologic factors suggest a possibility of exposure, immediate and periodic tuberculin skin testing should be considered. An initial Mantoux tuberculin skin test should be performed before initiation of immunosuppressive therapy in any child with an underlying condition that necessitates immunosuppressive therapy.

---

* BCG immunization is not a contraindication to tuberculin skin testing.
† Initial tuberculin skin testing is at the time of diagnosis or circumstance, beginning as early as at age 3 months.

Table 3.61. Commonly Used Drugs for the Treatment of Tuberculosis in Infants, Children, and Adolescents

Drugs	Dosage Forms	Daily Dose, mg/kg/d	Twice a Week Dose, mg/kg per dose	Maximum Dose	Adverse Reactions
Ethambutol	Tablets 100 mg 400 mg	15–25	50	2.5 g	Optic neuritis (usually reversible), decreased visual acuity, decreased red-green color discrimination, gastrointestinal disturbances, hypersensitivity
Isoniazid*	Scored tablets 100 mg 300 mg Syrup 10 mg/mL	10–15[†]	20–30	Daily, 300 mg Twice a week, 900 mg	Mild hepatic enzyme elevation, hepatitis,[†] peripheral neuritis, hypersensitivity
Pyrazinamide*	Scored tablets 500 mg	20–40	50	2 g	Hepatotoxicity, hyperuricemia
Rifampin*	Capsules 150 mg 300 mg Syrup formulated in syrup from capsules	10–20	10–20	600 mg	Orange discoloration of secretions/urine, staining contact lenses, vomiting, hepatitis, flu-like reaction, and thrombocytopenia; may render birth-control pills ineffective
Streptomycin (intramuscular administration)	Vials 1 g 4 g	20–40	20–40	1 g	Auditory and vestibular toxicity, nephrotoxicity, rash

* Rifamate is a capsule containing 150 mg of isoniazid and 300 mg of rifampin. Two capsules provide the usual adult (>50 kg body weight) daily doses of each drug. Rifater is a capsule containing 50 mg of isoniazid, 120 mg of rifampin, and 300 mg of pyrazinamide.

† When isoniazid in a dosage exceeding 10 mg/kg per day is used in combination with rifampin, the incidence of hepatotoxicity may be increased.

Rifampin is a bactericidal agent. It is metabolized by the liver and affects the pharmacokinetics of many other drugs, affecting their serum concentrations. *Mycobacterium tuberculosis*, initially resistant to rifampin, remains relatively uncommon in most areas of the United States. Rifampin is excreted in bile and urine and can cause orange urine, sweat, and tears. It can also cause discoloration of soft contact lenses and render oral contraceptives ineffective. Hepatotoxicity occurs rarely. Blood dyscrasia accompanied by influenza-like symptoms can occur if doses are taken sporadically

Table 3.62. Less Commonly Used Drugs for Treatment of Drug-Resistant Tuberculosis in Infants, Children, and Adolescents*

Drugs	Dosage Forms	Daily Dose, mg/kg/d	Maximum Dose	Adverse Reactions
Capreomycin	Vials, 1 g	15–30 (intramuscular administration)	1 g	Ototoxicity, nephrotoxicity
Ciprofloxacin[†]	Tablets 250 mg 500 mg 750 mg	Adults 500–1500 mg total per day (twice a day)	1.5 g	Theoretical effect on growing cartilage, gastrointestinal tract disturbances, rash, headache
Cycloserine	Capsules, 250 mg	10–20	1 g	Psychosis, personality changes, convulsions, rash
Ethionamide	Tablets, 250 mg	15–20 given in 2 or 3 divided doses	1 g	Gastrointestinal tract disturbances, hepatotoxicity, hypersensitive reactions
Kanamycin	Vials 75 mg/2 mL 500 mg/2 mL 1 g/3 mL	15–30 (intramuscular administration)	1 g	Auditory toxicity, nephrotoxicity, vestibular toxicity
Ofloxacin[†]	Tablets 200 mg 300 mg 400 mg	Adults 400–800 mg total per day (twice a day)	0.8 g	Theoretical effect on growing cartilage, gastrointestinal tract disturbances, rash, headache
Para-amino salicylic acid (PAS)	Tablets, 500 mg	200–300 (three or four times a day)	10 g	Gastrointestinal tract disturbances, hypersensitivity, hepatotoxicity

* These drugs should be used in consultation with a specialist in tuberculosis.
† Fluoroquinolones are not currently approved for use in persons younger than 18 years; their use in younger patients necessitates assessment of the potential risks and benefits (see Antimicrobials and Related Therapy, p 605).

or at intervals of 1 week or more. For infants and young children, the contents of the capsules can be suspended in wild cherry-flavored syrup or sprinkled on applesauce.

Pyrazinamide is bactericidal, attains therapeutic CSF concentrations, is detectable in macrophages, and is metabolized by the liver. In doses of 30 mg/kg per day or less, it is seldom hepatotoxic and is well tolerated by children.

Streptomycin is a bactericidal drug that is excreted by the kidneys. Resistance to streptomycin is relatively common, particularly among *M tuberculosis* isolates from developing areas such as Southeast Asia. Therapeutic CSF concentrations are achieved only in patients with meningitis. Streptomycin is usually prescribed for only 4 to 8 weeks and for no longer than 12 weeks because the incidence of vestibular and cochlear damage correlates with increasing total dose. If streptomycin is not available, kanamycin, capreomycin, or amikacin are alternatives.

Ethambutol is well absorbed, diffuses well throughout the body, and is excreted in the urine. At 15 mg/kg per day, it is bacteriostatic only and its primary therapeutic role is to prevent emergence of drug-resistant organisms. Because the population of tubercle bacilli is usually smaller in primary tuberculosis than in adult-type reactivation disease, development of secondary resistance during treatment of primary disease is rare. A dose of 25 mg/kg per day is necessary for bactericidal activity. Since ethambutol may cause reversible optic neuritis, recipients should be monitored monthly for visual acuity, visual fields, and red-green color discrimination. Because cooperation is essential for performance of these tests, use of ethambutol in young children whose visual acuity cannot be monitored requires careful consideration of the risks and benefits.

The less commonly used antituberculous drugs, their doses, and side effects are listed in Table 3.62 (p 550). Ethionamide is an antituberculous drug that is well tolerated by children, achieves therapeutic CSF concentrations, and may be useful in drug-resistant cases. Other drugs that have had limited usefulness because of minimal effectiveness, toxic properties, or both should be used only in consultation with a specialist. In cases of drug resistance or if patients cannot tolerate the commonly used drugs listed in Table 3.61 (p 549), drugs such as cycloserine, kanamycin, and capreomycin may be helpful (see Table 3.62, p 550). Fluoroquinolones (ofloxacin and ciprofloxacin) have antituberculous activity and can be used in special circumstances. Since these drugs are approved by the Food and Drug Administration for use only in persons 18 years of age and older, their use in younger patients necessitates careful assessment of the potential risks and benefits (see Antimicrobials and Related Therapy, p 605). In cases of multiple drug-resistant tuberculosis, these drugs should be considered for therapy.

All antituberculous agents can cause toxic effects. **The cautions listed in the product label for each drug should be followed.** Consultation with a tuberculosis specialist is advised when the nonconventional antituberculous regimens are considered.

Chemotherapy for Tuberculosis Infection (Preventive Therapy).

Isoniazid given to adults who have tuberculosis infection (ie, no clinical or roentgenographic manifestations) provides substantial protection (54% to 88% efficacy) against development of active disease for at least 20 years. Among children, efficacy approaches 100% with appropriate adherence to therapy. All infants, children, and adolescents who have a positive tuberculin test but no evidence of disease and who have never received antituberculous therapy should receive isoniazid alone unless resistance to the drug is suspected or a specific contraindication exists. Isoniazid in this circumstance is therapeutic for the infection and prevents development of disease. A chest roentgenogram should be obtained at the time preventive therapy is initiated; if this roentgenogram is normal, the child remains asymptomatic, and treatment is completed, it need not be repeated.

Contacts. Preventive isoniazid therapy is often indicated in recent contacts of persons with contagious tuberculosis when clinical disease has been excluded, even if the tuberculin skin test is negative, especially young children and those who are HIV-infected (see Preventive Therapy for Contacts, p 560).

Duration of Chemotherapy for Tuberculosis Infection. The optimal duration for preventive therapy remains unknown. In early studies, children received isoniazid for 1 year with excellent efficacy. Data in adults indicate that after 6 months of continuous medication, a 65% reduction in disease is achieved compared to a 75% reduction with 12 months of treatment. In non-HIV-infected adults, 6 months of therapy with isoniazid is now recommended in most cases.

In most infants and children, the recommended duration of isoniazid is at least 6 months of effective therapy. The exceptions are patients with HIV infection and other immunocompromising conditions for whom a minimum of 12 months is recommended. Isoniazid is given daily, 10 mg/kg (maximum, 300 mg), in a single dose. In situations where adherence with daily therapy cannot be assured, twice-a-week directly observed therapy with isoniazid can be considered, preferably after completion of 1 month of daily therapy. **Direct observation means that a health care worker or a trained third party (not a relative or friend) is present to document that the patient takes each dose of medication.** Each dose of isoniazid in the twice-a-week regimen is 20 to 30 mg/kg, not to exceed a daily maximum of 900 mg.

Therapy for Contacts of Patients With Isoniazid-Resistant M tuberculosis *Infection.* Possible isoniazid resistance always should be considered, particularly in children who are members of population in which the prevalence of drug-resistant tuberculosis is high (especially those born in countries with a high prevalence) or who have other risk factors listed in Table 3.63 (see p 553). For contacts who are infected by a source case with isoniazid-resistant but rifampin-susceptible organisms and in whom the consequences of the infection are likely to be severe (eg, children younger than 2 years), or those with HIV infection, rifampin should be given in addition to isoniazid until susceptibility test results on the isolate from the source case are available. If the source case is found to be excreting isoniazid-resistant organisms, isoniazid should be discontinued and rifampin given for a course of at least 6 months in total. Optimal therapy for children with tuberculosis infection caused by organisms with multiple drug resistance to isoniazid and rifampin is unknown. In these circumstances, multidrug regimens have been given. Drugs include pyrazinamide, a fluoroquinolone, and/or ethambutol. Consultation with a tuberculosis specialist is indicated.

Treatment of Active Disease. The goal of treatment is to achieve sterilization of the tuberculous lesion in the shortest possible time. Achievement of this goal reduces treatment cost and minimizes the possibility of development of resistant organisms. The major problem limiting successful treatment is poor adherence to prescribed treatment regimens. Directly observed therapy has been demonstrated to decrease relapse rates, treatment failures, and drug resistance rates. As a result, **directly observed therapy (DOT) is recommended for treatment of tuberculosis in the United States. Direct observation means that a health care worker or trained third party (not a relative or friend) is present to document that the patient takes each dose of medication.**

The encouraging results of 6- and 9-month treatment regimens in infants, children, and adolescents with both pulmonary and extrapulmonary tuberculosis have led to use of these shorter regimens. Shorter treatment regimens can be used in adolescents with adult-style disease, especially radiographic evidence of reactivation disease.

Table 3.63. **Patients at Increased Risk for Drug Resistance**

- Patients with a history of treatment for active tuberculosis (or whose source case for the contact was previously so treated)
- Contacts of a patient with drug-resistant tuberculosis
- Foreign-born persons
- Residents of areas where the prevalence of drug resistance is documented to be high (defined by most experts as including isoniazid resistance rates ≥4%)
- Patients or those whose source contact have positive smears or cultures after 2 months of antituberculous therapy.

A 6-month regimen consisting of isoniazid, rifampin, and pyrazinamide for the first 2 months and isoniazid and rifampin for the remaining 4 months as standard therapy is recommended for treatment of drug-susceptible *M tuberculosis* disease, including pulmonary, pulmonary with hilar adenopathy, and hilar adenopathy disease in infants, children, and adolescents. In children with hilar adenopathy in whom drug resistance is not a consideration, a 6-month regimen of only isoniazid and rifampin is adequate.

When initial drug resistance is suspected (see Table 3.63), a fourth drug, either ethambutol or streptomycin, should be added to the initial regimen until drug susceptibility results are available. If an isolate from the case under treatment is not available, drug susceptibilities of strains can be determined by susceptibility patterns of isolates from adult contacts and local endemic rates of single- and multiple-drug resistance. Data may not be available for foreign-born children or in circumstances of foreign travel. If the child likely was infected in an area of endemic drug resistance, a four-drug regimen is indicated.

In the 6-month regimen with triple-drug therapy, isoniazid, rifampin, and pyrazinamide are given once a day for the first 2 months. After this 2-month period, a regimen of isoniazid and rifampin given twice a week is acceptable if administration is directly observed (see Table 3.64, p 555, for doses). Several alternative regimens with differing durations of daily therapy and total therapy have been used successfully in adults. These alternative regimens should be prescribed and managed by or with a specialist in tuberculosis.

Chemotherapy for "Drug-Resistant" Disease. In the United States and Canada the incidence of drug resistance in previously untreated patients previously has been relatively low, but drug resistance rates are now higher. In certain areas, for example, the incidence of resistance to isoniazid can be as high as 10% to 20%. Drug resistance is most common in (1) foreign-born persons from high-risk areas such as Asia, Africa, and Latin America; (2) New York City and several other cities where hospital-based outbreaks of drug-resistant tuberculosis have been documented; (3) the homeless; (4) persons previously treated for tuberculosis; and (5) contacts, especially children with tuberculosis whose source case is a person from one of these groups (see also Table 3.63). If the child is at risk for isoniazid resistance, streptomycin or ethambutol should be added as previously described. **For all cases of drug-resistant tuberculosis, at least two drugs to which the isolate is susceptible should be**

given. For treatment of suspected cases of drug-resistant tuberculosis, a four-drug regimen should be prescribed. Treatment should include at least two bactericidal drugs, such as isoniazid, rifampin, streptomycin, other aminoglycosides, pyrazinamide, and high-dose ethambutol (25 mg/kg per day). In cases of tuberculosis with isoniazid- or rifampin-resistant strains, 6-month drug regimens are not recommended. Twice-a-week regimens also are not recommended for drug-resistant disease; 12 to 18 months of therapy are usually necessary to effect a cure. Directly observed therapy is critical to cure cases of drug-resistant tuberculosis and prevent the emergence of further resistance.

Extrapulmonary Tuberculosis. In general, extrapulmonary tuberculosis, including cervical lymphadenopathy, can be treated with the same regimens as pulmonary tuberculosis. Exceptions may be bone and joint disease, miliary disease, and meningitis, for which current data in children are inadequate to support a 6-month course of therapy. For these severe forms of drug-susceptible extrapulmonary tuberculosis, daily treatment with isoniazid, rifampin, pyrazinamide, and, usually, streptomycin for the first 1 or 2 months, followed by isoniazid and rifampin administered once a day or twice a week under direct observation, is recommended for a total of 12 months of therapy. For life-threatening tuberculosis, four drugs are given initially to protect against the possibility of drug resistance and the severe consequences of treatment failure (see Chemotherapy for "Drug-Resistant" Disease, p 553). Corticosteroid therapy is indicated in the initial treatment of meningitis.

Pyrazinamide is especially useful in disseminated and meningeal tuberculosis because it achieves better CSF concentrations than either streptomycin or ethambutol. In cases of severe tuberculosis with vomiting or obtundation, isoniazid or rifampin can be given parenterally. The dose is the same as that recommended for oral therapy.

Corticosteroids. Adjuvant treatment with corticosteroids in treating tuberculosis is controversial. Corticosteroids are indicated for children with tuberculous meningitis as dexamethasone has been demonstrated to lower mortality and long-term neurologic impairment. Corticosteroids also may be considered in children with pleural and pericardial effusions (to hasten reabsorption of fluid), severe miliary disease (to mitigate alveolocapillary block), and endobronchial disease (to relieve obstruction and atelectasis). Corticosteroids should be given only when accompanied by appropriate antituberculous therapy. Most experts consider 1 to 2 mg/kg per day of prednisone or its equivalent for 6 to 8 weeks to be appropriate.

Tuberculosis and HIV Infection. Adults and children with HIV infection have an increased incidence of tuberculosis. Hence, testing for HIV is indicated for all persons with tuberculosis disease. The clinical manifestations and roentgenographic appearance of tuberculosis in children with HIV infection tend to be similar to those in immunocompetent children, but manifestations in these patients can be unusual, including extrapulmonary involvement of multiple organs. In HIV-infected patients, a tuberculin skin test result of 5-mm induration or more is considered positive (see Table 3.59); however, a negative tuberculin test caused by HIV-related immunosuppression also can occur. Specimens for culture should be obtained in all suspected cases in children, since infection with nontuberculous mycobacteria also is common, and the results of mycobacterial drug susceptibility testing provide important information for therapeutic decisions. Appropriate specimens include lower respiratory

Table 3.64. Recommended Treatment Regimens for Drug-Susceptible Tuberculosis in Infants, Children, and Adolescents*

Infection or Disease Category	Regimen*	Remarks
Asymptomatic infection (positive skin test, no disease):		If daily therapy is not possible, therapy twice a week may be used for 6–9 mo. HIV-infected children should be treated for 12 mo.
—Isoniazid-susceptible	6–9 mo of isoniazid once a day	
—Isoniazid-resistant	6–9 mo of rifampin once a day	
—Isoniazid-rifampin-resistant*	Consult a tuberculosis specialist	
Pulmonary	**6-mo regimens** 2 mo of isoniazid, rifampin, and pyrazinamide once a day, followed by 4 mo of isoniazid and rifampin daily	If possible drug resistance is a concern (see text), another drug (ethambutol or streptomycin) is added to the initial 3-drug therapy until drug susceptibilities are determined.
	or 2 mo of isoniazid, rifampin, and pyrazinamide daily, followed by 4 mo of isoniazid and rifampin twice a week	Drugs can be given 2 or 3 times per wk under direct observation in the initial phase if nonadherence is likely.
	9-mo alternative regimens (for hilar adenopathy only): 9 mo of isoniazid and rifampin once a day **or** 1 mo of isoniazid and rifampin once a day, followed by 8 mo of isoniazid and rifampin twice a week	Regimens consisting of 6 mo of isoniazid and rifampin once a day, and 1 mo of isoniazid and rifampin once a day, followed by 5 mo of isoniazid and rifampin twice a week, have been successful in areas where drug resistance is rare.
Extrapulmonary meningitis, disseminated (miliary), bone/joint disease	2 mo of isoniazid, rifampin, pyrazinamide, and streptomycin once a day, followed by 10 mo of isoniazid and rifampin once a day (12 mo total)	Streptomycin is given with initial therapy until drug susceptibility is known.
	or 2 mo of isoniazid, rifampin, pyrazinamide, and streptomycin once a day, followed by 10 mo of isoniazid and rifampin twice a week (12 mo total)	For patients who may have acquired tuberculosis in geographic areas where resistance to streptomycin is common, capreomycin (15–30 mg/kg/d) or kanamycin (15-30 mg/kg/d) may be used instead of streptomycin.
Other (eg, cervical lymphadenopathy)	Same as for pulmonary disease.	See **Pulmonary.**

* Duration of therapy is longer in HIV-infected persons and additional drugs may be indicated (see p 554, Tuberculosis and HIV Infection).

tract secretions, gastric aspirates, blood, urine, stool, bone marrow, liver, lymph node, or other tissue as indicated clinically.

Most HIV-infected adult patients with drug-susceptible tuberculosis respond well to antituberculous drugs when appropriate therapy is given early. However, optimal therapy for tuberculosis in children with HIV infection has not yet been established. Therapy always should include at least three drugs initially and be continued for a minimum of 12 months. Isoniazid, rifampin, and pyrazinamide with or without ethambutol or an aminoglycoside should be given for at least the first 2 months. A fourth drug is indicated for disseminated disease and whenever drug-resistant disease is suspected. Consultation with a specialist who has experience in managing HIV-infected patients with tuberculosis is advised.

Evaluation and Monitoring of Therapy in Children and Adolescents. Careful monthly monitoring of the clinical and bacteriological responses to therapy is important. With directly observed therapy, clinical evaluation is an integral component of each visit for drug administration. Patients with pulmonary tuberculosis should have chest roentgenograms after 2 to 3 months of therapy to help evaluate response. Even with successful 6-month regimens, however, hilar adenopathy may require as long as 2 to 3 years for roentgenographic resolution, and a normal roentgenogram is not a necessary criterion to discontinue therapy. Follow-up roentgenograms beyond the termination of successful chemotherapy usually are not necessary unless clinical deterioration occurs.

If therapy has been interrupted, the date for its completion will need to be extended. Although guidelines cannot be provided for every situation, factors to consider in establishing the date for completion include the following: (1) the length of the interruption; (2) the time during therapy (early or late) in which interruption occurred; and (3) the patient's clinical, roentgenographic, and bacteriologic status before, during, and after interruption. Consultation with a specialist is advised.

Untoward effects of isoniazid therapy in children, including severe hepatitis, are rare. The incidence of hepatitis during isoniazid therapy is so low in otherwise healthy infants, children, and adolescents that routine determination of serum aminotransferase concentrations is not recommended. However, in children with severe tuberculosis, especially meningitis and disseminated disease, liver function should be monitored during the first several months of treatment. Other indications for liver function tests include (1) concurrent or recent liver disease; (2) high daily dose of isoniazid (more than 10 mg/kg per day) in combination with rifampin and/or pyrazinamide; (3) pregnancy or within 6 weeks postpartum; (4) clinical evidence of hepatotoxicity; or (5) hepatobiliary tract disease from other causes. In most other circumstances, monthly clinical evaluations for 3 months, followed by evaluation every 1 to 3 months to observe for signs or symptoms of hepatitis and other adverse effects of drug therapy, is an appropriate schedule for follow-up. Alternatively, some experts recommend routine clinical evaluation every 4 to 6 weeks throughout the course of therapy.

In all cases, frequent physician-patient contact to assess drug adherence, efficacy, and toxicity is an important aspect of management.

Immunizations. Patients who are receiving treatment for tuberculosis can be given measles and other live-virus vaccines, as otherwise indicated, unless they are receiving high-dose corticosteroids, are severely ill, or have other specific vaccine contraindications.

Tuberculosis in Pregnancy and Breastfeeding. Tuberculosis in pregnancy should be managed on a case-by-case basis due to the complexity of management decisions. During pregnancy, if active disease is diagnosed (by positive cultures or by compatible clinical or roentgenographic findings), isoniazid and rifampin, supplemented by ethambutol if isoniazid drug resistance is suspected, is recommended. Pyrazinamide is frequently used in a three- or four-drug regimen, but safety data in pregnancy have not been published. A course of therapy of at least 6 months is indicated for drug-susceptible disease. Prompt initiation of chemotherapy is mandatory to protect both the mother and fetus.

Asymptomatic pregnant women with a positive tuberculin skin test, a normal chest roentgenogram, and recent contact with an infectious person should receive isoniazid therapy. Duration is for 6 months if they are HIV-seronegative and for 12 months if they are HIV-seropositive. Therapy in these circumstances should begin after the first trimester. Although no harmful effects of isoniazid to the fetus have been observed, some experts would delay therapy until after delivery in the absence of these risk factors.

For all pregnant women receiving isoniazid, pyridoxine is indicated. Isoniazid, ethambutol, and rifampin appear to be relatively safe for the fetus. The benefit of ethambutol and rifampin for therapy of active disease in the mother outweighs the risk to the infant. Streptomycin should not be used unless administration is essential to treat the disease.

Women who are receiving isoniazid and are breastfeeding also should receive pyridoxine. While isoniazid is secreted in human milk, no adverse effects of isoniazid on nursing infants have been demonstrated (see Human Milk, p 73).

Congenital Tuberculosis. Women who have only pulmonary tuberculosis are not likely to infect the fetus until after delivery. Congenital tuberculosis is extremely rare, but in utero infections can occur after maternal *M tuberculosis* bacillemia. Miliary tuberculosis can infect the placenta and, thereby, gain access to the fetal circulation. In women with tuberculous endometritis, transmission of infection can result from fetal aspiration of *M tuberculosis* at the time of delivery. Ingestion of infected amniotic fluid in utero also can occur.

If a newborn is suspected of having congenital tuberculosis, a Mantoux skin test (5 TU PPD), chest roentgenogram, lumbar puncture, and appropriate cultures should be performed promptly. The skin test is usually negative in newborns with congenital or perinatally acquired infection. Hence, regardless of the skin test results, treatment of the infant should be initiated promptly with isoniazid, rifampin, pyrazinamide, and streptomycin or kanamycin. The placenta should be examined and cultured. The mother should be evaluated for the presence of pulmonary or extra-pulmonary, including uterine, tuberculosis. If the physical examination or chest roentgenogram support the diagnosis of tuberculosis, the newborn should be treated with regimens recommended for tuberculous meningitis, excluding corticosteroids.

If meningitis is confirmed, however, corticosteroids may be given (see Corticosteroids, p 554). The drug susceptibilities of the organism recovered from the mother and/or infant should be determined.

Management of the Newborn Infant Whose Mother (or Other Household Contact) Has Tuberculosis (Infection or Disease). Management of the newborn is based on categorization of the maternal (or household contact) infection. While protection of the infant from infection is of paramount importance, separation of the infant from the mother (or household contact) should be avoided when possible. Differing circumstances and resulting recommendations are as follows:

- *Mother (or household contact) has a negative roentgenogram.* If the mother (or household contact) is asymptomatic, no separation of mother and infant is required. The mother usually is a candidate for treatment of tuberculosis infection. The newborn needs no special evaluation or therapy. Because the positive tuberculin skin test could be a marker of an unrecognized case of contagious tuberculosis within the household, other household members should have Mantoux skin tests and further evaluation.

- *Mother (or household contact) has an abnormal chest roentgenogram.* If the roentgenogram is abnormal, the mother (or household contact) and infant should be separated until the mother (or household contact) has been evaluated, and if active tuberculosis disease is found, until she is receiving antituberculous therapy. Other household members should have skin tests and further evaluation.

- *Mother (or household contact) has an abnormal chest roentgenogram, but no evidence of active disease.* If the chest roentgenogram of the mother (or household contact)is abnormal, but the history, physical examination, sputum smear, and roentgenogram indicate no evidence of active disease, the infant can be assumed to be at low risk of *M tuberculosis* infection. The radiographic abnormality in this circumstance is probably due to another cause or a quiescent focus of tuberculosis. In the latter case, the mother may develop contagious, active tuberculosis, if untreated, and should receive appropriate therapy, if not previously treated. She and her infant should receive follow-up care. Other household members should have skin tests and further evaluation.

- *Mother (or household contact) has clinical or radiographic evidence of active, possibly contagious tuberculosis.* The mother (or household contact) should be reported immediately to the public health department so investigation of all household members can be performed within several days. All contacts should have a tuberculin skin test, chest roentgenogram, and physical examination. The infant should be evaluated for congenital tuberculosis (see Congenital Tuberculosis, p 557) and should be tested for HIV infection. The mother and infant should be separated until the infant and mother are receiving appropriate therapy and the mother is deemed to be noncontagious. Other household members should have skin tests and further evaluation.

If congenital tuberculosis is suspected, multiple drug therapy should be initiated (see Congenital Tuberculosis, p 557). If congenital tuberculosis is excluded (which is usually the case), isoniazid is given until the infant is 3 or 4 months of age, at which time the Mantoux skin test should be repeated. If the skin test is positive, the child should be reassessed for tuberculosis disease.

If disease is not present, isoniazid should be continued for a total of at least 6 months; HIV-infected children should be treated for 12 months. If the skin test is negative and the mother and other family members with tuberculosis have good adherence and response to treatment and are no longer infectious, isoniazid may be discontinued. The infant should be evaluated at monthly intervals during treatment.

If the mother (or household contact) has disease due to multiple-drug-resistant *M tuberculosis* or has poor adherence to treatment and directly observed therapy (DOT) is not possible, the infant should be separated from the ill family member and BCG vaccination may be considered for the infant. Since the response to the vaccine in infants may be delayed and inadequate for prevention of tuberculosis, DOT is preferred.

ISOLATION OF THE HOSPITALIZED PATIENT*: Most children with tuberculosis are not infectious and require only standard precautions. Airborne precautions are indicated for children with contagious pulmonary tuberculosis, ie, those with smear-positive sputum, until effective chemotherapy has been initiated, sputum smears demonstrate a diminishing number of organisms, and cough is abating. Children with no cough and negative sputum smears can be hospitalized on an open ward once effective chemotherapy has been initiated. Adolescent patients with pulmonary disease and/or cough should be isolated with airborne precautions, as is the case with adult patients. Infection control for hospital personnel include the use of personally "fitted" and "sealed" particulate respirators (that filter 1-mm or larger particles) at all times of patient contact.

The major concern in infection control relates to the adult family members and contacts who may be the source case. Appropriate evaluation with tuberculin skin testing and chest roentgenograms is warranted. Family and household members should be managed with airborne precautions when visiting until they are demonstrated not to have contagious tuberculosis. Nonadherent family members or contacts should be excluded from hospital visitation until evaluation is complete and tuberculosis is excluded or treatment has rendered the contacts noncontagious.

CONTROL MEASURES:

The control of tuberculosis in the United States necessitates access to health care, a thorough history taking of exposure(s) to persons with contagious tuberculosis, timely and effective contact investigations, proper interpretation of Mantoux skin tests, and appropriate use of therapy, including directly observed therapy. Variations in the epidemiology of tuberculosis in different locations reinforce the importance of communication with local public health officials and/or regional experts on tuberculosis.

Management of Contacts, Including Epidemiologic Investigation. Children with positive tuberculin skin tests or tuberculous disease should be the starting point for epidemiologic investigation, which is best accomplished with assistance from the local health department. Close contacts of the tuberculin-positive child should be skin tested, and persons with a positive reaction should be investigated for the presence of tuberculosis. Since children with primary tuberculosis are usually not conta-

---

* In addition to standard precautions.

gious, their contacts are not likely to be infected unless they also have been in contact with the same adult source. After the presumptive adult source of the child's disease is identified, other contacts of that person should be evaluated, including skin testing and chest roentgenograms for those whose skin tests are positive to identify those who need antituberculous therapy.

Preventive Therapy for Contacts. Persons recently exposed within the previous 3 months to a potentially contagious case of tuberculosis, especially those with impaired immunity (eg, HIV infected) and all household contacts younger than 4 years who are exposed to any adult with active tuberculosis, should undergo tuberculin skin testing, have a chest roentgenogram, and be given isoniazid preventive therapy even if the skin test is negative, once clinical disease is excluded (see Chemotherapy for Tuberculosis Infection, p 551). Candidates for preventive therapy if the skin test is negative include recent contacts, household contacts, and persons in possible contact who are known to be anergic, especially if from a population with a high prevalence of tuberculosis. Infected persons can have a negative skin test because tuberculin cellular reactivity has not yet developed or because of anergy. Persons who are not anergic should be retested 12 weeks after contact has been broken. If the skin test is still negative, isoniazid can be discontinued. If the skin test becomes positive, isoniazid is continued for a total of at least 6 months. For HIV-infected persons, the duration is 12 months.

Child Care and Schools. Children with tuberculous infection or disease can attend school or child care if they are receiving chemotherapy (see Children in Out-of-Home Child Care, p 80). They can return to regular activities as soon as effective chemotherapy has been instituted, adherence to therapy has been documented, clinical symptoms have disappeared, and an acceptable plan for completing the course of therapy has been developed.

Bacillus Calmette-Guerin (BCG) Vaccine. BCG is a live vaccine prepared from attenuated strains of *Mycobacterium bovis*. It is recommended by the Expanded Programme on Immunization (EPI) of the World Health Organization (WHO) for administration at birth (see Table 1.4, p 21), and currently is used in more than 100 countries, primarily in young infants, in an attempt to prevent disseminated and other life-threatening diseases caused by *M tuberculosis*. BCG, however, does not prevent infection with *M tuberculosis*. The various BCG vaccines used throughout the world differ because of genetic changes in the bacterial strains that have occurred over many years. Vaccine efficacy of the different BCG vaccines appears to be highly variable.

Two recent meta-analyses of published clinical trials and case-control studies concerning the efficacy of BCG vaccines concluded that BCG does have relatively high protective efficacy (approximately 80%) against meningeal and miliary tuberculosis in children. The protective efficacy against pulmonary tuberculosis, however, differed significantly among the studies, precluding a specific conclusion. Protection afforded by BCG in one of the meta-analyses was estimated to be 50%. One BCG vaccine, as of December 1996, is licensed in the United States (Tice strain), which last underwent efficacy field trials in 1955. A second vaccine, using a strain of *M bovis* maintained in Canada, is under consideration for licensure in the United States. Comparative evaluations of these and other BCG vaccines have not been performed.

Indications. In the United States, the administration of BCG should be considered only in limited and select circumstances, such as unavoidable risk of exposure to *M tuberculosis* and failure or infeasibility of other methods of prevention and control of tuberculosis. Recommendations for the use of BCG vaccination for the prevention and control of tuberculosis among children and health care workers have recently been published by the Advisory Committee on Immunization Practices (ACIP) of the Centers for Disease Control and Prevention (CDC).* In infants and children, BCG vaccination should be considered only for those with negative tuberculin skin tests and who are not infected with HIV in the following circumstances:

- The child is exposed continually to a person or persons with contagious pulmonary tuberculosis resistant to isoniazid and rifampin and cannot be removed from this exposure.
- The child is exposed continually to a person or persons with untreated or ineffectively treated contagious pulmonary tuberculosis and cannot be removed from such exposure or given antituberculous therapy.

BCG vaccination also should be considered for health care workers in certain high-risk settings (see ACIP recommendation*).

Careful assessment of the potential risks and benefits of BCG vaccine and consultation with personnel in local area control programs for tuberculosis is strongly recommended before use of BCG.

When the vaccine is given, care should be taken to observe the precautions and directions for administration in the product label. BCG may be given to healthy infants from birth to 2 months of age without tuberculin testing; thereafter, BCG is given only to children with negative Mantoux (5TU) skin tests.

Adverse Reactions. BCG can uncommonly (1% to 2%) result in local adverse reactions, such as subcutaneous abscess and lymphadenopathy, which generally are not serious. One rare complication, osteitis affecting the epiphysis of long bones, may occur as long as several years after the vaccination. Disseminated, fatal disease occurs rarely (≤2/1 000 000 persons), primarily in persons with impaired immune systems. Antituberculous therapy, except for pyrazinamide, is recommended to treat osteitis and disseminated disease caused by BCG. Some experts also recommend treatment of chronic suppurative lymphadenitis caused by BCG.

Contraindications. BCG should not be given to persons with burns, skin infections, and primary or secondary immunodeficiencies, including HIV infection. However, in populations of the world in which the risk of tuberculosis is high, the WHO recommends BCG vaccine for asymptomatic HIV-infected children. Use of BCG is also contraindicated in persons receiving immunosuppressive medication, including corticosteroids. Although no untoward effects of BCG on the fetus have been observed, vaccination during pregnancy is not recommended.

Interpretation of Mantoux Skin Tests in Persons Who Received BCG.
Following BCG vaccination, distinguishing between a positive skin test reaction (see Table 3.59, p 545) caused by *M tuberculosis* infection and that caused by the BCG can be difficult. The presence or size of a postvaccination tuberculin skin test reaction

---

* Centers for Disease Control and Prevention. The role of BCG vaccine in the prevention and control of tuberculosis in the United States: a joint statement by the Advisory Committee for the Elimination of Tuberculosis and the Advisory Committee on Immunization Practices. *MMWR.* 1996;45(No. RR-4);1-18.

does not predict the degree of protection against *M tuberculosis* provided by BCG vaccination. Skin test reactivity following receipt of BCG may not occur at all in some persons. When Mantoux skin test reactivity does occur following receipt of BCG, it is unlikely to persist at a size of 10 mm or greater for more than a few years postvaccination in the absence of exposure and infection with *M tuberculosis* or repeated tuberculin skin testing. The degree of reaction (ie, induration) on a Mantoux skin test following receipt of BCG is dependent on many factors, including age at vaccination, quality and strain of BCG used, number of doses of BCG received, the nutritional and immunological status of the vaccinee, the time interval elapsed since BCG vaccination, and the frequency of tuberculin skin tests. BCG vaccination given a few months or more after birth induces a larger reaction than when vaccination is given immediately after birth. A positive skin test reaction (10 mm or greater) from BCG alone is unlikely 5 or more years after a single BCG vaccination during infancy.

Infection with *M tuberculosis* should be strongly suspected in any symptomatic person with a positive skin test, regardless of the history of vaccination with BCG. When evaluating an asymptomatic child who has a positive skin test but who possibly received BCG, verification of prior vaccination by written documentation or identification of the typical BCG vaccination scar should be undertaken. While a positive skin test can never be proven to be due to BCG vaccination, certain factors such as documented receipt of multiple BCG vaccinations (as evidenced, eg, by multiple BCG scars) decrease the likelihood that the positive skin test reaction is due to infection. However, only few countries give multiple doses of BCG during infancy and childhood. Factors that increase the probability that a positive skin test reaction resulted from infection with *M tuberculosis* include known contact with a person with contagious tuberculosis, a family history of tuberculosis, immigration from a country with a high prevalence of tuberculosis, and a long interval since the last BCG vaccination.

Roentgenographic evaluation of all children with a positive Mantoux skin test reaction is required, regardless of the child's BCG vaccination status. In most situations, an asymptomatic BCG-vaccinated child with a positive Mantoux skin test will have a normal chest roentgenogram. Infection with *M tuberculosis* should be assumed in such children and antituberculous therapy initiated to prevent disease. In selected instances, such as a person recently vaccinated with BCG, documented multiple BCG vaccinations and/or immigration from a country with a low prevalence of tuberculosis, however, treatment may not be indicated. In such cases, follow-up evaluation of the patient is essential.

Consultation with a specialist in tuberculosis should be considered in many of these difficult circumstances of managing a child or adolescent who has a positive skin test and previously received BCG vaccine.

Reporting of Cases. Reporting of suspected as well as confirmed cases of tuberculosis is mandated by law in all states. **A diagnosis of tuberculosis infection or disease in a child is a sentinel event representing recent transmission of *M tuberculosis* in the community.** Physicians should assist in a search for a source case and others infected by the source case. Usually adults or adolescents, such as members of the household (including relatives, baby-sitters, boarders, servants, and frequent visitors) or other adults with whom the child has frequent contact are source cases.

Diseases Caused By Nontuberculous Mycobacteria
(Atypical Mycobacteria, Mycobacteria Other Than Tuberculosis)

CLINICAL MANIFESTATIONS: Several different syndromes are caused by nontuberculous mycobacteria (NTM). In children, the most common of these syndromes is cervical lymphadenitis. Less common infections are osteomyelitis, cutaneous infection, otitis media, and pulmonary disease. Disseminated infections are nearly always associated with severe acquired (or congenital) immunodeficiency characterized by impaired cell-mediated immunity, such as HIV infection. Manifestations include fever, night sweats, weight loss, abdominal pain, fatigue, diarrhea, and anemia.

ETIOLOGY: Of the many species of NTM that have been identified, only a small number account for most of the infections caused by these organisms. The species most frequently encountered in children are *Mycobacterium avium* complex (MAC) (including *M avium* and *M intracellulare**), *M scrofulaceum*, *M kansasii*, and *M marinum* (see Table 3.65, p 564). Infection in patients with HIV infection usually is caused by MAC. *Mycobacterium fortuitum*, *M chelonei*, and *M abscessus* frequently are referred to as "rapidly-growing" mycobacteria because they grow sufficiently in the laboratory to be identified within 7 days, whereas other NTM and *Mycobacterium tuberculosis* take weeks to grow. Rapidly growing mycobacteria occasionally have been implicated in wound, soft-tissue, bone, pulmonary, and middle-ear infections. Other mycobacterial species, which usually are not pathogenic, have caused infections in immunocompromised hosts or have been associated with the presence of a foreign body.

EPIDEMIOLOGY: Because infections caused by NTM are not reportable in most areas, systematic data concerning their incidence and distribution are fewer than data for infections caused by *M tuberculosis*. In the past, as the incidence of tuberculosis decreased, the relative proportion of mycobacterial infections caused by NTM increased. Since the epidemic of HIV infection, however, the incidences of both tuberculosis and MAC infections have increased.

Many NTM species are ubiquitous and are found in soil, food, water, and animals. Most infections appear to be acquired by aspiration or inoculation of the organisms from these natural sources. Skin testing surveys using purified protein derivative (PPD) antigens derived from various NTM indicate that infections occur worldwide. In the United States, a survey in the 1960s suggested that NTM infection is more common in the southeastern and south central areas, but it occurs in all regions. Although many persons are exposed to NTM, only a few of these exposures result in chronic infection or disease. *Mycobacterium avium* complex in the respiratory tract or gastrointestinal tract is common in persons with HIV infection. Nontuberculosis mycobacteria, usually MAC, can be recovered from 10% to 20% of adolescents and young adults with cystic fibrosis. The usual portals of entry for NTM infection are believed to be abrasions in the skin (eg, for the cutaneous lesions caused by *M marinum*); the oropharyngeal mucosa (the presumed portal for cervical lymphadenitis); the gastrointestinal or respiratory tracts for MAC; and the respiratory tract (including tympanostomy tubes) for otitis media and rare cases of mediastinal

---

* Formerly termed the Battey bacillus.

Table 3.65. Nontuberculous Mycobacterial Species That Most Commonly Cause Disease in Children

Organism	Syndrome
M avium complex (MAC)	Lymphadenitis, pulmonary infection, disseminated disease in HIV-infected and other immunocompromised hosts
M scrofulaceum	Lymphadenitis
M kansasii	Lymphadenitis, pulmonary infection
M marinum	Cutaneous infection ("swimming pool granuloma")
M fortuitum	Lymphadenitis, cutaneous infection
M chelonei	Cutaneous infection
M abscessus	Cutaneous infections, pulmonary infections, and otitis media

adenitis and of endobronchial disease. Most infections remain localized at the portal of entry or in regional lymph nodes. Severe pulmonary disease and dissemination to distal sites occur primarily in immunocompromised hosts, especially in persons with AIDS. No evidence for person-to-person transmission of NTM exists, but appropriate studies, especially in the case of HIV-infected and other immunosuppressed patients, have not been performed. Cases of otitis media caused by *M abscessus* have been associated with use of contaminated equipment and water. A water-borne route of transmission has been suspected for MAC infection in immunodeficient hosts.

The **incubation period** is not known.

DIAGNOSTIC TESTS: Definitive diagnosis of disease caused by NTM requires isolation and identification of the infecting organism. Caution must be exercised in the interpretation of cultures obtained from sites that are not necessarily sterile, such as from gastric washings, a draining sinus tract, or a single urine specimen. Caution in ascribing illness to an NTM isolate also is warranted if the species cultured is usually nonpathogenic (eg, *Mycobacterium gordonae*) and if only a few colonies are recovered from a single specimen. Repeated isolation of numerous colonies of a single species is more likely to indicate disease than transient colonization. Most reliable for diagnosis of infection is the recovery of NTM from sites that are otherwise sterile, such as cerebrospinal fluid, pleural fluid, bone marrow, blood, lymph node aspirates, middle ear or mastoid aspirates, or surgically excised tissue. With the radiometric broth or lysis-centrifugation techniques, blood cultures are highly sensitive in the recovery of MAC and other blood-borne NTM species.

Patients with NTM infection can have false-positive tuberculin skin tests, since tuberculin preparations (PPD) derived from *M tuberculosis* share a number of antigens with NTM species. These false-positive results occur in otherwise healthy children who have no history of exposure to *M tuberculosis* but may have been sensitized by exposure to NTM in the environment. Those cross-reactions that usually, but not always, result in Mantoux skin test reactions to PPD measuring less than 10 mm of induration can be more common than true-positive tuberculin reactions in populations with a low prevalence of tuberculosis and a high prevalence of NTM infections.

For both clinical and public health reasons, differentiating *M tuberculosis* infection from NTM infections is important. Studies in children have shown that dual Mantoux tests with standard PPD (for *M tuberculosis*) and PPD-Battey (for *M intracellulare*) are sometimes helpful in distinguishing tuberculous from nontuberculous infections. Skin tests using PPD derived from different NTM species, however, are not available commercially.

A reaction of 15 mm or greater to a standard intradermal Mantoux tuberculin skin test (5 TU PPD) is more indicative of infection with *M tuberculosis;* a reaction of less than 10 mm suggests NTM infection in the patient with cervical adenitis or other syndromes consistent with NTM disease, a normal chest roentgenogram, nonreactive PPD tests in other family members, and no likely exposure to a case of infectious tuberculosis. The identification of family members with positive tuberculin reactions increases the likelihood of *M tuberculosis* infection in the index case. Negative results on tuberculin skin testing, a normal chest roentgenogram, and no history of contact with persons with active tuberculosis are consistent with possible NTM infection.

Disseminated MAC disease should prompt a search for an underlying predisposing factor, usually HIV infection. Tests of immune function and a search for other opportunistic pathogens (eg, *Pneumocystis carinii*) are indicated. Patients with disseminated MAC disease should be evaluated for HIV infection.

TREATMENT: Many NTM are relatively resistant in vitro to antituberculosis drugs. In vitro resistance, however, does not necessarily correlate with clinical response. Only limited controlled therapeutic trials have been performed in NTM infections. The approach to therapy should consider the following factors: (1) the species causing the infection, (2) the results of drug-susceptibility testing, (3) the site(s) of infection, (4) the nature of the patient's underlying disease (if any), and (5) the frequent need to treat a patient presumptively for tuberculosis while awaiting culture reports that subsequently reveal NTM infection.

For the common problem of NTM lymphadenitis in otherwise healthy children, especially when the disease is caused by *M scrofulaceum* or MAC, surgical excision alone is frequently the most effective treatment. Antituberculosis chemotherapy usually offers little benefit, but clarithromycin may be of value in the treatment of some cases of NTM, especially when surgical excision is difficult.

Cutaneous infections with *M marinum* can require a combination of medical and surgical debridement. Minocycline has been used successfully for *M marinum* sporotrichoid skin infections; other tetracyclines also can be given. Tetracyclines, however, should not be given to children younger than 8 years unless the benefits of therapy are greater than the risks of dental staining (see Antimicrobials and Related Therapy, p 606). The combination of rifampin and ethambutol, clarithromycin, or trimethoprim-sulfamethoxazole given for a minimum of 3 months also may be effective.

Infections caused by *M kansasii* usually respond well to treatment with rifampin, ethambutol, and isoniazid, although the organism may be resistant in vitro to one or more of these agents. Ciprofloxacin is active in vitro against *M fortuitum* and, to a lesser extent, against MAC, and may have a role in treating some patients with infections caused by these organisms. Fluoroquinolones, however, should not be given to individuals younger than 18 years except in circumstances in which no other drug is available and the benefits of therapy are greater than the risks, such as in children with HIV infection who have disseminated infection (see Antimicrobials and Related Therapy, p 605).

Isolates of rapid-growing mycobacteria (*M fortuitum, M abscessus,* and *M chelonei*) should be tested in vitro against antituberculous agents, as well as against other drugs (such as amikacin, imipenem, cefoxitin, ciprofloxacin, clarithromycin, and doxycycline) to which they frequently are susceptible and which have been used with some success. Clarithromycin appears to be the drug of choice for cutaneous (disseminated) infections due to *M chelonei.* Details regarding choice of drugs, dosages, and duration should be reviewed with a consultant experienced in the management of these infections.

Additional information concerning treatment of NTM infections can be obtained from the Division of Bacterial and Mycotic Diseases, Centers for Disease Control and Prevention (see Directory of Telephone Numbers, p 667).

In patients with AIDS and in other immunocompromised persons with disseminated MAC infection, multidrug therapy is indicated. Single-dose therapy results in frequent development of antimicrobial resistance. Clinical isolates of MAC usually are resistant to many of the approved antituberculous drugs including isoniazid, but are often sensitive in vitro to clarithromycin, azithromycin, ethambutol, refabutin, rifampin, clofazimine, amikacin, and fluoroquinolones. The optimal regimen has to been determined. Based on available information at the time, the United States Public Health Service (USPHS) and the Infectious Diseases Society of America (IDSA) recommended in 1993 the following guidelines for therapy of disseminated MAC infection*:

- Treatment regimens, except in clinical trials, should include at least two drugs.
- Every regimen should contain either clarithromycin or azithromycin; many experts prefer ethambutol as a second drug. Many clinicians have added one or more of the following as second, third, or fourth agents: rifabutin, rifampin, clofazimine, ciprofloxacin, or, in some situations, amikacin.
- Patients receiving therapy should be monitored. Considerations are as follows:
  — Clinical manifestations of disseminated MAC infection, such as fever, weight loss, and night sweats, should be monitored several times during the initial weeks of therapy. Microbiologic response, as assessed by blood culture every 4 weeks during initial therapy, also can be helpful in interpreting the efficacy of a therapeutic regimen.
  — Most patients who ultimately respond show substantial clinical improvement in the first 4 to 6 weeks of therapy. Elimination of the organisms from blood cultures may take somewhat longer, often requiring 4 to 12 weeks.
  — Patients receiving clarithromycin plus rifabutin or high-dose rifabutin (with another drug) should be observed for the development of uveitis, polyarthralgias and pseudojaundice secondary to rifabutin.

---

* Centers for Disease Control and Prevention. Recommendations on prophylaxis and therapy for disseminated *Mycobacterium avium* complex for adults and adolescents infected with human immunodeficiency virus. *MMWR.* 1993;42(No. RR-9):17-20.

Since these recommendations were issued, the benefit of multiple drug therapy of MAC infection in adults with AIDS has been further evaluated. In a recent trial, enhanced resolution of bacteremia and improved survival was demonstrated in patients treated with a three-drug regimen of clarithromycin, ethambutol, and rifabutin in comparison to those treated with a four-drug regimen (rifampin, ethambutol, clofazimine, and ciprofloxacin) that did not include clarithromycin.

Therapy for disseminated MAC infection should continue for the lifetime of the patient, irrespective of the extent of clinical and microbiologic improvement.* A macrolide, usually clarithromycin, generally is recommended in conjunction with at least one other drug, such as ethambutol, clofazimine, or ciprofloxacin. Drug dosages should be the same as given for initial therapy.

Chemoprophylaxis. According to the 1995 guidelines of the USPHS/IDSA Prevention of Opportunistic Infections Working Group, prophylaxis with rifabutin should be considered for HIV-infected adults and adolescents with CD4+ T-lymphocyte counts of less than 75/µL.† Clarithromycin or azithromycin is an alternative and recommended by some experts. Disseminated MAC disease should be excluded by a negative blood culture before prophylaxis is initiated.

Prophylaxis with one of these drugs also should be considered for HIV-infected children younger than 12 years with low CD4+ T-lymphocyte counts. For those 6 to 12 years of age, a CD4+ count of less than 75/µL is a reasonable threshold for the initiation of chemoprophylaxis. Some adjustment for age is necessary in the interpretation of CD4+ counts in children less than 6 years of age (see HIV Infection, p 282).

Further information, including drug dosages for prophylaxis, is given in the 1995 USPHS/IDSA guidelines.* No pediatric formulation of rifabutin is currently available but a dosage of 5 mg/kg/per day has been used in pharmakokinetic studies.

These recommendations are subject to change because of clinical trials of prophylaxis in HIV-infected patients that have been completed since these guidelines were issued or are currently in progress.

ISOLATION OF THE HOSPITALIZED PATIENT: Standard precautions are recommended.

CONTROL MEASURES: The only control measures are chemoprophylaxis in certain patients with HIV infection (see Treatment, p 565) and use of sterile equipment for middle-ear instrumentation, including otoscopic equipment for prevention of *M abscessus* otitis media. Since MAC organisms are common in environmental sources such as food and water, current information does not support specific recommendations regarding avoidance of exposure for HIV-infected persons.

---

* Centers for Disease Control and Prevention. USPHS/IDSA guidelines for the prevention of opportunistic infections in persons infected with human immunodeficiency virus: a summary. *MMWR.* 1995;44(No. RR-8):11-12, 24-29.

† Centers for Disease Control and Prevention. Recommendations on prophylaxis and therapy for disseminated *Mycobacterium avium* complex for adults and adolescents infected with human immunodeficiency virus. *MMWR.* 1993;42(No. RR-9):17-20.

Tularemia

CLINICAL MANIFESTATIONS: Infection usually is characterized by fever and constitutional symptoms of chills, myalgia, and headache. Onset frequently is abrupt and conforms to one of the specific tularemic syndromes. The ulceroglandular syndrome, the most common, is characterized by (1) a primary, painful maculopapular lesion at the portal of entry, with subsequent ulceration and slow healing; and (2) painful, acutely inflamed lymph nodes, which may drain spontaneously. Other disease syndromes are the following: glandular (wherein no skin or mucous membrane lesion is present), oculoglandular (severe conjunctivitis and preauricular lymph node involvement), oropharyngeal (severe exudative pharyngitis), typhoidal (high fever, hepatomegaly, and splenomegaly), and pneumonic.

ETIOLOGY: *Francisella tularensis,* the causative agent, is a small, Gram-negative coccobacillus.

EPIDEMIOLOGY: Sources of the organism include approximately 100 species of wild mammals (eg, rabbits, hares, muskrats, squirrels, and deer); at least nine species of domestic animals (eg, sheep, cattle, and cats); blood-sucking arthropods that bite these animals (eg, ticks, deerflies, and mosquitoes); and water contaminated by infected animals. In the United States, rabbits and ticks are major sources of infection. Infected animals and arthropods are infective for prolonged periods: frozen, killed rabbits can remain infective for more than 3 years. Persons at risk are those with occupational or recreational exposure to infected animals or their habitat, such as rabbit hunters and trappers, those with tick or insect bites, and laboratory technicians working with *F tularensis* (which is a highly infectious agent in the laboratory). Ticks are the most important vectors. Transmission is by bites of infected arthropods, direct contact with infected animals, ingestion of contaminated water or inadequately cooked meat, or inhalation of contaminated particles. Person-to-person transmission has not been documented. Organisms may be present in the blood during the first 2 weeks of disease and in lesions for as long as 1 month if untreated.

The **incubation period** ranges from 1 to 21 days; most cases occur 3 to 5 days after exposure.

DIAGNOSTIC TESTS: Diagnosis is most frequently established by serological testing. A fourfold or greater rise in the serum *F tularensis* agglutinin titer frequently is evident after the second week of illness and is considered diagnostic. A single convalescent titer of 1:160 or greater is consistent with recent or past infection. Slide agglutination tests are less reliable than plate or tube agglutination tests; nonspecific cross-agglutination with *Brucella, Proteus,* and heterophile antibodies can cause false-positive antibody titers to *F tularensis.* The indirect fluorescent antibody test of ulcer exudate or aspirate material can be useful as a rapid and specific screening test. Isolation of the organism from blood, skin, ulcers, lymph node drainage, gastric washings, or respiratory tract secretions requires cysteine-enriched media or inoculation of laboratory mice (with subsequent passage). Some commercial supplemented chocolate agar or modified charcoal-yeast agar (used for culture of *Legionella*) can support growth of *F tularensis.* The laboratory always should be informed that *F tularensis* is suspected, because of the potential hazard to laboratory personnel and the need for special media. Culture should be attempted only by personnel who have been immunized against *F tularensis.*

TREATMENT: For many years, streptomycin has been the recommended drug of choice for treatment of tularemia. However, treatment with gentamicin also is highly effective and has the advantage that drug concentrations during therapy can be readily monitored. Duration of therapy is usually 6 to 10 days; the longer course is given for more severe illness.

Alternative drugs include a tetracycline (which ordinarily should not be given to children younger than 8 years or to pregnant women) and chloramphenicol. Clinical relapses are frequent, however, in patients treated with either of these drugs.

ISOLATION OF THE HOSPITALIZED PATIENT: Standard precautions are recommended for cutaneous and pulmonary infection.

CONTROL MEASURES:
- Persons should minimize opportunities for arthropod bites by wearing protective clothing, by frequent inspection for and removal of ticks from the skin and scalp, and by using insect repellents (see Control Measures for Prevention of Tick-Borne Infections, p 126).
- Children should be instructed not to handle any sick or dead animals.
- Rubber gloves should be worn by hunters, trappers, and food preparers when handling the carcasses of wild rabbits and other potentially infected animals.
- Game meats should be thoroughly cooked.
- Face masks and rubber gloves should be worn by those working with cultures or infective material in the laboratory, and the work should be performed in a biologic safety cabinet.
- Standard precautions should be used for handling clinical materials.
- Interstate or interarea shipment of infected animals should be prohibited.
- A live-attenuated vaccine is recommended for laboratory technicians who work with the organism. It is available from the US Army Medical Research and Material Command.*

Flea-Borne Typhus
(Murine Typhus, Endemic Typhus)

CLINICAL MANIFESTATIONS: Flea-borne typhus resembles louse-borne typhus but usually is milder, has a less acute onset, and has less severe systemic symptoms. In young children, the disease is mild. Fever can be accompanied by persistent headache and myalgias. The rash is typically macular or maculopapular, appears during days 3 to 5 of illness, lasts 4 to 8 days, and tends to remain discrete, with sparse lesions and no hemorrhage. The disease seldom lasts longer than 2 weeks, and visceral involvement usually does not occur. The disease rarely is fatal.

---

* Attn: SGRD-UMB, Fort Detrich, Frederick, MD 21702-5009.

ETIOLOGY: Flea-borne typhus is caused by *Rickettsia typhi* (formerly *Rickettsia mooseri*), an organism antigenically similar to *Rickettsia prowazekii.*

EPIDEMIOLOGY: Rats, in which infection is inapparent, are the natural hosts. Opossums also can be infected and serve as a reservoir. The vector for transmission among rats and to humans is the rat flea (usually *Xenopsylla cheopis*). The disease is worldwide in distribution, affects all races, tends to occur more commonly in adults and in males, and is most common during April to October. The disease is rare in the United States; most cases occur in focal areas in southern California, the south-eastern Gulf Coast and southern border states, and Hawaii. Exposure to rats and their fleas is the major risk factor, although a history of such exposure is frequently absent in infected patients.

The **incubation period** is 6 to 14 days.

DIAGNOSTIC TESTS: Serum agglutinins against *Proteus vulgaris* Ox-19 peak 2 to 3 weeks after the onset of disease, but these tests lack sensitivity and specificity. Indirect fluorescent antibody, latex agglutination, or complement fixation antibody concentrations peak at a similar or slightly later time. A fourfold titer change between acute and convalescent serum specimens is diagnostic but also can occur in patients with louse-borne typhus. Serologic differentiation between these diseases by antibody absorption is possible but is not available routinely. Isolation of the organism in culture is possible but is not attempted routinely because it is hazardous and requires specialized facilities.

TREATMENT: A single dose of doxycycline is the treatment of choice. Although repeated doses of doxycycline generally are not recommended for children younger than 8 years of age, the risk of dental staining from a single dose of doxycycline is minimal (see Antimicrobials and Related Therapy, p 606). Other tetracyclines and chloramphenicol also are effective drugs.

ISOLATION OF THE HOSPITALIZED PATIENT: Standard precautions are recommended.

CONTROL MEASURES: Rat fleas should be controlled by appropriate insecticides, preferably before the use of rodenticides, because the flea will seek alternate hosts when rats are not available. Rat populations should be controlled by appropriate means. A vaccine is no longer available in the United States. No treatment is recommended for exposed persons. The disease should be reported to public health departments.

Louse-Borne Typhus
(Epidemic Typhus)

CLINICAL MANIFESTATIONS: In epidemic louse-borne typhus, the onset of high fever, chills, and diffuse aching, accompanied by severe headache and malaise, is usually abrupt. Influenza-like illness frequently is suspected. The rash appears 4 to 7 days later, beginning on the trunk and spreading to the limbs. A concentrated eruption is present in the axillae. The rash is maculopapular, becomes petechial or hemorrhagic, then develops into brownish, pigmented areas. The face, palms, and soles usually are not affected. Changes in mental status are common, and delirium or coma can occur. Myocardial and renal failure occur when the disease is severe. Illness varies from moderately severe to fatal. When untreated, the illness typically lasts 2 weeks and ends by lysis of fever and subsidence of symptoms in those who recover. In untreated cases, mortality is uncommon in children but increases with advancing age, ranging from 10% to 40% in adults. Brill-Zinsser disease is a relapse of louse-borne typhus that occurs years after the initial episode. Stress or an unknown factor serves to reactivate the rickettsiae. The recrudescent illness is similar to the primary infection but generally is milder and of shorter duration.

ETIOLOGY: *Rickettsia prowazekii* is the cause.

EPIDEMIOLOGY: Humans are the major source of the organism, which is transmitted from person to person by the body louse, *Pediculus humanus* subspecies *corporis*. All ages and races and both sexes are affected. Poverty, crowding, poor sanitary conditions, lack of bathing, and poor personal hygiene contribute to the spread of lice, and, hence, the disease. Currently, cases of typhus rarely are reported but have occurred throughout the world, including Asia, Africa, some parts of Europe, and Central and South America. Typhus is common during the winter when conditions favor person-to-person transmission of the vector, the body louse. Rickettsiae are present in the blood and tissues of patients during the early febrile phase but are not found in secretions. Direct person-to-person spread of the disease does not occur in the absence of the vector. Cases in humans have been associated with contact with infected flying squirrels in the United States, their nests, or their ectoparasites. Squirrel-related disease appears to be a milder illness than louse-borne typhus.

The **incubation period** is 1 to 2 weeks.

DIAGNOSTIC TESTS: *Rickettsia prowazekii* can be isolated from blood by inoculation into guinea pigs and mice or the yolk sac of embryonated hens' eggs, but since isolation is dangerous, it is attempted rarely. Titers of serum agglutinins against *Proteus* Ox-19 peak 2 to 3 weeks after the onset of disease, but an indirect fluorescent antibody or complement fixation antibody test is preferred. A fourfold change in antibody titer between acute and convalescent serum specimens is diagnostic of either flea-borne or louse-borne typhus. An antibody absorption test can often differentiate the two diseases but is not available routinely.

TREATMENT: Tetracycline or chloramphenicol, given intravenously or orally, is the treatment of choice for louse-borne typhus. Therapy is given until the patient is afebrile for at least 7 days; the usual duration is 7 to 10 days. Repeated courses of tetracycline antibiotics generally are not recommended for children younger than 8 years but the risk of dental staining with a single course is minimal (see Antimicrobials and Related Therapy, p 606). Cream and gel pediculocides containing pyrethrins (0.16% to 0.33%), piperonyl butoxide (2% to 4%), crotamiton (10%), or lindane (1%) can be used for delousing. Convulsions have been reported in children receiving excessive doses of topical lindane.

ISOLATION OF THE HOSPITALIZED PATIENT: Standard precautions are recommended.

CONTROL MEASURES: Thorough delousing in epidemic situations, particularly among exposed contacts of cases, is recommended. Several applications may be needed because the lice eggs are resistant to most insecticides. Washing clothes in hot water kills lice and eggs. During epidemics, insecticides dusted onto the clothes of louse-infested populations are effective in louse control efforts. In some circumstances, preventing flying squirrels from living in human dwellings by sealing their access ports is recommended. A vaccine is no longer available in the United States. Cases should be reported to the regional public health department.

Ureaplasma urealyticum Infections

CLINICAL MANIFESTATIONS: The most common syndrome associated with *Ureaplasma urealyticum* infection is nongonococcal urethritis (NGU). While NGU is most frequently caused by *Chlamydia trachomatis, U urealyticum* appears to be responsible for a significant proportion of the remainder (20% to 30%). Without treatment, the disease usually resolves within 1 to 6 months, although asymptomatic infection may persist thereafter. In women, salpingitis, endometritis, and chorioamnionitis can occur. Prostatitis and epididymitis have been associated with *U urealyticum* infection in men.

Ureaplasma urealyticum has been isolated from the lower respiratory tract and lung biopsy specimens of preterm infants with pneumonia and chronic lung disease of prematurity. Although it also has been recovered from respiratory secretions of infants 3 months of age or younger with pneumonia, its role in the development of lower respiratory tract disease in otherwise healthy young infants, however, is controversial. *Ureaplasma urealyticum* is a rare cause of central nervous system infection in newborns and has been isolated in the cerebrospinal fluid in patients with meningitis, hydrocephalus, and intraventricular hemorrhage.

Isolated cases of *U urealyticum* arthritis, osteomyelitis, pericarditis, and progressive sinopulmonary disease in immunocompromised patients have been reported.

ETIOLOGY: Ureaplasmas and the mycoplasmas form the family *Mycoplasmataceae*. The genus *Ureaplasma* contains a single species, *U urealyticum*, which includes at least 16 serotypes.

EPIDEMIOLOGY: The principal reservoir of the human *U urealyticum* is the genital tract of sexually active adults. Colonization is found in approximately half of sexually active women; the incidence in sexually active men is lower. Colonization is uncommon in prepubertal children and in adolescents who are not sexually active. Transmission during delivery is likely from an asymptomatic colonized mother to her newborn. *Ureaplasma urealyticum* may colonize the throat, eyes, umbilicus and perineum of newborns, and persist for several months after birth.

The **incubation period** of NGU after sexual transmission is 10 to 20 days.

DIAGNOSTIC TESTS: The *U urealyticum* organism can be cultured in urea-containing broth. However, because *U urealyticum* is frequently isolated from the lower female genital tract and neonatal respiratory tract in the absence of disease, a positive culture does not establish its etiologic role in an acute infection. Accordingly, most experts do not recommend routine screening. If a culture is done, specific *Ureaplasma* transport media with refrigeration at 4°C is necessary. A rapid, sensitive polymerase chain reaction test for detection of *U urealyticum* has been developed, but is not routinely available. Serological testing for *U urealyticum* antibodies is of limited value and should not be used for routine diagnosis.

TREATMENT: For older children, adolescents, and adults, doxycycline (100 mg orally twice a day for 7 days) is the drug of choice. Recurrences are common. Erythromycin is the preferred antimicrobial agent for children younger than 8 years and for men with urethritis caused by tetracycline-resistant strains. Studies in adult men with NGU indicate that single-dose azithromycin (1 g orally in a single dose) also is effective. Antibiotic efficacy studies have been performed only in adult patients with NGU; definitive evidence of their efficacy in infants and children is lacking. A few infants with meningitis have been treated successfully with intravenous doxycycline, erythromycin, or chloramphenicol.

ISOLATION OF THE HOSPITALIZED PATIENT: Standard precautions are recommended.

CONTROL MEASURES: Partners of infected sexually active persons should be notified so they can be offered treatment.

Varicella-Zoster Infections

CLINICAL MANIFESTATIONS: Primary infection results in chickenpox, manifested by a generalized, pruritic, vesicular rash with mild fever and systemic symptoms. Complications include bacterial superinfection, thrombocytopenia, arthritis, hepatitis, encephalitis or meningitis, or glomerulonephritis. The disease can be more severe in adolescents and adults. Reye syndrome can also follow some cases of chickenpox. In immunocompromised children, progressive varicella characterized by continuing eruption of lesions and a high fever into the second week of the illness, and encephalitis, hepatitis, or pneumonia can develop. Chickenpox is often more severe in immunocompromised patients. Pneumonia is exceedingly rare in normal children but is the most common complication in older persons. Children with HIV infection can develop chronic or recurrent chickenpox with new lesions appearing for months.

The virus persists in a latent form after the primary infection. Reactivation results in herpes zoster ("shingles"). Grouped vesicular lesions appear in the distribution of one to three sensory dermatomes, sometimes accompanied by pain localized to the area. Systemic symptoms are few. Zoster occasionally can become generalized in immunocompromised patients, with lesions appearing outside the primary dermatomes and with visceral complications.

Fetal infection after maternal varicella in the first or early second trimester of pregnancy occasionally results in varicella embryopathy, which is characterized by limb atrophy and scarring of the skin of the extremity (the congenital varicella syndrome). Central nervous system and eye manifestations also can occur. Children who were exposed to varicella-zoster virus in utero can develop inapparent varicella and subsequent zoster early in life without having had extrauterine varicella. Severe varicella of the newborn infant with fatality rates as high as 30% can result when an infant's mother develops varicella from 5 days before to 2 days after delivery.

ETIOLOGY: Varicella-zoster virus (VZV) is a herpes virus.

EPIDEMIOLOGY: Humans are the only source of infection for this highly contagious virus. Person-to-person transmission occurs primarily by direct contact with patients with varicella or zoster, and occasionally occurs by air-borne spread from respiratory secretions and, rarely, from zoster lesions. In utero infection also can occur. Introduction of a VZV infection into a household usually results in infection of nearly all susceptible persons. Children who acquire their infection at home (secondary family cases) may have more severe disease than that in the index case. Nosocomial transmission is well documented in pediatric units, but transmission is extremely rare in newborn nurseries.

Varicella is most common during the late winter and early spring. Most reported cases of chickenpox in recent years occur in children younger than 10 years, but varicella in adolescents and young adults may be becoming more common. Immunity is generally lifelong. Symptomatic reinfection is rare in healthy persons, although asymptomatic reinfection does occur. Asymptomatic primary infection is unusual.

Immunocompromised individuals with either primary (varicella) or recurrent (zoster) infection are at increased risk of severe disease. Other groups of pediatric patients who may experience more severe or complicated disease include infants, adolescents, patients with chronic cutaneous or pulmonary disorders, and patients receiving systemic corticosteroids or chronic salicylate therapy. The attack rate for congenital varicella syndrome in infants born to mothers with chickenpox during the first trimester is 1.2%, based on aggregate prospective studies; it is greater (2%) when infection occurs between 13 and 20 weeks of gestation than between 0 and 12 weeks (0.4%). Zoster in infancy or early childhood, accordingly in one study, occurred in 0.8% of infants with intrauterine exposure to VZV between 13 and 24 weeks of gestation and in 1.7% of those with exposure between 25 and 36 weeks of gestation. Patients are most contagious for 1 to 2 days before and shortly after the onset of the rash. Contagiousness, however, can be for as long as 5 days after the onset of lesions, and in immunocompromised patients with progressive varicella, it probably lasts throughout the period of eruption of new lesions.

The **incubation period** is usually 14 to 16 days, occasionally as early as 10 or as late as 21 days after contact. It may be prolonged (for as long as 28 days) by the use of varicella-zoster immune globulin (VZIG) and shortened in immunocompromised patients. Varicella can develop between 1 and 16 days of life in infants born to mothers with active varicella; the usual interval from onset of rash in the mother to onset in the neonate is 9 to 15 days.

DIAGNOSTIC TESTS: Varicella-zoster virus can be isolated from vesicular lesions of otherwise healthy patients during the first 3 to 4 days of the eruption. Diagnosis can be accomplished by immunofluorescent staining of vesicular scrapings, using commercially available monoclonal antibodies that will distinguish between VZV and herpes simplex virus. The demonstration of multinucleated giant cells containing intranuclear inclusions in lesions (Tzanck smear) is less accurate than the immuno-fluorescent staining technique. Infection can be confirmed by testing acute- and convalescent-phase sera for VZV antibody. Serologic tests include enzyme immuno-assay (EIA), latex agglutination (LA) indirect fluorescent antibody (IFA), and fluores-cent antibody-to-membrane antigen (FAMA) assays. The LA test can be completed in 15 minutes and does not required special equipment; it has comparable sensitivity and specificity to the FAMA and other sensitive tests in detecting antibody response following infection. These tests are reliable in determining immune status in healthy hosts but are not necessarily reliable in immunocompromised persons (see Care of Exposed Persons, p 576). The complement fixation test is not sufficiently sensitive to be reliable in determining susceptibility in either case.

A highly sensitive enzyme-linked immunosorbent assay that utilizes purified VZV glycoproteins has been used in clinical trials for testing the immunogenicity of varicella vaccine, but it is not commercially available.

TREATMENT: Varicella and zoster may be treated with intravenous or oral acyclovir. Intravenous therapy is recommended for immunocompromised patients. Therapy initiated early in the course of the illness maximizes efficacy. Although Varicella-Zoster Immune Globulin (VZIG) given shortly after exposure can prevent or modify the course of disease, it is not effective once disease is established (see Care of Exposed Persons, p 576).

Oral acyclovir given to otherwise healthy children with varicella within 24 hours of the onset of rash results in a modest decrease in the duration and magnitude of fever and in the number and duration of skin lesions. However, therapy with oral acyclovir is not recommended routinely for treatment of uncomplicated varicella in the otherwise healthy child. This recommendation is based on the marginal thera-peutic effect, cost of the drug, difficulty in initiating the drug in the first 24 hours of illness, and potential unforeseen dangers of treating large numbers of children who are at low risk of developing complications. Oral acyclovir should be considered for otherwise healthy persons at increased risk of moderate to severe varicella, such as those older than 12 years, those with chronic cutaneous or pulmonary disorders, those receiving chronic salicylate therapy, and persons receiving short, intermittent, or aerosolized courses. For recommendations on dosage and duration of therapy, see Antiviral Drugs for Non-HIV Infections (p 634). Some experts also would consi-der use of oral acyclovir in secondary household cases in whom the disease is usually more severe.

Oral acyclovir is not recommended routinely in the pregnant adolescent or adult with uncomplicated varicella, since the risks and benefits to the fetus and mother are unknown. Some experts, however, recommend oral acyclovir for pregnant women with varicella, especially in the third trimester. Intravenous acyclovir is recommended for the pregnant patient with serious complications of varicella.* Oral acyclovir usu-

---

* Burroughs Welcome Company in conjunction with the Centers for Disease Control and Prevention maintains an Acyclovir in Pregnancy Registry to monitor fetal-maternal outcomes of pregnant women given systemic acyclovir. Physicians are encouraged to register pregnant women treated with acyclovir by calling 800-722-9292, ext 39437.

ally should not be used to treat immunocompromised children with varicella. However, some experts have used oral high-dose acyclovir in highly selected, immunocompromised patients perceived to be at lower risk of developing severe varicella, such as HIV-infected patients with relatively normal concentrations of CD4+ T-lymphocytes and children with leukemia in whom careful follow-up is assured.

Famciclovir and valacyclovir have recently been licensed for treatment of zoster in adults. No pediatric formulation is available and insufficient data currently exist on the use or dose of these drugs in children to recommend them for therapy in children.

Children with varicella should not receive salicylates because administration of salicylates to such children increases the risk of subsequent Reye syndrome. Acetaminophen may be used for control of fever.

ISOLATION OF THE HOSPITALIZED PATIENT*: Both airborne and contact precautions are recommended for patients with varicella for a minimum of 5 days after the onset of the rash and as long as the rash remains vesicular, which in immunocompromised patients can be a week or longer. For exposed, susceptible patients, airborne and contact precautions from 8 until 21 days after the onset of the rash in the index patient also are indicated; these precautions should be maintained until 28 days after exposure for those who received VZIG.

Airborne and contact precautions are recommended for neonates born to mothers with varicella and, if still hospitalized, continued until 21 days of age or 28 days if they received VZIG. Infants with varicella embryopathy do not require isolation.

Immunocompromised patients who have zoster (localized or disseminated) and normal patients with disseminated zoster require airborne and contact precautions for the duration of the illness. For normal patients with localized zoster, standard precautions are indicated until all lesions are crusted.

CONTROL MEASURES:

Child Care and School. Children with uncomplicated chickenpox who have been excluded from school or child care may return on the sixth day after the onset of the rash. In mild cases with only a few lesions and rapid resolution, children may return sooner if all lesions are crusted. Immunocompromised and other children with a prolonged course should be excluded for the duration of the vesicular eruption.

Exclusion of children with zoster whose lesions cannot be covered is based on similar criteria. Those who are excluded may return after the lesions have crusted. Lesions that are covered appear to pose little risk to susceptible individuals. Older children and staff members with zoster should be instructed to wash their hands if they touch potentially infectious lesions.

CARE OF EXPOSED PERSONS.

Hospital Exposure. If an inadvertent exposure in the hospital by an infected patient, health care worker, or visitor occurs, the following control measures are recommended:
 • Those personnel and patients who have been exposed (see Table 3.66, p 577) and are susceptible to varicella should be identified.

---

* In addition to standard precautions.

Table 3.66. **Types of Exposure to Varicella or Zoster for Which VZIG Is Indicated for Susceptible Persons*†**

- Household: Residing in the same household
- Playmate: Face-to-face‡ indoor play
- Hospital:

Varicella:	In same 2- to 4-bed room, or adjacent beds in a large ward, face-to-face‡ contact with an infectious staff member or patient, or visit by a person deemed contagious
Zoster:	Intimate contact (eg, touching or hugging) with a person deemed contagious.

- Newborn infant: Onset of varicella in the mother 5 d or less before delivery or within 48 h after delivery; VZIG is not indicated if the mother has zoster

---

* Patients should meet criteria of both significant exposure and candidacy for receiving varicella-zoster immune globulin (VZIG), as given in Table 3.67 (p 578).
† Varicella-zoster immune globulin should be administered as soon as possible, and no later than 96 hours after exposure.
‡ Experts differ in the duration of face-to-face contact that warrants the administration of VZIG. However, the contact should be nontransient. Some experts suggest a contact of 5 or more minutes as constituting significant exposure for this purpose; others define close contact as more than 1 hour.

- Varicella-zoster immune globulin should be administered to appropriate candidates (see Table 3.67, p 578).
- All exposed, susceptible patients should be discharged as soon as possible.
- All exposed, susceptible patients who cannot be discharged should be placed in strict isolation from day 8 to day 21 after exposure to the index patient. For those who have received VZIG, strict isolation should be continued until day 28.
- All susceptible, exposed staff should be either furloughed or excused from patient contact from day 8 to day 21 after exposure to an infectious patient. The interval is until day 28 for those who have received VZIG (see Active Immunization, p 581).
- For the management of vaccinated personnel, serological testing for immunity is not considered necessary because 99% of adults are seropositive after the second vaccine dose. However, since seroconversion does not always result in complete protection against disease, testing vaccinees for seropositivity immediately after exposure is a potentially effective strategy for identifying those who remain at risk for varicella. For more information, see the recommendations of the Advisory Committee on Immunization Practices of the Centers for Disease Control and Prevention.*

---

* Centers for Disease Control and Prevention. Prevention of varicella: recommendations of the Advisory Committee on Immunization Practices (ACIP). *MMWR.* 1996;45(No. RR-11):1-36.

Table 3.67. Candidates for VZIG, Provided Significant Exposure Has Occurred*

Immunocompromised children† without history of chickenpox‡

Susceptible, pregnant women

Newborn infant whose mother had onset of chickenpox within the 5 d before delivery or within the 48 h after delivery

Hospitalized premature infant (≥28 wk of gestation) whose mother has no history of chickenpox or seronegativity

Hospitalized premature infants (<28 wk of gestation or ≤1000 g), regardless of maternal history

---

* VZIG indicates varicella-zoster immune globulin. See text and Table 3.66 (p 577) for additional discussion.
† Including those who are HIV-infected.
‡ Immunocompromised adolescents and adults known to be susceptible also should receive VZIG.

- Varicella vaccination is recommended for susceptible staff if varicella does not develop from the exposure.

Postexposure Vaccination. The currently formulated varicella vaccine is not currently recommended for preventing the occurrence of varicella following exposure to varicella or zoster. However, studies with earlier product formulations indicate that the vaccine given within three days of exposure may prevent subsequent clinical illness in the contact. While postexposure prophylaxis is not an FDA-approved indication for varicella vaccine, its use for this purpose may be effective and confers little risk. If vaccine is given following exposure, parents should be informed regarding the possibility of chickenpox occurring in spite of vaccination.

Chemoprophylaxis. Oral acyclovir is not recommended. Prophylactic use to prevent acquisition of infection by a contact has not been studied adequately and could result in an alteration of the incubation period and/or of the immune response to VZV infection.

Passive Immunoprophylaxis. Susceptible individuals at high risk of developing severe varicella should be given VZIG within 96 hours; for maximum effectiveness, it should be given as soon as possible after exposure. VZIG can be obtained by contacting the local American Red Cross Blood Services.

The decision of whether to administer VZIG depends on the following three factors: (1) the likelihood that an individual will develop complications of varicella if infected; (2) the probability that a given exposure to varicella or zoster will result in infection; and (3) the likelihood that the exposed person is susceptible to varicella.

Household exposure to varicella poses an almost certain risk of infection; other types of exposure are less likely to result in infection. Exposure more than 5 days after the appearance of the first lesion in healthy patients poses a relatively low risk. Persons with a history of varicella are usually considered immune. However, persons without such a history may also be immune. In deciding whether a person with no history of varicella infection is likely to be susceptible, careful questioning about (1) history of varicella in other siblings (particularly younger siblings), (2) whether the patient attended an urban school, (3) previous exposure to patients with chicken-pox or zoster, and (4) other clues can be helpful.

In healthy persons, serologic testing to determine immune status is reliable. However, in immunocompromised patients, the use of serologic tests to determine immune status is not necessarily reliable. Children with malignancies receiving immunosuppressive therapy with no history of disease and who have low but mea-surable concentrations of serum VZV antibodies at the time of exposure have con-tracted varicella. Many of these patients, however, may have had passively acquired antibodies from recent transfusions of blood or blood products.

A carefully obtained history of chickenpox should be the primary consideration in the determination of immunity in immunocompromised patients. Administration of VZIG to exposed immunocompromised children with no history of varicella regardless of serologic results is usually advised. Some experts, however, do not recommend VZIG when the child is seropositive if determined by a sensitive assay (eg, LA or EIA) and has not received a blood product that could have provided the passive antibody.

Patients receiving monthly high-dose IGIV (mg/kg) are likely to be protected and probably do not require VZIG if the last dose was given 3 weeks or less before exposure.

Administration and Dose. VZIG is given by intramuscular injection. It contains between 10% and 18% globulin; thimerosal 1:10 000 is included as a preservative. One vial (approximate volume, 1.25 mL) containing 125 U is given for each 10 kg of body weight (and is the minimal dose). The suggested maximal dose is 625 U (ie, five vials).

Local discomfort after intramuscular injection, the most frequent adverse effect, is common, and can be lessened if the immune globulin is at room temperature when administered. Use of VZIG in patients with a bleeding diathesis should be avoided, as with other intramuscular injections, if possible. VZIG should never be given intravenously.

Indications. The following susceptible persons should receive VZIG (see also Tables 3.66 and 3.67, p 577 and p 578):

- ***Immunocompromised individuals, including those who are HIV-infected,*** should receive VZIG if they (1) have had a household exposure, (2) shared a hospital room containing four or fewer beds or adjacent beds in a larger ward with an infectious patient, (3) had a face-to-face contact with an infectious staff member or patient while an inpatient (see Table 3.66), or (4) played indoors with children who are contagious for chickenpox. Immunocompromised older adolescents and adults known to be susceptible also should receive VZIG. Hospitalized patients who have been exposed should be discharged before the eighth day after exposure, if possible. If discharge is not possible, they should be placed on precautions (see Isolation of the Hospitalized Patient).

- ***Pregnant women who are susceptible to varicella*** may be at higher risk for serious complications than adults in general. Hence, VZIG is indicated for these women after exposure. A major concern is the risk to the fetus of the congenital varicella syndrome when a woman acquires VZV infection, especially during the first half of pregnancy, but whether the fetus will be protected against the development of malformations if VZIG is given to a susceptible woman after exposure is unknown. VZIG conceivably could result in an asymptomatic maternal infection but not prevent VZV transmission to the fetus. Antibody administered to a pregnant woman in the 5 days before delivery is unlikely to be absorbed and transported across the placenta in sufficient quantities to protect the infant appreciably. Therefore, VZIG is recommended for the newborn even if the mother has received VZIG during this period.

- **Newborns.** Varicella-zoster immune globulin (125 U) should be given as soon as possible after delivery to infants whose mothers have had onset of varicella from 5 days before to 2 days after delivery. Approximately half of these infants can be expected to develop varicella even if VZIG is given, but the disease is often modified. Nevertheless, VZIG recipients should be followed closely.

  For healthy, full-term infants exposed postnatally to varicella, including those whose mother's rash developed more than 48 hours after delivery, VZIG is not indicated.

  Although nosocomial transmission of varicella in newborn nurseries is extremely rare, VZIG (125 U) is indicated for some hospitalized, preterm infants because of the poor transfer of antibody across the placenta early in pregnancy. These infants include (1) those born before 28 weeks of gestation (and/or who weigh less than 1000 g) who still require hospitalization for treatment of prematurity or related conditions and are exposed to varicella or zoster and (2) preterm infants born after 28 weeks of gestation who are exposed in the hospital and whose mothers have no history of infection and/ or are seronegative (see Table 3.67, p 578). Some experts also would advise use of VZIG for any susceptible newborn who has severe skin disease.

- **Healthy adults.** VZIG can be given to healthy, susceptible adults after exposure to varicella, but it is not routinely recommended in this circumstance. It was previously recommended for these persons because of the recognized increased severity of varicella in persons 13 years or older. However, acyclovir is now available, and recommended, for treating persons of this age with varicella. In adults with no histories of chickenpox or their histories are uncertain, most have a high probability of immunity.

- **Subsequent exposures and follow-up of VZIG recipients.** Since administration of VZIG can cause the infection to be asymptomatic, testing of recipients 2 months or later after administration of VZIG for infection from chickenpox to ascertain their immune status may be helpful in the event of subsequent exposure in a recipient in whom varicella did not develop. Some experts, however, would advise VZIG administration regardless of serologic results because of their possible unreliability in immunocompromised persons and the uncertainty about whether asymptomatic infection after VZIG administration confers lasting protection.

  The duration for which VZIG recipients are protected against chickenpox is unknown. If a second exposure occurs more than 3 weeks after administration of VZIG in a recipient in whom varicella did not develop, another dose of VZIG should be given.

Active Immunization.

Vaccine. It is a cell-free live-attenuated preparation of the wild Oka strain serially propagated and attenuated in human embryonic lung fibroblasts, guinea pig embryonic cells, and human diploid cell cultures. The product contains trace amounts of neomycin and gelatin.

Dose and Administration. The recommended dose of the vaccine is 0.5 mL, which contains not less than 1350 plaque-forming units of VZV. Subcutaneous administration is recommended, although intramuscular administration has been demonstrated to result in similar rates of seroconversion.

Immunogenicity. In healthy children 12 months to 12 years of age, a single dose of vaccine results in a seroconversion rate of 97% or more. Preexisting, presumably transplacental antibody, if present at 12 months, does not appear to interfere with antibody response.

In persons 13 years of age and older, seroconversion rates are 78% to 82% after one dose and 99% after two doses. The antibody response after vaccination is lower than that after natural disease.

In studies in the United States and Japan at a time in which wild-type virus continues to circulate, antibodies to VZV in vaccine recipients have been detected in more than 95% for as long as 8 to 20 years after immunization.

Efficacy. In a double-blind, placebo-controlled trial of children 1 to 14 years of age, using a high-titer experimental vaccine, the efficacy was 100% in the first year after vaccination. According to other unpublished studies from the manufacturer, the protection against any disease in vaccinees after household exposure was approximately 70%, and greater than 95% against more severe disease. Rates of protection are similar in adults. All studies demonstrate high rates of protection against severe disease. Varicella in vaccinees has been much milder than that occurring in unvaccinated children, with fewer skin lesions (median of 15 to 32), lower rate of fever (10% of temperature ≥102°F), and rapid recovery. At times, the disease is so mild that it is not easily recognizable as varicella because the skin lesions may resemble insect bites. Nevertheless, vaccine recipients with mild disease may be potentially infectious to susceptible persons.

Duration of Immunity. Waning immunity in vaccine recipients has not been demonstrated, at least in the context of continued VZV circulation. The rate of varicella after immunization during 7 years of study has averaged from less than 1% to 4.4% per year after exposure to wild virus whereas the comparative annual varicella rate in unvaccinated children is 7% to 8%. The rate has not increased with time after immunization.

Simultaneous Administration With Other Vaccines. Varicella vaccine may be given simultaneously with MMR vaccine, but separate syringes and injection sites must be used. If not given simultaneously, the interval between administration of varicella vaccine and MMR should be at least 1 month. Although further immunogenicity studies are needed on the use of varicella vaccine administered simultaneously with DTaP, DTP, poliovirus, hepatitis B, and/or *Haemophilus influenzae* type b vaccines, no reason exists to suspect that varicella vaccine will affect the immune response to these other vaccines. When necessary, varicella vaccine may be given simultaneously or at any interval after or before these vaccines.

Adverse Events. Adverse events following vaccination are minimal. Within
1 month of immunization, a mild vaccine-associated maculopapular or varicelliform
rash develops in approximately 7% of children and 8% of susceptible adolescents
and adults, with a median of two to five lesions, which may occur at the vaccine
injection site or elsewhere. Vaccine virus very rarely has been recovered from these
skin lesions. Approximately 20% of children and 25% to 35% of adolescents and
adults who have been vaccinated complain of transient pain, tenderness, or redness
at the injection site after each dose of vaccine. Immunization of persons immune to
varicella from natural disease or vaccine has not resulted in a significant increase in
adverse effects compared with immunization of susceptible persons.

Vaccine virus has been recovered from vaccine recipients with skin lesions, but
the spread of vaccine virus from healthy vaccinees to other persons, while documented, appears to be rare (less than 1%) and to occur only if the vaccinee develops
a rash. The risk of transmission of vaccine virus from children with leukemia in
whom a rash develops is higher. Contact cases with seroconversion have been asymptomatic or developed very mild illness, suggesting that the vaccine virus remains
attenuated when transmitted.

A zosterlike illness, marked by rash and minimal or absent systemic symptoms,
has been reported infrequently in healthy children immunized with varicella vaccine.
No cases have been severe. The incidence is no higher than that which occurs after
natural varicella. The frequency in vaccinated children after 7 years of follow up is
18 cases per 100 000 person-years; in comparison, zoster (which is unusual in childhood) is estimated to occur in a frequency of 77 cases per 100 000 person-years.
Moreover, in children with leukemia, zoster is less common after vaccination than
after natural varicella. During 11 to 13 years following the immunization of 500
adults in clinical trials, one case of zoster was reported from wild virus and none
from vaccine virus.

Storage. The lyophilized vaccine should be stored frozen at an average temperature of +5°F (−15°C) or colder. The diluent used for reconstitution should be stored
separately in a refrigerator or at room temperature. Once the vaccine has been reconstituted, it should be used within 30 minutes to maintain viral potency. For further
information, see the package insert.

Recommendations for Immunization.
Vaccine for universal use in early childhood
and immunization in susceptible older children and adolescents is recommended
based on the frequency of serious complications and deaths after infection with wild
varicella, the excess cost to the family and society incurred by varicella infection, and
the efficacy and safety of the live-attenuated varicella vaccine. Age-specific recommendations are as follows:

- **Age 12 months to the 13th birthday:**
  Age 12 to 18 months. One dose of varicella vaccine is recommended for
  universal immunization for all healthy children who lack a reliable history
  of varicella.

Age 19 months to the 13th birthday. Vaccination of susceptible children is recommended and may be given any time during childhood but before the 13th birthday because of the potential increased severity of natural varicella after this age. Susceptible is defined by either lack of proof of varicella vaccination or a reliable history of varicella. One dose is recommended.

- **Healthy adolescents and young adults.** Healthy adolescents past their 13th birthday who have not been immunized previously and have no history of varicella infection should be immunized against varicella by administration of two doses of vaccine 4 to 8 weeks apart. Longer intervals between doses do not necessitate a third dose, but may leave the individual unprotected during the intervening months.

- **Adults.** Recommendations for the use of varicella vaccine in adults have been issued by the Advisory Committee on Immunization Practices (ACIP) of the Centers for Disease Control and Prevention (CDC).* Varicella vaccination of susceptible adults is encouraged. Priority, according to the ACIP, should be given to vaccination of those who have close contact with persons at high risk for serious complications (eg, health care personnel and family contacts of immunocompromised persons), those at high risk of exposure, and non-pregnant women of child-bearing age.

Performing serologic tests to determine susceptibility, using a sensitive assay (eg, latex agglutination or enzyme immunoassay), before vaccination in healthy adolescents and adults with no history of varicella is optional, but is likely to not be cost-effective. If the test is positive, the vaccine is not indicated. In some individuals immunized with varicella vaccine, such as health care workers or others exposed to immunocompromised individuals, serological testing following exposure to varicella may help in the management of personnel assigned to high-risk areas.

Household Contacts of Immunocompromised Persons. Vaccination of household contacts of immunocompromised persons may pose a small risk of transmission of vaccine virus to the immunocompromised person. However, the risk appears to be very low, disease caused by vaccine virus in immunocompromised persons reported to date has been mild, and varicella due to wild virus in immunocompromised persons can be severe. Hence, the benefits of vaccinating household contacts of immunocompromised persons outweigh the potential risks.

Booster Immunization. Revaccination is not recommended currently, but the need for revaccination will be reassessed with time.

Contraindications and Precautions.

Intercurrent Illness. As with other vaccines, varicella vaccine should not be administered to individuals who have moderate or severe illnesses, with or without fever (see Vaccine Safety and Contraindications, p 26).

Immunocompromised Patients.

General recommendations. Varicella vaccine is contraindicated in immunocompromised individuals, such as those with congenital immunodeficiency, blood dyscrasias, leukemia, lymphoma, symptomatic HIV infection, and malignancy for

---

* Centers for Disease Control and Prevention. Prevention of varicella: recommendations of the Advisory Committee on Immunization Practices (ACIP). *MMWR* 1996;45(No. RR-11):1-36.

which they are receiving immunosuppressive therapy. The exceptions include children with acute lymphocytic leukemia to whom vaccine may be given in study conditions (see Acute Lymphocytic Leukemia, below). Asymptomatic HIV infection also is a contraindication for immunization, but since the risk in these persons is currently only theoretical, routine screening for HIV is not indicated. Immunodeficiency should be excluded prior to immunization in children with a family history of hereditary immunodeficiency. The presence of an immunodeficient or HIV-seropositive family member does not contraindicate vaccine use in other family members.

After cessation of immunosuppressive therapy, varicella vaccine in most circumstances is withheld for an interval of not less than 3 months (with the exception of corticosteroid recipients, see below). This interval is based on the assumption that immunologic responsiveness will have been restored in 3 months and the underlying disease for which immunosuppressive therapy was prescribed is in remission or under control. However, because the interval can vary with the intensity and type of immunosuppressive therapy, radiation therapy, underlying disease, and other factors, a definitive recommendation for an interval after cessation of immunosuppressive therapy when varicella vaccine can be safely and effectively administered often is not possible.

Children receiving corticosteroids. The potential risks of vaccination with the live-attenuated virus must be weighed against the potential risks of acquiring wild VZV infection, which has an increased risk of causing severe disease in immunocompromised patients.

Varicella vaccine should not be administered to persons who are receiving high doses of systemic corticosteroids (see Immunodeficient and Immunosuppressed Children, p 51). If these doses are given for 14 days or more, the recommended interval after discontinuation of therapy is at least 1 month.

Children with no history of varicella who are receiving systemic corticosteroids for conditions such as asthma or nephrotic syndrome may be immunized if they are receiving less than 2 mg/kg per day of prednisone (or its equivalent), or less than 20 mg/d if they weigh more than 10 kg and are not otherwise immunocompromised. Some experts, however, suggest discontinuing corticosteroid use for 2 weeks after immunization if possible. Most experts agree that immunization of children receiving only inhaled corticosteroids does not increase the risk of disease from varicella vaccine, although no studies in such children have not been performed.

Households with potential contact with immunocompromised persons. Transmission of vaccine-type VZV from healthy persons has been documented, albeit rarely (see Adverse Events, p 582). Even in families with immunocompromised persons, including those with HIV infection, no precautions are needed after vaccination of healthy children in whom a rash does not develop. Vaccinees in whom a rash develops should avoid direct contact with immunocompromised, susceptible hosts for the duration of the rash. If contact inadvertently occurs, the routine use of VZIG is not recommended currently because transmission is rare and disease, if it develops, would be expected to be mild.

Acute lymphocytic leukemia (ALL). Although the current vaccine is not licensed for routine use in children with malignancies, immunization should be considered when a child with ALL has been in continuous remission for at least 1 year and has a lymphocyte count greater than 700/μL and platelet count greater than 100 000/μL 24 hours prior to vaccination. Immunization has been demonstrated to be safe, immunogenic, and effective in these children, and the vaccine may be obtained free for use in a research protocol. This protocol requires approval by the appropriate institutional review board as well as monitoring for safety. To immunize a child with ALL, the following should be contacted: The Varivax Coordinating Center, Bio-Pharm Clinical Services, Inc, 4 Valley Square, Blue Bell, PA 19422 (215-283-0897).

Pregnancy and Lactation. Varicella vaccine should not be administered to pregnant women, since the possible effects on fetal development are unknown.* When postpubertal females are immunized, pregnancy should be avoided for at least 1 month following immunization.

A pregnant mother or other household member is not a contraindication for vaccination of the child. Transmission of vaccine virus is rare; more than 90% of adults are immune, and vaccination of the child will likely protect the mother from exposure to wild VZV. If the pregnant woman is known to be susceptible, however, some experts would defer immunization of the child until the third trimester or until after delivery, if feasible.

Whether vaccine-acquired VZV is secreted in human milk and its infectiousness to infants are unknown. Varicella vaccine may be considered for a susceptible nursing mother, if risk of exposure to natural VZV is high.

Immune Globulin. Whether administration of immune globulin can interfere with the immunological response to varicella vaccination is not known. However, immune globulin administration can interfere with the response to other live-virus vaccines, such as measles vaccine, and because of the potential inhibition of the response to varicella vaccination by passively transferred antibodies, varicella vaccine should not be given for at least 5 months after the administration of immune globulins, VZIG, blood products (except washed red blood cells), or plasma transfusions. Infants and children receiving RSV-IGIV should not receive varicella vaccine until 9 months after the last dose.

If possible, immune globulin preparations should not be administered for 3 weeks after vaccination. If an immune globulin is given in the interval before vaccination, the recipient either should be revaccinated 5 months later or tested for varicella immunity 6 months later and revaccinated if seronegative.

Salicylates. Whether Reye syndrome results from the administration of salicylates after vaccination for varicella in children is unknown. No cases have been reported. The vaccine manufacturer, however, recommends that salicylates should not be administered for 6 weeks after the varicella vaccine has been given because of the association between Reye syndrome, natural varicella, and salicylates. Physicians need to weigh the theoretical risks associated with varicella vaccine against the known risks of the wild type virus in children receiving long-term salicylate therapy.

Allergy to vaccine component. Varicella vaccine should not be administered to persons who have had an anaphylactic-type reaction to any component of the vaccine, including gelatin and neomycin. Most persons with allergy to neomycin have contact dermatitis, which is not a contraindication to vaccination.

---

* The manufacturer, in collaboration with the CDC, has established the VARIVAX Pregnancy Registry to monitor the maternal and fetal outcomes of women who are inadvertently given varicella vaccine 3 months before or at any time during pregnancy. Reporting cases is encouraged and may be done by telephone (800-986-8999).

VIBRIO INFECTIONS

Cholera
(*Vibrio cholerae*)

CLINICAL MANIFESTATIONS: Cholera is characterized by painless, voluminous diarrhea without abdominal cramps or fever. Dehydration, hypokalemia, metabolic acidosis, and, occasionally, hypovolemic shock can occur in 4 to 12 hours if fluid losses are not replaced. Coma, convulsions, and hypoglycemia also can occur, particularly in children. Typical stools are colorless, with small flecks of mucus ("rice-water"), and contain high concentrations of sodium, potassium, chloride, and bicarbonate. However, most infected persons with toxigenic *Vibrio cholerae* 01 have no symptoms and some have only mild-to-moderate diarrhea, whereas less than 5% have severe watery diarrhea, vomiting, and dehydration (cholera gravis).

ETIOLOGY: *Vibrio cholerae* is a Gram-negative, curved, motile bacillus with many serogroups. Until recently, only enterotoxin-producing organisms of serogroup 01 have caused epidemics. *Vibrio cholerae* 01 is divided into two serotypes, Inaba and Ogawa, and two biotypes, classical and E1 Tor. The current predominant biotype is E1 Tor. Beginning in 1992, toxicogenic *V cholerae* serogroup 0139 (a non-01, toxicogenic strain) has caused epidemic cholera in the Indian subcontinent and southeast Asia. Serogroups of *V cholerae* other than 01 and 0139 and nontoxicogenic strains of *V cholerae* 01 can cause sporadic diarrheal illness, but do not cause epidemics.

EPIDEMIOLOGY: In the last three decades, *V cholerae* 01, biotype El Tor has spread from India and Southeast Asia to Africa, the Middle East, Southern Europe, and the Western Pacific Islands (Oceania). In 1991, epidemic cholera caused by toxicogenic *V cholerae* 01, serotype Inaba, biotype El Tor, appeared in Peru. It has spread to most countries in South and North America. In the United States, cases resulting from travel to Latin America or Asia and with ingestion of contaminated food transported from Latin America or Asia have been reported. In addition, the Gulf Coast of Louisiana and Texas has an endemic focus of a unique strain of toxicogenic *V cholerae* 01. Most cases of disease from this strain have resulted from consumption of raw or undercooked shellfish. Humans are the only documented natural host, but free-living *V cholerae* organisms can exist in the aquatic environment. The usual mode of infection is ingestion of contaminated water or food (particularly raw or undercooked shellfish), moist grains held at ambient temperature, and raw or partially dried fish. The boiling of water or treating it with chlorine or iodine and adequate cooking of food kills the organism. Direct person-to-person spread by contact has not been documented. Persons with low gastric acidity are at increased risk for cholera infection. The period of communicability is unknown but presumably is related to the duration of carriage.

The **incubation period** is usually 1 to 3 days, with a range of a few hours to 5 days.

DIAGNOSTIC TESTS: *Vibrio cholerae* can be cultured from stool or a rectal swab that is placed in transport media and plated on appropriate selective media. Suspect colonies are confirmed serologically by agglutination with specific antisera. Because most laboratories in the United States do not routinely culture for *V cholerae* or other vibrios, clinicians should request appropriate cultures for clinically suspected cases. Isolates of *V cholerae* should be sent to a state health department laboratory for serogrouping; those of serogroup 01 or 0139 are then sent to the Centers for Disease Control and Prevention for testing for production of cholera toxin. A fourfold rise in vibriocidal antibody titers between acute and convalescent serum samples or a fourfold decline in vibriocidal titers between early and late convalescent (more than a 2-month interval) sera can confirm the diagnosis retrospectively.

TREATMENT: Oral or parenteral rehydration therapy to correct dehydration and electrolyte abnormalities is the most important modality of therapy and should be initiated as soon as the diagnosis is suspected.* Oral rehydration is preferred unless the patient is in shock, is obtunded, or has intestinal ileus.

Antimicrobial therapy results in prompt eradication of vibrios, reduces the duration of diarrhea, and reduces requirements for fluid replacement. It should be considered for persons who are moderately to severely ill. Oral tetracycline (50 mg/kg per day, maximum 2 g/d, in four divided doses) for 3 days or doxycycline (6 mg/kg, maximum 300 mg) as a single dose are the drugs of choice for cholera. The use of tetracyclines generally is not recommended for children younger than 8 years, but in cases of severe cholera, the benefits may offset the risk of staining of developing teeth (see Antimicrobials and Related Therapy, p 606). If strains are resistant to tetracyclines, trimethoprim-sulfamethoxazole (8 mg/kg per day of trimethoprim and 40 mg/kg per day of sulfamethoxazole), erythromycin (40 mg/kg per day, maximum 1000 mg), or furazolidone (5 to 8 mg/kg per day, maximum 400 mg) may be used. However, *Vibrio cholerae* 0139 strains are not susceptible to trimethoprim-sulfamethoxazole or furazolidone. Ciprofloxacin or ofloxacin are effective therapeutic agents for both *V cholerae* 01 and 0139 infection, but generally should only be used in persons at least 18 years old (see Antimicrobials and Related Therapy, p 605). Antimicrobial susceptibilities of newly isolated organisms should be determined.

ISOLATION OF THE HOSPITALIZED PATIENT†: Contact precautions are indicated for diapered and/or incontinent children for the duration of illness.

CONTROL MEASURES:

Hygiene. Because cholera spreads by contaminated food or water, and infection frequently requires ingestion of large numbers of organisms, disinfection or boiling of water will prevent transmission. Thoroughly cooking crabs, oysters, and other shellfish from the Gulf Coast before eating also is recommended to reduce the likelihood of transmission. Foods such as fish, rice, or grain gruels should be refrigerated

---

* For further information and detailed recommendations, see Duggan C, Santosham M, Glass RI. The management of acute diarrhea in children: oral rehydration, maintenance, nutritional therapy. *MMWR.* 1992;41(No. RR-16):1-20.

† In addition to standard precautions.

promptly after use. Appropriate hand washing after defecating and before preparing or eating food is important in preventing transmission.

Treatment of Contacts. The administration of tetracycline, doxycycline, or trimethoprim-sulfamethoxazole within 24 hours of identification of the index case may be effective in preventing coprimary and secondary cases of cholera among household contacts if the household secondary rate is high. The use of tetracyclines generally is not recommended for children younger than 8 years (see Antimicrobials and Related Therapy, p 606). Chemoprophylaxis is not recommended in the United States, since secondary spread is rare, unless unusual sanitary and hygienic conditions indicate that the rate of secondary transmission could be high.

Vaccine. The only currently available vaccine in the United States is of limited value. It protects approximately 50% of those immunized for only 3 to 6 months, does not prevent *Vibrio* excretion or inapparent infection, and is unrelated serologically to serotype 0139 and, therefore, is unlikely to provide protection against this strain (see Etiology, p 586). Furthermore, travelers using appropriate precautions are at a low risk of infection in countries with cholera. Cholera vaccination is not required for travelers entering the United States from cholera-affected areas, and the World Health Organization no longer recommends vaccination for travel to or from cholera-infected areas. No country currently requires cholera vaccine for entry. The vaccine should not be administered to contacts of patients with cholera or used to control the spread of infection, and it is not generally recommended for international travelers. Several recently developed, orally administered vaccines have demonstrated improved efficacy with fewer side effects than the currently available parenterally administered vaccine.

Reporting. Cases of cholera must be reported to health authorities in any country in which they occur or were contracted. State health departments should be notified immediately of presumed or known cases of cholera.

Other *Vibrio* Infections

CLINICAL MANIFESTATIONS: *Vibrio* species are associated with the following three major syndromes: diarrhea, septicemia, and wound infection. Diarrhea is most frequent, characterized by acute onset of watery stools and crampy, abdominal pain. Approximately half of those afflicted will have low-grade fever, headache, and chills; about 30% will have vomiting. Spontaneous recovery follows in 2 to 5 days. Bacteremia is rare.

Infection can develop in contaminated wounds. Skin infections in compromised patients can cause extensive and rapid tissue necrosis. Patients with immunodeficiency or liver disease are susceptible to septicemia from bowel or skin infections, often resulting in shock, bullous or necrotic skin lesions, and death.

ETIOLOGY: Vibrios are facultatively anaerobic, motile, Gram-negative bacilli that are tolerant of salt. The most important noncholera *Vibrio* species associated with diarrhea are *V parahaemolyticus, V cholerae* non-01, *V mimicus, V hollisae, V fluvialis,* and *V furnissii. Vibrio vulnificus* causes septicemia and wound infections in immunocompromised patients, especially those with liver disease. *Vibrio parahaemolyticus,*

V damsela, and *V alginolyticus* also are associated with wound infections. *Vibrio alginolyticus* has been associated with otitis externa.

EPIDEMIOLOGY: Noncholera vibrios commonly are found in seawater, increasing quantitatively during the summer. Most infections occur during the summer and fall. Enteritis usually is acquired from seafood that is eaten raw or undercooked, especially oysters, crabs, and shrimp. The disease is probably not communicable from person to person. Wound infections commonly result from exposure of abrasions to contaminated seawater or from punctures resulting from handling of contaminated shellfish. Persons with increased susceptibility to infection with *Vibrio* species include those with liver disease, low gastric acidity, and immunodeficiency, including persons with HIV infection.

The median **incubation period** of enteritis is 23 hours, with a range of 5 to 92 hours.

DIAGNOSTIC TESTS: These organisms can be isolated from stool or vomitus of patients with diarrhea, from blood, and from wound exudates. Because identification of the organism requires special techniques, laboratory personnel should be notified when *Vibrio* infection is suspected.

TREATMENT: Most episodes of diarrhea are mild and self-limited and do not require treatment other than oral rehydration. Antibiotic therapy may benefit those with severe diarrhea or wound infections. Most organisms are susceptible to tetracycline (which usually should not be given to patients younger than 8 years), cefotaxime, gentamicin and chloramphenicol.

ISOLATION OF THE HOSPITALIZED PATIENT*: Contact precautions are recommended for diapered and/or incontinent children.

CONTROL MEASURES: Seafood should be cooked adequately, and if not ingested immediately, it should be refrigerated. Uncooked mollusks and crustaceans should be handled with care. Abrasions suffered by ocean bathers should be rinsed with clean, fresh water. Persons with liver disease or immunodeficiency should be warned to avoid eating raw oysters or clams.

Yersinia enterocolitica and *Yersinia pseudotuberculosis* Infections
(Enteritis and Other Illnesses)

CLINICAL MANIFESTATIONS: *Yersinia* cause several age-specific syndromes as well as a variety of uncommon presentations. The most common manifestation of infection with *Y enterocolitica* is enterocolitis with fever and diarrhea; stools often contains leukocytes, blood, and mucus. This syndrome occurs most often in young children. A pseudoappendicitis syndrome (fever, abdominal pain, right

---

* In addition to standard precautions

lower quadrant tenderness, and leukocytosis) occurs primarily in older children and young adults. Focal infections, abscess formation (such as hepatic and splenic), and bacteremia occur most often in patients with predisposing conditions such as excessive iron storage. Other manifestations of infection include pharyngitis, meningitis, osteomyelitis, pyomyositis, conjunctivitis, pneumonia, acute proliferative glomerulonephritis and primary cutaneous infection. Postinfectious sequelae observed with *Y enterocolitica* include erythema nodosum and reactive arthritis, and occur most often in adults.

The major triad of infection caused by *Y pseudotuberculosis* is fever, rash, and abdominal symptoms. Acute abdominal pain syndromes are most common, resulting from mesenteric adenitis, appendicitis or terminal ileitis. Other findings include diarrhea, erythema nodosum, septicemia, and sterile pleural and joint effusions. The rash usually is scarlatiniform. Clinical features can mimic those of Kawasaki disease.

ETIOLOGY: *Yersinia enterocolitica* and *Y pseudotuberculosis* are Gram-negative bacilli; 34 serotypes of *Y enterocolitica* and five serotypes of *Y pseudotuberculosis* are recognized. Differences in virulence exist among various serotypes of *Y enterocolitica*; 0:3 and 0:9 are the most common causes of diarrhea.

EPIDEMIOLOGY: The reservoirs of the organisms are animals, including rodents (*Y pseudotuberculosis)* and swine (*Y enterocolitica*). Infection is believed to be transmitted by ingestion of contaminated food, especially uncooked pork products and unpasteurized milk, or contaminated water; by direct or indirect contact with animals; by transfusion with packed red blood cells; and possibly by fecal-oral, person-to-person transmission. Bottle-fed infants can be infected if their caregivers simultaneously are handling raw pork intestines (chitterlings). *Yersinia enterocolitica* is isolated more frequently in cooler climates and more frequently in winter than in summer. Patients with excessive iron storage syndromes, as well as those receiving deferoxamine for iron overload, have unusual susceptibility to *Yersinia* bacteremia. The period of communicability is unknown; it is probably for the duration of excretion of the specific organisms, which averages 6 weeks after diagnosis.

The **incubation period** is typically 4 to 6 days, varying from 1 to 14 days.

DIAGNOSTIC TESTS: *Yersinia enterocolitica* and *Y pseudotuberculosis* can be recovered from throat swabs, mesenteric lymph nodes, peritoneal fluid, and blood. Stool cultures are generally positive during the first 2 weeks of illness, regardless of the nature of the gastrointestinal tract manifestations. *Yersinia enterocolitica* also has been isolated from synovial fluid, bile, urine, cerebrospinal fluid, sputum, and wounds. Because laboratory identification of organisms from stool requires special techniques, laboratory personnel should be notified that *Yersinia* infection is suspected. Pathogenic strains of *Y enterocolitica* are usually pyrazinamidase-negative. Infection can be confirmed by demonstrating serum antibody titer rises after infection, but these tests generally are available only in reference or research laboratories. Cross-reactions of these antibodies with *Brucella, Vibrio, Salmonella,* and *Rickettsia* species and *Escherichia coli* lead to false-positive *Y enterocolitica* and *Y pseudotuberculosis* titers. In patients with thyroid disease, persistently elevated *Y enterocolitica* antibody titers can result from antigenic similarity of the organism with antigens of the thyroid epithelial cell membrane.

TREATMENT: Both *Y enterocolitica* and *Y pseudotuberculosis* are susceptible to aminoglycosides, cefotaxime, tetracycline (which usually should not be given to children younger than 8 years of age), chloramphenicol, and trimethoprim-sulfamethoxazole. *Yersinia enterocolitica* isolates typically are resistant to first-generation cephalosporins and to most penicillins. Patients with septicemia or sites of infection other than the gastrointestinal tract and compromised hosts with enterocolitis should receive antibiotic therapy. Benefit from antibiotic therapy in patients with enterocolitis, the pseudoappendicitis syndrome, or mesenteric adenitis, other than reduced duration of excretion of the organism in stool, has not been established.

ISOLATION OF THE HOSPITALIZED PATIENT*: Contact precautions are indicated for diapered and/or incontinent children with enterocolitis for the duration of illness.

CONTROL MEASURES: Ingestion of uncooked meat, contaminated water, or unpasteurized milk should be avoided. Persons handling pork intestines should wash their hands after contact.

---

* In addition to standard precautions.

Antimicrobial Prophylaxis

ANTIMICROBIAL PROPHYLAXIS

Antimicrobial agents are commonly prescribed to prevent infections in infants and children. The efficacy of the prophylactic use of these agents has been documented for some conditions but is unsubstantiated for most. Chemoprophylaxis is directed at different, but not mutually exclusive, targets: specific pathogens, infection-prone body sites, and vulnerable patients. Effective prophylaxis is more readily achieved with specific pathogens and certain body sites. In any situation where prophylactic antimicrobial therapy is considered, the long-term risk of selective pressure of the emergence of resistant organisms must be weighed against the potential benefits. Antimicrobial prophylaxis should have as narrow a spectrum of action as possible and should be used for as brief a period of time as is necessary.

Specific Pathogens

Prophylaxis is feasible if the physician can recognize situations associated with an increased risk of serious infection with a specific pathogen and select an antimicrobial agent that will eliminate the pathogen from persons at risk with minimal adverse effects. For some pathogens that initially colonize the upper respiratory tract, elimination of the carrier state can be difficult and requires the use of an antibiotic, such as rifampin, which achieves effective concentrations in nasopharyngeal secretions. In this circumstance, this property is lacking among antibiotics ordinarily used to treat infections caused by such pathogens. Table 4.1 (p 594) lists examples of pathogens amenable to antimicrobial prophylaxis in children and provides information about documented efficacy. In cases where prophylaxis is recommended, the regimen is described in the disease-specific chapter in Section 3.

Infection-Prone Body Sites

Prevention of infection of vulnerable body sites may be possible if (1) the period of risk is defined and brief, (2) the expected pathogens have predictable antibiotic susceptibility, and (3) the site is accessible to antibiotics. Examples of infection-prone body sites amenable to chemoprophylaxis are listed in Table 4.2 (p 596). More detailed discussions of the prevention of surgical wound infection, and neonatal ophthalmia are given where relevant in Section 4.

Otitis media recurs less frequently in otitis-prone children treated prophylactically with antibiotics. Studies have demonstrated that either amoxicillin or sulfisoxazole is effective. However antibiotic prophylaxis may alter the nasopharyngeal flora and foster colonization with resistant organisms, compromising long-term efficacy of the prophylactic drug.

Protection afforded the urinary tract by chemoprophylaxis is critically dependent on the rate of emergence of antibiotic resistance in the gastrointestinal tract flora, the

Table 4.1. Examples of Specific Pathogens Amenable to Antimicrobial Prophylaxis

Pathogen	Diseases To Be Prevented	Antimicrobial Agent	Efficacy
Bacteria			
Bordetella pertussis	Secondary cases of pertussis in household contacts	Erythromycin	Established
Calymmato-bacterium granulomatis	Urogenital infection in exposed persons	Tetracycline, trimethoprim-sulfamethoxazole	Proposed
Chlamydia trachomatis	Urogenital or neonatal infections in exposed persons	Tetracycline,* doxycycline,* erythromycin, azithromycin	Proposed
Coryne-bacterium diphtheriae	Diphtheria in unimmunized contacts	Penicillin, erythromycin	Proposed
Haemophilus ducreyi	Urogenital infection in exposed persons	Ceftriaxone, azithromycin, amoxicillin-clavulanate, ciprofloxacin[†]	Proposed
Haemophilus influenzae type b	Secondary cases of systemic infection in close contacts <1 y and those aged 12 to 47 mo who are not fully immunized	Rifampin	Established for household contacts
Mycobac-terium tuberculosis	Pulmonary or metastatic disease	Isoniazid Rifampin, others	Established Proposed
Mycobac-terium avium complex	Infection in HIV-infected host	Clarithromycin, azithromycin, rifabutin	Established (data in adults only)
Neisseria gonorrhoeae	Urogenital or neonatal infections in exposed persons	Ceftriaxone	Established
Neisseria meningitidis	Meningococcemia in exposed, susceptible persons	Rifampin, ceftriaxone, ciprofloxacin[†]	Established
Streptococcus pneumoniae	Fulminant pneumococcal infection in persons with functional or anatomic asplenia	Penicillin, amoxicillin	Established for penicillin V in children with sickle cell disease
Group A streptococcus	Recurrent rheumatic fever	Penicillin, sulfonamide	Established
Group B streptococcus	Neonatal infection	Ampicillin, penicillin	Established
Treponema pallidum	Syphilis in exposed persons	Penicillin	Established

Table 4.1. **Examples of Specific Pathogens
Amenable to Antimicrobial Prophylaxis, continued**

Pathogen	Diseases To Be Prevented	Antimicrobial Agent	Efficacy
Vibrio cholerae	Cholera in close contacts of a case	Tetracycline*	Proposed
Yersinia pestis	Plague in household contacts or those exposed to pneumonic disease	Tetracycline,* trimethoprim-sulfamethoxazole	Proposed
Fungi			
Pneumocystis carinii	Pneumonia in compromised host	Trimethoprim-sulfamethoxazole, pentamidine aerosol	Established (data in adults only)
Parasites			
Plasmodium species (malaria)	Overt infection in endemic areas	Chloroquine	Established
		Mefloquine	Proposed
		Doxycycline*	Proposed
Viruses			
Influenza A	Influenza in persons at risk for complications	Amantadine, rimantadine	Established
Herpes simplex	Recurrent genital lesions	Acyclovir	Established (during continuous use only)
Varicella-zoster	Varicella in persons at risk of complications	Acyclovir	Proposed
HIV	Congenital infection	Zidovudine	Established

* Tetracyclines can cause dental staining in children younger than 8 years.
† Not recommended for persons younger than 18 years.

usual source of bacteria that invade the bladder. The long-term effectiveness of nitrofurantoin and trimethoprim-sulfamethoxazole is explained by the minimal effect of these drugs on the development of resistant flora. Both drugs are concentrated in urine, and adequate inhibitory activity can be obtained with less than the usual therapeutic dose. Use of a single dose at bedtime has been successful.

Chemoprophylaxis of human and animal bite wounds has become common practice even though dog bites, the most common wound, become infected in only 5% of cases (see Bite Wounds, p 122, for recommendations).

Vulnerable Hosts

Most attempts to prevent infection in vulnerable patients have been foiled by the rapid replacement of initial bacteria by others resistant to antibiotics. Table 4.3 (p 596) lists circumstances in which antibiotics are frequently given to prevent infection.

Table 4.2. **Examples of Infection-Prone Body Sites Amenable to Antimicrobial Prophylaxis**

Body Site	Infection To Be Prevented	Agents Used	Efficacy
Conjunctivae	Neonatal gono-coccal ophthalmia	Topical, 1% silver nitrate,* 0.5% erythromycin*; 1% tetracycline*; penicillin (if susceptible)	Established
		Ceftriaxone, penicillin (if susceptible)	Established
		Topical 2.5% povidine-iodine	Proposed
Abnormal heart valve	Bacterial endocar-ditis (ie, after dental extraction)	Amoxicillin, others	Proposed
Surgical wound	Postoperative wound infection	Appropriate for expected contaminants	See Antimicrobial Prophylaxis in Pediatric Surgical Patients (p 597)
Middle ear	Recurrent otitis media	Sulfisoxazole, ampicillin	Established
Urinary tract	Recurrent urinary infection	Sulfonamides, trimetho-prim-sulfamethoxazole, nitrofurantoin	Established
Human/animal bite wound	Wound infection, cellulitis	Penicillin, amoxicillin-clavulanate	Proposed

*Topical administration.

Table 4.3. **Examples of Chemoprophylaxis for the Vulnerable Host**

Infection To Be Prevented	Agents Used	Efficacy
Pneumocystis carinii pneumonia in immunocompromised host	Trimethoprim-sulfametho-xazole, pentamidine aerosol	Established (data in adults only)
Mycobacterium avium complex	Rifabutin, azithromycin, clarithromycin	Established (data in adults only)
Oral and esophageal candidiasis in patients with HIV infection	Nystatin, fluconazole, ketoconazole	Proposed
Fulminant bacteremia in persons with anatomic or functional asplenia	Penicillin, amoxicillin	Established for penicillin V in children with sickle cell anemia
Bacterial infection in persons with chronic granulomatous disease	Trimethoprim-sulfamethoxazole	Proposed
Mycoplasma pneumoniae pneumonia in persons with sickle cell hemoglobinopathy	Tetracycline	Proposed (limited data)
	Erythromycin	Proposed

ANTIMICROBIAL PROPHYLAXIS IN PEDIATRIC SURGICAL PATIENTS*

A major use of antimicrobial agents in hospitalized children is for prophylaxis against postoperative wound infections. In view of this frequent use and the emerging consensus on recommendations for prevention of surgical wound infections, guidelines for surgical antimicrobial prophylaxis in children have been developed. Prophylaxis is defined as the use of antimicrobial drugs in the absence of suspected or documented infection to reduce the incidence of infection.

Frequency of Antimicrobial Prophylaxis

In hospitalized patients, antimicrobial drugs commonly are initiated for prophylaxis of infection after surgery or an invasive procedure such as cystoscopy or cardiac catheterization. The frequency and reasons for antimicrobial use have been studied primarily in general hospitals, but the patterns of use in children are similar to those in adults. Two studies demonstrated that prophylaxis accounts for approximately 75% of the use of antibiotics on pediatric surgical services. The efficacy of antimicrobial agents in lowering the incidence of postoperative infection after certain types of surgery has been amply demonstrated in controlled clinical trials. These and earlier studies in experimental animals have delineated the principles for effective use of antimicrobial agents in prophylaxis of wound infections, including choice of drugs and when and how long they are to be given.

Inappropriate Antimicrobial Prophylaxis

Prophylaxis has been identified as a major cause of inappropriate use of antimicrobial agents in both adults and children. In a study of children younger than 6 years undergoing surgery, in which appropriateness of use was assessed on the basis of commonly accepted guidelines at that time, prophylactic antimicrobials were administered inappropriately to 42% of children receiving preoperative antimicrobial(s), 67% receiving intraoperative antimicrobial(s), and 55% receiving postoperative antimicrobial(s). Similarly, in a large teaching hospital, 66% of antimicrobial use in children on surgical services was considered inappropriate for reasons of wrong drug, dose, time of initiation, duration, or lack of indication. These studies suggest that the use of antimicrobial agents in children undergoing surgery and other invasive procedures should be subject to periodic review.

Guidelines for Appropriate Use

Studies documenting that systemic prophylaxis reduces the incidence of surgical wound infections have been performed primarily in adults. Because the pathogenesis of these infections is the same in children, the principles of surgical prophylaxis in children should be similar. In the absence of studies in children, guidelines recom-

---

* Adapted from American Academy of Pediatrics, Committee on Infectious Diseases, Committee on Drugs, and Section on Surgery. Antimicrobial prophylaxis in pediatric surgical patients. *Pediatrics.* 1984;74:437-439.

mended by *The Medical Letter,** the American College of Surgeons, and the Surgical Infection Society[†] provide standards for use of systemic prophylactic antibiotics in pediatric surgical patients. The following general principles are recommended as guidelines, with the understanding that studies in children may result in changes and that factors unique to children may justify exceptions.

Indications for Prophylaxis

Systemic prophylaxis is indicated when the benefits of preventing wound infection outweigh the risks of drug reactions and the emergence of resistant bacteria. The latter poses a potential risk not only to the recipient but also to other hospitalized patients, who may develop a nosocomial infection caused by antibiotic-resistant organisms. Procedures in which the benefits justify the risks incurred in antimicrobial prophylaxis are those associated with a significant risk of postoperative infection, and those in which the likelihood of infection may not be great but the consequence of infection is extreme morbidity or mortality.

A major determinant of the probability of surgical wound infection is the number of microorganisms in the wound at the completion of the procedure. This fact allows the classification of surgical procedures (see the Addendum, p 600), based on an estimation of bacterial contamination and the risk of subsequent infection, into the four following categories: (1) clean wounds, (2) clean-contaminated wounds, (3) contaminated wounds, and (4) dirty and infected wounds. Within these categories, however, variation in the risk of infection is considerable. Risk factors include operations on the abdomen, operations lasting more than 2 hours, and the presence of at least three medical diagnoses. The use of a patient risk index, which in addition to classifying wounds as contaminated or dirty and infected also considers the American Society of Anesthesiologists preoperative assessment score and the duration of the operation, has been demonstrated to be a better predictor of postoperative wound infection than this classification.[‡]

CLEAN WOUNDS.

In clean wound procedures, the benefits of systemic antimicrobial prophylaxis may not justify the potential risks associated with antimicrobial use, except in circumstances in which the consequences of infection may be major and life threatening, such as with implantation of a prosthetic foreign body (eg, insertion of a prosthetic heart valve), open-heart surgery for repair of structural defects, compromised immune status (such as patients receiving high doses of corticosteroids or chemotherapy for a malignancy, or those with prior splenectomy), and body cavity exploration in neonates. Prophylaxis has been given in these circumstances, although studies establishing efficacy have not been performed. Prophylaxis also is justified in patients with two or more of the risk factors previously listed. Systemic antimicrobial agents have also been empirically recommended for clean procedures in patients with infection at another site.

---

* Antimicrobial prophylaxis in surgery. *The Medical Letter.* 1995;37:79-82.
† Page CP, Bohnen JMA, Fletcher JR, et al. Antimicrobial prophylaxis for surgical wounds: guidelines for clinical care. *Arch Surg.* 1993;128:79-88.
‡ Culver DH, Horan TC, Gaynes RP, et al. Surgical wound infection rates by wound class, operative procedure, and patient risk index. *Am J Med.* 1991;91(suppl 3B):152S-157S.

CLEAN-CONTAMINATED WOUNDS.

In clean-contaminated wound procedures, the degree of contamination is variable, and prophylaxis is limited to procedures with significant risk of wound contamination and infection. Based on data from adults, indications for prophylaxis for pediatric patients include the following: (1) many alimentary tract procedures, (2) selected biliary tract operations (eg, with obstructive jaundice), and (3) urinary tract surgery or instrumentation in the presence of bacteriuria or obstructive uropathy.

CONTAMINATED DIRTY AND INFECTED WOUNDS.

In contaminated and in dirty and infected wound procedures, such as those for a perforated abdominal viscus or a compound fracture, or if a major break in sterile technique has occurred, antimicrobial therapy is indicated and is considered treatment rather than prophylaxis.

When Should Prophylactic Antibiotics Be Given?

Prophylaxis of infection requires effective drug concentrations in tissues during surgical procedures because bacterial contamination occurs intraoperatively. Except in patients undergoing cesarean section, the antimicrobial agent should be administered just before (within 30 minutes of) the surgical incision to ensure adequate tissue concentration at the time of possible contamination. For patients with cesarean section, it should be given after the umbilical cord is clamped.

For How Long Should Antibiotics Be Given?

A single antimicrobial dose that provides adequate tissue concentration throughout the procedure usually is sufficient. When surgery is prolonged or massive blood loss occurs, a second dose is advisable during the procedure. Postoperative doses of prophylactic drugs generally are unnecessary. These recommendations are based on studies in adults and may not necessarily apply to all pediatric patients, particularly neonates. However, inasmuch as the pathogenesis of wound infection does not differ with age, the recommendation for brief duration of prophylaxis is probably applicable to patients of all ages.

Which Antibiotics Should Be Given?

The choice of an antimicrobial is based on knowledge of the common bacteria causing infectious complications after the specific procedure, bacterial susceptibility to the drug, proved efficacy of the drug selected, and the safety of the drug. New, costly antimicrobial agents generally should not be used unless prophylactic efficacy has been proven superior to that of drugs of established benefit. The drugs should be active against the most likely pathogens. They do not have to be active against every potential organism, since effective prophylaxis appears to correlate with a decrease in the total number of pathogens rather than eradication of all organisms. Recommended doses and route of administration are based on the need to achieve therapeutic blood and tissue concentrations throughout the procedure; parenteral (usually intravenous) administration is usually necessary. For antimicrobial prophylaxis of patients undergoing colonic procedures, additional oral antibiotic prophylaxis should be given before the procedure but is not a substitute for adequate mechanical bowel preparation.

Physicians should be aware of potential interactions and/or adverse effects associated with prophylactic antimicrobials and other medications that the patient is receiving.

Conclusions

These guidelines for antimicrobial prophylaxis of surgical wound infections in children were originally developed by the Committee in collaboration with the Committee on Drugs and the Section on Surgery of the American Academy of Pediatrics in 1984.* They have been modified in accordance with recent data and recommendations. Because the benefit of systemic antimicrobial prophylaxis in many pediatric surgical procedures has not been established, additional studies in commonly performed surgical procedures in children (eg, insertion of neurosurgical shunts and orthopedic procedures) are needed. Pediatricians, pediatric surgeons, and surgical subspecialists should review the prophylactic use of antimicrobial agents as part of the monitoring of antibiotic use in their hospitals, and they should use the guidelines given here to develop standards for antimicrobial use.

Addendum

Definitions of surgical wounds in the classification scheme are as follows:

CLEAN WOUNDS.

Clean wounds are uninfected operative wounds in which no inflammation is encountered, and the respiratory, alimentary, or genitourinary tract or oropharyngeal cavity is not entered. The operative procedures are elective and the wounds are closed primarily, and, if necessary, drained with closed drainage. No break in technique occurs. Operative incisional wounds that follow nonpenetrating (blunt) trauma should be included in this category if they meet the criteria.

CLEAN-CONTAMINATED WOUNDS.

In clean-contaminated operative wounds, the respiratory, alimentary, or genitourinary tract is entered under controlled conditions and without unusual contamination. Operations involving the biliary tract, appendix, vagina, and oropharynx and urgent or emergency surgery in an otherwise clean procedure are included in this category, provided that no evidence of infection is encountered and no major break in technique occurs.

CONTAMINATED WOUNDS.

Contaminated wounds include open, fresh, accidental wounds; operative wounds in the setting of major breaks in sterile technique or gross spillage from the gastrointestinal tract; penetrating trauma less than 4 hours before; and incisions in which acute, nonpurulent inflammation is encountered.

---

* See American Academy of Pediatrics, Committee on Infectious Diseases, Committee on Drugs, and Section on Surgery. Antimicrobial prophylaxis in pediatric surgical patients. *Pediatrics.* 1984;74:437-439.

DIRTY AND INFECTED WOUNDS.

Dirty and infected wounds include penetrating traumatic wounds more than 4 hours before, those with retained devitalized tissue, and wounds involving existing clinical infection or perforated viscera. This definition suggests that the organisms causing postoperative infection were present in the operative field before surgery.

PREVENTION OF BACTERIAL ENDOCARDITIS

The Committee on Rheumatic Fever, Endocarditis and Kawasaki Disease of the American Heart Association (AHA) issues detailed recommendations on the rationale, indications, and antibiotic regimens for the prevention of bacterial endocarditis for persons at increased risk. In previous editions of the *Red Book*, these AHA recommendations have been given. New guidelines, superseding those originally published in 1990 and later in the *Red Book*, have been prepared by AHA Committee and are expected to be published in 1997. Health care providers should consult the current recommendations in the 1994 *Red Book* (pp 525–533) until the new AHA guidelines are published.

PREVENTION OF NEONATAL OPHTHALMIA

Topical 1% silver nitrate, 0.5% erythromycin, and 1% tetracycline are considered equally effective for prophylaxis of ocular gonorrheal infection in newborn infants. Each is available in single-dose tubes. Recent studies indicate that 2.5% povidone-iodine solution also may be useful in preventing neonatal ophthalmia, but a product for this purpose currently is not available in the United States. Silver nitrate causes more chemical conjunctivitis than the other agents but appears to be the best one in areas where the incidence of penicillinase-producing *Neisseria gonorrhoeae* (PPNG) is appreciable. Published data on the efficacy of erythromycin or povidone-iodine prophylaxis against PPNG are not available, and only one study has demonstrated effectiveness of prophylactic tetracycline in an area with a high incidence of PPNG infections. Silver nitrate, povidone-iodine, and probably erythromycin are effective in preventing nongonococcal, nonchlamydial conjunctivitis in the first 2 weeks of life.

Neonatal chlamydial ophthalmia, although not as severe as gonococcal conjunctivitis, is common in the United States. In most areas, its frequency far surpasses that of gonococcal ophthalmia. The results of studies on the clinical efficacy of erythromycin and of tetracycline ointment in the prophylaxis of chlamydial conjunctivitis have been conflicting. Topical antibiotics, silver nitrate, and 2.5% povidone-iodine do not have proven efficacy in preventing conjunctivitis or nasopharyngeal colonization.

Specific recommendations for the prevention of neonatal ophthalmia are as follows:

- *Choice of drugs.* For prophylaxis of gonococcal ophthalmia neonatorum, a 1% silver nitrate solution in single-dose ampules or single-use tubes of an ophthalmic ointment containing 0.5% erythromycin or 1% tetracycline are each effective and acceptable.

- **Administration.** Before administering local prophylaxis, each eyelid should be wiped gently with sterile cotton. Two drops of a 1% silver nitrate solution or a 1-cm ribbon of antibiotic ointment are placed in each lower conjunctival sac. The eyelids should then be massaged gently to spread the ointment. After 1 minute, excess solution or ointment can be wiped away with sterile cotton. None of the prophylactic agents should be flushed from the eye after instillation. Comparative studies of the efficacy of silver nitrate prophylaxis with and without flushing are lacking, but anecdotal reports suggest that flushing may reduce the efficacy of prophylaxis without reducing the incidence of chemical conjunctivitis.

  Infants born by cesarean section should receive prophylaxis against neonatal gonococcal ophthalmia. Although gonococcal and chlamydial infections are usually transmitted to the infant during passage through the birth canal, infection by the ascending route also occurs. The risk of these infections occurring in untreated infants born by cesarean section has not been determined.

  Prophylaxis should be given shortly after birth. Although some suggest that prophylaxis may be administered more effectively in the nursery than in the delivery room, the efficacy of delaying prophylaxis has not been studied. However, delaying prophylaxis for as long as 1 hour after birth to facilitate parent-infant bonding is unlikely to influence efficacy. **Hospitals in which prophylaxis is delayed should establish a check system to ensure that all infants are treated.**

- **Pregnant women with gonococcal infections.** Identification and treatment of women who have gonococcal infection is essential. These infections in pregnant women, including those who are asymptomatic, have been associated with septic abortion, early and prolonged rupture of membranes, premature labor, and delivery of low-birth-weight infants. In addition to conjunctivitis, *N gonorrhea* also can cause scalp abscesses in infants receiving intrauterine fetal monitoring as well as disseminated neonatal gonococcal infection. Failure to treat an infected woman before or at delivery can result in postnatal transmission of gonococcal infection to infants.

- **Neonates whose mothers have gonorrhea.** In addition to ophthalmic prophylaxis, newborn infants whose mothers have gonorrhea at the time of delivery should receive a single dose of ceftriaxone (125 mg; for low-birth-weight infants, 25 to 50 mg/kg, not to exceed 125 mg) intravenously or intramuscularly. Cefotaxime in a single dose (100 mg/kg given intravenously or intramuscularly) is an alternative. Gonococcal ophthalmia, or disseminated infection, occasionally has occurred in infants managed by any of the current modes of topical prophylaxis.

- **Neonates with gonococcal ophthalmia or disseminated infection.** Newborns with clinical evidence of gonococcal ophthalmia or complicated (disseminated) gonococcal infection should be hospitalized and treated appropriately (see Gonococcal Infections, p 212).

- **Neonates whose mothers were treated for chlamydial cervicitis (see Chlamydia trachomatis, p 170).** Treatment of pregnant women who have chlamydial cervicitis can prevent neonatal chlamydial infection; oral erythromycin is the preferred treatment (see *Chlamydia trachomatis,* p 170). Infants born to women who received appropriate therapy for chlamydia cervicitis do not need to receive prophylaxis unless reason exists to believe that the woman has been reinfected.

- *Neonates whose mothers have untreated chlamydial infection.* Newborn infants whose mothers have untreated chlamydial infection at the time of delivery should be treated with oral erythromycin for 14 days (see *Chlamydia trachomatis,* p 170). Erythromycin may be poorly tolerated in neonates, in which case therapy with an oral sulfonamide after the immediate newborn period is an acceptable alternative.
- *Identification of Chlamydia-infected women (see* **Chlamydia trachomatis,** *p 170).* *Chlamydia* infections can be identified by screening with one of several antigen or nucleic acid detection tests. Testing is warranted in women at high risk for *C trachomatis* infection (eg, those younger than 25 years or those with new or multiple sex partners), in areas of high prevalence, and in women found to have other sexually transmitted diseases. Some experts advocate universal screening of pregnant women for infection with *Chlamydia* species.

Antimicrobials and Related Therapy

•••••••••••••••••••••••••••••••

INTRODUCTION

In some instances, drugs are recommended for specific indications other than those in the product label (package insert) approved by the Food and Drug Administration (FDA). An FDA-approved indication means that adequate and well-controlled studies were conducted and reviewed by the FDA. However, accepted medical practice often includes drug use that is not reflected in approved drug labeling. Lack of approval does not necessarily mean lack of effectiveness, but only that the appropriate studies have not been performed or data have not been submitted to the FDA for approval for that indication. Unapproved use does not imply improper use, provided that reasonable medical evidence justifies doing so and the use is deemed in the best interests of the patient. The decision to prescribe a drug rests with the physician who must weigh the risks and benefits of using the drug, whether or not it has full FDA approval.

Some antimicrobials with proven therapeutic benefit in humans are not approved by the FDA for use in pediatric patients or are considered contraindicated in children because of possible toxicity. However, some of these drugs, such as the fluoroquinolones and tetracyclines (in those younger than 8 years of age), may be used in special circumstances after careful assessment of the risks and benefits. Obtaining informed consent before use is prudent. The following delineates general principles for the use of these classes of drugs.

Fluoroquinolones

Use of fluoroquinolones (for example, ciprofloxacin, enoxacin, lomefloxacin, norfloxacin, and ofloxacin) is generally contraindicated, according to FDA-approved product labeling, in children and adolescents younger than 18 years as of December 1996 because they can cause cartilage damage in immature animals. The available data, however, indicate that these drugs are well tolerated, do not cause arthropathy in humans, and are effective in pediatric patients. Accordingly, in special circumstances in which alternative drugs are either not available or less effective, and after careful assessment of the risks and benefits for the individual patient, use of a fluoroquinolone can be justified. Circumstances in which fluoroquinolones may be useful include those in which (1) no oral agent is available, necessitating an alternative drug given parenterally; and (2) infection is caused by multiresistant, Gram-negative, and other pathogens, such as certain *Pseudomonas* strains and *Mycobacterium tuberculosis*. Possible uses, accordingly, include the following:

- Urinary tract infection
- Chronic suppurative otitis media
- Chronic osteomyelitis
- Exacerbation of cystic fibrosis
- *Mycobacterium tuberculosis* infections
- Other Gram-negative bacterial infections in immunocompromised hosts in which prolonged oral therapy is desired

Approval of one or more fluoroquinolones for use in children, and with limited indications, may occur. Until then, however, if use of a fluoroquinolone is recommended for a patient younger than 18 years, the risks and benefits should be explained to the parents or caregivers.

Tetracyclines

Use of these drugs in children has been limited because they can cause permanent dental discoloration in children younger than 8 years of age. Published studies have documented that tetracyclines and their colored degradation products that are bound to teeth are readily observed in the dentin and incorporated diffusely in the enamel. The period of odontogenesis to completion of the formation of enamel in permanent teeth appears to be the critical time for the effects of these drugs and is virtually complete by 8 years of age, at which time the drug can be given without concern for dental staining. The degree of staining appears to be dependent upon dosage and duration of therapy, and the total dosage received is the most important factor. In addition to dental discoloration, tetracyclines also may cause enamel hypoplasia and reversible delay in rate of bone growth.

These possible adverse events have resulted in the use of alternative, equally effective antimicrobials in most circumstances in young children in which tetracyclines are likely to be effective. However, in some cases the benefits of therapy with a tetracycline will exceed the risks, particularly if the alternative drugs are associated with significant adverse effects or may be less effective, and the use of tetracyclines in young children is justified. Examples include life-threatening rickettsial infections such as Rocky Mountain spotted fever (see p 452) and ehrlichiosis (see p 196). Doxycycline is usually the agent of choice in such children because the risk of dental staining is less with this product than that with other tetracyclines. In addition, the drug is given twice a day in contrast to the more frequent dosing regimen of other tetracyclines.

TABLES OF ANTIBACTERIAL DRUG DOSAGES

The recommended dosages for antimicrobials commonly used for newborn infants (see Table 5.1, p 607) and for older infants and children (see Table 5.2, p 609) are given separately because of the physiologic immaturity of the newborn infant and resulting different pharmacokinetics. The table for newborn infants is divided by postnatal age and birth weight because all infections in this age group are considered severe.

The recommended dosages are not absolute and are intended only as a guide. Clinical judgment about the disease, alterations in renal or hepatic function, and other factors affecting pharmacokinetics, patient response, and laboratory results may dictate modifications of these recommendations in the individual patient. In some cases, monitoring of serum drug concentrations is recommended to avoid toxicity and to ensure therapeutic efficacy.

Product label information should be consulted for such details as the diluent for reconstitution of injectable preparations, measures to be taken to avoid incompatibilities, drug interactions, and other precautions.

Table 5.1. Antibacterial Drugs for Newborn Infants: Dose* (mg/kg or Units [U]/kg) and Frequency of Administration†

Drug	Route	Infants 0–4 wk BW <1200 g	Infants <1 wk old BW 1200–2000 g	Infants <1 wk old BW >2000 g	Infants ≥1 wk old BW 1200–2000 g	Infants ≥1 wk old BW >2000 g
Aminoglycosides‡§						
Amikacin	IV, IM	7.5 every 18 h	7.5 every 12 h	7.5–10 every 12 h	7.5–10 every 8 or 12 h	10 every 8 h
Gentamicin	IV, IM	2.5 every 18 h	2.5 every 12 h	2.5 every 12 h	2.5 every 8 or 12 h	2.5 every 8 h
Kanamycin	IV, IM	7.5 every 18 h	7.5 every 12 h	7.5–10 every 12 h	7.5–10 every 8 or 12 h	10 every 8 h
Neomycin	PO only	25 every 6 h	25 every 6 h	25 every 6 h	25 every 6 h	25 every 6 h
Tobramycin	IV, IM	2.5 every 18 h	2.5 every 12 h	2.5 every 12 h	2.5 every 8 or 12 h	2.5 every 8 h
Antistaphylococcal penicillins‖						
Methicillin	IV, IM	25 every 12 h	25 every 12 h	25 every 8 h	25 every 8 h	25 every 6 h
Nafcillin	IV, IM	25 every 12 h	25 every 12 h	25 every 8 h	25 every 8 h	25 every 6 h
Oxacillin	IV, IM	25 every 12 h	25 every 12 h	25 every 8 h	25 every 8 h	25 every 6 h
Aztreonam§	IV, IM	30 every 12 h	30 every 12 h	30 every 8 h	30 every 8 h	30 every 6 h
Cephalosporins						
Cefotaxime	IV, IM	50 every 12 h	50 every 12 h	50 every 8 or 12 h	50 every 8 h	50 every 6 or 8 h
Ceftazidime	IV, IM	50 every 12 h	50 every 12 h	50 every 8 or 12 h	50 every 8 h	50 every 8 h
Ceftriaxone#	IV, IM	50 every 24 h	50 every 24 h	50 every 24 h	50 every 24 h	50–75 every 24 h
Chloramphenicol‖	IV, PO	25 every 24 h	25 every 24 h	25 every 24 h	25 every 24 h	25 every 12 h
Clindamycin	IV, IM, PO	5 every 12 h	5 every 12 g	5 every 8 h	5 every 8 h	5 every 6 h
Erythromycin	PO	10 every 12 h	10 every 12 h	10 every 12 h	10 every 8 h	10 every 8 h
Metronidazole**	IV, PO	7.5 every 48 h	7.5 every 24 h	7.5 every 12 h	7.5 every 8 h	15 every 12 h

Table 5.1. Antibacterial Drugs for Newborn Infants: Dose (mg/kg or Units [U]/kg*) and Frequency of Administration,† continued

Drug	Route	Infants 0–4 wk BW <1200 g	Infants <1 wk old BW ≤1200–2000 g	Infants <1 wk old BW >2000 g	Infants ≥1 wk old BW ≤1200–2000 g	Infants ≥1 wk old BW >2000 g
Penicillins						
Ampicillin‡‖	IV, IM	25 every 12 h	25 every 12 h	25 every 8 h	25 every 8 h	25 every 6 h
Mezlocillin	IV, IM	75 every 12 h	75 every 12 h	75 every 8 h	75 every 8 or 12 h	75 every 6 h
Penicillin G, ‡‖ aqueous	IV, IM	25 000 U every 12 h	25 000 U every 12 h	25 000 U every 8 h	25 000 U every 8 h	25 000 U every 6 h
Penicillin G, procaine	IM	50 000 U every 24 h	50 000 U every 24 h	50 000 U every 24 h	50 000 U every 24 h	50 000 U every 24 h
Ticarcillin	IV, IM	75 every 12 h	75 every 12 h			
Vancomycin‡	IV	15 every 24 h	10–15 every 12–18 h	10–15 every 8–12 h	10–15 every 8–12 h	15–20 every 8 h

* Unless otherwise listed, dosages are given as mg/kg.
† BW indicates body weight; IV, intravenous; IM, intramuscular; PO, oral.
‡ Optimal dosage should be based on determination of serum concentrations, especially in low-birth-weight (<1500 g) infants. In very-low-birth-weight infants (<1200 g) every 18 to 24 hour dosing may be appropriate in the first week of life.
§ Dosages for the aminoglycosides may differ from those recommended by the manufacturer in the package insert.
‖ For meningitis, the recommended dosage should be doubled.
¶ Food and Drug Administration approval is pending as of December 1996.
# Drug should not be administered to hyperbilirubinemic neonates, especially those born prematurely.
** Safety in infants and children has not been established.
‡‡ Higher doses are recommended for the treatment of group B streptococcal meningitis (see Group B Streptococcal Infections, p 495).

Table 5.2. Antibacterial Drugs for Pediatric Patients Beyond the Newborn Period

Drug, Generic (Trade Name)	Route	Dosage per kg/d		Comments
		Mild to Moderate Infections	Severe Infections	
Aminoglycosides*				
Amikacin (Amikin)	IV, IM	Inappropriate	15–22.5 mg in 3 doses (daily adult dose, 15 mg/kg; maximum, 1.5 g)	30 mg in 3 doses is recommended by some consultants
Gentamicin (Garamycin)	IV, IM	Inappropriate	3–7.5 mg in 3 doses (daily adult dose is the same)	
Kanamycin (Kantrex)	IV, IM	Inappropriate	15–22.5 mg in 3 doses (daily adult dose, 1–1.5 g)	30 mg in 3 doses is recommended by some consultants
Neomycin (numerous types)	PO only	100 mg in 4 doses	100 mg in 4 doses	For some enteric infections
Netilmicin (Netromycin)	IV, IM	Inappropriate	3–7.5 mg in 3 doses (daily adult dose is the same)	…
Paromomycin (Humatin)	PO	30 mg in 3 doses (maximum daily adult dose, 4 g)	Inappropriate	
Tobramycin (Nebcin)	IV, IM	Inappropriate	3–7.5 mg in 3 doses (daily adult dose, 3–5 mg in 3 doses)	…
Aztreonam† (Azactam)	IV, IM	90 mg in 3 doses (daily adult dose, 3 g)	120 mg in 4 doses (maximum daily adult dose, 8 g)	FDA approval pending for use in infants and children, as of December 1996
Cephalosporins†				
Cefaclor (Ceclor)	PO	20–40 mg in 2 or 3 doses (daily adult dose, 750 mg–1.5 g)	Inappropriate	A twice-daily regimen has been demonstrated to be effective for treatment of acute otitis media

Table 5.2. Antibacterial Drugs for Pediatric Patients Beyond the Newborn Period, continued

Drug, Generic (Trade Name)	Route	Dosage per kg/d		Comments
		Mild to Moderate Infections	Severe Infections	
Cephalosporins,[†] continued				
Cefadroxil (Duricef, Utracef)	PO	30 mg in 2 doses (maximum daily adult dose, 2 g)	Inappropriate	...
Cefazolin (Kefzol, Ancef)	IV, IM	25–50 mg in 3 doses (daily adult dose, 750 mg–2 g)	50–100 mg in 3 doses (maximum adult dose 4–6 g)	...
Cefepime[‖] (Maxipime)	IV, IM	1–2 g in 2 doses (daily adult dose)	2–4 g in 2 doses (daily adult dose)	Not approved for therapy of meningitis
Cefixime (Suprax)	PO	8 mg in 1 or 2 doses (daily adult dose, 400 mg)	Inappropriate	Diarrhea occurs in 10%–15% of patients
Cefonicid (Monocid)	IV, IM	20–40 mg in 1 dose (maximum daily adult dose, 2 g)	No data available	Not approved for children
Cefoperazone (Cefobid)	IV, IM	100–150 mg in 2 or 3 doses (maximum daily adult dose, 4 g)	No data available	Not approved for children
Cefotaxime (Claforan)	IV, IM	75–100 mg in 3 or 4 doses (daily adult dose, 4–6 g)	150–300 mg in 3 or 4 doses (daily adult dose, 8–10 g)	A regimen of 75 mg/kg 3 times a day has been successfully used for therapy of meningitis
Cefoxitin (Mefoxin)	IV, IM	80–100 mg in 3–4 doses (daily adult dose, 3–4 g)	80–160 mg in 4–6 doses (daily adult dose, 6–12 g)	...
Cefpodoxime proxetil (Vantin)	PO	10 mg in 2 doses (maximum daily adult dose, 800 mg)	Inappropriate	...
Cefprozil (Cefzil)	PO	15–30 mg in 2 doses (maximum daily adult dose, 1 g)	Inappropriate	30–mg dosage recommended for treatment of acute otitis media

Table 5.2. Antibacterial Drugs for Pediatric Patients Beyond the Newborn Period, continued

Drug, Generic (Trade Name)	Route	Dosage per kg/d		Comments
		Mild to Moderate Infections	Severe Infections	
Cephalosporins,[†] continued				
Ceftazidime (Fortaz, Tazicef, Tazidime)	IV, IM	75–100 mg in 3 doses (daily adult dose, 3 g)	125–150 mg in 3 doses (daily adult dose, 6 g)	Only cephalosporin with anti–*Pseudomonas* activity that has been approved for use in children
Ceftibuten (Cedax)	PO	9 mg in 1 dose (maximum daily adult dose: see package insert)	Inappropriate	⋯
Ceftizoxime (Cefizox)	IV, IM	100–150 mg in 3 doses (daily adult dose, 3–4 g)	150–200 mg in 3 doses (daily adult dose, 4–6 g)	⋯
Ceftriaxone (Rocephin)	IV, IM	50–75 mg in 1 or 2 doses (daily adult dose, 2 g)	80–100 mg in 1 or 2 doses (daily adult dose, 4 g)	⋯
Cefuroxime (Zinacef)	IV, IM	75–100 mg in 3 doses (daily adult dose, 2–4 g)	100–150 mg in 3 doses (daily adult dose, 4–6 g)	200–240-mg dosage recommended for meningitis
Cefuroxime axetil (Ceftin)	PO	20–30 mg in 2 doses (daily adult dose, 1–2 g)	Inappropriate	Higher dosage recommended for treatment of otitis media
Cephalexin (Keflex)	PO	25–50 mg in 4 doses (daily adult dose, 1–4 g)	Inappropriate	⋯
Cephalothin (Keflin)	IV, IM	80–100 mg in 4 doses (daily adult dose, 2–4 g)	100–150 mg in 4–6 doses (daily adult dose, 8–12 g)	⋯
Cephapirin (Cefadyl)	IV, IM	40 mg in 4 doses (daily adult dose, 2 g)	40–80 mg in 4 doses (daily adult dose, 4–12 g)	⋯
Cephradine (Anspor)	PO	25–50 mg in 2–4 doses (daily adult dose, 1–4 g)	Inappropriate	⋯

Table 5.2. Antibacterial Drugs for Pediatric Patients Beyond the Newborn Period, continued

Drug, Generic (Trade Name)	Route	Dosage per kg/d		Comments
		Mild to Moderate Infections	Severe Infections	
Cephalosporins,† continued				
(Velosef)	IV, IM	50–100 mg in 4 doses (daily adult dose, 2–8 g)	100 mg/kg in 4 doses (daily adult dose, 6–8 g)	…
Loracarbef (Lorabid)	PO	30 mg for otitis media and 15 mg for other indications in 2 doses (maximum daily adult dose, 800 mg)	Inappropriate	…
Chloramphenicol (Chloromycetin)				
Chloramphenicol palmitate‡	PO	Inappropriate	50–100 mg in 4 doses (daily adult dose, 1–2 g)	Optimal dosage is determined by measurement of serum concentrations with resulting modifications to achieve therapeutic concentrations. Use only for serious infections because of the rare occurrence of aplastic anemia after administration.
Chloramphenicol succinate	IV	Inappropriate	50–100 mg in 4 doses (daily adult dose, 2–4 g)	
Clindamycin (Cleocin)	IM, IV	15–25 mg in 3–4 doses (daily adult dose, 600 mg–3.6 g)	25–40 mg in 3–4 doses (daily adult dose, 1.2–2.7 g)	Active against anaerobes, especially *Bacteroides* species. Active against many multidrug resistant pneumococci.
	PO	10–20 mg in 3–4 doses (daily adult dose, 600 mg–1.8 g)	Inappropriate	…

Table 5.2. Antibacterial Drugs for Pediatric Patients Beyond the Newborn Period, continued

Drug, Generic (Trade Name)	Route	Dosage per kg/d Mild to Moderate Infections	Severe Infections	Comments
Fluoroquinolones[‡]				
Ciprofloxacin (Cipro)	PO	20–30 mg in 2 doses (daily adult dose, 0.5–1.5 mg)	30 mg in 2 doses (daily adult dose, 1.0–1.5 g)	Not approved for use in persons younger than 18 years old, as of December 1996.[‡] However, drug has selective indications in children and adolescents (see p 605).[§‖]
	IV	Inappropriate	Daily adult dose, 400–800 mg in 2 doses	
Imipenem[†§] (Primaxin)	IV, IM	40–60 mg in 4 doses (daily adult dose, 1–2 g)	60 mg in 4 doses (daily adult dose, 2–4 g)	Caution in use for therapy of meningitis because of possible seizures
Macrolides				
Erythromycins (numerous types)	PO	20–50 mg in 2–4 doses (daily adult dose, 1–2 g)	Inappropriate	Available in base, stearate, ethyl succinate, and estolate preparations
	IV	Inappropriate	15–50 mg in 4 doses (daily adult dose, 1–4 g)	Administer in a continuous drip or by slow infusion over 60 min or longer. May cause cardiac arrhythmia.
Azithromycin (Zithromax)	PO	5–12 mg/kg once daily (maximum daily adult dose, 600 mg)	Inappropriate	Otitis: 10 mg/kg on first day, 5 mg/kg/d for additional 4 d Pharyngitis: 12 mg/kg/d for 5 days Recently approved for treatment of *Helicobacter pylori* infection
Clarithromycin (Biaxin)	PO	7.5 mg in 2 doses (maximum daily adult dose, 1 g)	Inappropriate	

Table 5.2. Antibacterial Drugs for Pediatric Patients Beyond the Newborn Period, continued

Drug. Generic (Trade Name)	Route	Dosage per kg/d		Comments
		Mild to Moderate Infections	Severe Infections	
Meropenem[†] (Merrem)	IV	60 mg in 3 doses (maximum daily adult dose, 3 g)	60–120 mg in 3 doses (maximum daily adult dose, 6 g)	Approved for use in patients ≥ 3 months of age, including those with meningitis (in which case higher dose is indicated)
Methenamine mandelate (Mandelamine)	PO	50–75 mg in 3–4 doses (daily adult dose, 2–4 g)	Inappropriate	Should not be used for infants; urine pH must be adjusted to 5–5.5
Metronidazole (Flagyl)	PO	15–35 mg in 3 doses (maximum daily adult dose, 1–2 g)	Inappropriate	Safety in infants and children has not been established
Nitrofurantoin (Furadantin)	PO	5–7 mg in 4 doses (daily adult dose, 200–400 mg)	Inappropriate	Should not be used for young infants; prophylactic dose is 1–2 mg/kg/d in one dose
PENICILLINS[†] **Broad–spectrum penicillins**				
Ampicillin (numerous types)	IV, IM	100–150 mg in 4 doses (daily adult dose, 2–4 g)	200–300 mg in 4 doses (daily adult dose, 6–12 g)	Ineffective against ß-lactamase–producing organisms. Diarrhea occurs in approximately 20%
	PO	50–100 mg in 4 doses (daily adult dose, 2–4 g)	Inappropriate	Diarrhea occurs in approximately 20% of recipients

Table 5.2. Antibacterial Drugs for Pediatric Patients Beyond the Newborn Period, continued

Drug, Generic (Trade Name)	Route	Dosage per kg/d Mild to Moderate Infections	Severe Infections	Comments
PENICILLINS, continued				
Ampicillin–sulbactam (Unasyn)‖	IV	100–150 mg of ampicillin in 4 doses	200–300 mg of ampicillin in 4 doses (daily adult dose, 6–12 g)	...
Amoxicillin (numerous types)	PO	25–50 mg in 3 doses (daily adult dose, 750 mg–1.5 g)	Inappropriate	...
Amoxicillin–clavulanate (Augmentin)	PO	20–45 mg of amoxicillin in 2–3 doses, depending on the formulation (daily adult dose, 750 mg–1.5 g)	Inappropriate	For use of the newly approved 7:1 amoxicillin–clavulanate formulation, 45 mg/kg dosage of amoxicillin in 2 doses
Bacampicillin (Spectrobid)	PO	25–50 mg in 2 doses (daily adult dose, 1–2 g)	Inappropriate	Prodrug of ampicillin with excellent bioavailability
Mezlocillin (Mezlin)	IV, IM	100–150 mg in 4 doses (daily adult dose, 6–8 g)	200–300 mg in 4–6 doses (daily adult dose, 12–18 g)	Contains 1.85 mEq of Na per gram
Piperacillin‖ (Pipracil)	IV, IM	100–150 mg in 4 doses (daily adult dose, 6–8 g)	200–300 mg in 4–6 doses (daily adult dose, 12–18 g)	Contains 1.85 mEq of Na per gram
Piperacillin/tazobactam‖ (Zosyn)	IV	Inappropriate	240 mg of piperacillin in 3 doses	...
Ticarcillin (Ticar)	IV, IM	100–200 mg in 4 doses (daily adult dose, 4–6 g)	200–300 mg in 4–6 doses (daily adult dose, 12–24 g)	Contains 5.2 mEq of Na per gram
Ticarcillin–clavulanate (Timentin)	IV, IM	100–200 mg of ticarcillin in 4 doses (4–6 g)	200–300 mg of ticarcillin in 4 doses (12–24 g)	...

Table 5.2. **Antibacterial Drugs for Pediatric Patients Beyond the Newborn Period, continued**

Drug, Generic (Trade Name)	Route	Dosage per kg/d		Comments
		Mild to Moderate Infections	Severe Infections	
PENICILLINS, continued				
Penicillin G and V[‖]				
Penicillin G, crystalline K or Na (numerous types)	IV, IM	25 000–50 000 U in 4 doses	250 000–400 000 U in 4–6 doses	1.68 mEq K or Na per 1 000 000 U; use Na salt for large IV doses
Penicillin G, procaine (numerous types)	IM	25 000–50 000 U in 1–2 doses	Inappropriate	Contraindicated in procaine allergy
Penicillin G, benzathine (Bicillin, Permapen)	IM	<27.3 kg (60 lb): 600 000 U ≥27.3 kg: 1 200 000 U	Inappropriate	Major use is prevention of rheumatic fever by treatment and prophylaxis of streptococcal infections
Penicillin G, potassium oral (numerous types)	PO	25 000–50 000 U in 3 or 4 doses	Inappropriate	Variable absorption; optimal to administer unbuffered penicillin G at least 1 h before, or 2 h after meals
Penicillin V (numerous types)	PO	25 000–50 000 U in 3 or 4 doses	Inappropriate	1600 U is equivalent to 1 mg; optimal to administer on an empty stomach
Penicillinase-resistant penicillins[†]				
Methicillin (Staphcillin)	IV, IM	100–150 mg in 4 doses (daily adult dose, 4–8 g)	150–200 mg in 4–6 doses (daily adult dose, 4–12 g)	Methicillin-resistant staphylococci are usually resistant to all other semisynthetic antistaphylococcal cephalosporins. Interstitial nephritis (ie, hematuria) occurs in 0%–4% of patients

Table 5.2. Antibacterial Drugs for Pediatric Patients Beyond the Newborn Period, continued

Drug, Generic (Trade Name)	Route	Dosage per kg/d		Comments
		Mild to Moderate Infections	Severe Infections	
PENICILLINS, continued				
Penicillinase–resistant penicillins,[†] **continued**				
Oxacillin (Prostaphlin, Bactocill)	IV, IM	100–150 mg in 4 doses (daily adult dose, 2–4 g)	150–200 mg in 4–6 doses (daily adult dose, 4–12 g)	…
	PO	50–100 mg in 4 doses (daily adult dose, 2–4 g)	Inappropriate	Absorption of oral preparations is variable; administer at least 1 h before or 2 h after meals
Nafcillin (Unipen, Nafcil)	IV, IM	50–100 mg in 4 doses (daily adult dose, 2–4 g)	150–200 mg in 4–6 doses (daily adult dose, 4–12 g)	Serum concentrations after oral administration are low compared with those after other orally administered antistaphylococcal drugs
	PO	50–100 mg in 4 doses (daily adult dose, 2–4 g)	Inappropriate	…
Cloxacillin (Tegopen, Cloxapen)	PO	50–100 mg in 4 doses (daily adult dose, 2–4 g)	Inappropriate	…
Dicloxacillin (Dynapen, Pathocil)	PO	25–50 mg in 4 doses (daily adult dose, 1–2 g)	Inappropriate	Excellent serum concentrations after oral administration
Rifampin (numerous types)	PO	10–20 mg/kg in 1–2 doses (daily adult dose, 600 mg)	20 mg/kg in 2 doses	Should not be used as monotherapy except when given for prophylaxis

Table 5.2. Antibacterial Drugs for Pediatric Patients Beyond the Newborn Period, continued

Drug, Generic (Trade Name)	Route	Dosage per kg/d		Comments
		Mild to Moderate Infections	Severe Infections	
Rifampin, continued	IV	10–20 mg/kg in 1–2 doses (daily adult dose, 600 mg)	20 mg/kg in 2 doses	...
Sulfonamides				
Sulfadiazine¶	PO	100–150 mg in 4 doses	100–150 mg in 4–6 doses	...
Sulfisoxazole (Gantrisin)	PO	120–150 mg in 4–6 doses	120–150 mg in 4–6 doses	...
Triple sulfonamides (numerous types)	PO	120–150 mg in 4 doses	120–150 mg in 4 doses	...
Trimethoprim–sulfamethoxazole (Bactrim, Septra)	PO	8–12 mg trimethoprim—40–60 mg sulfamethoxazole in 2 doses (daily adult dose, 320 mg trimethoprim—1.6 g sulfamethoxazole)	20 mg trimethoprim—100 mg sulfamethoxazole in 4 doses (for use only in *Pneumocystis carinii* pneumonia)	For prophylaxis in immunocompromised patients, recommended daily dose is 5 mg trimethoprim—25 mg sulfamethoxazole per kg/d in 2 doses
	IV	Inappropriate	8–12 mg trimethoprim—40–60 mg sulfamethoxazole in 4 doses **or** 20 mg trimethoprim—100 mg sulfamethoxazole in 4 doses (for treatment of *Pneumocystis* infection)	Use intravenous formulation when oral formulation cannot be administered ...

Table 5.2. Antibacterial Drugs for Pediatric Patients Beyond the Newborn Period, continued

Drug, Generic (Trade Name)	Route	Dosage per kg/d		Comments
		Mild to Moderate Infections	Severe Infections	
Tetracyclines (numerous types)	IV	Inappropriate	10–25 mg in 2–4 doses (daily adult dose, 1–2 g)	Responsible for staining of developing teeth; use only in children 8 y or older except in circumstances in which the benefits of therapy exceed the risks and alternative drugs are less effective or more toxic (see p 606).
	PO	20–50 mg in 4 doses (daily adult dose, 1–2 g)	Inappropriate	...
Doxycycline (numerous types)	PO, IV	2–4 mg in 1–2 doses (daily adult dose, 100–200 mg)	Inappropriate	Side effects similar to those of other tetracycline products except that risk of dental staining in children less than 8 y is less
Vancomycin (Vancocin, Vancoled, Vancor)	IV	40 mg in 3–4 doses (daily adult dose,# 1–2 g)	40–60 mg in 4 doses (daily adult dose,# 2–4 g)	In meningitis, 60 mg/kg dose should be given during at least 60 min; routine monitoring of serum concentrations is unnecessary

* Dosages for the aminoglycosides may differ from those recommended by the manufacturers (see package insert).
† In patients with history of allergy to penicillin or one of its many congeners, alternative drugs are recommended. In some circumstances, a cephalosporin or other β-lactam class drug may be acceptable. However, these drugs should not be used in patients with an immediate hypersensitivity (anaphylaxis) to penicillin because approximately 5% to 15% of penicillin-allergic patients will also be allergic to the cephalosporins.
‡ Not approved for use in patients younger than 18 years, as of December 1996; however, approval of ciprofloxacin for treatment of acute respiratory exacerbations on patients with cystic fibrosis is pending.
§ Not approved for use in patients younger than 12 years.
‖ Patients with a history of allergy to penicillin G or V should be considered for subsequent skin testing. Many such patients can be treated safely with penicillin, since only 10% of children with such history are proven allergic when skin-tested.
¶ Available from Eon Labs, Laurelton, NY (800–526–0225).
# In adults, daily dose is given in 2 to 4 divided doses.

DEXAMETHASONE THERAPY FOR BACTERIAL MENINGITIS IN INFANTS AND CHILDREN

Case fatality rates for bacterial meningitis in infants and children in the United States are from 5% to 10%. As many as 20% of survivors have long-term sequelae, the most common of which is hearing impairment. The reported incidence of hearing loss after meningitis has ranged from 5% to 31%, depending on the selection of patients, techniques used to assess hearing and etiology. These sequelae of bacterial meningitis are attributable, at least in part, to inflammation. Cytokines, including tumor necrosis factor-α (TNF-α) interleukin-1β (IL-1β), and platelet activating factor (PAF), produced by endothelial and mononuclear cells in response to activation by highly inflammatory bacterial cell wall products appear to be responsible for initiating the inflammatory response in meningitis. Bacterial cell wall fragments are created when bacteria are lysed by antibiotics. The pathophysiologic events believed to be medicated by cytokines include alteration of cerebral capillary endothelial cells that comprise the blood-brain barrier, cytotoxic and vasogenic cerebral edema, and increased intracranial pressure. These events can lead to decreased cerebral perfusion pressure, resulting in diminution in cerebral blood flow and subsequent regional hypoxia and focal ischemia of brain tissue. The pathogenesis of the sensorineural hearing loss, the most common neurologic sequela, may be different as the degree of hearing loss does not in general correlate with disease severity. In the animal model, hearing loss appears to be the result of entry of inflammatory cells and mediators from the cerebrospinal fluid (CSF) into the inner ear via the cochlear aqueduct.

Since dexamethasone is a potent inhibitor of TNF-α and IL-1β production, adjunctive therapy with dexamethasone has been evaluated in experimental meningitis and in infants and children with meningitis. Dexamethasone results in a significant increase in cerebral perfusion and decreases in intracranial pressure, brain edema, and lactate concentrations in CSF in experimental *Haemophilus influenzae* type b and *Streptococcus pneumoniae* meningitis when administered shortly before antibiotics are given. Dexamethasone administration also has been associated with lowered mortality and neurologic sequelae in rabbits with experimental pneumococcal meningitis.

In infants and children, results of double-blind, placebo-controlled trials of dexamethasone therapy for bacterial meningitis demonstrate decreased hearing loss and/or neurologic sequelae in dexamethasone recipients with *H influenzae* type b infection. In these studies, this organism accounted for approximately 75% of the cases of meningitis. Beneficial effects of dexamethasone on neurologic and audiologic outcome have not been demonstrated in prospective studies of patients infected with *S pneumoniae* or *Neisseria meningitis* as the limited number of patients with these infections was insufficient to determine efficacy. With the substantial decline in the incidence of *H influenzae* type b disease since the introduction of effective vaccination, the total number of cases of bacterial meningitis in infants and children has decreased and, as a result, the relative proportion of cases of bacterial meningitis caused by pneumococci and meningococci has increased substantially. In all studies, however, the frequency of neurologic sequelae has been decreased (but with varying degrees of statistical significance) when dexamethasone-treated patients with bacterial meningitis are compared to those who did not receive this adjunctive therapy.

Administration of dexamethasone shortly before or at the time of antibiotic administration, ie, before bacterial lypis results in release of cell wall fragments, appears to be an important factor in the effect of dexamethasone on inflammatory mediators. However, adjunctive dexamethasone therapy in children with suspected pneumococcal or meningococcal meningitis has been controversial for several reasons. In addition to lack of proven efficacy in prospective placebo-controlled trials, concerns have included possible decreased CSF concentrations of antimicrobials, increased mortality in adults with septic shock due to Gram-negative bacilli who were treated with corticosteroids, and possible different mechanisms of inflammation in pneumococcal meningitis than that in *H influenzae* meningitis. Another consideration is that dexamethasone results in rapid defervescence of fever and general clinical improvement, which may be present in spite of persistence of bacteria growth in the CSF. Since neurologic sequelae have been correlated with the timing of CSF sterilization, this phenomenon could result in increased risk of sequelae, particularly in meningitis caused by antimicrobial-resistant bacteria. However, long-term deleterious sequelae of dexamethasone administration have not been demonstrated.

Adverse Effects

Dexamethasone therapy was not associated with delayed sterilization of CSF cultures in the double-blind, placebo-controlled trials of dexamethasone therapy performed before the marked increase in the incidence of antimicrobial-resistant *S pneumoniae* infection occurred. In approximately one-fifth to two-thirds of patients in these studies, secondary and low-grade fever occurred 24 to 48 hours after discontinuation of dexamethasone and lasted 24 to 36 hours. Rarely, dexamethasone recipients have developed gastrointestinal bleeding requiring blood transfusions on the second and third days of corticosteroid treatment. However, whether the bleeding resulted from dexamethasone therapy is uncertain. No complications of therapy have developed in patients with aseptic meningitis treated with dexamethasone for suspected bacterial meningitis.

Recommendations

- Dexamethasone therapy should be considered when bacterial meningitis in infants and children 6 weeks and older is diagnosed or strongly suspected on the basis of the CSF tests, including Gram-stained smears, after the physician has weighed the benefits and possible risks and before the etiology has been established.
- Dexamethasone is recommended for treatment of infants and children with *H influenzae* type b meningitis.
- Dexamethasone should be considered for the treatment of infants and children with pneumococcal or meningococcal meningitis. However, its efficacy for these infections is unproven, and some experts do not recommend its use.
- The recommended dexamethasone regimen is 0.6 mg/kg per day in four divided doses, given intravenously, for the first 2 days of antibiotic treatment. A regimen of 0.8 mg/kg per day in two divided doses also is appropriate.

- If dexamethasone is given, it should be administered as early as possible, preferably at the time of, or shortly before, the first dose of antibacterial therapy. Dexamethasone when initiated 4 or more hours after administration of parenteral antimicrobial therapy is unlikely to be effective. Some experts consider that an interval of more than 1 or 2 hours precludes possible effectiveness.
- If dexamethasone is given to patients with pneumococcal meningitis, a repeat lumbar puncture should be considered after 24 to 48 hours to assess the response to therapy (see Pneumococcal Infections, p 412).
- Dexamethasone should not be used for suspected or proven nonbacterial meningitis. If dexamethasone had been started before the diagnosis of nonbacterial meningitis was made, it should be discontinued.
- "Partially treated" meningitis with negative cultures is not an indication for continued dexamethasone therapy.
- The decision to give dexamethasone in patients with presumed bacterial meningitis should not be based on severity of the presenting illness.
- No data are currently available on which to base a recommendation concerning the use of dexamethasone for treatment of bacterial meningitis in infants younger than 6 weeks, or of meningitis in those with congenital or acquired abnormalities of the central nervous system, with or without a prosthetic device.

SEXUALLY TRANSMITTED DISEASES

Table 5.3. Guidelines for Treatment of Sexually Transmitted Diseases (STDs) in Children and Adolescents According to Syndrome

Preferred regimens (as of December 1996) are listed. For further information concerning other acceptable regimens and diseases not included, see specific recommendations in disease-specific chapters in Section 3.*† In addition, revised recommendations on the treatment of STDs are likely to be issued by the Centers for Disease Control and Prevention in late 1997 or early 1998.

Syndrome	Organism(s)/Diagnoses	Treatment of Adolescent†	Treatment for Infant/Child
Urethritis: Inflammation of urethra with mucoid, mucopurulent, or purulent discharge	Neisseria gonorrhoeae, Chlamydia trachomatis	Ceftriaxone, 125 mg IM, single dose **or** Cefixime, 400 mg orally, single dose **PLUS** Doxycycline, 100 mg orally every 12 h for 7 d **or** Azithromycin, 1 g orally, single dose	Ceftriaxone, 125 mg IM, single dose **PLUS** Erythromycin, 40 mg/kg/d orally, in 4 divided doses (maximum 2 g/d) for 7 d **or** Azithromycin, 10 mg/kg orally, single dose
Mucopurulent cervicitis: Inflammation of cervix with muco-purulent or purulent cervical discharge. Cervicitis occurs very rarely in prepubertal girls (see Prepubertal vaginitis)	N gonorrhoeae, C trachomatis	Ceftriaxone, 125 mg IM, single dose **or** Cefixime, 400 mg orally, single dose **PLUS** Doxycycline, 100 mg orally every 12 h for 7 d **or** Azithromycin, 1 g, single dose	See Prepubertal vaginitis
Pelvic inflammatory disease (PID)‡§	N gonorrhoeae, C trachomatis, anaerobes, coliform bacteria, genital Mycoplasma species, Streptococcus species	Hospitalization‖: _Regimen A:_ Cefoxitin, 2 g IV every 6 h **or** Cefotetan, 2 g IV every 12 h **PLUS** Doxycycline, 200 mg IV or orally every 12 h and continued to complete a 14-d course	PID occurs rarely, if at all, in prepubertal girls

Table 5.3. Guidelines for Treatment of Sexually Transmitted Diseases in Children and Adolescents According to Syndrome, continued

Syndrome	Organism(s)/Diagnoses	Treatment of Adolescent	Treatment for Infant/Child
Pelvic inflammatory disease (PID), continued		**OR**	
		Regimen B: Clindamycin, 900 mg IV every 8 h **PLUS**	
		Gentamicin, 2 mg/kg IV every 8 h followed by doxycycline, 200 mg orally every 12 h for 14 d	
		Outpatient: Cefoxitin, 2 g IM, single dose, with concurrent administration of probenicid, 1 g orally, single dose	
		or	
		Ceftriaxone, 250 mg IM, single dose **PLUS**	
		Doxycycline, 100 mg orally every 12 h for 14 d	
Prepubertal vaginitis (STD-related): Inflammation of the vagina with a mucopurulent or purulent vaginal discharge	*N gonorrhoeae*	...	Ceftriaxone, 125 mg, single dose
	C trachomatis	...	Erythromycin, 40 mg/kg orally, in 4 divided doses (maximum 2 g/d) for 7 d
	Trichomonas vaginalis	...	Metronidazole, 15 mg/kg/d orally in 3 divided doses (maximum 2 g/d) for 7 d
	Bacterial vaginosis	...	Metronidazole, 15 mg/kg/d orally in 2 divided doses (maximum 1 g/d) for 7 d
	Herpes simplex virus — primary infection	...	Acyclovir, 80 mg/kg/d orally in 3 divided doses (maximum 1.2 g/d) for 7–10 d

Table 5.3. Guidelines for Treatment of Sexually Transmitted Diseases in Children and Adolescents According to Syndrome, continued

Syndrome	Organism(s)/Diagnoses	Treatment of Adolescent†	Treatment for Infant/Child
Adolescent vulvovaginitis	T vaginalis Bacterial vaginosis	Metronidazole, 2 g orally, single dose Metronidazole, 1 g/d orally in 2 divided doses for 7 d	… …
	Candida species	or Metronidazole, 2 g orally, single dose Clotrimazole, 500 mg intravaginally, single dose	…
		or Miconazole or clotrimazole, 200 mg intravaginally for 3 d	…
	Herpes simplex virus — primary infection	Acyclovir, 1.0 g/d orally in 5 divided doses for 7–10 d or 1.2 g/d in 3 divided doses for 7–10 d	…
Syphilis	Treponema pallidum	Primary and secondary syphilis: Benzathine penicillin G, 2.4 million U IM, single dose

Latent syphilis: Early: benzathine penicillin G, 2.4 million U IM, single dose Late or unknown duration (except neurosyphilis§): benzathine penicillin G, 2.4 million U, single dose, every 7 d IM for 3 wk | Same as for congenital syphilis (see p 509, Table 3.57, p 510) |

Table 5.3. Guidelines for Treatment of Sexually Transmitted Diseases in Children and Adolescents According to Syndrome, continued

Syndrome	Organism(s)/Diagnoses	Treatment of Adolescent†	Treatment for Infant/Child
Genital ulcer disease	*T pallidum*	Same as for syphilis	Same as for congenital syphilis (see p 509 , Table 3.57, p 510)
	Herpes simplex virus — primary infection	Acyclovir, 1.0 g/d orally in 5 divided doses for 7–10 d	Acyclovir, 80 mg/kg/d orally in 3 divided doses (maximum 1.2 g/d) for 7–10 d
	Haemophilus ducreyi (chancroid)	**or** 1.2 g/d in 3 divided doses for 7–10 d Azithromycin, 1 g orally, single dose **or** Ceftriaxone, 250 mg IM, single dose	Ceftriaxone, 50 mg/kg IM, single dose **or** Azithromycin, 20 mg/kg, single dose (maximum 1 g) ...
Sexually acquired epididymitis	*C trachomatis, N gonorrhoeae,* Gram-negative enteric organisms	Ceftriaxone, 250 mg IM, single dose **or** Cefixime, 400 mg orally, single dose **PLUS** Doxycycline, 100 mg orally every 12 h for 10 d **or** Azithromycin, 1 g orally, single dose	
Anogenital warts	Human papillomavirus	Podophyllin,# podofilox,# cryotherapy, trichloracetic acid, electrocautery, laser surgery, or surgical excision	Same as for adolescents

* For additional information and recommendations, see the following; Centers for Disease Control and Prevention. 1993 sexually transmitted diseases treatment guidelines. *MMWR.* 1993; 42 (No. RR-14):1-102. IM indicates intramuscularly; IV, intravenously; and STD, sexually transmitted disease.

† Some regimens are not indicated for pregnant adolescents. For a more complete listing of acceptable treatment regimens, consult the reference in preceding footnote.

‡ Many experts recommend hospitalization for all patients with PID, particularly adolescents.

§ Other treatment regimens for PID may be acceptable (see Pelvic Inflammatory Disease, p 393).

‖ For at least 48 hours after significant clinical improvement.

¶ For treatment of neurosyphilis, see Syphilis, p 512.

\# Not tested for safety in children and contraindicated in pregnancy.

DRUGS OF CHOICE FOR INVASIVE AND OTHER SERIOUS FUNGAL INFECTIONS IN CHILDREN

Table 5.4. Drugs of Choice for Invasive and Other Serious Fungal Infections*

Disease	Intravenous	Oral, Absorbable		Intravenous or Oral	
	Amphotericin B	Flucytosine	Ketoconazole	Itraconazole†	Fluconazole
Aspergillosis	P, S	S	...	A, M	...
Blastomycosis	P	...	A, M	A, M	...
Candidiasis:					
Chronic, mucocutaneous	A, S	S	P	...	A
Oropharyngeal, gastrointestinal	A (severe cases)	S	P	A	A, (P)
Systemic	P, S	S	...	...	A
Coccidioidomycosis	P	...	...	A, M	A, M
Cryptococcosis	C	C	...	A	A
Histoplasmosis	P	...	A, M	A, M	A, M
Mucormycosis (phycomycosis, zygomycosis)	P	...	...	...	...
Paracoccidioidomycosis (South American blastomycosis)	P‡ (severe cases)	...	P (nonsevere cases)	A, (P) (nonsevere cases)	...
Sporotrichosis	P	...	...	A, (P)	...

* P indicates preferred treatment in most cases (parentheses indicate drug is considered preferred treatment by some experts); M, for mild and moderately severe cases; A, efficacy less well established or alternative drug; C, combination recommended; S, combination recommended if infection is severe or central nervous system is involved.

† Efficacy and safety have not been established for children.

‡ Usually in combination with a sulfonamide or azole, such as ketoconazole or itraconazole.

RECOMMENDED DOSES OF PARENTERAL AND ORAL ANTIFUNGAL DRUGS

Table 5.5. **Recommended Doses of Parenteral and Oral Antifungal Drugs**

Drug	Route*	Dose (per day)	Adverse Reactions‡
Amphotericin B (see Systemic Treatment With Amphotericin B, p 630, for detailed information)	IV	0.25 mg/kg (after test dose) initially, increase as tolerated to 0.5-1 mg/kg; infuse as single dose during 4-6 h	Fever, chills, hypotension, renal dysfunction hypokalemia, anemia, cardiac arrhythmias, anaphylaxis, gastrointestinal symptoms, headache
	IT	0.025 mg, increase to 0.5 mg twice a week	Headache, gastrointestinal symptoms, arachnoiditis/radiculitis
Amphotericin B Lipid Complex§	IV	5 mg/kg given as single infusion at rate of 2.5 mg/kg/h	Fever, chills, other reactions associated with amphotericin B
Clotrimazole	PO	10-mg tablet 5 times a day (dissolved slowly in mouth)	Gastrointestinal symptoms, hepatotoxicity
Fluconazole	IV PO	Children‖: 3-6 mg/kg/d, single dose Adults: 200 mg once, followed by 100 mg/d for oropharyngeal, esophageal candidiasis; 400 mg once, followed by 200-400 mg/d for other invasive fungal infections; 200 mg/d for suppressive therapy in HIV-infected patients with cryptococcal meningitis	Rash, gastrointestinal symptoms, headache, probable hepatotoxicity
Flucytosine	PO	50 to 150 mg/kg in 4 doses at 6-h intervals (adjust dose if renal dysfunction)	Cardiorespiratory arrest, bone marrow suppression, renal dysfunction, hypokalemia, gastrointestinal symptoms, rash, neuropathy
Griseofulvin	PO	Ultramicrosize: 5-10 mg/kg, single dose; maximum dose, 750 mg. Microsize: 10-20 mg/kg/d divided in 2 doses; maximum dose, 1000 g	Rash, paresthesias, leukopenia, gastrointestinal symptoms, proteinuria, hepatotoxicity, mental confusion

Table 5.5. Recommended Doses of Parenteral and Oral Antifungal Drugs, continued

Drug	Route*	Dose (per day)	Adverse Reactions†‡
Itraconazole	PO	Children: dose not established; 3- to 16-y-old children have been treated with 100 mg/d Adults: 200 mg once or twice a day	Gastrointestinal symptoms, rash, edema, headache, hypokalemia, hepatotoxicity, hypertension
Ketoconazole	PO	Children¶: 3.3–6.6 mg/kg/d, single dose Adults: 200–400 mg once a day	Hepatotoxicity, gastrointestinal symptoms, rash, anaphylaxis, fever, thrombocytopenia, hemolytic anemia, gynecomastia, adrenal insufficiency
Nystatin	PO	Infants: 200 000 U, 4 times a day, after meals Children and adults: 400 000–600 000 U, 3 times a day, after meals	Gastrointestinal symptoms, rash

* IV indicates intravenous; IT, intrathecal; PO, oral.
† See package insert or listing in current edition of the *Physicians' Desk Reference.* Montvale, NJ: Medical Economics.
‡ Interactions with other drugs are common. Consult the *Physicians' Desk Reference*, a drug interaction reference or database, or a pharmacist before prescribing these medications.
§ Experience with drug in children is limited, but no serious adverse events have been reported.
‖ Limited or no information about use in newborns is available.
¶ For children 2 years and younger, the daily dose has not been established.

SYSTEMIC TREATMENT WITH AMPHOTERICIN B

Amphotericin B is the most important antifungal drug. However, because it causes many major and minor adverse reactions, particularly renal toxic effects, its parenteral use is primarily restricted to selected, potentially fatal fungal infections. Before using amphotericin B, the physician should consult the manufacturer's package insert for specific precautions, adverse reactions, and infusion information.

Amphotericin is administered in 5% or 10% dextrose in water at a concentration of 0.5 mg/mL for delivery through a central venous catheter, or at a concentration of 0.1 mg/mL for delivery through a peripheral venous catheter. Dilution of amphotericin B with solutions of high ionic strength may cause drug aggregation and should be avoided. Solutions that become turbid when amphotericin B is added should be discarded.

Amphotericin B is initially administered intravenously in a single test dose of 0.1 mg/kg (maximum, 1 mg) given during a 20-minute to 1-hour period to assess the patient's febrile and hemodynamic responses. Temperature, pulse, respiration, and blood pressure should be carefully monitored during the infusion. If no serious adverse effects are noted, therapeutic doses of 0.4/mg/kg or more can be given, beginning the same day as the test dose. The infusions usually are given during a 2- to 6-hour interval. Shorter infusion times of approximately 1 hour have not resulted in undue adverse reactions, but experience is insufficient to recommend routinely this procedure. The use of a test dose has also been challenged because of the improved formulation of amphotericin B and the lack of data on its predictive reliability, but controlled studies have not been performed.

Low doses of amphotericin B (eg, 0.1 to 0.3 kg/d) have been used successfully in infections such as esophagitis caused by *Candida* species. Conversely, doses of 1.25 to 1.5 mg/kg in some illnesses may be necessary and have been given. The proper dose for preterm and newborn infants has not been determined, but the aforementioned doses have been used successfully.

The serum concentration is not significantly increased in patients with impaired renal function. Hemodialysis and peritoneal dialysis do not significantly lower serum concentrations of the drug.

After completing 1 week of daily therapy, adequate serum concentrations of the drug usually can be maintained by administering double the daily dose (maximum, 1.5 mg/kg) on alternate days.

The duration of therapy depends on the type and extent of the specific fungal infection.

Commonly observed adverse reactions include the following: fever (sometimes with shaking chills), nausea and vomiting, headache, generalized body pains, pain at the intravenous administration site (phlebitis), abnormal renal function (eg, hypokalemia, elevated serum creatinine and blood urea nitrogen concentrations, decreased creatinine clearance rate, a diminished ability to concentrate urine, and renal tubular acidosis), and normochromic, normocytic anemia. Less common severe reactions include anuria, oliguria, thrombocytopenia, mild leukopenia, hypomagnesemia, cardiovascular toxicity (eg, arrhythmias, hypertension, and hypotension), anaphylactoid reactions, and convulsions and other neurologic symptoms. An irreversible reduction in the glomerular filtration rate often follows a therapeutic course of amphotericin B.

Nephrotoxicity can be prevented or reduced through the use of sodium loading. Multiple regimens have been used to attempt to prevent infusion-related reactions, but few have been studied in controlled clinical trials. Renal toxic effects may be enhanced with the concomitant administration of amphotericin B and aminoglycosides, cyclosporine, cisplatin, nitrogen mustard compounds, and acetazolamide. Pretreatment with antipyretics (eg, acetaminophen), alone or combined with diphenhydramine, may alleviate febrile reactions (although these reactions appear to be less common in children than in adults). Hydrocortisone (25 to 50 mg in adults) also can be added to the infusion to reduce febrile and other systemic reactions. Tolerance to the febrile reactions develops with time, allowing tapering and eventual discontinuation of the hydrocortisone. Both meperidine and ibuprofen have been effective in treating fever and chills. Some experts add heparin (500 to 1000 units) to the infusion to decrease phlebitis, although using lower concentrations of amphotericin B (less than 0.1 mg/mL), pediatric scalp-vein needles, venous-site rotation, and slow infusion rates are probably as effective.

Amphotericin B-lipid formulations have been under investigation in the United States and, as of 1996, only one, amphotericin B lipid complex (ABLC), has been approved for use. These formulations are less nephrotoxic than is amphotericin B and have a role in patients whose tolerance for amphotericin B is limited by nephrotoxicity. Originally ABLC was approved by the Food and Drug Administration only for the treatment of aspergillosis in adults, but the indication recently has been expanded to the treatment of invasive fungal infections in patients who are refractory to or intolerant of conventional amphotericin B therapy. Use in children in these circumstances also should be considered. These lipid formulations are currently undergoing clinical evaluation for treatment of other fungal infections and for use in children.

For patients with central nervous system fungal infections who do not experience the desired response to intravenous therapy, consideration should be given to the concomitant administration of amphotericin B intrathecally, intraventricularly, or intracisternally. Injections preferably should be given into the lateral ventricles through a cisternal Ommaya reservoir. The value of this approach has been clearly established only in coccidioidal meningitis, but it may be justified in the patient with other fungal infections that do not respond to treatment, as cerebrospinal fluid (CSF) concentrations of the drug are low or undetectable after intravenous administration of the drug. Amphotericin B may be administered twice weekly or more frequently in the lumbar, cisternal, or ventricular areas. The usual starting dose in adults is 0.025 mg three times a week; subsequent doses are increased by doubling until a maintenance dose of 0.5 mg is reached. Hydrocortisone (10 to 15 mg in adults) is added as required to relieve headaches. The solution should be freshly prepared and diluted with 2 to 10 mL of sterile 5% dextrose in water (10% dextrose in water for intralumbar injections) without preservatives. Before injection, the solution should be further diluted with CSF so that the final concentration per milliliter is one tenth the dose. Duration of therapy depends on the clinical and mycologic responses. Nausea, vomiting, urinary retention, leg and back pain, headache, transitory radiculitis, sensory loss, and foot drop have been observed as a result of intrathecal therapy; permanent changes have also occurred.

TOPICAL DRUGS FOR SUPERFICIAL FUNGAL INFECTIONS

Table 5.6. **Topical Drugs for Superficial Fungal Infections**

Drug	Strength	Formulation*†	Trade Name(s) (Examples)‡	Application(s) per Day	Adverse Reactions/Notes†
Amphotericin B	3%	C, L, O	Fungizone	2–4	Drying, local irritation, erythema, pruritus, burning; more effective topical preparations are now available
Ciclopirox	1%	C, L	Loprox	2	Irritation, erythema, burning
Clotrimazole	1%	C, L, S, Su	Desenex,§ Lotrimin,§ Mycelex§	2	Erythema, stinging, blistering, peeling, edema, pruritus, hives, burning
Econazole	1%	C	Spectazole	1–2	Burning, pruritus, stinging, erythema
Ketaconazole	2%	C, Sh	Nizoral	1	Irritation, pruritus, stinging
Miconazole	2%	C, P, S, Su	Desenex,§ Fungoid,§ Micatin,§ Monistat-Derm, Monistat-3	1–2	Irritation, dermatitis, pruritus
Nafifine	1%	C	Naftin	1	Burning, stinging, erythema, pruritus, irritation; fungicidal agent
Nystatin	100 000 U/mL or 100 000 U/g	C, L, P, O, Su	Mycolog, Mycostatin, Mytrex, Nilstat, Nystatin	2–3	Rare adverse reactions; effective against yeast only
Oxiconazole	1%	C	Oxistat	1	Pruritus, burning, irritation, erythema, folliculitis
Sulconazole	1%	C, S	Exelderm	1–2	Pruritus, burning, stinging
Terbinafine	1%	C	Lamisil	1–2	Pruritus, irritation, burning

Table 5.6. Topical Drugs for Superficial Fungal Infections

Drug	Strength	Formulation*	Trade Name(s) (Examples)‡	Application(s) per Day	Adverse Reactions/Notes†
Tolnaftate	1%	C, P, S	Desenex,§ Tinactin,§ Ting§	2	Rare adverse reactions
Undecylenate	10%–20%	P, C, O, L	Caldesene,§ Cruex,§ Desenex§	2	Irritation
Other Remedies					
Benzoic acid (6%) and salicylic acid (3%)	...	S, O	Whitfield's ointment§	2	Irritation, burning; potent keratolytic agent
Castellani's paint	...	S	...	1–2	Local irritation (contains basic fuchsin, phenol, resorcinol, acetone, alcohol)
Gentian violet‡	1%–2%	S	...	2	Staining
Selenium sulfide	2.5%	L, Sh	Exsel§	1	For tinea capitis,[‖][¶] tinea versicolor
	1%	Sh	Head & Shoulders,§ Selsun Blue§	1	For tinea capitis,[‖][¶] tinea versicolor[¶]
Sodium thiosulfate	25%	L	Tinver§	1–2	For tinea versicolor

* C indicates cream; F, foam; L, lotion; O, ointment; P, powder; S, solution; Sh, shampoo; Su, suppositories.

† For use in pregnancy, see package insert.

‡ Other products of these drugs also may be available.

§ Nonprescription drug.

‖ Reduces transmission only; primary therapy is oral griseofulvin. For further information, see Tinea Capitis, p 523.

¶ 1% shampoo may be used as a lotion for treatment. For further information, see Tinea Versicolor, p 529.

ANTIVIRAL DRUGS FOR NON-HIV INFECTIONS

Table 5.7 lists major antiviral drugs for children and adolescents, their indications, and dosages, exclusive of antiretroviral drugs. For indications and dosages of antiretroviral drugs, see HIV Infection, p 289 and p 290.

Table 5.7. Antiviral Drugs for Non-HIV Infections

Generic (Trade Name)	Indication	Route	Usually Recommended Dosage
Acyclovir* (Zovirax)	Genital herpes simplex virus (HSV) infection, first episode	Oral:	1000 mg/d in 5 divided doses or 1200 mg/d in 3 divided doses for 7–10 d†
		IV:	15 mg/kg/d in 3 divided doses for 5–7 d
	Genital HSV infection, recurrence	Oral:	1000 mg/d in 5 divided doses or 1200 mg/d in 3 divided doses or 1600 mg/d in 2 divided doses for 5 d†
	Genital HSV infection, chronic suppression	Oral:	1200 mg/d in 3 divided doses†
	Recurrent genital HSV episodes in patient with frequent recurrences, chronic suppressive therapy	Oral:	800–1000 mg/d in 2–5 divided doses for as long as 12 continuous months†
	HSV in immunocompromised host (localized, progressive, or disseminated)‡	IV:	For children <1 y, except neonates (see Neonatal HSV, p 266): 15–30 mg/kg/d in 3 divided doses for 7–14 d; some experts also recommend this dose for children ≥1 y
		IV:	For children ≥1 y: 750 mg/M²/d in 3 divided doses for 7–14 d; some experts recommend 1500 mg/M²/d in 3 divided doses
	Prophylaxis of HSV in immunocompromised HSV-seropositive patients‡	Oral:	1000 mg/d in 3–5 divided doses for 7–14 d†
		Oral:	600–1000 mg/d in 3–5 divided doses during risk period†
		IV:	750 mg/M²/d in 3 divided doses during risk period
	HSV encephalitis‡	IV:	For children <1 y: 30 mg/kg/d in 3 divided doses for a minimum of 14 d; some experts also recommend this dose for children ≥1 y

Table 5.7. Antiviral Drugs for Non-HIV Infections, continued

Generic (Trade Name)	Indication	Route	Usually Recommended Dosage
		IV:	For children ≥1 y: 1500 mg/M^2/d in 3 divided doses for 14–21 d; some experts also recommend this dose for children <1 y
	Neonatal HSV[‡]	IV:	30 mg/kg/d in 3 divided doses for 14–21 d; some experts recommend 45–60 mg/kg/d in 3 divided doses for term infants; for premature infants, 20 mg/kg/d in 2 divided doses is recommended for 14–21 d
	Varicella or zoster in immunocompromised host	IV:	For children <1 y: 30 mg/kg/d in 3 divided doses; some experts also recommend this dose for children ≥1 y
		IV:	For children ≥1 y: 1500 mg/M^2/d in 3 divided doses for 7–10 d
	Zoster in immuno-competent host[‡]	IV:	Same as for zoster in immunocompromised host
		Oral:	4000 mg/d in 5 divided doses for 5–7 d for patients ≥12 y[†]
	Varicella in immuno-competent host[§]	Oral:	80 mg/kg/d in 4 divided doses for 5 d; maximum dose, 3200 mg/d
	Prophylaxis of cyto-megalovirus (CMV) infection in immuno-compromised host (eg, transplant recipient)[‡]	Oral:	800–3200 mg/d in 1–4 divided doses during risk period[*†]
		IV:	1500 mg/M^2/d in 3 divided doses during risk period
Amantadine (Symmetrel)	Influenza A: treatment and prophylaxis	Oral:	See Influenza (p 314), including Table 3.32 (p 311)

Table 5.7. Antiviral Drugs for Non-HIV Infections, continued

Generic (Trade Name)	Indication	Route	Usually Recommended Dosage
Foscarnet* (Foscavir)	CMV retinitis in patients with AIDS	IV:	180 mg/kg/d in 2–3 divided doses for 14–21 d, then 90–120 mg/kg once a day as maintenance dose
	HSV infection resistant to acyclovir in immuno-compromised host‡	IV:	120 mg/kg/d in 3 divided doses until resolution of infection
Ganciclovir* (Cytovene)	Acquired CMV retinitis in immunocompromised host‖	IV:	10 mg/kg/d in 2 divided doses for 14–21 d; for long-term suppression, 5 mg/kg/d for 5–7 d/wk
	Prophylaxis of CMV in high-risk host‡	IV:	10 mg/kg/d in 2 divided doses for 1 wk, then 5 mg/kg/d in 1 dose for 100 d
Ribavirin (Virazole)	Treatment of respiratory syncytial virus (RSV) infection	Aerosol:	Given by a small-particle generator, in a solution of 6 g in 300 mL sterile water (20 mg/mL), for 12–20 h/d for 1–7 d; longer treatment may be necessary in some patient
Rimantadine (Flumadine)	Influenza A: treatment and prophylaxis	Oral:	See Influenza (p 314), including Table 3.32 (p 311)

* Dose should be decreased in patients with impaired renal function.
† Oral dosage of acyclovir in children should not exceed 80 mg/kg/d.
‡ Drug is not licensed for this indication or is investigational, as of December 1996.
§ Selective indications; see Varicella-Zoster Infections (p 573).
‖ Some experts use ganciclovir in immunocompromised host with CMV gastrointestinal disease and CMV pneumonitis (with or without CMV Immune Globulin Intravenous).

DRUGS FOR PARASITIC INFECTIONS

The following tables (5.8, 5.9, and 5.10) are reproduced from *The Medical Letter* (1995;37:99-108).* They provide recommendations that are likely to be consistent in many cases with those of the Committee on Infectious Diseases, as given in the chapters on specific diseases in Section 3. However, because *The Medical Letter* recommendations are developed independently and were issued in 1995, these recommendations occasionally may differ from those of the Committee. Accordingly, both should be consulted. The Committee thanks *The Medical Letter* for their courtesy in allowing this information to be reprinted.

In Table 5.8 (p 638), first-choice and alternative drugs with recommended adult and pediatric dosages for most parasitic infections are given. In each case, the need for treatment must be weighed against the toxic effects of the drug. A decision to withhold therapy often may be correct, particularly when the drugs can cause severe adverse effects. When the first-choice drug is initially ineffective and the alternative is more hazardous, a second course of treatment with the first drug before giving the alternative may be prudent. Adverse effects of some antiparasitic drugs are listed in Table 5.10 (p 661).

Several drugs recommended in Table 5.8 have not been approved by the Food and Drug Administration and, thus, are investigational (see footnotes). When prescribing an unapproved drug, the physician should inform the patient of the investigational status and adverse effects of the drug.

These recommendations are periodically (usually every other year) updated by *The Medical Letter* and, thus, are likely to be superseded by new ones before the next edition of the *Red Book* is published.

---

* Reprinted with permission from *The Medical Letter.*

Table 5.8. Drugs for Treatment of Parasitic Infections

Infection	Drug	Adult dosage*	Pediatric dosage*
AMEBIASIS (Entamoeba histolytica)[1]			
asymptomatic			
Drug of choice:	Iodoquinol[2]	650 mg tid × 20d	30–40 mg/kg/d in 3 doses x 20d
OR	Paromomycin	25–35 mg/kg/d in 3 doses x 7d	25–35 mg/kg/d in 3 doses x 7d
Alternative:	Diloxanide furoate[3]	500 mg tid × 10d	20 mg/kg/d in 3 doses × 10d
mild to moderate intestinal disease			
Drug of choice[4]:	Metronidazole	750 mg tid × 10d	35–50 mg/kd/d in 3 doses × 10d
OR	Tinidazole[5]	2 grams/d × 3d	50 mg/kg (max. 2 grams) qd × 3d
severe intestinal disease, hepatic abscess			
Drug of choice[4]:	Metronidazole	750 mg tid × 10d	35–50 mg/kd/d in 3 doses × 10d
OR	Tinidazole[5]	600 mg bid or 800 mg tid × 5d	50 mg/kg or 60 mg/kg (max. 2 grams) qd × 3d
AMEBIC (Acanthamoeba) keratitis			
Drug of choice:	See footnote 6		
AMEBIC MENINGOENCEPHALITIS, PRIMARY			
Naegleria			
Drug of choice:	Amphotericin B[7, 8]	1 mg/kg/d IV, uncertain duration	1 mg/kg/d IV, uncertain duration
Acanthamoeba			
Drug of choice:	See footnote 9		
ANCYLOSTOMA caninum (Eosinophilic enterocolitis)			
Drug of choice:	Mebendazole	100 mg bid × 3d	100 mg bid × 3d
OR	Pyrantel pamoate[8]	11 mg/kg (max. 1 gram) × 3d	11 mg/kg (max. 1 gram) × 3d
OR	Albendazole	400 mg once	400 mg once
Ancylostoma duodenale, see HOOKWORM			

ANGIOSTRONGYLIASIS

Angiostrongylus cantonensis
Drug of choice[10]:

Mebendazole[8]	100 mg bid × 5d	100 mg bid × 5d

Angiostrongylus costaricensis
Drug of choice:

Thiabendazole[8]	75 mg/kg/d in 3 doses × 3d (max. 3 grams/d)[11]	75 mg/kg/d in 3 doses x 3d (max. 3 grams/d)[11]

Alternative:

Mebendazole	200–400 mg tid × 10d	200–400 mg tid × 10d

* The letter d stands for day.

1 Entamoeba histolytica and E. dispar, until recently termed "pathogenic" and "nonpathogenic" E. histolytica, respectively, are morphologically indistinguishable.

2 Dosage and duration of administration should not be exceeded because of possibility of causing optic neuritis; maximum dosage is 2 grams/day.

3 In the USA, this drug is available from the CDC Drug Service, Centers for Disease Control and Prevention, Atlanta, Georgia 30333; telephone: 404-639-3670 (evenings, weekends, and holidays: 404-639-2888).

4 Treatment should be followed by a course of iodoquinol or one of the other intraluminal drugs used to treat asymptomatic amebiasis.

5 A nitro-imidazole similar to metronidazole, but not marketed in the USA; tinidazole appears to be at least as effective as metronidazole and better tolerated. Ornidazole, a similar drug, is also used outside the USA. Higher dosage is for hepatic abscess.

6 Trophozoites and cysts of *Acanthamoeba* from infected corneas, contact lenses and their cases are susceptible *in vitro* to chlorhexidine, polyhexamethylene biguanide, propamidine, pentamidine, diminazine and neomycin and, especially, to combinations of these drugs (J Hay et al, Eye, 8:555, 1994). For treatment of iritic keratitis plus topical miconazole, have been successful (MB Moore et al, Br J Ophthalmol, 73:271, 1989; Y Ishabashi et al, Am J Ophthalmol, 109:121, 1990). Recently, 0.02% topical polyhexamethylene biguanide (PHMB) has been used successfully in a large number of patients (MJ Elder et al, Lancet, 345:791, 1995). PHMB is available as Baquacil (ICI America), a swimming pool disinfectant (E Yee and TK Winarko, Am J Hosp Pharm, 50:2523, 1993).

7 Naegleria infections have been treated successfully with amphotericin B, rifampin and chloramphenicol (A Wang et al, Clin Neurol Neurosurg, 95:249, 1993), amphotericin B, oral rifampin and oral ketoconazole (N Poungvarin et al, J Med Assoc Thailand, 74:112, 1991), and amphotericin B alone (RL Brown, Arch Intern Med, 152:1330, 1992).

8 An approved drug, but considered investigational for this condition by the U.S. Food and Drug Administration.

9 Strains of *Acanthamoeba* isolated from fatal granulomatous amebic encephalitis are usually susceptible *in vitro* to pentamidine, ketoconazole *(Nizoral)*, flucytosine and (less so) to amphotericin B. One patient with disseminated infection was treated successfully with intravenous pentamidine isethionate, topical chlorhexidine and 2% ketoconazole cream, followed by oral itraconazole (CA Slater et al, N Engl J Med, 331:85, 1994).

10 Most patients recover spontaneously without antiparasitic drug therapy. Analgesics, corticosteroids, and careful removal of CSF at frequent intervals can relieve symptoms (J Koo et al, Rev Infect Dis, 10:1155, 1988). Albendazole, levamisole *(Ergamisol)*, or ivermectin has also been used successfully in animals.

11 This dose is likely to be toxic and may have to be decreased.

Table 5.8. Drugs for Treatment of Parasitic Infections, continued

Infection	Drug	Adult dosage*	Pediatric dosage*
ANISAKIASIS (Anisakis)			
Treatment of choice:	Surgical or endo-scopic removal		
ASCARIASIS (Ascaris lumbricoides, roundworm)			
Drug of choice:	Mebendazole	100 mg bid × 3d	100 mg bid × 3d
OR	Pyrantel pamoate	11 mg/kg once (max. 1 gram)	11 mg/kg once (max. 1 gram)
OR	Albendazole	400 mg once	400 mg once
BABESIOSIS (Babesia spp.)			
Drugs of choice[12]:	Clindamycin[8]	1.2 grams bid IV or 500 mg tid PO × 7d	20-40 mg/kg/d in 3 doses × 7d
	plus quinine	650 mg tid PO × 7d	25 mg/kg/d in 3 doses × 7d
BALANTIDIASIS (Balantidium coli)			
Drug of choice:	Tetracyclin[8]	500 mg qid × 10d	40 mg/kg/d in 4 doses × 10d (max. 2 grams/d)[13]
Alternatives:	Iodoquinol[2,8]	650 mg tid × 20d	40 mg/kg/d in 3 doses × 20d
	Metronidazole[8]	750 mg tid × 5d	35-50 mg/kg/d in 3 doses × 5d
BAYLISASCARIASIS (Baylisascaris procyonis)			
Drug of choice:	See footnote 14		
BLASTOCYSTIS hominis infection			
Drug of choice:	See footnote 15		
CAPILLARIASIS (Capillaria philippinensis)			
Drug of choice:	Mebendazole[8]	200 mg bid × 20d	200 mg bid × 20d
Alternatives:	Albendazole	200 mg bid × 10d	200 mg bid × 10d
	Thiabendazole[8]	25 mg/kg/d in 2 doses × 30d	25 mg/kg/d in 2 doses × 30d

Chagas' disease, see TRYPANOSOMIASIS

Clonorchis sinensis, see FLUKE infection

CRYPTOSPORIDIOSIS (*Cryptosporidium*)

Drug of choice[16]:	Paromomycin	500–750 mg qid

CUTANEOUS LARVA MIGRANS (creeping eruption, dog and cat hookworm)

Drug of choice[17]:	Thiabendazole	Topically ± 50 mg/kg/d PO in 2 doses (max. 3 grams/d) × 2–5d[11]	Topically ± 50 mg/kg/d PO in 2 doses (max. 3 grams/d) × 2–5[11]
OR	Ivermectin	150–200 µg/kg once	150–200 µg/kg once
OR	Albendazole	200 mg bid × 3d	200 mg bid × 3d

CYCLOSPORA infection

Drug of choice:	Trimethoprim-sulfamethoxazole[18]	TMP 160 mg, SMX 800 mg bid x 7 days	TMP 5 mg/kg, SMX 25 mg/kg bid x 7 days

CYSTICERCOSIS, see TAPEWORM infection

12 Atovaquone suspension, 750 mg b.i.d., plus azithromycin, 500 to 1000 mg daily, may be effective when quinine and clindamycin fail. Exchange transfusion has been used in severely ill patients with high (>10%) parasitemia (V Iacopino and T Earnhart, Arch Intern Med. 150:1527, 1990). One report indicates that azithromycin (*Zithromax*), 500–1000 mg daily, plus quinine may also be effective (LM Weiss et al, J Infect Dis, 168:1289, 1993). Concurrent use of pentamidine and trimethoprim-sulfamethoxazole has been reported to cure an infection with *B. divergens* (D Raoult et al, Ann Intern Med, 107:944, 1987).

13 Not recommended for use in children less than eight years old.

14 Drugs that could be tried include albendazole, mebendazole, thiabendazole, levamisole (*Ergamisol*) and ivermectin. Steroid therapy may be helpful, especially in eye and CNS infections. Ocular baylisascariasis has been treated successfully using laser photocoagulation therapy to destroy the intraretinal larvae.

15 Clinical significance of these organisms is controversial, but metronidazole 750 mg tid × 10 d or iodoquinol 650 mg tid × 20d anecdotally has been reported to be effective (PFL Borehamand D Stenzel, Adv Parasitol, 32:2, 1993; JS Keystone, EK Markell, Clin Infect Dis, 21:102 and 104, July 1995).

16 Infection is self-limited in immunocompetent patients. In HIV-infected patients paromomycin has limited effectiveness (AC White et al, J Infect Dis. 170:419, 1994; F Bissuel, Clin Infect Dis, 18:447, 1994). In unpublished clinical trials, azithromycin 1250 mg daily for two weeks followed by 500 mg daily, has apparently been effective in some patients.

17 E Caumes et al, Am J Trop Med Hyg. 49:641, 1993; P Wolf et al, Hautarzt, 44:462, 1993; HD Davies et al, Arch Dermatol, 129:588, 1993.

18 HIV-infected patients may need higher dosage and long-term maintenance (JW Pape et al, Ann Intern Med. 121:654, 1994).

Table 5.8. **Drugs for Treatment of Parasitic Infections, continued**

Infection	Drug	Adult dosage*	Pediatric dosage*
DIENTAMOEBA *fragilis* infection			
Drug of choice:	Iodoquinol[2]	650 mg tid × 20d	40 mg/kg/d in 3 doses × 20d
OR	Paromomycin	25–30 mg/kg/d in 3 doses × 7d	25–30 mg/kg/d in 3 doses × 7d
OR	Tetracycline[8]	500 mg qid × 10d	40 mg/kg/d (max. 2 grams/d) in 4 doses × 10d[13]
Diphyllobothrium latum, see TAPEWORM infection			
DRACUNCULUS medinensis (guinea worm) infection			
Drug of choice:	Metronidazole[8, 19]	250 mg tid × 10d	25 mg/kg/d (max. 750 mg/d) in 3 doses × 10d
Alternative:	Thiabendazole[8, 19]	50–75 mg/kg/d in 2 doses × 3d[11]	
Echinococcus, see TAPEWORM infection			
Entamoeba histolytica, see AMEBIASIS			
ENTAMOEBA polecki infection			
Drug of choice:	Metronidazole[8]	750 mg tid × 10d	35-50 mg/kg/d in 3 doses × 10d
ENTEROBIUS vermicularis (pinworm) infection			
Drug of choice:	Pyrantel pamoate	11 mg/kg once (max. 1 gram); repeat after 2 weeks	11 mg/kg once (max. 1 gram); repeat after 2 weeks
OR	Mebendazole	A single dose of 100 mg; repeat after 2 weeks	A single dose of 100 mg; repeat after 2 weeks
OR	Albendazole	400 mg once; repeat in 2 weeks	400 mg once; repeat in 2 weeks
Fasciola hepatica, see FLUKE infection			
FILARIASIS			
Wuchereria bancrofti, Brugia malayi			
Drug of choice[20]:	Diethylcarbamazine[21]	Day 1: 50 mg, p.c.	Day 1: 1 mg, p.c.

Infection / Drug		Adult dosage	Pediatric dosage
		Day 2: 50 mg tid Day 3: 100 mg tid Days 4 through 21: 6 mg/kg/d in 3 doses[22]	Day 2: 1 mg tid Day 3: 1–2 mg tid Days 4 through 21: 6 mg/kg/d in 3 doses[22]
Loa loa Drug of choice[23]:	Diethylcarbamazine[21]	Day 1: 50 mg, oral, p.c. Day 2: 50 mg tid Day 3: 100 mg tid Days 4 through 21: 9 mg/kg/d in 3 doses[22]	Day 1: 1 mg, oral, p.c. Day 2: 1 mg tid Day 3: 1–2 mg tid Days 4 through 21: 9 mg/kg/d in 3 doses[22]
Mansonella ozzardi Drug of choice:	See footnote 24		
Mansonella perstans Drug of choice:	Mebendazole[8]	100 mg bid × 30d	100 mg bid × 30d
Tropical Pulmonary Eosinophilia (TPE) Drug of choice:	Diethylcarbamazine	6 mg/kg/d in 3 doses × 21d	6 mg/kg/d in 3 doses × 21d
Onchocerca volvulus Drug of choice:	Ivermectin[3]	150 µ/kg once, repeated every 3 to 12 months	150 µg/kg once, repeated every 3 to 12 months

19 Not curative, but decreases inflammation and facilitates removing the worm. Mebendazole 400-800 mg/d for 6d has been reported to kill the worm directly.

20 A single dose of ivermectin, 20-200 µg/kg, has been reported to be effective for treatment of microfilaremia (SK Kar et al, Southeast Asian J Trop Med Public Health, 24:80, 1993).

21 Antihistamines or corticosteroids may be required to decrease allergic reactions due to disintegration of microfilariae in treatment of filarial infections, especially those caused by *Loa loa*.

22 For patients with no microfilariae in the blood, full doses can be given from day one.

23 Diethylcarbamazine should be administered with special caution in heavy infections with *Loa loa* because rapid killing of microfilariae can provoke an encephalopathy. Ivermectin or albendazole has been used to reduce microfilaremia (Y Martin-Prevel et al, Am J Trop Med Hyg, 48:186, 1993; AD Klion et al, J Infect Dis, 168:202, 1993). Apheresis has been reported to be effective in lowering microfilarial counts in patients heavily infected with *Loa loa* (EA Ottesen, Infect Dis Clin North Am, 7:619, 1993). Diethylcarbamazine, 300 mg once weekly, has been recommended for prevention of loiasis (TB Nutman et al, N Engl J Med, 319:752, 1988).

24 Diethylcarbamazine has no effect. Ivermectin, 150 µg/kg, may be effective (TB Nutman et al, J Infect Dis, 156:622, 1987).

Table 5.8. Drugs for Treatment of Parasitic Infections, continued

Infection	Drug	Adult dosage*	Pediatric dosage*
FLUKE, hermaphroditic, infection			
***Clonorchis sinensis* (Chinese liver fluke)**			
Drug of choice:	Praziquantel	75 mg/kg/d in 3 doses × 1d	75 mg/kg/d in 3 doses × 1d
OR	Albendazole	10 mg/kg × 7d	
***Fasciola hepatica* (sheep liver fluke)**			
Drug of choice[25]:	Bithionol[3]	30–50 mg/kg on alternate days × 10–15 doses	30–50 mg/kg on alternate days × 10–15 doses
***Fasciolopsis buski* (intestinal fluke)**			
Drug of choice:	Praziquantel[8]	75 mg/kg/d in 3 doses × 1d	75 mg/kg/d in 3 doses × 1d
***Heterophyes heterophyes* (intestinal fluke)**			
Drug of choice:	Praziquantel[8]	75 mg/kg/d in 3 doses × 1d	75 mg/kg/d in 3 doses × 1d
***Metagonimus yokogawai* (intestinal fluke)**			
Drug of choice:	Praziquantel[8]	75 mg/kg/d in 3 doses × 1d	75 mg/kg/d in 3 doses × 1d
Nanophyetus salmincola			
Drug of choice:	Praziquantel[8]	60 mg/kg/d in 3 doses × 1d	60 mg/kg/d in 3 doses × 1d
***Opisthorchis viverrini* (liver fluke)**			
Drug of choice:	Praziquantel	75 mg/kg/d in 3 doses × 1d	75 mg/kg/d in 3 doses × 1d
***Paragonimus westermani* (lung fluke)**			
Drug of choice:	Praziquantel[8]	75 mg/kg/d in 3 doses × 2d	75 mg/kg/d in 3 doses × 2d
Alternative[26]:	Bithionol[3]	30–50 mg/kg on alternate days × 10–15 doses	30–50 mg/kg on alternate days × 10–15 doses

GIARDIASIS (Giardia lamblia)

Drug of choice[27]:		
	Metronidazole[8]	250 mg tid × 5d
Alternatives[27]:		
	Tinidazole[5]	2 grams once
	Furazolidone	100 mg qid × 7–10d
	Paromomycin[28]	25–35 mg/kg/d in 3 doses × 7d

GNATHOSTOMIASIS (Gnathostoma spinigerum)

Treatment of choice[29]:	Surgical removal	
	plus	
	Albendazole[30]	400–800 mg qd × 21d

HOOKWORM infection (Ancylostoma duodenale, Necator americanus)

Drug of choice:	Mebendazole	100 mg bid × 3d
OR	Pyrantel pamoate[8]	11 mg/kg (max. 1 gram) × 3d
OR	Albendazole	400 mg once

Hydatid cyst, see TAPEWORM infection

Hymenolepis nana, see TAPEWORM infection

ISOSPORIASIS (Isospora belli)

Drug of choice:	Trimethoprim-sulfamethoxazole[8,31]	160 mg TMP, 800 mg SMX qid × 10d, then bid × 3 wks

---

25 Unlike infections with other flukes, *Fasciola hepatica* infections may not respond to praziquantel. Recent data indicate that triclabendazole (*Fasinex*), a veterinary fasciolide, is safe and effective in a single oral dose of 10 mg/kg (W Apt et al, Am J Trop Med Hyg, 52:532, 1995).

26 Unpublished data indicate triclabendazole (*Fasinex*), a veterinary fasciolide, may be effective in a dosage of 5 mg/kg once daily for 3 days or 10 mg/kg twice in one day.

27 Furazolidone has been reported to be mutagenic and carcinogenic. Albendazole 400 mg daily × 5d may be effective (A Hall and Q Nahar, Trans R Soc Trop Med Hyg, 87:84, 1993). Bacitracin zinc or bacitracin 120,000 U bid for 10 days may also be effective (BJ Andrews et al, Am J Trop Med Hyg, 52:318, 1995).

28 Not absorbed and not highly effective, but may be useful for treatment of giardiasis in pregnancy.

29 Ivermectin has been reported to be effective in animals (MT Anantaphruti et al, Trop Med Parasitol, 43:65, 1992).

30 P Kraivichian et al, Trans R Soc Trop Med Hyg, 86:418, 1992.

31 In sulfonamide-sensitive patients, such as some HIV-infected patients, pyrimethamine 50–75 mg daily has been effective (LM Weiss et al, Ann Intern Med, 109:474, 1988). In immunocompromised patients, it may be necessary to continue therapy indefinitely.

Table 5.8. Drugs for Treatment of Parasitic Infections, continued

Infection	Drug	Adult dosage*	Pediatric dosage*
LEISHMANIASIS (L. mexicana, L. tropica, L. major, L. braziliensis, L. donovani [Kala-azar])			
Drug of choice:	Sodium stibogluconate[3]	20 mg Sb/kg/d IV or IM × 20–28d[32]	20 mg Sb/kg/d IV or IM × 20–28d[32]
OR	Meglumine antimonate	20 mg Sb/kg/d × 20–28d[32]	20 mg Sb/kg/d × 20–28d[32]
Alternatives[33]:	Amphotericin B[8]	0.25 to 1 mg/kg by slow infusion daily or every 2d for up to 8 wks	0.25 to 1 mg/kg by slow infusion daily or every 2d for up to 8 wks
	Pentamidine isethionate[8]	2–4 mg/kg daily or every 2d IM for up to 15 doses[32]	2–4 mg/kg daily or every 2 d IM for up to 15 doses[32]
LICE infestation (Pediculus humanus, capitis, Phthirus pubis)[34]			
Drug of choice:	1% Permethrin[35]	Topically	Topically
OR	0.5% Malathion	Topically	Topically
Alternative:	Pyrethrins with piperonyl butoxide	Topically[36]	Topically[36]
Loa loa, see FILARIASIS			
MALARIA, Treatment of (Plasmodium falciparum, P. ovale, P. vivax, and P. malariae)			
Chloroquine-resistant P. falciparum[37]			
ORAL			
Drugs of choice:	Quinine sulfate	650 mg q8h × 3–7d[38]	25 mg/kg/d in 3 doses × 3–7d[38]
plus	pyrimethamine-sulfaxodoxine[39]	3 tablets at once on last day of quinine	<1 yr: ¼ tablet 1–3 yrs: ½ tablet 4–8 yrs: 1 tablet 9–14 yrs: 2 tablets
	plus tetracycline[8]	250 mg qid × 7d	20 mg/kg/d in 4 doses x 7d[13]
OR	plus clindamycin[8]	900 mg tid × 3–5d	20-40 mg/kg/d in 3 doses × 3–5d

Alternatives:[41]		
OR[40]		
Mefloquine[42,43]	1250 mg[44]	25 mg/kg once[45] (<45 kg)
Halofantrine[46]	500 mg q6h × 3 doses; repeat in 1 week	8 mg/kg q6h × 3 doses (<40 kg); repeat in 1 week

32 May be repeated or continued. A longer duration may be needed for some forms of visceral leishmaniasis.

33 Limited data indicate that ketoconazole (Nizoral), 400 to 600 mg daily for four to eight weeks, may be effective for treatment of cutaneous leishmaniasis (RE Saenz et al, Am J Med, 89:147, 1990). Some studies indicate that L. donovani resistant to sodium stibogluconate or meglumine antimonate may respond to recombinant human gamma interferon in addition to antimony (R Badaro and WD Johnson, J Infect Dis, 167 suppl 1:S13, 1993), or pentamidine followed by a course of antimony (CP Thakur et al, Am J Trop Med Hyg, 45:435, 1991). Liposomal encapsulated amphoterici B (AmBisome, Vestar, San Dimas, CA) has been used successfully to treat multiple-drug-resistant visceral leishmaniasis (RN Davidson et al, Q J Med, 87:75, 1994; R Dietze et al, Clin Infect Dis, 17:981, 1993). Recently the combination of aminosidine (chemically identical to paromomycin) and sodium stibogluconate has been used to decrease the time to clinical cure of kala-azar (CP Thakur et al, Trans R Soc Trop Med Hyg, 89:219, 1995) and to cure diffuse cutaneous leishmaniasis caused by L. aethiopica (S Teklemariam et al, Trans R Soc Trop med Hyg, 88:334, 1994). In addition, preliminary studies suggest that aminosidine ointment appears to be effective in the treatment of cutaneous Old World leishmaniasis (ADM Bryceson et al, Trans R Soc Trop Med Hyg, 88:226, 1994).

34 For infestation of eyelashes with crab lice use petrolatum.

35 FDA-approved only for head lice.

36 Some consultants recommend a second application one week later to kill hatching progeny.

37 Chloroquine-resistant P. falciparum infections occur in all malarious areas except Central America west of the Panama Canal Zone, Mexico, Haiti, the Dominican Republic, and most of the Middle East (chloroquine resistance has been reported in Yemen, Oman and Iran).

38 In Southeast Asia and possibly in other areas, such as South America, relative resistance to quinine has increased and the treatment should be continued for seven days.

39 Fansidar tablets contain 25 mg of pyrimethamine and 500 mg of sulfadoxine. Resistance to pyrimethamine-sulfadoxine has been reported from Southeast Asia, the Amazon basin, East Africa, Bangladesh and Oceania.

40 In pregnancy.

41 For treatment of multiple-drug-resistant P. falciparum in Southeast Asia, especially Thailand, where resistance to mefloquine and halofantrine frequently occur, a 7-day course of quinine and tetracycline is recommended (G Watt et al, Am J Trop Med Hyg, 47:108, 1992). Combinations of artesunate plus mefloquine (C Luxemburger et al, Trans R Soc Trop Med Hyg, 88:213, 1994), aretemether plus mefloquine (J Karbwang et al, Trans R Soc Trop Med Hyg, 89:296, 1995) or mefloquine plus tetracycline are also used to treat multiple-drug-resistant P. falciparum.

42 At this dosage, adverse effects including nausea, vomiting, diarrhea, dizziness, disturbed sense of balance, toxic psychosis and seizures can occur. Mefloquine is teratogenic in animals and it has not been approved for use in pregnancy, but mefloquine prophylaxis has been reported to be safe and effective when used during the second half of pregnancy (F Nosten et al, J Infect Dis, 169:595, 1994). Limited studies also have demonstrated its efficacy in treating P. falciparum malaria during pregnancy (K Na Bangchang et al, Trans R Soc Trop Med Hyg, 88:321, 1994). It should not be given together with quinine or quinidine, and caution is required in using quinine or quinidine to treat patients with malaria who have taken mefloquine for prophylaxis. The pediatric dosage has not bee approved by the FDA. Resistance to mefloquine has been reported in some areas, such as the Thailand-Myanmar border and the Amazon region, where 25 mg/kg should be used.

43 In the USA, a 250-mg tablet of mefloquine contains 228 mg of mefloquine base. Outside the USA, each 275-mg tablet contains 250 mg base.

44 750 mg followed 6–8 hours later by 500 mg.

Table 5.8. **Drugs for Treatment of Parasitic Infections, continued**

Infection	Drug	Adult dosage*	Pediatric dosage*
PARENTERAL Drug of choice[47,48]:	Quinidine gluconate[49,50]	10 mg/kg loading dose (max. 600 mg) in normal saline slowly over 1 to 2 hrs, followed by continuous infusion of 0.02 mg/kg/min until oral therapy can be started	Same as adult dose
OR	Quinine dihydrochloride[50,51]	20 mg/kg loading dose in 10 mg/kg 5% dextrose over 4 hrs, followed by 10 mg/kg over 2–4 hrs q8h (max. 1800 mg/d) until oral therapy can be started	Same as adult dose

All Plasmodium except Chloroquine-resistant *P. falciparum*[37]

Infection	Drug	Adult dosage*	Pediatric dosage*
ORAL Drug of choice:	Chloroquine phosphate[52,53]	1 gram (600 mg base), then 500 mg (300 mg base) 6 hrs later, then 500 mg (300 mg base) at 24 and 48 hrs	10 mg base/kg (max. 600 mg base), then 5 mg base/kg 6 hrs later, then 5 mg base/kg at 24 and 48 hrs
PARENTERAL Drug of choice[48]:	Quinidine gluconate[49,50]	same as above	same as above
OR	Quinine dihydrochloride[50,51]	same as above	same as above

Prevention of relapses: *P. vivax* and *P. ovale* only

Drug of choice: Primaquine phosphate[54,55]

26.3 mg (15 mg base)/d × 14d or 79 mg (45 mg base)/wk x 8 wks

0.3 mg base/kg/d × 14d

---

45 NJ White, Eur J Clin Pharmacol, 34:1, 1988.

46 May be effective in multiple-drug-resistant *P. falciparum* malaria, but treatment failures and resistance have been reported, and the drug causes consistent dose-related lengthening of the PR and Qtc intervals (A Castot et al, Lancet, 341:1541, 1993). Several patients have developed first degree block (F Nosten et al, Lancet 341:1054, 1993). The micronized form of halofantrine has improved its bioavailability, but variability in absorption remains an important problem (J Karbwang et al, Clin Pharmacokinet, 27:104, 1994). It should not be taken one hour before to three hours after meals and should not be used for patients with cardiac conduction defects. Cardiac monitoring is recommended.

47 One study found artemether, a Chinese drug, effective for parenteral treatment of severe malaria in children (NJ White et al, Lancet, 339:317, 1992).

48 Exchange transfusion has been helpful for some patients with high-density (>10%) parasitemia, altered mental status, pulmonary edema or renal complications (JR Zucker and CC Campbell, Infect Dis Clin North Am, 7:547, 1993).

49 Continuous EKG, blood pressure and glucose monitoring are recommended.

50 Quinidine may have greater antimalarial activity than quinine. The loading dose should be decreased or omitted in those patients who have received quinine or mefloquine. If more than 48 hours of parenteral treatment is required, the quinine or quinidine dose should be reduced by ⅓ to ½.

51 Not available in the USA. With IV administration of quinine dihydrochloride, monitoring of EKG and blood pressure is recommended. Use of parenteral quinine or quinidine may also lead to severe hypoglycemia; blood glucose should be monitored.

52 If chloroquine phosphate is not available, hydroxychloroquine sulfate is as effective; 400 mg of hydroxychloroquine sulfate is equivalent to 500 mg of chloroquine phosphate.

53 In *P. falciparum* malaria, if the patient has not shown a response to conventional doses of chloroquine in 48-72 hours, parasitic resistance to this drug should be considered. *P. vivax* with decreased susceptibility to chloroquine has been reported from Papua-New Guinea, Brazil, Myanmar, India, Colombia, and Indonesia; a single dose of mefloquine, 15 mg/kg, has been recommended to treat these infections.

54 Some relapses have been reported with this regimen; relapses should be treated with chloroquine plus primaquine, 22.5 to 30 mg base/d x 14 days.

55 Primaquine phosphate can cause hemolytic anemia, especially in patients whose red cells are deficient in glucose-6-phosphate dehydrogenase. This deficiency is most common in Africa, Asia, and Mediterranean peoples. Patients should be screened for G-6-PD deficiency before treatment. Primaquine should not be used during pregnancy.

Table 5.8. Drugs for Treatment of Parasitic Infections, continued

Infection	Drug	Adult dosage*	Pediatric dosage*
MALARIA, Prevention of			
Chloroquine-sensitive areas			
Drug of choice:	Chloroquine phosphate[58]	500 mg (300 mg base), once/week[59]	5 mg/kg base once/week, up to adult dose of 300 mg base
Chloroquine-resistant areas[37]			
Drug of choice:	Mefloquine[53,58,61]	250 mg once/week[59]	15–19 kg: ¼ tablet 20–30 kg: ½ tablet 31–45 kg: ¾ tablet >45 kg: 1 tablet
	Doxycycline[58,62]	100 mg daily[62]	>8 years of age: 2 mg/kg/d, up to 100 mg/day
Alternatives: OR	Chloroquine phosphate[58] **plus**	same as above	same as above
	Pyrimethamine-sulfadoxine[39] for presumptive treatment	Carry a single dose (3 tablets) for self-treatment of febrile illness when medical care is not immediately available	<1 yr: ¼ tablet 1–3 yrs: ½ tablet 4–8 yrs: 1 tablet 9–14 yrs: 2 tablets
	or **plus** proguanil[63] (in Africa south of the Sahara)	200 mg daily	<2 yrs: 50 mg daily 2–6 yrs: 100 mg daily 7–10 yrs: 150 mg daily >10 yrs: 200 mg daily

MICROSPORIDIOSIS

Ocular (*Encephalitozoon bellem, Vittaforma corneae [Nosema corneum]*)
Drug of choice: See footnote 64

Intestinal (*Enterocytozoon bieneusi, Septata [Encephalitozoon] intestinalis*)

Drug of choice: See footnote 65

Disseminated (*Encephalitozoon hellem, Encephalitozoon cuniculi, Pleistophora sp.*)

Drug of choice: See footnote 66

Mites, see SCABIES

56 No drug regimen guarantees protection against malaria. If fever develops within a year (particularly within the first two months) after travel to malarious areas, travelers should be advised to seek medical attention. Insect repellents, insecticide-impregnated bed nets and proper clothing are important adjuncts for malaria prophylaxis.

57 In pregnancy, chloroquine prophylaxis has been used extensively and safely, but the safety of other prophylactic antimalarial agents in pregnancy is unclear. Therefore, travel during pregnancy to chloroquine-resistant areas should be discouraged. (See footnote 42.)

58 For prevention of attack after departure from areas where *P. vivax* and *P. ovale* are endemic, which includes almost all areas where malaria is found (except Haiti), some experts prescribe in addition primaquine phosphate 15 mg base (26.3 mg)/d or, for children, 0.3 mg base/kd/g during the last two weeks of prophylaxis. Others prefer to avoid the toxicity of primaquine and rely on surveillance to detect cases when they occur, particularly when exposure was limited or doubtful. See also footnote 54 and 55.

59 Beginning one week before travel and continuing weekly for the duration of stay and for four weeks after leaving.

60 Several recent studies have shown that daily primaquine provides effective prophylaxis against chloroquine-resistant *P. falciparum* (WR Weiss et al, J Infect Dis, 171:1569, June 1995).

61 The pediatric dosage has not been approved by the FDA, and the drug has not been approved for use during pregnancy. Women should take contraceptive precautions while taking mefloquine and for two months after the last dose. Mefloquine is not recommended for patients with cardiac conduction abnormalities. Patients with a history of seizures or psychiatric disorders and those whose occupation requires fine coordination or spatial discrimination should probably avoid mefloquine (Medical Letter, 32:13, 1990). Resistance to mefloquine has been reported in some areas, such as Thailand; in these areas, doxycycline should be used for prophylaxis.

62 Beginning one day before travel and continuing for the duration of stay and for four weeks after leaving. Use of tetracyclines is contraindicated in pregnancy and in children less than eight years old. Doxycycline can cause gastrointestinal disturbances, vaginal moniliasis and photosensitivity reactions.

63 Proguanil (*Paludrine*—Ayerst, Canada; ICI, England), which is not available in the USA but is widely available overseas, is recommended mainly for use in Africa south of the Sahara. Prophylaxis is recommended during exposure and for four weeks afterwards. Failures in prophylaxis with chloroquine and proguanil have been reported in travelers to Kenya (AJ Barnes, Lancet, 338:1338, 1991).

64 Ocular lesions due to *E. hellem* in HIV-infected patients have responded to fumagillin eyedrops prepared from *Fumidil-B*, a commercial product used to control a microsporidial disease of honey bees, available from Mid-Continent Agrimarketing, Inc., Lenexa, Kansas 66215 (MC Diesenhouse, Am J Ophthalmol, 115:293, in an HIV-infected patient was treated successfully with surgical debridement, topical antibiotics and itraconazole (RW Yee et al, Ophthalmology, 97:953, 1990).

65 Albendazole, 400 mg bid may be effective for *S. intestinalis* infections (C Blanshard et al, AIDS, 6:311, 1992) and may be helpful for *E. bieneusi* infections (DT Dieterich et al, J Infect Dis, 169:178, 1994). Octreotide (*Sandostatin*) has provided symptomatic relief in some patients with large volume diarrhea.

66 Albendazole 400 mg bid may be effective for *E. hellem* and *E. cuniculi*. There is no established treatment for *Pleistophora*.

Table 5.8. Drugs for Treatment of Parasitic Infections, continued

Infection	Drug	Adult dosage*	Pediatric dosage*
MONILIFORMIS moniliformis infection			
Drug of choice:	Pyrantel pamoate[8]	11 mg/kg once, repeat twice 2 wks apart	11 mg/kg once, repeat twice, 2 wks apart
Naegleria species, see AMEBIC MENINGOENCEPHALITIS, PRIMARY			
Necator americanus, see HOOKWORM infection			
OESOPHAGOSTOMUM bifurcum			
Drug of choice:	See footnote 67		
Onchocerca volvulus, see FILARIASIS			
Opisthorchis viverrini, see FLUKE infection			
Paragonimus westermani, see FLUKE infection			
Pediculus capitis, humanus, Phthirus pubis, see LICE			
Pinworm, see ENTEROBIUS			
PNEUMOCYSTIS carinii pneumonia[68]			
Drug of choice:	Trimethoprim-sulfamethoxazole	TMP 15 mg/kg/d, SMX 75 mg/kg/d, oral or IV in 3 or 4 doses × 14–21d[69]	Same as adult dose
Alternatives[70]:	Pentamidine	3–4 mg/kg IV qd × 14–21 days[69]	Same as adult dose
	Trimetrexate **plus** folinic acid	45 mg/m² IV qd × 21 days 20 mg/m² PO or IV q6h × 21 days	
	Trimethoprim[8] **plus** dapsone[8]	5 mg/kg PO tid × 21 days 100 mg PO qd × 21 days	
	Atovaquone suspension	750 mg bid PO × 21 d	
	Primaquine[8,55] **plus** clindamycin[8]	600 mg IV q6h × 21 days, or 300–450 mg PO q6h × 21 days	

Primary and secondary prophylaxis

Drug of choice:	Trimethoprim-sulfamethoxazole	1 DS tab PO qc or 3×/week	TMP 150 mg, SMX 750 mg in 2 doses PO 3×/week
Alternatives:	Dapsone[8]	50–100 mg PO qd, or 100 mg PO 2×/week	2 mg/kg PO qd
	±Pyrimethamine[71]	50 mg PO 2×/week	
	Aerosol pentamidine	300 mg inhaled monthly via *Respirgard II* nebulizer	>5 yrs: same as adult dose

Roundworm, see ASCARIASIS

SCABIES (Sarcoptes scabiei)

Drug of choice:	5% Permethrin	Topically	Topically
Alternatives:	Ivermectin	200 µg/kg PO once	200 µg/kg PO once
	10% Crotamiton	Topically	Topically

SCHISTOSOMIASIS (Bilharziasis)

S. haematobium

Drug of choice:	Praziquantel	40 mg/kg/d in 2 doses × 1d	40 mg/kg/d in 2 doses × 1d

S. japonicum

Drug of choice:	Praziquantel	50 mg/kg/d in 3 doses × 1d	50 mg/kg/d in 3 doses × 1d

---

67 Albendazole or pyrantel pamoate may be effective (HP Krepel et al, Trans R Soc Trop Med Hyg, 87:87, 1993).

68 In severe disease with room air Po2≤70 mmHg or Aa gradient ≥35 mmHg, prednisone should also be used (see Medical Letter, 37:89, Oct 13, 1995).

69 HIV-infected patients should be treated for 21 days.

70 For patients who have failed or are intolerant to trimethoprim-sulfamethoxazole.

71 Plus folinic acid, 10 mg, with each dose of pyrimethamine.

Table 5.8. Drugs for Treatment of Parasitic Infections, continued

Infection	Drug	Adult dosage*	Pediatric dosage*
S. mansoni			
Drug of choice:	Praziquantel	40 mg/kg/d in 2 doses × 1d	40 mg/kg/d in 2 doses × 1d
	Oxamniquine[72]	15 mg/kg once[73]	20 mg/kg once[73]
S. mekongi			
Drug of choice:	Praziquantel	60 mg/kg/d in 3 doses × 1d	60 mg/kg/d in 3 doses × 1d

Sleeping sickness, see TRYPANOSOMIASIS

STRONGYLOIDIASIS (*Strongyloides stercoralis*)

Drug of choice:[74]	Thiabendazole	50 mg/kg/d in 2 doses (max. 3 grams/d) × 2d[11,75]	50 mg/kg/d in 2 doses (max. 3 grams/d) × 2d[11,75]
OR	Ivermectin[76]	200 µg/kg/d × 1-2d	200 µg/kg/d × 1-2d

TAPEWORM infection—Adult (intestinal stage)

***Diphyllobothrium latum* (fish), *Taenia saginata* (beef), *Taenia solium* (pork), *Dipylidium caninum* (dog)**

Drug of choice:	Praziquantel[8]	5-10 mg/kg once	5-10 mg/kg once

***Hymenolepis nana* (dwarf tapeworm)**

Drug of choice:	Praziquantel[8]	25 mg/kg once	25 mg/kg once

***Echinococcus granulosus* (hydatid cyst)**
 —Larval (tissue stage)

Drug of choice:	Albendazole[77,78]	400 mg bid × 28 days, repeated as necessary	15 mg/kg/d × 28 days, repeated as necessary

Echinococcus multilocularis

Treatment of choice:	See footnote[7]	

***Crysticercus cellulosae* (cysticercosis)**

Drug of choice:	Albendazole[81]	15 mg/kg/d in 2-3 doses × 8-28d, repeated as necessary	15 mg/kg/d in 2-3 doses × 8-28d, repeated as necessary

Praziquantel[8]   50 mg/kg/d in 3 doses   50 mg/kg/d in 3 doses × 15d
× 15d

OR

Alternative: Surgery

Toxocariasis, see VISCERAL LARVA MIGRANS

[72] Neuropsychiatric disturbances and seizures have been reported in some patients (H Stokvis et al, Am J Trop Med Hyg, 35:330, 1986).

[73] In East Africa, the dose should be increased to 30 mg/kg, and in Egypt and South Africa, 30 mg/kg/d × 2d. Some experts recommend 40-60 mg/kg over 2–3 days in all of Africa (KC Shekhar, Drugs, 42:379, 1991).

[74] In immunocompromised patients, it may be necessary to prolong therapy or use other agents.

[75] In disseminated strongyloidiasis, thiabendazole therapy should be continued for at least five days.

[76] C Naquira et al, Am J Trop Med Hyg, 40:304, 1989; M Lyagoubi et al, Trans R Soc Trop Med Hyg, 86:541, 1992; PH Gann et al, J Infect Dis, 169:1076, 1994.

[77] With a fatty meal to enhance absorption. Some patients may benefit from or require surgical resection of cysts (RK Tompkins, Mayo Clinic Proc, 66:1281, 1991). Praziquantel may also be useful preoperatively or in case of spill during surgery.

[78] Percutaneous drainage with ultrasound guidance plus albendazole therapy has been effective for management of hepatic hydatid cyst disease (MS Khuroo et al, Gastroenterology, 104:1452, 1993).

[79] Surgical excision is the only reliable means of treatment, although some reports have suggested use of albendazole or mebendazole (W Hao et al, Trans R Soc Trop Med Hyg, 88:340, 1994).

[80] Corticosteroids should be given for two to three days before and during drug therapy for neurocysticercosis. Any cysticercocidal drug may cause irreparable damage when used to treat ocular or spinal cysts, even when corticosteroids are used.

[81] Albendazole should be taken with a fatty meal to enhance absorption.

Table 5.8. Drugs for Treatment of Parasitic Infections, continued

Infection	Drug	Adult dosage*	Pediatric dosage*
TOXOPLASMOSIS (*Toxoplasma gondii*)[82]			
Drugs of choice[83]:	Pyrimethamine[71]	25–100 mg/d × 3-4 wks	2 mg/kg/d × 3d, then 1 mg/kg/d (max. 25 mg/d) x 4 wks[84]
	plus sulfadiazine	1–1.5 grams qid × 3-4 wks	100–200 mg/kg/d × 3–4 wks
Alternative:	Spiramycin[85]	3–4 grams/d	50–100 mg/kg/d × 3–4 wks
TRICHINOSIS (*Trichinella spiralis*)			
Drugs of choice:	Steroids for severe symptoms		
	plus mebendazole[8,86]	200–400 mg tid × 3d, then 400–500 mg tid × 10d	
TRICHOMONIASIS (*Trichomonas vaginalis*)			
Drug of choice[87]:	Metronidazole	2 grams once or 250 mg tid or 375 mg bid PO × 7d	15 mg/kg/d orally in 3 doses × 7d
OR	Tinidazole[5]	2 grams once	50 mg/kg once (max. 2 grams)
***TRICHOSTRONGYLUS* infection**			
Drug of choice:	Pyrantel pamoate[8]	11 mg/kg once (max. 1 gram)	11 mg/kg once (max. 1 gram)
Alternative:	Mebendazole[8]	100 mg bid × 3d	100 mg bid × 3d
OR	Albendazole	400 mg once	400 mg once
TRICHURIASIS (*Trichuris trichiura*, whipworm)			
Drug of choice:	Mebendazole	100 mg bid × 3d	100 mg bid × 3d
OR	Albendazole	400 mg once[88]	400 mg once[88]

TRYPANOSOMIASIS

T. cruzi (American trypanosomiasis, Chagas' disease)

Drug of choice:	Nifurtimox[3,89]	1–10 yrs: 15–20 mg/kg/d in 4 doses × 90d;
		11–16 yrs: 12.5–15 mg/kg/d in 4 doses × 90d
		8–10 mg/kg/d in 4 doses × 120d
Alternative:	Benznidazole[90]	5–7 mg/kg/d × 30–120d

82 In ocular toxoplasmosis, corticosteroids should also be used for an anti-inflammatory effect on the eyes.

83 To treat CNS toxoplasmosis in HIV-infected patients, some clinicians have used pyrimethamine 50 to 100 mg daily after a loading dose of 200 mg with a sulfonamide and, when sulfonamide sensitivity developed, have given clindamycin 1.8 to 2.4 g/d in divided doses instead of the sulfonamide (JS Remington et al, Lancet, 338:1142, 1991; BJ Luft et al, N Engl J Med, 329:995, 1993). Atovaquone plus pyrimethamine appears to be an effective alternative in sulfa-intolerant patients (JA Kovacs et al, Lancet, 340:637, 1992). Dapsone-pyrimethamine can prevent first episodes of toxoplasmosis (P-M Girard et al, N Engl J Med, 328:1514, 1993).

84 Congenitally infected newborns should be treated with pyrimethamine every two or three days and a sulfonamide daily for about one year (JS Remington and G Desmonts in JS Remington and JO Klein, eds, *Infectious Disease of the Fetus and Newborn Infant*, 4th ed, Philadelphia: Saunders, 1995, page 140).

85 For use during pregnancy, continue the drug until delivery. If it has been determined that transmission has occurred *in utero*, then therapy with pyrimethamine and sulfadiazine should be started.

86 Albendazole or flubendazole (not available in the USA) may also be effective.

87 Sexual partners should be treated simultaneously. Outside the USA, ornidazole has also been used for this condition. Metronidazole-resistant strains have been reported; higher doses of metronidazole for longer periods are sometimes effective against these strains (J Lossick, Rev Infect Dis, 12:S665, 1990). Experimental studies suggest that bacitracin and bacitracin zinc have microbicidal activity against multiple isolates of *T. vaginalis* (BJ Andrews et al, Trans R Soc Trop Med Hyg, 88:704, 1994).

88 In heavy infection it may be necessary to extend therapy for 3 days.

89 The addition of gamma interferon to nifurtimox for 20 days in a limited number of patients and in experimental animals appears to have shortened the acute phase of Chagas' disease (RE McCabe et al, J Infect Dis, 163:912, 1991).

90 Limited data.

Table 5.8. Drugs for Treatment of Parasitic Infections, continued

T. brucei gambiense; T.b. rhodesiense (African trypanosomiasis, sleeping sickness) hemolymphatic stage

Infection	Drug	Adult dosage*	Pediatric dosage*
Drug of choice:	Suramin[3]	100–200 mg (test dose) IV, then 1 gram IV on days 1,3,7,14, and 21 See footnote 91	20 mg/kg on days 1,3,7,14, and 21
OR	Eflornithine		
Alternative:	Pentamidine isethionate[8]	4 mg/kg/d IM × 10d	4 mg/kg/d IM × 10d
late disease with CNS involvement			
Drug of choice:	Melarsoprol[3,92]	2–3.6 mg/kg/d IV × 3d; after 1 wk 3.6 mg/kg per day IV × 3d; repeat again after 10–21 days	18–25 mg/kg total over 1 month; initial dose of 0.36 mg/kg IV, increasing gradually to max. 3.6 mg/kg at intervals 1–5d for total of 9–10 doses
OR	Eflornithine	See footnote 91	
Alternatives: (*T.b. gambiense* only)	Tryparasamide	One injection of 30 mg/kg (max. 2g) IV every 5d to total of 12 injections; may be repeated after 1 month	
	plus suramin[3]	One injection of 10 mg/kg IV every 5 d to total of 12 injections; may be repeated after 1 month	

VISCERAL LARVA MIGRANS[93] (*Toxocariasis*)

Infection	Drug	Adult dosage*	Pediatric dosage*
Drug of choice:	Diethylcarbamazine[8]	6 mg/kg/d in 3 doses × 7–10d	6 mg/kg/d in 3 doses × 7–10d
Alternatives:	Albendazole[8]	400 mg bid × 3–5d	400 mg bid × 3–5d
	Mebendazole[8]	100–200 mg bid × 5d	100–200 mg bid × 5d

Whipworm, see TRICHURIASIS

Wuchereria bancrofti, see FILARIASIS

91 In *T.b. gambiense* infections, eflornithine is highly effective in both the hemolymphatic and CNS stages. Its effectiveness in *T.b. rhodesiense* infections has been variable. Some clinicians have given 400 mg/kg/d IV in 4 divided doses for 14 days, followed by oral treatment with 300 mg/kg/d for 3–4 wks (F Milord et al, Lancet, 340:652, 1992).

92 In frail patients, begin with as little as 18 mg and increase the dose progressively. Pretreatment with suramin has been advocated for debilitated patients. Corticosteroids have been used to prevent arsenical encephalopathy (J Pepin et al, Trans R Soc Trop Med Hyg, 89:92, 1995).

93 For severe symptoms or eye involvement, corticosteroids can be used in addition.

Table 5.9. Manufacturers of Antiparasitic Drugs

* albendazole—*Zentel* (SmithKline Beecham)
** aminosidine (paromomycin)
atovaquone—*Mepron* (Glaxo-Wellcome)
bacitracin—many manufacturers
** bacitracin-zinc (Apothekernes Laboratorium A.S., Oslo, Norway‡)

benznidazole—*Rochagan* (Roche, Brazil)

† bithionol—*Bitin* (Tanabe, Japan)
chloroquine—*Aralen* (Sanofi Winthrop), others
crotamiton—*Eurax* (Westwood-Squibb)
Dapsone (Jacobus)
* diethylcarbamazine—*Hetrazan* (Wyeth-Ayerst)
† diloxanide furoate—*Furamide* (Boots, England)
* eflornithine (difluoromethylornithine, DFMO)—*Ornidyl* (Merrell Dow)
** flubendazole—(Janssen)
furazolidone—*Furoxone* (Roberts)
** halofantrine—*Halfan* (SmithKline Beecham)
hydroxychloroquine—*Plaquenil* (Sanofi Winthrop) iodoquinol (diiodohydroxyquin) —*Yodoxin* (Glenwood), others
† ivermectin—*Mectizan* (Merck)
malathion—*Prioderm*
mebendazole—*Vermox* (Janssen)
mefloquine—*Lariam* (Roche)
** meglumine antimonate—*Glucantime* (Rhône-Poulenc Rorer, France)
† melarsoprol—*Arsobal* (Rhône-Poulenc Rorer, France)
metronidazole—*Flagyl* (Searle), others

† nifurtimox—*Lampit* (Bayer, Germany)
** ornidazole—*Tiberal* (Hoffman-LaRoche, Switzerland)
oxamniquine—*Vansil* (Pfizer)
paromomycin—*Humatin* (Parke-Davis)
pentamidine isethionate—*Pentam 300* (Fujisawa), *NebuPent* (Fujisawa)
permethrin—*Nix* (Glaxo-Wellcome), *Elimite* (Herbert), Lyclear (Canada)
praziquantel—*Biltricide* (Miles)
primaquine phosphate—(Sanofi Winthrop)
** proguanil—*Paludrine* (Ayerst, Canada, ICI, England)
pyrantel pamoate—*Antiminth* (Pfizer)
pyrethrins and piperonyl butoxide—*RID* (Pfizer), others
pyrimethamine—*Daraprim* (Glaxo-Wellcome)
pyrimethamine-sulfadoxine—*Fansidar* (Roche)
quinidine gluconate—(Lilly)
quinine dihydrochloride
quinine sulfate—many manufacturers
** sodium stibogluconate (antimony sodium gluconate) — *Pentostam* (Glaxo-Wellcome, England)
* spiraycin—*Rovamycine* (Rhône-Poulenc Rorer)
sulfadiazine—(Eon Labs, and others)
† suramin—(Bayer, Germany)
thiabendazole—*Mintezol* (Merck)
** tinidazole—*Fasigyn* (Pfizer)
** triclabendazole (Ciba-Geigy)
trimetrexate—*Neutrexin* (US Bioscience)
** tryparsamide

* Available in the USA only from the manufacturer.
** Not available in the USA.
† Available from the CDC Drug Service, Centers for Disease Control and Prevention, Atlanta, Georgia 30333; 404-639-3670 (evenings, weekends, or holidays: 404-639-2888).

Table 5.10. Adverse Effects of Some Antiparasitic Drugs*

ALBENDAZOLE (*Zentel*)
Occasional: diarrhea; abdominal pain; migration of *ascaris* through mouth and nose
Rare: leukopenia; alopecia; increased serum transaminase activity

AMINOSIDINE—See Paromomycin

ATOVAQUONE (*Mepron*)
Frequent: rash, nausea
Occasional: diarrhea

BACITRACIN
Frequent: nephorotxicity
Occasional: rash
Rare: anaphylaxis

BENZNIDAZOLE (*Rochagan*)
Frequent: allergic rash; dose-dependent polyneuropathy; gastrointestinal disturbances; psychic disturbances

BITHIONOL (*Bitin*)
Frequent: photosensitivity reactions; vomiting; diarrhea; abdominal pain; urticaria
Rare: leukopenia; toxic hepatitis

CHLOROQUINE HCl and CHLOROQUINE PHOSPHATE (*Aralen*, and others)
Occasional: pruritis; vomiting; headache; confusion; depigmentation of hair; skin eruptions; corneal opacity; weigh loss; partial alopecia; extraocular muscle palsies; exacerbation of psoriasis, eczema, and other exfoliative dermatoses; myalgias; photophobia

Rare: irreversible retinal injury (especially when total dosage exceeds 100 grams); discoloration of nails and mucus membranes; nerve-type deafness; peripheral neuropathy and myopathy; heart block; blood dyscrasias; hematemesis

CROTAMITON (*Eurax*)
Occasional: rash, conjunctivitis

DAPSONE
Frequent: rash; transient headache; GI irritation; anorexia; infectious mononucleosis-like syndrome
Occasional: cyanosis due to methemoglobinemia and sulfhemoglobinemia; other blood dyscrasias, including hemolytic anemia; nephrotic syndrome; liver damage; peripheral neuropathy; hypersensitivity reactions; increased risk of lepra reactions; insomnia; irritability; uncoordinated speech; agitation; acute psychosis
Rare: renal papillary necrosis; severe hypoalbuminemia; epidermal necrolysis; optic atrophy; agranulocytosis; neonatal hyperbilirubinemia after use in pregnancy

DIETHYLCARBAMAZINE CITRATE USP (*Hetrazan*)
Frequent: flatulence
Occasional: nausea; vomiting; diarrhea
Rare: diplopia; dizziness; urticaria; pruritus

EFLORNITHINE (Difluoromethylornithine, DFMO, *Ornidyl*)
Frequent: anemia; leukopenia
Occasional: diarrhea; thrombocytopenia; seizures
Rare: hearing loss

---

* Drug interactions are generally not included here; see the current edition of *The Medical Letter Handbook of Adverse Drug Interactions*.

Table 5.10. Adverse Effects of Some Antiparasitic Drugs,* continued

FLUBENDAZOLE—similar to mebendazole

FURAZOLIDONE *(Furoxone)*
Frequent: nausea; vomiting
Occasional: allergic reactions, including pulmonary infiltration, hypotension, urticaria, fever, vesicular rash; hypoglycemia; headache
Rare: hemolytic anemia in G-6-PD deficiency and neonates; disulfiram-like reaction with alcohol; MAO-inhibitor interactions; polyneuritis

HALOFANTRINE *(Halfan)*
Occasional: diarrhea; abdominal pain; pruritus; prolongation of Qtc and PR interval

IODOQUINOL *(Yodoxin)*
Occasional: rash; acne; slight enlargement of the thyroid gland; nausea; diarrhea; cramps; anal pruritus
Rare: optic neuritis; optic atrophy, loss of vision, peripheral neuropathy after prolonged use in high dosage (for months); iodine sensitivity

IVERMECTIN *(Mectizan)*
Occasional: Mazzotti-type reaction seen in onchocerciasis, including fever, pruritus, tender lymph nodes, headache, and joint and bone pain
Rare: hypotension

MALATHION *(Prioderm)*
Occasional: local irritation

MEBENDAZOLE *(Vermox)*
Occasional: diarrhea; abdominal pain; migration of ascaris through mouth and nose
Rare: leukopenia; agranulocytosis; hypospermia

MEFLOQUINE *(Lariam)*
Frequent: vertigo; lightheadedness; nausea; other gastrointestinal disturbances; nightmares; visual disturbances; headache
Occasional: confusion
Rare: psychosis; hypotension; convulsions; coma; paresthesias

MEGLUMINE ANTIMONATE *(Glucantime)* Similar to sodium stibogluconate

MELARSOPROL *(Arsobal)*
Frequent: nausea; headache; dry mouth; metallic taste
Occasional: vomiting; diarrhea; insomnia; weakness; stomatitis; vertigo; tinnitus; paresthesias; rash; dark urine; urethral burning; disulfiram-like reaction with alcohol
Rare: seizures; encephalopathy; pseudomembranous colitis; ataxia; leukopenia; peripheral neuropathy; pancreatitis

NIFURTIMOX *(Lampit)*
Frequent: anorexia; vomiting; weight loss; loss of memory; sleep disorders; tremor; paresthesias; weakness; polyneuritis
Rare: convulsions; fever; pulmonary infiltrates and pleural effusion

ORNIDAZOLE *(Tiberal)*
Occasional: dizziness; headache; gastrointestinal disturbances
Rare: reversible peripheral neuropathy

OXAMNIQUINE *(Vansil)*
Occasional: headache; fever; dizziness; somnolence; nausea; diarrhea; rash; insomnia; hepatic enzyme changes; ECG changes; EEG changes; orange-red discoloration of urine
Rare: seizures; neuropsychiatric disturbances

PAROMOMYCIN; (aminosidine; *Humatin*)
Frequent: GI disturbances with oral use
Occasional: eighth-nerve damage (mainly auditory) and renal damage when aminosidine is given IV; vertigo; pancreatitis

PENTAMIDINE ISETHIONATE (*Pentam 300, NebuPent*)
Frequent: hypotension; hypoglycemia often followed by diabetes mellitus; vomiting; blood dyscrasias; renal damage; pain at injection site; GI disturbances
Occasional: may aggravate diabetes; shock; hypocalcemia; liver damage; cardiotoxicity; delirium; rash
Rare: Herxheimer-type reaction; anaphylaxis; acute pancreatitis; hyperkalemia

PERMETHRIN (*Nix, Elimite*)
Occasional: burning; stinging; numbness; increased pruritus; pain; edema; erythema; rash

PRAZIQUANTEL (*Biltricide*)
Frequent: malaise; headache; dizziness
Occasional: sedation; abdominal discomfort; fever; sweating; nausea; eosinophilia; fatigue
Rare: pruritus; rash

PRIMAQUINE PHOSPHATE USP
Frequent: hemolytic anemia in G-6-PD deficiency
Occasional: neutropenia; GI disturbances; methemoglobinemia
Rare: CNS symptoms; hypertension; arrhythmias

PROGUANIL (*Paludrine*)
Occasional: oral ulceration; hair loss; scaling of palms and soles; urticaria

Rare: hematuria (with large doses); vomiting; abdominal pain; diarrhea (with large doses); thrombocytopenia

PYRANTEL PAMOATE (*Antiminth*)
Occasional: GI disturbances; headache; dizziness; rash; fever

PYRETHRINS and PIPERONYL BUTOXIDE (*RID*, others)
Occasional: allergic reactions

PYRIMETHAMINE USP (*Daraprim*)
Occasional: blood dyscrasias; folic acid deficiency
Rare: rash; vomiting; convulsions; shock; possibly pulmonary eosinophilia; fatal cutaneous reactions with **pyrimethamine-sulfadoxine** (*Fansidar*)

QUININE DIHYDROCHLORIDE and SULFATE
Frequent: cinchonism (tinnitus, headache, nausea, abdominal pain, visual disturbance)
Occasional: deafness; hemolytic anemia; other blood dyscrasias; photosensitivity reactions; hypoglycemia; arrhythmias; hypotension; drug fever
Rare: blindness; sudden death if injected too rapidly

SODIUM STIBOGLUCONATE (*Pentostam*)
Frequent: muscle and joint pain; fatigue; nausea; transaminase elevations; T-wave flattening or inversion; pancreatitis
Occasional: weakness; abdominal pain; liver damage; bradycardia; leukopenia; thrombocytopenia; rash; vomiting
Rare: diarrhea; pruritus; myocardial damage; hemolytic anemia; renal damage; shock; sudden death

* Drug interactions are generally not included here; **see the current edition of** *The Medical Letter Handbook of Adverse Drug Interactions.*

Table 5.10. Adverse Effects of Some Antiparasitic Drugs,* continued

SPIRAMYCIN (*Rovamycine*)
  Occasional: GI disturbances
  Rare: allergic reactions

SURAMIN SODIUM
  Frequent: vomiting; pruritus; urticaria; paresthesias; hyperesthesia of hands and feet; photophobia; peripheral neuropathy
  Occasional: kidney damage; blood dyscrasias; shock; optic atrophy

THIABENDAZOLE (*Mintezol*)
  Frequent: nausea; vomiting; vertigo; headache; drowsiness; pruritus
  Occasional: leukopenia; crystalluria; rash; hallucination and other psychiatric reactions; visual and olfactory disturbance; erythema multiforme
  Rare: shock; tinnitus; intrahepatic cholestasis; convulsions; angioneurotic edema; Stevens-Johnson syndrome

TINIDAZOLE (*Fasigyn*)
  Occasional: metallic taste; nausea; vomiting; rash

TRIMETREXATE (with "leucovorin rescue")
  Occasional: rash; peripheral neuropathy; bone marrow depression; increased serum aminotransferase activity

TRYPARSAMIDE
  Frequent: nausea; vomiting
  Occasional: impaired vision; optic atrophy; fever; exfoliative dermatitis; allergic reactions; tinnitus

* Drug interactions are generally not included here; see the current edition of *The Medical Letter Handbook of Adverse Drug Interactions*.

MEDWATCH — MEDICAL PRODUCTS REPORTING PROGRAM

MEDWATCH, the Food and Drug Administration (FDA) Medical Products Reporting Program, is an educational and promotional initiative to enhance the effectiveness of postmarking surveillance of all medical products regulated by the FDA, including drugs and biologics as well as medical devices and special nutritional products such as medical foods, dietary supplements, and infant formulas. Physicians and other health professionals are in the best position to recognize problems and deficiencies arising from the use of medical products. The FDA and the manufacturer are very dependent on the clinicians to monitor for and report adverse events and other problems with products. Accordingly, the FDA strongly encourages reporting of serious adverse events and problems, ie, those types of events with potentially the most significant public health impact.

The program, MEDWATCH, has the four following general goals: (1) to increase awareness of drug- and device-induced disease; (2) to clarify what should (and should not) be reported to the agency; (3) to make reporting easier, and (4) to provide regulating information to the health care community about safety issues involving medical products.

Reporting is facilitated by a one-page, postage-paid, voluntary form (see Fig 5.1, p 666) for health professionals to report directly to the agency and/or the manufacturer. A 24-hour toll-free number (800-FDA-1088) is also available for health professionals to report by telephone, to request forms either via fax or mail, or to obtain a copy of the *FDA Desk Guide to Adverse Event and Product Problem Reporting*, which includes examples of events to report, completed sample forms, and also blank forms with instructions. Providers may also report to the FDA on-line (800-FDA-7737), or by fax (800-FDA-0178). The only exception is vaccines. Adverse events and problems associated with vaccines should be reported to the Vaccine Adverse Events Reporting System (VAERS) (see Reporting of Adverse Events, p 27).

Fig 5.1. Medwatch reporting form.

MEDWATCH

THE FDA MEDICAL PRODUCTS REPORTING PROGRAM

For VOLUNTARY reporting by health professionals of adverse events and product problems

Page ___ of ___

Form Approved: OMB No. 0910-0291 Expires: 4/30/96
See OMB statement on reverse

FDA Use Only

Triage unit sequence #

PLEASE TYPE OR USE BLACK INK

A. Patient information

1. Patient identifier ______ In confidence
2. Age at time of event: ______ or Date of birth:
3. Sex ☐ female ☐ male
4. Weight ____ lbs or ____ kgs

B. Adverse event or product problem

1. ☐ Adverse event and/or ☐ Product problem (e.g., defects/malfunctions)
2. Outcomes attributed to adverse event (check all that apply)
   - ☐ death ______ (mo/day/yr)
   - ☐ life-threatening
   - ☐ hospitalization – initial or prolonged
   - ☐ disability
   - ☐ congenital anomaly
   - ☐ required intervention to prevent permanent impairment/damage
   - ☐ other: ______
3. Date of event (mo/day/yr)
4. Date of this report (mo/day/yr)
5. Describe event or problem
6. Relevant tests/laboratory data, including dates
7. Other relevant history, including preexisting medical conditions (e.g., allergies, race, pregnancy, smoking and alcohol use, hepatic/renal dysfunction, etc.)

C. Suspect medication(s)

1. Name (give labeled strength & mfr/labeler, if known)
   #1
   #2
2. Dose, frequency & route used
   #1
   #2
3. Therapy dates (if unknown, give duration) from/to (or best estimate)
   #1
   #2
4. Diagnosis for use (indication)
   #1
   #2
5. Event abated after use stopped or dose reduced
   #1 ☐ yes ☐ no ☐ doesn't apply
   #2 ☐ yes ☐ no ☐ doesn't apply
6. Lot # (if known)
   #1
   #2
7. Exp. date (if known)
   #1
   #2
8. Event reappeared after reintroduction
   #1 ☐ yes ☐ no ☐ doesn't apply
   #2 ☐ yes ☐ no ☐ doesn't apply
9. NDC # (for product problems only)
10. Concomitant medical products and therapy dates (exclude treatment of event)

D. Suspect medical device

1. Brand name
2. Type of device
3. Manufacturer name & address
4. Operator of device
   - ☐ health professional
   - ☐ lay user/patient
   - ☐ other: ______
5. Expiration date (mo/day/yr)
6. model # ______
   catalog # ______
   serial # ______
   lot # ______
   other # ______
7. If implanted, give date (mo/day/yr)
8. If explanted, give date (mo/day/yr)
9. Device available for evaluation? (Do not send to FDA)
   ☐ yes ☐ no ☐ returned to manufacturer on ______ (mo/day/yr)
10. Concomitant medical products and therapy dates (exclude treatment of event)

E. Reporter (see confidentiality section on back)

1. Name & address
   phone #
2. Health professional? ☐ yes ☐ no
3. Occupation
4. Also reported to
   - ☐ manufacturer
   - ☐ user facility
   - ☐ distributor
5. If you do NOT want your identity disclosed to the manufacturer, place an " X " in this box. ☐

FDA

Mail to: MEDWATCH
5600 Fishers Lane
Rockville, MD 20852-9787

or FAX to:
1-800-FDA-0178

FDA Form 3500 1/96)

Submission of a report does not constitute an admission that medical personnel or the product caused or contributed to the event.

•••••••••••••••••••••
APPENDIX I.

Directory of Telephone Numbers

ORGANIZATION OR SOURCE	TELEPHONE NUMBER
American Academy of Pediatrics	847-228-5005
AIDS/HIV Treatment Information Service	800-HIV-0440
Centers for Disease Control and Prevention (CDC)	404-639-3311
• 24 Hour Service	404-332-4555
• Division of Bacterial and Mycotic Diseases	404-639-1603
• Division of Parasitic Diseases	770-488-7760
• Division of Tuberculosis Control	404-639-8120
• Division of Viral Diseases	404-639-3574
• Drug Service (weekdays, 8 to 4:30 E.T.)	404-639-3670
• Drug Service (weekends, nights, holidays)	404-639-2888
• Fax Information Service (including international travel and immunization)	404-332-4565
• Hepatitis Branch	404-639-2709
• Immunization, Infectious Diseases, and Other Health Information—Voice Information System	800-232-SHOT
• International Traveler's Hotline	404-332-4559
• National Center for Infectious Diseases	404-639-3401
• National HIV and AIDS Hotline	800-342-AIDS
• National Immunization Program	404-639-8200
• Public Inquiries	404-639-3534
• Publications	404-639-8614 (fax)
• Vector-Borne Infectious Diseases	970-221-6400
Food and Drug Administration:	
• Center for Biologics Evaluation and Research	301-827-0372
• Center for Drug Evaluation and Research	301-594-6740
• MEDWATCH	800-FDA-1088
Michigan Biologic Products Institute	517-335-8120
National Vaccine Injury Compensation Program (for information on filing claims)	800-338-2382
National Vaccine Program Office	404-639-4450
Pediatric AIDS Drug Trials—Information:	
• Pediatric Branch, National Cancer Institute	301-402-0696
• Pediatric Clinical Trials Group (NIAID-sponsored)	800-TRIALS-A
Vaccine Adverse Events Reporting System (VAERS)	800-822-7967

•••••••••••••••••••••••••

APPENDIX II.

Standards for Pediatric Immunization Practices*

Recommended by the
National Vaccine Advisory Committee
April 1992

Approved by the
United States Public Health Service
May 1992

Endorsed by the
American Academy of Pediatrics
May 1992

The Standards represent the consensus of the National Vaccine Advisory Committee (NVAC) and of a broad group of medical and public health experts about what constitute the most desirable immunization practices. The NVAC recognizes that not all of the current immunization practices of public and private providers are in compliance with the Standards. Nevertheless, the Standards should be useful as a means of helping providers to identify needed changes, to obtain resources if necessary, and to actually implement the desirable immunization practices in the future.

Standards for Pediatric Immunization Practices

PREAMBLE

Ideally, immunizations should be given as part of comprehensive child health care. This is the ultimate goal toward which the nation must strive if all of America's children are to benefit from the best primary disease prevention our health care system has to offer.

Overall improvement in our primary care delivery system requires intensive effort and will take time. However, we should not wait for changes in this system before providing immunizations more effectively to our children. Current health care policies and practices in all settings result in the failure to deliver vaccines on schedule to many of our vulnerable preschool-aged children. This failure is due primarily to barriers that impede vaccine delivery and to missed opportunities during clinic visits. Changes in policies and practices can immediately improve coverage. The present system should be geared to "user-friendly," family-centered, culturally sensitive, and comprehensive primary health care that can provide rapid,

---

* Modified from *Standards for Pediatric Immunization Practices.* Atlanta, Ga: Centers for Disease Control and Prevention; 1993. US Dept of Health and Human Services. The major change is an update in the list of vaccine contraindications and precautions to be consistent with 1997 recommendations of the Centers for Disease Control and Prevention.

efficient, and consumer-oriented services to the users, ie, children and their parents. The failure to do so is evidenced by the recent resurgence of measles and measles-related childhood mortality, which may be an omen of other vaccine-preventable disease outbreaks.

Present childhood immunization practices must be changed if we wish to protect the nation's children and immunize 90% of two-year-olds by the year 2000.

The following standards for pediatric immunization practices address these issues. These standards are recommended for use by **all** health professionals in the public and private sector who administer vaccines to or manage immunization services for infants and children. These **Standards** represent the most desirable immunization practices which health care providers should strive to achieve to the extent possible. By adopting these **Standards**, providers can begin to enhance and change their own policies and practices. While not all providers will have the funds necessary to fully implement the **Standards** immediately, those providers and programs lacking the resources to implement the **Standards** fully should find them a useful tool in better delineating immunization needs and in obtaining additional resources in the future in order to achieve the Healthy People 2000 immunization objective.

STANDARDS

Standard 1. Immunization services are **readily available.**

Standard 2. **No barriers** or **unnecessary prerequisites** to the receipt of vaccines exist.

Standard 3. Immunization services are available **free** or for a minimal fee.

Standard 4. Providers utilize all clinical encounters to **screen** and, when indicated, **immunize** children.

Standard 5. Providers **educate** parents and guardians about immunization in general terms.

Standard 6. Providers **question** parents or guardians about **contraindications** and, before immunizing a child, **inform** them in specific terms about the risks and benefits of the immunizations their child is to receive.

Standard 7. Providers follow only true **contraindications.**

Standard 8. Providers administer **simultaneously** all vaccine doses for which a child is eligible at the time of each visit.

Standard 9. Providers use accurate and complete **recording procedures.**

Standard 10. Providers **co-schedule** immunization appointments in conjunction with appointments for other child health services.

Standard 11. Providers **report adverse events** following immunization promptly, accurately and completely.

Standard 12. Providers operate a **tracking system.**

Standard 13. Providers adhere to appropriate procedures for **vaccine management.**

Standard 14. Providers conduct semi-annual **audits** to assess immunization coverage levels and to review immunization records in the patient populations they serve.

Standard 15. Providers maintain up-to-date, easily retrievable **medical protocols** at all locations where vaccines are administered.

Standard 16. Providers operate with **patient-oriented** and **community-based** approaches.

Standard 17. Vaccines are administered by **properly trained** individuals.

Standard 18. Providers receive **ongoing education** and **training** on current immunization recommendations.

DISCUSSION

1. **Immunization services are *readily available.***

Immunization services should be responsive to the needs of patients. For example, in large urban areas, public immunization clinic services should be available daily, 8 hours per day. In smaller cities and rural areas, clinics may operate less frequently. To be fully responsive, providers in many locations should consider offering immunization services each working day as well as during some off-hours (eg, weekends, evenings, early mornings, or lunch-hours). Immunization services should be considered for all days and at all hours that other child health services in the same site are offered (eg, Special Supplemental Food Program for Women, Infants, and Children [WIC]). Private providers who offer primary care to infants and children should always include immunization services as a routine part of that care.

Ready availability of immunization services also requires that the supply of vaccines be adequate at all times.

2. ***No barriers* or *unnecessary prerequisites* to the receipt of vaccines exist.**

Appointment-only systems often serve as barriers to immunization in both public and private settings. Thus, immunization services should also be available on a walk-in basis at all times for both routine and new enrollee visits. Waiting time should be minimized and generally not exceed 30 minutes. Furthermore, administration of needed vaccines should not be contingent on enrollment in a well-baby program unless enrollment is immediately available. Children presenting only for immunizations should be rapidly and efficiently screened without requiring other comprehensive health services. However, children receiving immunizations in such an "express lane" fashion and found not to have a primary care provider should be referred to one.

Physical examinations and temperature measurements prior to immunization should not be required if they delay or impede the timely receipt of immunizations (eg, appointments for physical examination in some facilities may take weeks to months). A reliable decision to vaccinate can be based exclusively on the information elicited from a parent or guardian and on the provider's observations and judgment about the child's wellness at the time of vaccination. At a minimum, children should have pre-immunization assessments, including (a) observing the child's general state of health, (b) asking the parent or guardian if the child is well, and (c) questioning the parent or guardian about potential contraindications (see Table, p 676).

In public clinic settings, the administration of vaccines should not be dependent on individual written orders or on a referral from a primary care provider. Rather, standing orders should be developed and implemented.

3. **Immunization services are available *free* or for a minimal fee.**
   In the public sector, immunizations should be free of charge. If fees must be collected, they should be kept to a minimum. In the private sector, charges should include the cost of the vaccine, and a reasonable administration fee. Affordable vaccinations will limit the fragmentation of care and help assure the immunization of the greatest number of children. Public and private providers charging a fee to administer vaccines obtained through a consolidated federal contract should prominently display a state approved sign indicating that no one will be denied immunization services because of inability to pay the fee.

4. **Providers utilize all clinical encounters to *screen* for needed vaccines and, when indicated, *immunize* children.**
   Each encounter with a health care provider, including an emergency room visit or hospitalization, is an opportunity to screen the immunization status and, if indicated, administer needed vaccines. Before discharge from the hospital, children should receive immunizations for which they are eligible by age and/or health status. The child's regular health care provider should be informed about the immunizations administered. Implementation of this standard minimizes the number of missed opportunities to vaccinate.

   In addition, children accompanying parents or siblings who are seeking any service should also be screened and, when indicated, given needed vaccines.

   Providers in subspecialty clinics (eg, oncology) who care for children should pay particular attention to the immunization status of their patients and vaccinate or refer them to immunization services or primary health care providers as appropriate.

   Providers in other specialties should also note the immunization status of children and refer or immunize as appropriate.

5. **Providers *educate* parents and guardians about immunization in general terms.**
   Providers should educate parents and guardians in a culturally sensitive way, preferably in their own language, about the importance of immunizations, the diseases they prevent, the recommended immunization schedules, the need to receive immunizations at recommended ages and the importance of bringing their child's immunization record to each visit. Parents should be encouraged to take responsibility for ensuring that their child completes the full series. Providers should answer all questions parents and guardians may have and provide appropriate educational materials at suitable reading levels in pertinent languages.

6. **Providers *question* parents or guardians about *contraindications* and, before immunizing a child, *inform* them in specific terms about the risks and benefits of the immunizations their child is to receive.**
   Minimal acceptable screening procedures for precautions and contraindications include asking questions to elicit a possible history of adverse events following prior immunizations and determining any existing precautions or contraindications (see Table, p 676).

The Vaccine Information Statements required by federal regulation to be used universally for measles, mumps, rubella, diphtheria, tetanus, pertussis, and polio by all providers administering vaccine, including those who purchase their own vaccines, should be provided and reviewed with parents or guardians. Similar information contained in the Important Information Statements for other vaccines (eg, hepatitis B and *Haemophilus influenzae* type b) should be provided to all parents or guardians in public clinics and use of these statements should be considered by private providers. Providers should ensure that information materials are current and available in appropriate languages. Providers should ask parents or guardians if they have questions about what they have read and should ensure that they receive satisfactory answers to their questions.

Providers should explain where and how to obtain medical care during day- and night-time hours in case of an adverse event following vaccination.

7. **Providers follow only true *contraindications*.**

Accepting conditions which are not true contraindications as being true contraindications (see Table, p 676) often results in the needless deferment of indicated immunizations. The table of true contraindications is based on the recommendations of the Advisory Committee on Immunization Practices (ACIP) and the recommendations of the Committee on Infectious Diseases of the American Academy of Pediatrics (AAP). Sometimes these recommendations may vary from those contained in the manufacturer's package inserts. For more detailed information, providers should consult the published recommendations of the ACIP, the AAP, the American Academy of Family Physicians (AAFP), and the manufacturer's package inserts.

8. **Providers administer *simultaneously* all vaccine doses for which a child is eligible at the time of each visit.**

Available evidence suggests that the simultaneous administration of childhood immunizations is safe and effective. In addition, evidence suggests that the simultaneous administration of multiple needed vaccines can potentially raise immunization coverage by 9%–17%. If providers elect not to administer a needed vaccine simultaneously with others (based either on their judgment that this action will not compromise the timely immunization of the child or on a request by the parent or guardian), they should document such actions and the reasons why the vaccine was not administered. The record should be flagged with an automatic recall for an appointment to receive the needed vaccine(s). This next appointment should be discussed with the parent or guardian of the child.

Measles, mumps, rubella (MMR) vaccine should always be used in combined form when providing routine childhood immunizations.

9. **Providers use accurate and complete *recording procedures*.**

Providers are required by statute to record what vaccine was given, the date the vaccine was given (month, day, year), the name of the manufacturer of the vaccine, the lot number, the signature and title of the person who gave the vaccine, and the address where the vaccine was given. In addition, providers should record on the child's personal immunization record card (preferably the official state version) what vaccine was given, the date the vaccine was given and the name of the provider. Providers should encourage parents or guardians to maintain a copy of their child's personal immunization record card. This card should be updated at each visit for immunizations. If a parent fails to bring their child's card, a new one should be issued containing all previous immunizations and designated as a replacement record card. When accepting immunization record data from parents, providers should confirm that prior doses of vaccines have actually been administered, either by reviewing immunization record cards or by contacting former providers and entering this verified information onto their records. When a provider who does not routinely vaccinate or care for a child administers a vaccine to that child, the regular provider should be informed.

Providers with manual record-keeping systems should maintain separate or easily retrievable files of the immunization records of preschoolers to facilitate assessment of coverage as well as the identification and recall of children who miss appointments. In addition, pre-schooler immunization files should be sorted periodically, with inactive records placed into a separate file. Providers should indicate in their records, or in an appropriately identified place, all primary care services that each child receives in order to facilitate co-scheduling with other services.

10. **Providers *co-schedule* immunization appointments in conjunction with appointments for other child health services.**
Providers of immunization-only services which require an appointment should co-schedule immunization appointments with other needed health care services such as WIC, dental exams or developmental screening **provided such scheduling does not create a barrier** by delaying needed immunizations.

11. **Providers *report adverse* events following immunization promptly, accurately, and completely.**
Providers should encourage parents or legal guardians to inform them of adverse events following immunization. Providers should report all such clinically significant events, including those required by law, to the Vaccine Adverse Event Reporting System (VAERS), regardless of whether or not they believe the events are caused by the vaccines. Report forms and assistance are available by calling 800-822-7967. Providers should document fully the adverse event in the medical record at the time of the event or as soon as possible thereafter.

12. **Providers operate a *tracking system*.**
A tracking system should produce reminders of upcoming immunizations as well as recalls for children who are overdue. A system may be automated or manual and may include mailed or telephone messages. In the public sector, health department staff may also make home visits. All providers should identify, for additional intensive tracking efforts, children considered at high risk of failing to complete the immunization series on schedule (eg, children who start their series late).

13. **Providers adhere to appropriate procedures for *vaccine management*.**
Vaccines should be handled and stored as recommended in the manufacturer's package inserts. The temperatures at which vaccines are stored and transported should be monitored daily and the expiration date for each vaccine should be noted.

Providers using publicly purchased vaccine should periodically report usage, wastage, loss and inventory as required by state or local public health authorities.

14. Providers conduct semi-annual *audits* to assess immunization coverage levels and to review immunization records in the patient populations they serve.
In both the public and private sector, the assessment of immunization services for pre-school-aged patients should include audits of immunization records or inspection of a random sample of records (1) to determine the immunization coverage level (ie, the percentage of children that are up-to-date by their second birthday), (2) to identify how frequently opportunities for simultaneous immunization are missed and (3) to assess the quality of documentation. The results of such assessments should be discussed by providers as part of their ongoing quality assurance reviews and used to develop solutions to the problems identified.

15. Providers maintain up-to-date, easily retrievable *medical protocols* at all locations where vaccines are administered.
Providers administering vaccines should maintain a protocol which, at a minimum, discusses the appropriate vaccine dosage, vaccine contraindications, the recommended sites and techniques for vaccine administration as well as possible adverse events and their emergency management. Such protocols should specify the necessary emergency medical equipment, drugs (including dosage) and personnel to safely and competently deal with any medical emergency which may arise after the administration of a vaccine. All providers should be familiar with the content of these protocols, their location and how to follow them. Vaccines can be administered in any setting (eg, schools, churches) where providers can adhere to these protocols.

16. Providers practice *patient-oriented* and *community-based* approaches.
Public providers should routinely seek the input of their patients on specific approaches to better serve their immunization needs and implement the changes necessary to provide more user-friendly services.

Public providers should adopt a community-based approach to the provision of immunization services which calls for reaching high coverage levels in their catchment area populations and not only in the active patient populations they serve. Such a community-based approach requires all public providers to publicize the availability of their immunization services and to conduct community outreach activities to increase demand for immunization services. Private providers should cooperate with local health officials in their efforts to assure high coverage levels throughout the community. Without high immunization coverage levels, no community is completely protected against vaccine-preventable diseases. All providers share in the responsibility to achieve the highest possible degree of community protection.

17. Vaccines are administered by *properly trained* individuals.

Only properly trained individuals should administer vaccines. However, the task of administering vaccines need not be assigned exclusively to physicians and nurses. With appropriate training, including the management of emergency situations, and under professional supervision, other personnel can skillfully and safely administer vaccines. In some jurisdictions, statutory requirements may limit the administration of vaccines to licensed physicians and/or nurses which could therefore create barriers to immunization. If so, legal opinion should be sought locally to determine the necessary steps to overcome this barrier.

18. Providers receive *ongoing education* and *training* on current immunization recommendations.

Providers include all individuals who are involved in the administration of vaccines, the management of immunization clinics, or the support of these functions. Training and education should cover current guidelines and recommendations of the ACIP, AAP and the AAFP, as well as the Standards for Pediatric Immunization Practices and other immunization information sources such as the manufacturer's package inserts. Providers should also receive information about ongoing national efforts to reach the year 2000 goal of 90% series complete immunization by the second birthday.

Table. Guide to Contraindications and Precautions to Immunizations, January 1997

Note. This information is based on the recommendations of the Advisory Committee on Immunization Practices (ACIP) and of the Committee on Infectious Diseases of the American Academy of Pediatrics (AAP). Sometimes these recommendations vary from those in the manufacturers' product label. For more detailed information, providers should consult the published recommendations of the ACIP, AAP, and the manufacturers' package inserts.

These guidelines, originally issued in 1993 and revised by the US Public Health Service in January 1996, have been updated to give 1997 recommendations (based on information available as of January 1997).

Vaccine	True Contraindications and Precautions	Not True (Vaccines may be given)
GENERAL FOR ALL VACCINES (DTP/DTaP, OPV, IPV, MMR, Hib, HBV, Var)	Anaphylactic reaction to a vaccine contra-indicates further doses of that vaccine Anaphylactic reaction to a vaccine constituent contraindicates the use of vaccines containing that substance Moderate or severe illnesses with or without a fever	Mild to moderate local reaction (soreness, redness, swelling) following a dose of an injectable antigen Low-grade or moderate fever following a prior vaccine dose Mild acute illness with or without low-grade fever Current antimicrobial therapy Convalescent phase of illnesses Prematurity (same dosage and indications as for normal, full-term infants) Recent exposure to an infectious disease History of penicillin or other nonspecific allergies or fact that relatives have such allergies Pregnancy of mother or household contact Unvaccinated household contact

Table. **Guide to Contraindications and Precautions to Immunizations, January 1997, continued**

Vaccine	True Contraindications and Precautions	Not True (Vaccines may be given)
DTP/DTaP[1]	Encephalopathy within 7 days of administration of previous dose of DTP/DTaP	Family history of convulsions[2]
		Family history of sudden infant death syndrome
		Family history of an adverse event following DTP/DTaP administration
	Precautions[1] Fever of $\geq 40.5°C$ (105°F) within 48 hrs after vaccination with a prior dose of DTP/DTaP	
	Collapse or shocklike state (hypotonic-hyporesponsive episode) within 48 hrs of receiving a prior dose of DTP/DTaP	
	Seizures within 3 days of receiving a prior dose of DTP/DTaP (see footnote 2 regarding management of children with a personal history of seizures at any time)	
	Persistent, inconsolable crying lasting ≥ 3 hrs, within 48 hrs of receiving a prior dose of DTP/DTaP	
	Guillain-Barré syndrome (GBS) within 6 weeks after a dose[3]	

Table. Guide to Contraindications and Precautions to Immunizations, January 1997, continued

Vaccine	True Contraindications and Precautions	Not True (Vaccines may be given)
OPV[4]	Infection with HIV or a household contact with HIV	Breastfeeding
	Known altered immunodeficiency (hematologic and solid tumors; congenital immunodeficiency; and long-term immunosuppressive therapy)	Current antimicrobial therapy; Mild diarrhea
	Immunodeficient household contact	
	Precaution[1]: Pregnancy	
IPV[1]	Anaphylactic reaction to neomycin or streptomycin	
	Precaution[1]: Pregnancy	
MMR[1]	Anaphylactic reactions to neomycin	Tuberculosis or positive PPD
	Pregnancy	Simultaneous tuberculin skin testing[5]
	Known altered immunodeficiency (hematologic and solid tumors; congenital immunodeficiency; severe HIV infection and long-term immunosuppressive therapy)	Breastfeeding
	Anaphylactic reaction to gelatin	Pregnancy of mother of recipient
	Precautions[1, 6]: Recent (within 3 to 11 months, depending on product and dose) immune globulin administration	Immunodeficient family member or household contact
		Infection with HIV
		Nonanaphylactic reactions to eggs or neomycin
	Thrombocytopenia or history of thrombocytopenic purpura[7]	

Table. **Guide to Contraindications and Precautions to Immunizations, January 1997,** continued

Vaccine	True Contraindications and Precautions	Not True (Vaccines may be given)
Hib	None	
Hepatitis B	Anaphylactic reaction to baker's yeast	Pregnancy
Varicella	Anaphylactic reaction to neomycin and to gelatin Infection with HIV Known altered immunodeficiency (hematologic and solid tumors; congenital immunodeficiency; and long-term immunosuppressive therapy) Precaution[1]: Recent (within 5 months) IG administration[8] Family history of immunodeficiency[9]	Immunodeficiency in a household contact Household contact with HIV

[1] The events or conditions listed as precautions, although not contraindications, should be carefully reviewed. The benefits and risks of administering a specific vaccine to an individual under the circumstances should be considered. If the risks are believed to outweigh the benefits, the immunization should be withheld; if the benefits are believed to outweigh the risks (for example, during an outbreak or foreign travel), the immunization should be given. Whether and when to administer DTaP or DTP to children with proven or suspected underlying neurologic disorders should be decided on an individual basis. On theoretical grounds, to avoid vaccinating pregnant women is prudent. However, if immediate protection against poliomyelitis is needed, OPV, nor IPV, is recommended.

[2] Acetaminophen given prior to administering DTaP or DTP and thereafter every 4 hours for 24 hours should be considered for children with a personal or with a family history of convulsions in siblings or parents.

[3] The decision to give additional doses of DTaP or DTP should be based on consideration of the benefit of further vaccination vs. the risk of recurrence of GBS. For example, completion of the primary series in children is justified.

Table. Guide to Contraindications and Precautions to Immunizations, January 1997, continued

4 A theoretical risk exists that the administration of multiple live virus vaccines (eg, OPV and MMR) within 30 days (4 weeks) of one another if not given on the same day will result in suboptimal immune response. No data substantiates this risk, however.

5 Measles vaccination may temporarily suppress tuberculin reactivity. MMR vaccine may be given after, or on the same day as, TB testing. If MMR has been given recently, postpone the TB test until 4–6 weeks after administration of MMR. If giving MMR simultaneously with tuberculin skin test, use the Mantoux test and not multiple puncture tests, because the latter require confirmation if positive, which would have to be postponed 4–6 weeks.

6 An anaphylactic reaction to egg ingestion formerly was considered a contraindication unless skin testing and, if indicated, desensitization had been performed. However, skin testing is no longer recommended. For further information, see recommendations of AAP in the 1997 *Red Book* and of ACIP.

7 The decision to vaccinate should be based on consideration of the benefits of immunity to measles, mumps, and rubella vs. the risk of recurrence or exacerbation of thrombocytopenia following vaccination, or from natural infections of measles or rubella. In most instances, the benefits of vaccination will be much greater than the potential risks and justify giving MMR, particularly in view of the even greater risk of thrombocytopenia following measles or rubella disease. However, if a prior episode of thrombocytopenia occurred in close temporal proximity to vaccination, not giving a subsequent dose may be prudent.

8 Varicella vaccine should not be given for at least 5 months after administration of blood (except washed red blood cells), or plasma transfusions, immune globulin, or VZIG. Immune globulin or VZIG should not be given for 3 weeks following vaccination unless the benefits exceed those of the vaccination. In such cases, the vaccinee should either be revaccinated 5 months later and tested for immunity 6 months later and revaccinated if seronegative.

9 Varicella vaccine should not be given to a member of a household with a family history of immunodeficiency until the immune status of the recipient and other children in the family is documented.

APPENDIX III.

National Vaccine Injury Compensation Program—Vaccine Injury Table

As of March 24, 1997, compensation is provided for the following vaccination-associated events in which the initial manifestation occurred within the specified time period. For further information, see Vaccine Injury Compensation (p 27).

Vaccine Injury Table
(Effective March 24, 1997)

Vaccine	Illness, Disability, Injury or Condition Covered	Time Period for First Symptom or Manifestation of Onset or of Significant Aggravation After Vaccine Administration
I. Vaccines containing tetanus toxoid (eg, DTaP, DTP, DT, Td, or TT)	A. Anaphylaxis or anaphylactic shock	4 hours
	B. Brachial neuritis	2–28 days
	C. Any acute complication sequela (including death) of an illness, disability, injury, or condition referred to above which illness, disability, injury, or condition arose within the time period prescribed	Not applicable
II. Vaccines containing whole-cell pertussis bacteria, extracted or partial cell pertussis bacteria, or specific pertussis antigen(s) (eg, DTP, DTaP, P, DTP-Hib)	A. Anaphylaxis or anaphylactic shock	4 hours
	B. Encephalopathy (or encephalitis)	72 hours
	C. Any acute complication or sequela (including death) of an illness, disability, injury, or condition referred to above which illness, disability, injury, or condition arose within the time period prescribed.	Not applicable
III. Measles, mumps, and rubella vaccine or any of its components (eg, MMR, MR, M, R)	A. Anaphylaxis or anaphylactic shock	4 hours
	B. Encephalopathy (or encephalitis)	5-15 days (not less than 5 days and not more than 15 days) for measles, mumps, rubella, or any vaccine containing any of the foregoing as a component.
	C. Any acute complication or sequela (including death) of an illness, disability, injury, or condition referred to above which illness, disability, injury, or condition arose within the time period prescribed.	Not applicable

Vaccine Injury Table, continued

Vaccine	Illness, Disability, Injury or Condition Covered	Time Period for First Symptom or Manifestation of Onset or of Significant Aggravation After Vaccine Administration
IV. Vaccines containing rubella virus (eg, MMR, MR, R)	A. Chronic arthritis	42 days
	B. Any acute complication or sequela (including death) of an illness, disability, injury, or condition referred to above which illness, disability, injury, or condition arose within the time period prescribed.	Not applicable
V. Vaccines containing measles virus (eg, MMR, MR, M)	A. Thrombocytopenic purpura	7–30 days
	B. Vaccine-strain measles viral infection in an immunodeficient recipient	6 months
	C. Any acute complication or sequela (including death) of an illness, disability, injury, or condition referred to above which illness, disability, injury, or condition arose within the time period prescribed.	Not applicable
VI. Vaccines containing polio live virus (OPV)	A. Paralytic polio	
	—in a non-immunodeficient recipient	30 days
	—in an immunodeficient recipient	6 months
	—in a vaccine associated community case	Not applicable
	B. Vaccine-strain polio viral infection	
	—in a non-immunodeficient recipient	30 days
	—in an immunodeficient recipient	6 months
	—in a vaccine associated community case	Not applicable
	C. Any acute complication or sequela (including death) of an illness, disability, injury, or condition referred to above which illness, disability, injury, or condition arose within the time period prescribed	Not applicable

Vaccine Injury Table, continued

Vaccine	Illness, Disability, Injury or Condition Covered	Time Period for First Symptom or Manifestation of Onset or of Significant Aggravation After Vaccine Administration
VII. Vaccines containing polio inactivated virus (eg, IPV)	A. Anaphylaxis or anaphylactic shock	4 hours
	B. Any acute complication or sequela (including death) of an illness, disability, injury, or condition referred to above which illness, disability, injury, or condition arose within the time period prescribed	Not applicable
VIII. Hepatitis B vaccines	A. Anaphylaxis or anaphylactic shock	4 hours
	B. Any acute complication or sequela (including death) of an illness, disability, injury, or condition referred to above which illness, disability, injury, or condition arose within the time period prescribed	Not applicable
IX. *Haemophilus influenzae* type b polysaccharide vaccines (unconjugated, PRP vaccines)	A. Early-onset Hib disease	7 days
	B. Any acute complication or sequela (including death) of an illness, disability, injury, or condition referred to above which illness, disability, injury, or condition arose within the time period prescribed	Not applicable
X. *Haemophilus influenzae* type b polysaccharide conjugate vaccines	No condition specified	
XI. Varicella vaccine	No condition specified	
XII. Any new vaccine recommended by the Centers for Disease Control and Prevention for routine administration to children, after publication by the Secretary of a notice of coverage	No condition specified	

Qualifications and Aids to Interpretation.

(1) *Anaphylaxis and anaphylactic shock* mean an acute, severe, and potentially lethal systemic allergic reaction. Most cases resolve without sequelae. Signs and symptoms begin minutes to a few hours after exposure. Death, if it occurs, usually results from airway obstruction caused by laryngeal edema or bronchospasm and may be associated with cardiovascular collapse. Other significant clinical signs and symptoms may include the following: Cyanosis, hypotension, bradycardia, tachycardia, arrhythmia, edema of the pharynx and/or trachea and/or larynx with stridor and dyspnea. Autopsy findings may include acute emphysema which results from lower respiratory tract obstruction, edema of the hypopharynx, epiglottis, larynx, or trachea and minimal findings of eosinophilia in the liver, spleen and lungs. When death occurs within minutes of exposure and without signs of respiratory distress, there may not be significant pathologic findings.

(2) *Encephalopathy.* For purposes of the Vaccine Injury Table, a vaccine recipient shall be considered to have suffered an encephalopathy only if such recipient manifests, within the applicable period, an injury meeting the description below of an acute encephalopathy, and then a chronic encephalopathy persists in such person for more than 6 months beyond the date of vaccination.

   (i) An *acute encephalopathy* is one that is sufficiently severe so as to require hospitalization (whether or not hospitalization occurred).

   (A) *For children less than 18 months of age* who present without an associated seizure event, an acute encephalopathy is indicated by a "significantly decreased level of consciousness" (see "D" below) lasting for at least 24 hours. Those children less than 18 months of age who present following a seizure shall be viewed as having an acute encephalopathy if their significantly decreased level of consciousness persists beyond 24 hours and cannot be attributed to a postictal state (seizure) or medication.

   (B) *For adults and children 18 months of age or older,* an acute encephalopathy is one that persists for at least 24 hours and characterized by at least two of the following:

       (1) A significant change in mental status that is not medication related; specifically a confusional state, or a delirium, or a psychosis;

       (2) A significantly decreased level of consciousness, which is independent of a seizure and cannot be attributed to the effects of medication; and

       (3) A seizure associated with loss of consciousness.

   (C) Increased intracranial pressure may be a clinical feature of acute encephalopathy in any age group.

   (D) A "significantly decreased level of consciousness" is indicated by the presence of at least one of the following clinical signs for at least 24 hours or greater (see paragraphs (2)(i)(A) and (2)(i)(B) of this section for applicable time frames):

       (1) Decreased or absent response to environment (responds, if at all, only to loud voice or painful stimuli);

       (2) Decreased or absent eye contact (does not fix gaze upon family members or other individuals); or

       (3) Inconsistent or absent responses to external stimuli (does not recognize familiar people or things).

Qualifications and Aids to Interpretation, continued

(E) The following clinical features alone, or in combination, do not demonstrate an acute encephalopathy or a significant change in either mental status or level of consciousness as described above: Sleepiness, irritability (fussiness), high-pitched and unusual screaming, persistent inconsolable crying, and bulging fontanelle. Seizures in themselves are not sufficient to constitute a diagnosis of encephalopathy. In the absence of other evidence of an acute encephalopathy, seizures shall not be viewed as the first symptom or manifestation of the onset of an acute encephalopathy.

(ii) *Chronic encephalopathy* occurs when a change in mental or neurologic status, first manifested during the applicable time period, persists for a period of at least 6 months from the date of vaccination. Individuals who return to a normal neurologic state after the acute encephalopathy shall not be presumed to have suffered residual neurologic damage from that event; any subsequent chronic encephalopathy shall not be presumed to be a sequela of the acute encephalopathy. If a preponderance of the evidence indicates that a child's chronic encephalopathy is secondary to genetic, prenatal or perinatal factors, that chronic encephalopathy shall not be considered to be a condition set forth in the Table.

(iii) An encephalopathy shall not be considered to be a condition set forth in the Table if in a proceeding on a petition, it is shown by a preponderance of the evidence that the encephalopathy was caused by an infection, a toxin, a metabolic disturbance, a structural lesion, a genetic disorder or trauma (without regard to whether the cause of the infection, toxin, trauma, metabolic disturbance, structural lesion or genetic disorder is known). If at the time a decision is made on a petition filed under section 2111(b) of the Act for a vaccine-related injury or death, it is not possible to determine the cause by a preponderance of the evidence of an encephalopathy, the encephalopathy shall be considered to be a condition set forth in the Table.

(iv) In determining whether or not an encephalopathy is a condition set forth in the Table, the Court shall consider the entire medical record.

(3) *Residual Seizure Disorder.* A petitioner may be considered to have suffered a residual seizure disorder for purposes of the Vaccine Injury Table, if the first seizure or convulsion occurred 5–15 days (not less than 5 days and not more than 15 days) after administration of the vaccine and 2 or more additional distinct seizure or convulsion episodes occurred within 1 year after the administration of the vaccine which were unaccompanied by fever (defined as a rectal temperature equal to or greater than 101.0 degrees Fahrenheit or an oral temperature equal to or greater than 100.0 degrees Fahrenheit). A distinct seizure or convulsion episode is ordinarily defined as including all seizure or convulsive activity occurring within a 24-hour period, unless competent and qualified expert neurological testimony is presented to the contrary in a particular case.

For purposes of the Vaccine Injury Table, a petitioner shall not be considered to have suffered a residual seizure disorder, if the petitioner suffered a seizure or convulsion unaccompanied by fever (as defined above) before the fifth day after the administration of the vaccine involved.

(4) *Seizure and convulsion.* For purposes of paragraphs (2) and (3) of this section, the terms, "seizure" and "convulsion" include myoclonic, generalized tonic-clonic (grand mal), and simple and complex partial seizures. Absence (petit mal) seizures shall not be considered to be a condition set forth in the Table. Jerking movements or staring episodes alone are not necessarily an indication of seizure activity.

Qualifications and Aids to Interpretation, continued

(5) *Sequela.* The term "sequela" means a condition or event which was actually caused by a condition listed in the Vaccine Injury Table.

(6) *Chronic Arthritis.* For purposes of the Vaccine Injury Table, chronic arthritis may be found in a person with no history in the 3 years prior to vaccination of arthropathy (joint disease) on the basis of:

(A) Medical documentation, recorded within 30 days after the onset, of objective signs of acute arthritis (joint swelling) that occurred between 7 and 42 days after a rubella vaccination;

(B) Medical documentation (recorded within 3 years after the onset of acute arthritis) of the persistence of objective signs of intermittent or continuous arthritis for more than 6 months following vaccination;

(C) Medical documentation of an antibody response to the rubella virus.

For purposes of the Vaccine Injury Table, the following shall not be considered as chronic arthritis: Musculoskeletal disorders such as diffuse connective tissue diseases (including but not limited to rheumatoid arthritis, juvenile rheumatoid arthritis, systemic lupus erythematosus, systemic sclerosis, mixed connective tissue disease, polymyositis/dermatomyositis, fibromyalgia, necrotizing vasculitis and vasculopathies and Sjogren's Syndrome), degenerative joint disease, infectious agents other than rubella (whether by direct invasion or as an immune reaction), metabolic and endocrine diseases, trauma, neoplasms, neuropathic disorders, bone and cartilage disorders and arthritis associated with ankylosing spondylitis, psoriasis, inflammatory bowel disease, Reiter's syndrome, or blood disorders.

Arthralgia (joint pain) or stiffness without joint swelling shall not be viewed as chronic arthritis for purposes of the Vaccine Injury Table.

(7) *Brachial neuritis* is defined as dysfunction limited to the upper extremity nerve plexus (ie, its trunks, divisions, or cords) without involvement of other peripheral (eg, nerve roots or a single peripheral nerve) or central (eg, spinal cord) nervous system structures. A deep, steady, often severe aching pain in the shoulder and upper arm usually heralds onset of the condition. The pain is followed in days or weeks by weakness and atrophy in upper extremity muscle groups. Sensory loss may accompany the motor deficits, but is generally a less notable clinical feature. The neuritis, or plexopathy, may be present on the same side as or the opposite side of the injection; it is sometimes bilateral, affecting both upper extremities. Weakness is required before the diagnosis can be made. Motor, sensory, and reflex findings on physical examination and the results of nerve conduction and electromyographic studies must be consistent in confirming that dysfunction is attributable to the brachial plexus. The condition should thereby be distinguishable from conditions that may give rise to dysfunction of nerve roots (ie, radiculopathies) and peripheral nerves (ie, including multiple mononeuropathies), as well as other peripheral and central nervous system structures (eg, cranial neuropathies and myelopathies).

Qualifications and Aids to Interpretation, continued

(8) *Thrombocytopenic purpura* is defined by a serum platelet count less than 50,000/mm³. Thrombocytopenic purpura does not include cases of thrombocytopenia associated with other causes such as hypersplenism, autoimmune disorders (including alloantibodies from previous transfusions) myelodysplasias, lymphoproliferative disorders, congenital thrombocytopenia or hemolytic uremic syndrome. This does not include cases of immune (formerly called idiopathic) thrombocytopenic purpura (ITP) that are mediated, for example, by viral or fungal infections, toxins or drugs. Thrombocytopenic purpura does not include cases of thrombocytopenia associated with disseminated intravascular coagulation, as observed with bacterial and viral infections. Viral infections include, for example, those infections secondary to Epstein Barr virus, cytomegalovirus, hepatitis A and B, rhinovirus, human immunodeficiency virus (HIV), adenovirus, and dengue virus. An antecedent viral infection may be demonstrated by clinical signs and symptoms and need not be confirmed by culture or serologic testing. Bone marrow examination, if performed, must reveal a normal or an increased number of megakaryocytes in an otherwise normal marrow.

(9) *Vaccine-strain measles viral infection* is defined as a disease caused by the vaccine-strain that should be determined by vaccine-specific monoclonal antibody or polymerase chain reaction tests.

(10) *Vaccine-strain polio viral infection* is defined as a disease caused by poliovirus that is isolated from the affected tissue and should be determined to be the vaccine-strain by oligonucleotide or polymerase chain reaction. Isolation of poliovirus from the stool is not sufficient to establish a tissue specific infection or disease caused by vaccine-strain poliovirus.

(11) *Early-onset Hib disease* is defined as invasive bacterial illness associated with the presence of Hib organism on culture of normally sterile body fluids or tissue, or clinical findings consistent with the diagnosis of epiglottitis. Hib pneumonia qualifies as invasive Hib disease when radiographic findings consistent with the diagnosis of pneumonitis are accompanied by a blood culture positive for the Hib organism. Otitis media, in the absence of the above findings, does not qualify as invasive bacterial disease. A child is considered to have suffered this injury only if the vaccine was the first Hib immunization received by the child.

APPENDIX IV.

Clinical Syndromes Associated With Food-Borne Diseases

Food-borne disease is a major cause of morbidity and mortality in children and adults in developed countries. The epidemiology of food-borne disease is complex due to the number of organisms associated with illness, recent changes in food production, rapid international distribution of food, changes in dietary habits, the potential for extraintestinal manifestations of disease caused by many food-associated pathogens, and the susceptibility of certain immunocompromised individuals to severe and prolonged disease.

The diagnosis of food-borne disease should be considered when two or more persons who have shared a meal develop an acute illness characterized by nausea, vomiting, diarrhea, neurologic symptoms, and/or, occasionally, other extraintestinal manifestations. The diagnosis of the specific etiologic agent is suggested by the clinical syndrome, incubation period, and epidemiologic dues. To aid in the diagnosis, syndromes of food-borne diseases are categorized by incubation period and cause and foods commonly associated with specific causes are listed. The diagnosis can be confirmed by laboratory testing of stool, emesis, food and/or blood.

Table. Clinical Syndromes Associated With Food-Borne Diseases

Clinical Syndromes	Incubation Period	Causes	Commonly Associated Vehicles
Nausea and vomiting	< 1–6 h	*Staphylococcus aureus* (preformed toxins, A, B, C, D, E)	Ham, poultry, cream-filled pastries, potato and egg salad, mushrooms
		Bacillus cereus (emetic toxin)	Fried rice, pork
		Heavy metals (copper, tin, cadmium, zinc)	Acidic beverages
Histamine response and gastrointestinal (GI) tract	< 1 h	Histamine (scombroid)	Fish (bluefish, bonito, mackerel, mahi-mahi, tuna)
Neurologic, including parasthesia and GI tract	0–6 h	Tetrodotoxin, ciguatera	Puffer fish
			Fish (amberjack, barracuda, grouper, snapper)
		Paralytic compounds	Shellfish (clams, mussels, oysters, scallops, other mollusks)
		Neurotoxic compounds	Shellfish
		Domoic acid	Mussels
		Monosodium glutamate	Chinese food
Neurologic and GI tract manifestations	0–2 h	Mushroom toxins (early onset)	Mushrooms
Moderate-to-severe abdominal cramps and watery diarrhea	8–16 h	*B cereus* enterotoxin	Beef, pork, chicken, vanilla sauce
		Clostridium perfringens enterotoxin	Beef, poultry, gravy
	16–48 h	Caliciviruses	Shellfish, salads, ice
		Enterotoxigenic *Escherichia coli*	Fruits, vegetables
		Vibrio cholerae 01 and 0139	Shellfish
		V cholerae non-01	Shellfish
Diarrhea, fever, abdominal cramps, blood and mucus in stools	16–72 h	*Salmonella*	Poultry, pork, eggs, dairy products, including ice cream, vegetables, fruit
		Shigella	Egg salad, vegetables
		Campylobacter jejuni	Poultry, raw milk
		Invasive *E coli*	Vegetables

Table. Clinical Syndromes Associated With Food-Borne Diseases, continued

Clinical Syndromes	Incubation Period	Causes	Commonly Associated Vehicles
Bloody diarrhea, abdominal cramps	72–120 h	Yersinia enterocolitica	Pork chitterlings, tofu, raw milk
		Vibrio parahaemolyticus	Fish, shellfish
		Enterohemorrhagic E coli	Beef (hamburger), raw milk, roast beef, salami, salad dressings
Methemoglobin poisoning	6–12 h	Mushrooms (late onset)	Mushrooms
Hepatorenal failure	6–24 h	Mushrooms (late onset)	Mushrooms
Gastrointestinal then blurred vision, dry mouth, dysarthria, diplopia, descending paralysis	18–36 h	Clostridium botulinum	Canned vegetables, fruits and fish, salted fish, bottled garlic
Extraintestinal manifestations	Varied	Brainerd disease	Unpasteurized milk
		Brucella	Cheese, raw milk
		Group A streptococcus	Egg and potato salad
		Listeria monocytogenes	Cheese, raw milk, hot dogs, cole slaw, cold cuts
		Trichinella spiralis	Pork
		Vibrio vulnificus	Shellfish

····················

APPENDIX V.

Diseases Transmitted by Animals

The transmission of diseases of animals to humans is of special interest in the care of children who may share a household with pets or unwanted rodents or who are otherwise in contact with animals. Important zoonoses that may be encountered in North America and that are reviewed in the *Red Book* (see disease-specific chapters in Section 3 for further information) are given in the following table, which also gives primary modes of animal transmission. Other modes of spread, including human-to-human, also may occur. For a more complete listing of these diseases, one or more of the following resources may be consulted:

- *The Zoonoses* prepared jointly by the US Department of Health and Human Services, the US Public Health Service, the Centers for Disease Control and Prevention, the Centers for Infectious Diseases, and the Office of Biosafety, Atlanta, GA 30333; and the University of Texas, School of Public Health, Science Center, Houston, TX 77025.
- Acha PM, Szyfres B. *Zoonoses and Communicable Diseases Common to Man and Animals.* ed 2. Scientific Publication No 503, 1987, Pan American Health Organization, Pan American Sanitary Bureau, Regional Offices of the World Health Organization, 525 23rd Street, NW, Washington, DC 20037.
- Beran GW, Steele JH. *Handbook of Zoonoses.* ed 2. Boca Raton, Fla: CRC Press Inc; 1994.
- Chomel BB. Zoonoses of house pets other than dogs, cats, and birds. *Pediatr Infect Dis J.* 1992;11:479-487.
- Weinberg AN, Weber DJ, eds. Animal associated human infections. *Infect Dis Clin North Am.* 1991;5:1-175, 649-731.

Morbidity resulting from zoonotic diseases in the United States is reported annually by the Centers for Disease Control and Prevention (see *Summary of Notifiable Diseases*).

Table. Diseases Transmitted by Animals

Disease and/or Organism	Common Animal Sources	Vector or Means of Spread
BACTERIAL DISEASES		
Borreliosis		
Lyme disease (*Borrelia burgdorferi*)	Deer, wild rodents	Tick bite
Relapsing fever (*Borrelia* species)	Wild rodents	Tick bite
Brucellosis (*Brucella* species)	Cattle, goats, sheep, swine, rarely dogs	Direct contact with birth products, ingestion of contaminated milk, inhalation of aerosols
Campylobacteriosis (*Campylobacter jejuni*)	Poultry, dogs, cats, ferrets	Ingestion of contaminated food, direct contact, (particularly with diarrhetic animals)
Capnocytophaga caninmorsus	Dogs, rarely cats	Bites, contact
Cat-scratch disease (*Bartonella henselae*)	Cats, infrequently other animals (<10%)	Scratches, bites
Hemolytic-uremic syndrome (*Escherichia coli* 0157:H7)	Cattle	Ingestion of contaminated food or water
Leptospirosis (*Leptospira* species)	Dogs, rats, livestock	Contact with urine, particularly in contaminated water
Mycobacteriosis (*Mycobacteria marianum*, others)	Fish, aquaria	Wound infection
Pasteurella multocida	Cats, infrequently dogs	Bites, scratches
Plague (*Yersinia pestis*)	Wild rodents, wild rabbits, cats	Bite of rodent fleas, direct contact with infected animals

Table. **Diseases Transmitted by Animals, continued**

Disease and/or Organism	Common Animal Sources	Vector or Means of Spread
Rat-bite fever (*Streptobacillus moniliformis, Spirillum minus*)	Rodents (particularly rats)	Bites
Salmonellosis (*Salmonella* species)	Poultry, reptiles, dogs, cats, rodents, ferrets, turtles, other wild and domestic animals	Ingestion of contaminated food, direct contact
Tetanus (*Clostridium tetani*)	Any animal, usually indirect via soil	Wound infection, contaminated bites
Tularemia (*Francisella tularensis*)	Wild rabbits, rodents, cats	Tick bite, occasionally deerfly bite, direct contact with infected animal, ingestion of contaminated water, mechanical transmission from claws or teeth (cats)
Yersiniosis (*Yersinia enterocolitica*)	Swine; rarely dogs, cats, rodents	Ingestion of contaminated food or water, rarely direct contact
FUNGAL DISEASES		
Cryptococcosis (*Cryptococcus neoformans*)	Birds, particularly pigeons	Inhalation of aerosols from accumulations of pigeon feces
Histoplasmosis (*Histoplasma capsulatum*)	Bats, birds, particularly starlings	Inhalation of aerosols from accumulations of bat and bird feces
Ringworm (*Microsporum* and *Trichophyton* species)	Cats, dogs, rabbits, rodents	Direct contact
Sporotrichosis (*Sporotrichium schenkii*)	Cats	Direct contact

PARASITIC DISEASES

Disease	Reservoir	Transmission
Anisakiasis (*Anisakis* species)	Saltwater and anadromous fish	Ingestion of undercooked or raw fish (eg, sushi)
Babesiosis (*Babesia* species)	Wild rodents	Tick bite
Dwarf tapeworm (*Hymenolepis nana*)	Hamsters, rodents	Ingestion of eggs from feces (contaminated food, water)
Cryptosporidiosis (*Cryptosporidium* species)	Domestic animals, particularly cattle	Ingestion of oocysts shed in feces
Cutaneous larva migrans (*Ancylostoma species*)	Dogs, cats	Penetration of skin by larvae, which develop in soil contaminated with eggs shed in feces
Cysticercosis (*Taenia solium*)	Swine (intermediate host)	Ingestion of eggs from fecal-oral contact or contaminated food, water
Dog tapeworm (*Dipylidium caninum*)	Dogs, cats	Ingestion of fleas infected with larvae
Echinococcosis, hydatid disease (*Echinococcus* species)	Dogs, foxes, possibly other carnivores	Ingestion of eggs shed in feces
Fish tapeworm (*Diphyllobothrium* latum)	Saltwater and freshwater fish	Ingestion of larvae in raw or undercooked fish
Giardiasis (*Giardia lamblia*)	Wild and domestic animals, including dogs, cats, beavers	Ingestion of cysts from fecal-oral contact or in contaminated food, water
Beef, pork tapeworm, taeniasis (*Taenia saginata and solium*)	Cattle, swine	Ingestion of larvae in undercooked beef or pork
Toxoplasmosis (*Toxoplasma gondii*)	Cats, livestock	Ingestion of oocysts from infected cat feces, consumption of insufficiently cooked meat, contact with birth products of sheep, goats

Table. Diseases Transmitted by Animals, continued

Disease and/or Organism	Common Animal Sources	Vector or Means of Spread
Trichinosis (Trichinella spiralis)	Swine, bears, possibly other wild carnivores	Ingestion of larvae in raw or undercooked meat
Visceral larva migrans (Toxocara canis and cati)	Dogs, cats	Ingestion of eggs, usually from soil contaminated by feces
CHLAMYDIAL AND RICKETTSIAL DISEASES		
Ehrlichiosis (Ehrlichia species)	Unknown	Tick bite
Psittacosis (Chlamydia psittaci)	Psittacine and domestic birds	Inhalation of aerosols from feces
Q fever (Coxiella burnetii)	Sheep, other livestock, wild rodents, rabbits	Direct contact and aerosols from birth products, ingestion of contaminated milk, occasionally tick bite
Rickettsialpox (Rickettsia akari)	House mouse	Mite bite
Rocky Mountain spotted fever (Rickettsia rickettsii)	Dogs, wild rodents, rabbits	Tick bite
Typhus, flea-borne endemic typhus (Rickettsia typhi)	Rats, opossums	Flea feces scratched into abrasions
Typhus, louse-borne* epidemic typhus (Rickettsia prowazekii)	Flying squirrels	Contact with squirrels, their nests, or ectoparasites

VIRAL DISEASES

Disease	Reservoir	Transmission
Colorado tick fever	Wild rodents, particularly squirrels	Tick bite
Encephalitis		
California	Wild rodents	Mosquito bite
Eastern equine	Wild birds, poultry, horses	Mosquito bite
Western equine	Wild birds, poultry, horses	Mosquito bite
St Louis	Wild birds, poultry	Mosquito bite
Venezuelan equine	Horses	Mosquito bites
Powassan	Rodents, rabbits	Mosquito bite
		Tick bite
Hantaviruses	Rodents	Inhalation of aerosols of infected secreta and excreta
Lymphocytic choriomeningitis	Rodents, particularly hamsters, mice	Direct contact, inhalation of aerosols, ingestion of contaminated food
Rabies	Dogs, cats, ferrets, bats, skunks, foxes, woodchucks	Bites

* Disease is usually transmitted from person to person (see Louse-Borne Typhus, p 570).

······························

APPENDIX VI.

Raw Milk*

Serious systemic infections due to *Salmonella* species, *Campylobacter* species, and *Escherichia coli* 0157:H7 have been attributed to the consumption of raw milk, including certified raw milk. The American Academy of Pediatrics strongly recommends that parents and public health officials should be fully informed of the important risks inherent in the consumption of all raw milk, and endorses the use of pasteurized milk.

---

* Interstate sale of raw milk is banned by the Food and Drug Administration.

APPENDIX VII.

State Immunization Requirements for School Attendance

All states require immunization of children at the time of entry into school and most states require immunization for entry into licensed child care. In addition, many states have regulations requiring immunization of older children in upper grades as well as those entering college. The most up-to-date information about which vaccines are required in a specific state can be obtained from the immunization program manager of each state health department, as well as from a number of local health departments.

The Centers for Disease Control and Prevention collects and publishes data on current school entry laws, child care and Head Start immunization regulations, and college immunization requirements in effect in the various states. This survey of school laws is usually published annually. Copies of the latest survey, "State Immunization Requirements for School Attendance," may be obtained by sending a request for single copies to the following: Centers for Disease Control and Prevention, National Immunization Program, Mailstop E-52, Atlanta, GA 30333.

•••••••••••••••••••••••••••••••

APPENDIX VIII.

Nationally Notifiable Infectious Diseases in the United States

Public health officials at state health departments and the Centers for Disease Control and Prevention (CDC) collaborate in determining which diseases should be nationally notifiable (see Table). The Council of State and Territorial Epidemiologists, with advice from the CDC, makes recommendations annually for additions and deletions to the list of nationally notifiable diseases. A disease may be added to the list as a new pathogen emerges or a disease may be deleted as its incidence declines. However, reporting of nationally notifiable diseases to the CDC by the states is voluntary. Reporting is currently mandated (ie, by state legislation or regulation) only by the individual states. The list of diseases that are considered notifiable, therefore, varies slightly by state. Additional and specific requirements should be obtained from the appropriate state health department. All states generally report the internationally quarantinable diseases (ie, cholera, plague, and yellow fever) in compliance with the World Health Organization's International Health Regulations.

When health care providers suspect or diagnose a case of a disease considered notifiable in the state, they should report the case by telephone or by mail to the local, county, or state health department. Clinical laboratories also report results consistent with reportable diseases. Staff members in the county health department implement disease control measures as needed. The written case report is forwarded to the state health department.

The CDC acts as a common agent for the states and territories in the collection and reporting of nationally notifiable diseases. Reports of the occurrences of nationally notifiable diseases are transmitted to the CDC each week from the 50 states, 2 cities and 5 territories. Provisional data are published weekly in the *Morbidity and Mortality Weekly Report;* final data are published each year in the annual *Summary of Notifiable Diseases, United States,* published by the CDC. The timelines of the provisional weekly reports provide information which the CDC and state or local epidemiologists use to detect and more effectively interrupt outbreaks. Reporting also provides the timely information needed to measure and demonstrate the impact of changed immunization laws or a new therapeutic modality. The finalized annual data also provide information on reported disease incidence which is necessary for the study of epidemiologic trends and the development of disease prevention policies. The CDC is the sole repository for these data, which are widely used by schools of medicine and public health, communications media, and pharmaceutical or other companies producing health-related products as well as by local, state, and federal health agencies and other agencies or persons concerned with the trends of reportable conditions in the United States.

Table. Infectious Diseases Designated as Notifiable at the National Level*—United States, 1997

Acquired immunodeficiency syndrome
Anthrax
Botulism[†]
Brucellosis
Chancroid[†]
Chlamydia trachomatis, genital infection
Cholera
Coccidioidomycosis[†]
Congenital rubella syndrome
Congenital syphilis
Cryptosporidiosis
Diphtheria
Encephalitis, California
Encephalitis, eastern equine
Encephalitis, St Louis
Encephalitis, western equine
Escherichia coli O157:H7
Gonorrhea

Haemophilus influenzae, invasive disease
Hansen disease (Leprosy)
Hantavirus pulmonary syndrome
Hemolytic-uremic syndrome, post-diarrheal[†]
Hepatitis A
Hepatitis B
Hepatitis, C/non-A, non-B
HIV infection, pediatric
Legionellosis
Lyme disease
Malaria
Measles
Meningococcal disease
Mumps
Pertussis
Plague
Poliomyelitis, paralytic
Psittacosis

Rabies, animal
Rabies, human
Rocky Mountain spotted fever
Rubella
Salmonellosis[†]
Shigellosis[†]
Streptococcal disease, invasive, group A[†]
Streptococcus pneumoniae, drug-resistant[†]
Streptococcal toxic-shock syndrome
Syphilis
Tetanus
Toxic-shock syndrome
Trichinosis
Tuberculosis
Typhoid fever
Yellow fever[†]

* Although varicella is not a nationally notifiable disease, the Council of State and Territorial Epidemiologists recommends reporting of cases of this disease to the Centers for Disease Control and Prevention.
† Not currently published in the weekly tables.

•••••••••••••••••••••••••••

APPENDIX IX.

Services of the Centers for Disease Control and Prevention (CDC)

The Centers for Disease Control and Prevention (US Public Health Service, Department of Health and Human Services, Atlanta, Ga) is the federal agency charged with protecting the public health of the nation by preventing disease and other disabling conditions. The CDC administers national programs for the prevention and control of (1) infectious diseases, (2) occupational diseases and injury, (3) chronic diseases, and (4) environment-related injury and illness. The CDC also provides consultation to other nations and participates with international agencies in the control of preventable diseases. In addition, the CDC directs and enforces foreign quarantine activities and regulations, and it provides consultation and assistance in upgrading the performance of clinical laboratories.

The CDC provides a number of services related to infectious disease management and control. Although the CDC is principally a resource for state and local health departments, it also offers direct and indirect services to hospitals and practicing physicians. The range of services includes reference laboratory diagnosis and epidemiologic consultation, both usually arranged through the state health department. In addition, the CDC Drug Service supplies some specific prophylactic or therapeutic drugs and biologic agents.

Specific immunobiologic products available include botulinal equine (trivalent, ABE) antitoxin, diphtheria equine antitoxin, vaccinia immune globulin (VIG), botulinus pentavalent toxoid, and vaccinia vaccine.

In addition, several drugs for the treatment of parasitic disease, which are not currently licensed for use in the United States, are handled under an Investigational New Drug (IND) permit. These antiparasitic drugs include suramin, nifurtimox, bithionol, dehydroemetine, ivermectin, melarsoprol, and stibogluconate sodium.

Requests for biologic products, antiparasitic drugs, and related information should be directed to the CDC Drug Service (see Directory of Telephone Numbers, p 667).

Index

Page numbers in boldface indicate a main discussion, "t" indicates a table, and "f" indicates a figure.

F

Face shields, in standard precautions, 101
Famciclovir, for herpes simplex virus, 270
Fasciitis, necrotizing
    Bacteroides and *Prevotella*, 150
    streptococcal, 483, 485
        treatment, 490
Fascioliasis *(Fasciola hepatica)*, 382t
    treatment, 644t
Fasciolopsiasis *(Fasciolopsis buski)*, 382t
    treatment, 644t
Febrile reactions, to animal sera, 44
Fecal-oral transmission
    adenoviruses, 130
    Ascaris, 143
    astroviruses, 145
    Balantidium coli, 152
    Blastocystis hominis, 153
    caliciviruses, 159
    Campylobacter from, 160–161
    in child care settings, 81t, 91
    Clostridium difficile, 177
    enteroviruses, 198, 199
    Escherichia coli, 206, 208
    Giardia lamblia, 210, 212
    hepatitis A, 237
    hepatitis E, 265
    isosporiasis, 315
    pinworm infestation, 407
    poliovirus, 424
    rotavirus, 454
    Salmonella, 463
    in school-age children, 98
    Shigella, 472
    tapeworms, 515
    toxocariasis, 530
    toxoplasmosis, 532, 535
Fever
    arboviral hemorrhagic, 140t
    arenaviral hemorrhagic, 232–234
    boutonneuse, 450
    Colorado tick, 137, 138, 138t, 140t
    from DTP vaccine, 402
    Haverhill, 442–443
    and immunization, 31
    Katayama, 470
    of malaria, 335
    Q, 433–435
    rat-bite, 442–443
    relapsing louse- and tick-borne, **155–157**
    of rickettsial diseases, 449, 452–454
    Rocky Mountain spotted, 452–454

trench, 165
    yellow, **137–141**, 138t, 140t
Fifth disease, **383–385.** *See also* Parvovirus B19
Filariasis
    Bancroftian, Malayan, and Timorian,
        209–210
        clinical manifestations, 209
        control measures, 210
        diagnosis, 209
        epidemiology, 209
        etiology, 209
        isolation measures, 210
        treatment, 210, 642t–643t
    river blindness, 373–374. *See also*
        Onchocerciasis
Fish tapeworm, 517, 695t
Fitz-Hugh–Curtis syndrome. *See* Perihepatitis
Flat warts, 374–376
Flea-borne infections
    plague, 408
    typhus, 450, **569–570**
Flubendazole, adverse effects, 662t
Fluconazole
    for candidiasis, 163, 164
    for coccidioidomycosis, 182
    for cryptococcosis, 185
    dosages and adverse reactions, 628t
    for histoplasmosis, 278
    indications, 627t
Flucytosine
    for aspergillosis, 145
    for candidiasis, 164
    for *Cryptococcus neoformans,* 185
    dosages and adverse reactions, 628t
    indications, 627t
Flukes. *See also specific parasites*
    treatment, 644t
Fluorescent antibody-to-membrane antigen
    (FAMA) assay, for varicella, 575
Fluoroquinolones, **605–606**, 613t. *See also*
        individual drugs
    contraindications, 605
    dosages, beyond newborn period, 613t
    indications, 605
    for nontuberculous mycobacteria, 566
    for Q fever, 435
    for *Salmonella,* 464
Fly-borne infections, onchocerciasis, 373, 374
Folinic acid, for toxoplasmosis, 534
Food and Drug Administration (FDA),
        telephone numbers, 667
Food-borne disease, **689**, 690t–691t
    Bacillus cereus, 147, 148
    Balantidium coli, 152

N

Naegleria fowleri, meningoencephalitis and keratitis, **134–135**
treatment, 638t
Nafcillin
dosages
beyond newborn period, 617t
for newborns, 607t
for staphylococcal infections, 478
Naftifine, 632t
for tinea, 525, 527
Nalidixic acid, contraindicated in breast-feeding, 78t
Nanophyetus salmincola, treatment, 644t
Nasopharyngeal carcinoma, Epstein-Barr virus and, 200
Nasopharyngitis, diphtheria, 191
National Childhood Vaccine Injury Act of 1986, 3, 25, 27
National Vaccine Advisory Committee (NVAC), Standards for Pediatric Immunization Practices, **668–680**
National Vaccine Injury Compensation Program, 27, 681, 682t–688t
address, 28
telephone number, 667
vaccine injury table, **682t–688t**
National Vaccine Program Office, telephone number, 667
Nausea and vomiting, from food-borne diseases, **690t**
Necator, **304–306.** *See also* Hookworm infections
Needles, injuries from discarded, 120–122
Neisseria gonorrhoeae, **212–219.** *See also* Gonococcal infections (gonorrhea)
Neisseria meningitidis, **357–362.** *See also* Meningococcal infections
Neomycin dosages
beyond newborn period, 609t
for newborns, 607t
Neonatal infections. *See* Perinatal transmission; Pregnancy; Transplacental transmission
Neoplasms. *See also specific neoplasms*
and HIV infection, 279
Nephropathia epidemica, 234
Nephrotic syndrome, from malaria, 335
Netilmicin dosages, beyond newborn period, 609t
Neurocysticercosis, 515

Neurologic disorders. *See also specific disorders*
cysticercosis, 515
DTaP vaccine and, 405–407
DTP vaccine and, 403–404, 405–407
rubella, 456
Neurosyphilis, 505
diagnosis, 506
treatment, 512–513
Nifurtimox
adverse effects, 662t
for trypanosomiasis, 541, 657t
Nitrofurantoin, **614t**
contraindicated in breastfeeding, 78t
dosages, beyond newborn period, 614t
prophylactic use, 595
Nocardiosis, **372–373**
clinical manifestations, 372
diagnosis, 372
epidemiology, 372
etiology, 372
isolation measures, 373
treatment, 372–373
Nontreponemal tests, for syphilis, 506, 507, 508t, 513
Norfloxacin, 605
contraindicated in breastfeeding, 77, 78t
North Queensland tick typhus, 450
Norwalk-like virus, 159–160
Norwegian scabies, 468
Notifiable infectious diseases, **700, 701t**
Nurseries. *See also* Child care centers
epidemic staphylococcal disease in, 480
Nystatin
for candidiasis, 163
dosages and adverse reactions, 629t, 632t

O

Ocular larva migrans, **530–531**
Oculoglandular tularemia, 568
Ofloxacin, 605
for cholera, 587
contraindications, 605
breastfeeding, 77, 78t
for gonococcal infections, 216t
for leprosy, 325
for pelvic inflammatory disease, 392t
for *Shigella,* 473
for tuberculosis, 551
dosage and adverse reactions, 550t
Omphalitis
Bacteroides and *Prevotella,* 150
streptococcal, 483

Treponema pallidum, 504–514. *See also*
 Syphilis
Trichinosis *(Trichinella spiralis),* 535–536
 clinical manifestations, 535
 control measures, 536
 diagnosis, 536
 epidemiology, 535–536, 696t
 incubation period, 536
 isolation measures, 536
 treatment, 536, 656t
Trichomonas vaginalis (trichomoniasis),
 536–537
 clinical manifestations, 536
 control measures, 537
 diagnosis, 537
 epidemiology, 537
 incubation period, 537
 isolation measures, 537
 sexual abuse and, 112
 testing for, 115, 115t
 treatment, 537, 656t
Trichophyton, 523, 525, 526, 527, 694t. *See
 also* Tinea
Trichostrongylus infection, treatment, 656t
Trichuriasis (whipworm infection), 537–538
 clinical manifestations, 537
 control measures, 538
 diagnosis, 538
 epidemiology, 538
 isolation measures, 538
 treatment, 538, 656t
Trimethoprim-sulfamethoxazole (TMP-SMX)
 for brucellosis, 158
 for cholera, 587, 588
 for *Cyclospora* infections, 640t
 dosages, beyond newborn period, 618t
 for *Escherichia coli,* 207
 for gonococcal infections, 215
 for isosporiasis, 316, 645t
 for nocardiosis, 373
 for nontuberculous mycobacteria, 565
 for pertussis, 396
 for *Pneumocystis carinii,* 420, 423t,
 652t–653t
 dosages, 652t–653t
 prophylactic use, 595
 for Q fever, 435
 for *Salmonella,* 464
 for *Shigella,* 473
 for toxoplasmosis, 534
Trimetrexate, adverse effects, 664t
Tropical pulmonary eosinophilia (TPE),
 treatment, 643t

Trypanosomiasis *(Trypanosoma)*
 African (sleeping sickness), 538–539
 clinical manifestations, 538
 control measures, 539
 diagnosis, 539
 epidemiology, 539
 etiology, 539
 incubation period, 539
 isolation measures, 539
 treatment, 539, 659t
 American (Chagas' disease), 540–541
 clinical manifestations, 540
 control measures, 541
 diagnosis, 540
 etiology, 540
 incubation period, 540
 isolation measures, 541
 treatment, 541, 658t–659t
 cruzi, 540–541
 gambiense, 538–539
 treatment, 658t–659t
Tryparsamide
 adverse effects, 664t
 for trypanosomiasis, 658t
Tsetse fly, and trypanosomiasis, 538, 539
TSS. *See* Toxic shock syndrome
Tuberculin testing, 541, 543, 544–547, 548t,
 559, 560
 BCG vaccine and, 546, 561–562
 for congenital disease, 557
 for contacts, 559, 560, 561
 definitions of positive, 545t
 false positives for nontuberculous species,
 564–565
 and foreign travel, 71
 and HIV infection, 545, 545t, 547, 548t,
 554, 558–559, 560, 561
 interpretation, 546
 measles vaccine and, 354
 recommendations for, 546–547, 548t
 vaccine administration and, 24
Tuberculosis, 541–562
 airborne precautions, 102
 and breastfeeding, 74
 chemoprophylaxis, 594t
 in child care centers, 83, 84, 85–86
 clinical manifestations, 541–542
 control measures, 559–562
 BCG vaccine, 560–562. *See also*
 Bacillus Calmette-Guerin vaccine
 child care and schools, 560
 epidemiologic investigation, 559–560
 management of contacts, 559–560